THE PNEUMONIAS

Clinical Approaches to Infectious Diseases of the Lower Respiratory Tract

Edited by
Matthew E. Levison

John Wright • PSG Inc
Boston Bristol London
1984

Library of Congress in Publication Data
Main entry under title:

The Pneumonias : clinical approaches to infectious
diseases of the lower respiratory tract.

Bibliography: p.
Includes index.
1. Pneumonia. I. Levison, Matthew E., 1938–
[DNLM: 1. Pneumonia. WC 202 P737]
RC771.P685 1984 616.2′41 83-10473
ISBN 0-7236-7020-X

Published simultaneously by:
John Wright • PSG Inc, 545 Great Road, Littleton,
Massachusetts 01460, U.S.A.
John Wright & Sons Ltd, 823–825 Bath Road,
Bristol BS4 5NU, England

Medicine is an ever-changing science. As new research and clinical experience broaden our knowledge, changes in treatment and drug therapy are required. The author and the publisher of this work have made very effort to ensure that the treatment and drug dosage schedules herein are accurate and in accord with the standards accepted at the time of publication. Readers are advised, however, to check the product information sheet included in the package of each drug they plan to administer to be certain that changes have not been made in the recommended dose or in the indications and contraindications for administration. This recommendation is of particular importance in regard to new or infrequently used drugs.

Printed in the United States of America.

International Standard Book Number: 0-7236-7020-X

Library of Congress Catalog Card Number: 83-10473

Contributors

Elias Abrutyn, MD
Professor and Assistant Chairman
Department of Medicine
Division of Infectious Diseases
The Medical College of Pennsylvania
Assistant Chief of Medicine and
Chief, Infectious Diseases
V.A. Hospital of Philadelphia
Philadelphia, Pennsylvania

Stephen Baumgart, MD
Assistant Professor of Pediatrics
The University of Pennsylvania
School of Medicine
Philadelphia, Pennsylvania

Jerome Boscia, MD
Assistant Professor of Medicine
Division of Infectious Diseases
The Medical College of Pennsylvania
Philadelphia, Pennsylvania

Jaime Carrizosa, MD,
Altamonte Springs, Florida
(Formerly with the Division of
Infectious Diseases,
The Medical College of Pennsylvania)

Paul E. Epstein, MD
Associate Professor of Medicine
The University of Pennsylvania
Chief, Pulmonary Medicine
Graduate Hospital
Philadelphia, Pennsylvania

Harvey M. Friedman, MD
Associate Professor of Medicine
The University of Pennsylvania
Director, Diagnostic Virology
Laboratory
Children's Hospital
Philadelphia, Pennsylvania

Richard Gilpin, PhD
Associate Professor of Microbiology
and Immunology
The Medical College of Pennsylvania
Philadelphia, Pennsylvania

Linda Griska, MD
Associate Professor
Department of Radiology
The Medical College of Pennsylvania
Philadelphia, Pennsylvania

Donald Kaye, MD
Professor and Chairman
Department of Medicine
The Medical College of Pennsylvania
Philadelphia, Pennsylvania

Oksana M. Korzeniowski, MD
Assistant Professor of Medicine
Division of Infectious Diseases
The Medical College of Pennsylvania
Philadelphia, Pennsylvania

Jack L. LeFrock, MD
Professor of Medicine and Chief
Division of Infectious Diseases and
Clinical Microbiology
Hahnemann University School of
Medicine
Philadelphia, Pennsylvania

Arnold Lentnek, MD
Group Director, Anti-Infective
Products
Medical Affairs Department
Smith Kline & French Laboratories

Matthew E. Levison, MD
Professor of Medicine and Chief
Division of Infectious Diseases
The Medical College of Pennsylvania
Philadelphia, Pennsylvania

Bennett Lorber, MD
Professor of Medicine
Chief, Section of Infectious Diseases
Temple University Health Sciences Center
Philadelphia, Pennsylvania

Rob Roy MacGregor, MD
Associate Professor of Medicine
Chief of the Infectious Diseases Section
The University of Pennsylvania School of Medicine
Philadelphia, Pennsylvania

Paul L. Marino, MD
Assistant Professor of Medicine
Graduate Hospital and Hospital of the University of Pennsylvania
Philadelphia, Pennsylvania

Richard V. McCloskey, MD
Associate Director
Department of Medical Research
Hoffman-LaRoche, Inc.
Nutley, New Jersey

William B. McNamee, Jr., MD
Director of Infectious Diseases
Mercy Catholic Medical Center
Philadelphia, Pennsylvania
(Formerly with the Division of Infectious Diseases
The Medical College of Pennsylvania)

Abdolghader Molavi, MD
Associate Professor of Medicine
Division of Infectious Diseases and Clinical Microbiology
Hahnemann University School of Medicine
Philadelphia, Pennsylvania

Sheila Ann Murphey, MD
Clinical Associate Professor of Medicine
Director, Division of Infectious Diseases
Jefferson Medical College of Thomas Jefferson University
Philadelphia, Pennsylvania

Richard A. Polin, MD
Assistant Professor of Pediatrics
University of Pennsylvania School of Medicine
The Children's Hospital of Philadelphia
Philadelphia, Pennsylvania

George A. Poporad, MD
Clinical Assistant Professor of Medicine
The Medical College of Pennsylvania
Co-Head of the Section of Infectious Diseases
Frankford Hospital
Philadelphia, Pennsylvania
(Formerly with the Division of Infectious Diseases
The Medical College of Pennsylvania)

Jerome Santoro, MD
Clinical Associate Professor of Medicine
Jefferson Medical College of Thomas Jefferson University
Philadelphia, Pennsylvania
(Formerly with the Division of Infectious Diseases
The Medical College of Pennsylvania)

Richard Snepar, MD
Clinical Instructor of Medicine
Rutgers Medical School-U.M.D.N.J.
Piscataway, New Jersey
(Formerly with the Division of Infectious Diseases
The Medical College of Pennsylvania)

Jack D. Sobel, MD
Associate Professor of Medicine
Division of Infectious Diseases
The Medical College of Pennsylvania
Philadelphia, Pennsylvania

Alan R. Spitzer, MD
Assistant Professor of Pediatrics and Obstetrics and Gynecology
University of Pennsylvania School of Medicine
Philadelphia, Pennsylvania

George H. Talbot, MD
Assistant Professor of Medicine
Hospital Epidemiologist
The Hospital of the University of Pennsylvania
Philadelphia, Pennsylvania

Clifford G. Wlodaver, MD
Clinical Instructor in Medicine at the University of Oklahoma
Health Science Center
College of Medicine
Oklahoma City, Oklahoma

Contents

PATHOGENS
Bacteria

Viruses

Fungi

Protozoa and Helminths

Preface

Pneumonia remains one of the most common infections seen in both the community and among hospitalized patients and its mortality is still high despite improvements in diagnostic methods and new antimicrobial agents developed over the past decade.

The impact of pneumonia on the population can be documented in several ways. A National Health Survey of households for acute illness and injuries found that pneumonia afflicted 3,178,000 persons between July 1977 and June 1978, and resulted in a period of restricted activity of approximately 14.8 days, including an average of 9.4 days confined to bed. By contrast, other acute conditions resulted in an average of only 4.5 days of restricted activity and 2.0 days of bed rest. Similarly, a study by the National Center for Health Statistics found that pneumonia accounted for 2% of all principal hospital discharge diagnoses in 1978 and the average length of hospitalization for pneumonia was 8.8 days. This was the same frequency as was found in 1970, but the number of hospitalized patients had increased by approximately 22% in the interval. In addition, pneumonia was the second most common indication for antibiotic therapy among the over 15% of hospitalized patients who received an antimicrobial for an infectious disease indication in a study of 20 randomly selected Pennsylvania hospitals (Shapiro et al, 1979).

Patients are particularly susceptible to pneumonia acquired after admission to a hospital. Pneumonia accounts for 8% to 33% of all nosocomial infections, and it is the third most common nosocomial infection after urinary tract and surgical wound infection. The reported incidence of nosocomial pneumonia ranges from 0.5% to 5.0% of hospital discharges. The incidence of such infections varies with the inpatient service and type of hospital. For example, on obstetrical services in community hospitals, nosocomial pneumonia is uncommon, but it is more common on surgical or medical services and in teaching hospitals. Nosocomial pneumonia is frequently a postoperative infection, especially for operations that involve the chest or abdomen. Also, it is frequently caused by facultative gram-negative bacilli and this type of infection is fatal more than 50% of the time.

The elderly, who are becoming a larger portion of the population, are especially at risk of morbidity and mortality from pneumonia. A National Center for Health Statistics study found that although pneumonia was seen in a larger percentage of patients aged 15 years or younger, the length of hospital stay due to pneumonia increased steadily with increasing age. Those 65 years or older accounted for almost half the hospital days due to pneumonia. In addition to the elderly, patients who are at risk of pneumonia as a result of being compromised immunologically or in other ways are increasing in number. This has occurred because of more aggressive management of underlying diseases and advances in life-support technology.

Pneumonia and influenza have continued to rank fifth among the 15 leading causes of death in the United States during the past decade. However, over this period of time, the age-adjusted death rate attributed to pneumonia and influenza has steadily declined, and in 1979 was the lowest recorded for the United States, in part a reflection of the absence of an influenza epidemic in 1979. Septicemia, the next most frequent infection on the list of leading causes of death, continued an upward trend to become 15th in rank in 1977–1981, but its death rate was only approximately one-fifth that for pneumonia and influenza during this period of time.

During the past few years, several new etiologic agents of pneumonia (such as the *Legionella* group of organisms) have been recognized. Other etiologic agents, such as *Pneumocystis*, have emerged as dominant pathogens in patients with a newly described immunodeficiency state (AIDS). Certain organisms, such as the pneumococcus, have developed resistance to antimicrobials to which they had been uniformly susceptible. Also, as broad spectrum antibiotics are increasingly used, more and more of the hospital-acquired pneumonias are caused by antibiotic-resistant organisms. Because international travel has become commonplace, travelers may present in the United States with pneumonic illnesses due to exotic organisms acquired abroad. As a result of all these factors, our approach to the diagnosis and treatment of pulmonary infection has changed appreciably.

The intent of this book is to aid both students and those who care for patients with pneumonia in understanding its pathogenesis, diagnosis and therapy. Because pneumonia traverses the usual boundaries established by medical specialists, pneumonia requires the attention of many different types of practitioners, including the internist, surgeon, general practitioner, emergency room physician, physician's assistant, pediatrician, public health physician, obstetrician-gynecologist, infection control officer, house officer, microbiologist and respiratory technician. Each of these groups requires emphasis of different topics at different depths of discussion.

For this reason, the format of this book approaches pneumonia in several different ways. The introductory section covers general principles necessary for a clear understanding of pathogenesis, diagnosis and management. Pneumonia, when it occurs in certain distinct clinical or epidemiologic settings, is more likely to be caused by one of a group of microorganisms than others. Recognition of these patterns by which groups of infectious agents present aids in rapid formulation of an etiologic diagnosis and initiation of appropriate therapy. Therefore, the second section emphasizes patterns of presentation. The final section approaches pneumonia by describing the various microorganisms that can infect the lung. An attempt has been made for each of the chapters dealing with etiologic agents and those dealing with patterns of presentation to be complete. Therefore, some repetition was unavoidable. However, cross-reference was made frequently between the appropriate sections. References given at the end of each chapter are for the most part limited to reviews that contain comprehensive bibliographies and to certain articles which document specific or controversial data quoted in the text.

For their contributions to this book, I am grateful to the authors for their willingness to cooperate in this joint venture. We all want to express our special appreciation to our office staffs for their efforts in typing portions of the manuscript, and I wish to especially thank Vivian G. Sharp for typing and retyping most of the manuscript for this book.

We also all want to thank our respective families for their patience and perseverance during the immense amount of time the formulation of this book required.

REFERENCES

National Center for Health Statistics: *Acute Conditions. Incidence and Associated Disability, United States, July 1977–June 1978*. Series 10, No 132. Hyattsville, MD, DHEW Publication PHS-79-1560, September 1979.

National Center for Health Statistics: Advance report of final mortality statistics, 1979. *Monthly Vital Statistics Report* September 30, 1982;31(6)(suppl).

National Center for Health Statistics: Annual summary of births, deaths, marriages and divorces: United States, 1980. *Monthly Vital Statistics Report* September 17, 1981;29(13).

National Center for Health Statistics: Annual summary of births, deaths, marriages and divorces: United States, 1981. *Monthly Vital Statistics Report* December 20, 1982;30(13).

National Center for Health Statistics: *Vital Statistics of the United States, 1973–1978*. Vol 2, Mortality, Part A, Rockville, MD, 1977–1982.

National Center for Health Statistics: *Utilization of Short-Stay Hospitals. Annual Summary for the United States, 1978*. Series 13, No 46. Hyattsville, MD, DHEW Publication PHS 80-1797.

Shapiro M, Townsend TR, Rosner B, et al: Use of antimicrobial drugs in general hospitals. II. Analysis of patterns of use. *J Infect Dis* 1979;139:698–706.

1 *Pathogenesis of Pneumonia*

Matthew E. Levison
Jerome Boscia

MODES OF TRANSMISSION

Infectious agents may be transmitted to the lower respiratory tract by one of five mechanisms: 1) inhalation of small airborne infectious particles; 2) aspiration of resident naso-oropharyngeal flora or large airborne infectious particles after deposition in the naso-oropharynx; 3) hematogenous spread to the lung from another site of infection; 4) direct extension from a contiguous site of infection; or 5) exogenous penetration and contamination of lung parenchyma. Inhalation and aspiration are by far the most common mechanisms.

Airborne Transmission

Pneumonia as a consequence of inhalation of small airborne infectious particles occurs, for example, with tuberculosis, influenza, *Mycoplasma* pneumonia, the respiratory mycoses, measles, smallpox, psittacosis, brucellosis, anthrax and Q fever pneumonia. However, some respiratory pathogens do not seem to spread well through the air. For example, Gwaltney et al (1978) found that rhinovirus, when transferred by fingers to nasal or conjunctival mucosa from contaminated surfaces, regularly resulted in infection and illness, whereas face-to-face exposure of susceptible volunteers to infected volunteers who coughed and sneezed did not result in infection (large particle exposure), nor did exposure in a room in which susceptibles were separated from infected subjects by a wire mesh barrier result in infection (small particle aerosol exposure). These findings from volunteer studies suggest that rhinovirus spreads by contact.

Several conditions must be met for diseases to be transmitted by air: 1) the infectious agent must be present in sufficient numbers at the site of particle production; 2) some mechanism must occur to cause the particle to become airborne; 3) the organisms must remain alive and infectious while in transit in the air; and 4) the organisms must be deposited on susceptible tissue in the new host. The high velocity of air passing over the respiratory tract mucosa during sneezes and coughs, as well as other exhalatory activities, produces a large population of organism-bearing airborne particles of various sizes which can serve as vehicles of airborne transmission. Each large particle may contain large numbers of organisms, while the smallest particles may contain none or, at most, one or two organisms.

As particles $< 100\ \mu m$ in diameter fall through air, evaporation rapidly occurs. In this way, the particle becomes smaller and lighter in weight. After evaporation is complete, the residual particle contains any organism originally present and is called a droplet nucleus. These droplet nuclei, usually less than 5 μm in diameter, are so buoyant that they disperse rapidly and remain suspended in air for a prolonged time by gentle air currents, unless removed by ventilation or inhalation.

Particles that are greater than 100 μm in diameter, called droplets, will settle out of the air by gravity in a relatively short time and within a relatively short distance from their source before significant evaporation can take place. On the ground they become mixed with other debris in dust. Infectious particles in dust gradually dry and may survive for long periods, to be resuspended when the dust is disturbed. Some of these resuspended particles are presumably small enough to have aerodynamic characteristics similar to droplet nuclei.

Airborne particles can reach the tissues of a new host either by direct sedimentation or by inhalation. Droplets ejected from the respiratory tract may be projected directly onto the skin or mucous membranes of the conjunctiva, lips, or possibly the anterior nares. Inhaled particles are deposited at variable sites along the respiratory tract depending upon the size of the particle. The larger particles are removed in the upper respiratory tract. Small particles, on the other hand, are carried wherever the air goes. Most particles the size of droplet nuclei penetrate deeply into the peripheral regions of the lung where the alveoli and alveolar ducts are located. The effect of gravity causes settling of the lightweight particles at a slow rate which, because of the small size of the pulmonary air spaces, is nevertheless adequate to account for their deposition in the alveoli. The fate of a particle also depends very much on whether or not it is hygroscopic. Accretion of water from the humid air in the airways can substantially increase the particle size and thereby increase the rate of settling. Factors other than particle size that influence penetration and the site of deposition include differences in breathing patterns (eg, breathing during exercise, mouth breathing), the distribution of alveolar ventilation and the state of the airways. For example, a greater proportion of alveolar ventilation is distributed to the lower lobes which should result in greater deposition of aerosolized particles in that area. Also, in smokers central deposition is favored over deeper penetration of particles.

Certain types of large infectious particles impacting on the mucosa of the upper respiratory tract may nevertheless reach the lung indirectly. If sufficiently virulent, organisms can penetrate the upper respiratory tract mucosa, appear in the lymphatics and, after variable periods of time, reach the lung by the lympho-hematogenous route. Another mechanism by which large airborne infectious particles could reach the lung would be aspiration of upper respiratory secretions after deposition and multiplication on the naso-oropharyngeal mucosa.

The number of organisms that is required to initiate infection must allow for elimination of organisms in transit between the source and the susceptible locus in the new host. If the susceptible tissue is the lung, a much larger number of organisms, if mostly in the form of large particles, would be required because of losses in the atmosphere and the upper respiratory tract, than if the organisms were in the form of droplet nuclei. If the susceptible tissue is the nasal mucosa, then airborne organisms in the form of large particles would be more efficient transmitters of infection than droplet nuclei.

The size of the airborne infectious particle also has epidemiologic consequences. The occurrence of explosive outbreaks of respiratory illness, as have been described for tuberculosis, influenza and measles, are often best explained by a common source of exposure. Such an exposure might occur if one or only a few infected patients were particularly good producers of small aerosolized infectious particles that can disperse widely and remain suspended in a poorly ventilated enclosed space filled with a large number of susceptibles. Although large airborne particles are formed by coughing and sneezing, because of rapid settling they can ordinarily transmit infection only in near proximity to a patient, making it difficult to distinguish this route of transmission from contact spread of infection. The number of person-to-person contacts required to disseminate the organism rapidly enough by means of large airborne particles between patients and susceptibles would be too great to realistically account for explosive outbreaks of respiratory illness.

Transmission by the airborne route usually will occur indoors, especially if ventilation is poor, because of rapid dispersion of inocula outdoors. Similarly, inocula may not persist for more than several hours indoors if ventilation is good. However, aerosols created outdoors can also transmit infection, perhaps because small inocula can be sufficient to cause infection if the airborne particle is small and if the susceptible tissue is the lung. Organisms in soil, aerosolized by wind storms, farming or construction have caused sporadic and epidemic occurrrences of histoplasmosis and coccidioidomycosis. Organisms in polluted ocean water adsorb to bubbles in the surf which, on bursting at the sea surface, form aeorsols. These are carried great distances by onshore breezes. Aerosolized organisms from the outdoors also can be fed directly into intakes of forced air ventilation systems, and in this way have caused outbreaks of legionellosis and histoplasmosis. Aerosols created by industrial activity, for example, in abattoirs have been associated with brucellosis and Q fever.

These considerations suggest the following ways by which the transmission of airborne infection can be interrupted: 1) elimination of sources; 2) elimination of infectious particles in air; 3) protection of susceptibles; and 4) reduction of the numbers of susceptibles.

Environmental sources of infectious aerosols can be eliminated, as has been done to control outbreaks of legionellosis. Patients who are producing aerosols from infected sites on their respiratory tract during coughing or sneezing can be excluded from the presence of susceptibles until cured or on effective therapy. Increasing the distance between a patient and susceptibles may decrease transmission of larger infectious particles that are projected only a short distance from the patient. Masks worn by patients can decrease shedding of infectious droplets, but their efficacy in preventing inhalation of droplet nuclei when worn by susceptibles is open to question. On the other hand, infectious droplet nuclei can be removed from air indoors by ventilation, or killed by use of ultraviolet lights. The efficacy of any one of these attempts to specifically interrupt airborne transmission may be limited by the fact that agents may be transmitted in more than one way, and tactics that interrupt airborne transmission may still allow transmission by other routes, for example, by direct contact. Reduction of susceptibles can be achieved by immunization, as discussed in Chapter 20 on prevention of pneumococcal pneumonia. However, the efficacy of immunization is often limited due, for example, to antigenic variation (eg, influenza) or large numbers of infectious agents (eg, adenoviruses).

Other Modes of Transmission

Aspiration of oropharyngeal secretions is a common event that is said to occur in normal individuals during sleep as well as in patients with depressed consciousness. Because upper respiratory secretions contain large numbers of organisms (10^7 to 10^{10}/mL), the aspiration of as little as 0.01 mL of upper respiratory tract secretions could deliver a large enough inoculum of organisms, if sufficiently virulent, to cause pneumonia. Organisms involved are either the normal commensals of the oropharynx (mixture of anaerobes), or potential pathogens that have colonized the oropharynx during exposure to infected patients (pneumococci, *Staphylococcus aureus*, Enterobacteriaceae or *Pseudomonas aeruginosa*) or to a highly contaminated environment, eg, a hospital. Aspiration is discussed in more detail in Chapter 9.

Hematogenous spread from another site of infection can occur, for example, with tricuspid valve endocarditis (usually caused by *S. aureus*), or septic pelvic or jugular thrombophlebitis (usually due to anaerobic bacteria, such as *Bacteroides* sp). The distribution in the lungs of hematogenous pneumonia differs from bronchogenic infection. When numerous, metastatic lesions have a uniform and bilateral distribution not seen in bronchogenic pneumonia. If larger pulmonary arteries are obstructed by septic emboli, infarction may occur, with subsequent spread of infection into the site of infarction. Pneumonia evolving by direct extension from a contiguous site of infection can occur, for example, with amebic liver abscess. Pneumonia also can develop following exogenous penetration and contamination of lung parenchyma, eg, following accidental trauma or surgery.

FATE OF MICROORGANISMS IN THE BODY

Influenza virus progressively infects the epithelial cells of the respiratory tract. Usually, damage is confined to the epithelium of the trachea and bronchi, but in cases of viral pneumonia, foci of infection occur in the epithelial cells of the bronchioles and alveoli, and in alveolar macrophages. Necrosis and desquamation of the respiratory epithelium and hemorrhagic pneumonitis results. Because of extensive loss of respiratory defense mechanisms, the danger of secondary bacterial pneumonia by way of aspiration is greatly increased. A similar propensity for secondary bacterial pneumonia occurs following measles.

Organisms that penetrate the alveolar spaces by inhalation or aspiration are, for the most part, taken up by phagocytes. Phagocytes, with their contained particles, can move up the bronchial tree on the mucous blanket, but the exact mechanism by which they move from the alveoli to the ciliated bronchioles is not known. Some alveolar phagocytes containing small particles penetrate the alveolar epithelium and enter the lymphatic system. Some particles penetrate the alveolar epithelium without previously being phagocytized, and the lymphatics readily become permeable to these small particles introduced into intercellular tissue spaces. The particles are then carried to the regional lymph nodes.

Avirulent organisms that have little ability to multiply in tissues can remain localized to the portal of entry or the regional lymphatics, and are subsequently cleared. Virulent organisms in a susceptible host multiply faster than they can be disposed. A local inflammatory reaction may then intensify in the alveolus, with continued exudation of humoral and cellular antibacterial elements. Certain organisms (eg, *S. pneumoniae*) can be carried in the exudate from one alveolus to another, passing directly through the pores of Kohn and, in this way, involve an entire lobe. Other lobules and lobes may be involved via the airways. With some organisms, necrosis of the lung (abscess formation) may occur more frequently (*S. aureus*) than with others (*S. pneumoniae*).

The pneumonic process in a subpleural location may result in a serofibrinous exudation in the pleural space. If the pleura becomes heavily infected, the exudate becomes frankly purulent. In other types of infection, there may be no evidence whatsoever related to the deposition of infectious particles in the lung, yet the lung may well be the portal of entry for the infection. In some cases, the organisms that have caused no apparent reaction in the lung may nevertheless cause a lymphadenitis, which becomes the initial and major site of involvement (eg, massive hemorrhagic mediastinitis in inhalation anthrax). In other cases, the organisms that have caused no apparent reaction in the lung may fail to be localized to the regional lymphatics and become disseminated via the bloodstream, as may occur in blastomycosis. In these cases, the place where clinical symptoms appear or where multiplication of organisms occurs may bear no obvious relation to the portal of entry.

Infectious agents rarely enter the bloodstream directly from tissue, the passage being mainly by way of lymphatics, except when gross trauma to blood vessels is present. Organisms in the bloodstream, either free or inside phagocytes, are cleared by tissue macrophages predominantly in the liver and spleen. Circulating polymorphonuclear leukocytes may also contribute to their clearance. In blood, infectious agents may be aggregated into larger masses, sometimes mixed with platelets, and as such are filtered from the circulation in finer capillaries, accompanied by a local accumulation of granulocytes. In this way, the number of circulating leukocytes may be rapidly decreased in early stages of bacteremia, as they are sequestered in various organs where they phagocytize the trapped microorganisms.

Pathogens trapped in tissues either may be cleared or remain alive for variable periods. In more chronic infections, such as tuberculosis, they can persist for years. If the microorganism is sufficiently virulent or host defense mechanisms are inadequate, microbial growth can continue in the lymph nodes, liver, spleen and other tissue foci, such as the lung, and produce secondary bacteremia and additional tissue foci of infection. In a similar manner, bacteremia arising from primary infection at sites other than the lung may secondarily establish infection in the lung.

Once antibody is formed, there may be more rapid elimination of microorganisms, especially those that are encapsulated. When opsonized by antibody and complement, encapsulated organisms are rapidly phagocytized. Some organisms are rapidly killed once taken up by phagocytes; other organisms have the capacity to multiply within cells of the host. These facultative intracellular organisms continue to multiply intracellularly, may thus kill the phagocyte and then parasitize new phagocytes. These agents include *M. tuberculosis*, *Brucella* sp, *Salmonella* sp; *Listeria monocytogenes*; fungi such as *H. capsulatum*, *Coccidioides immitis*, and *Blastomyces*; *Chlamydia*; *Rickettsia*; protozoa such as *Toxoplasma*; and viruses. A granulomatous inflammatory reaction develops around these foci of organisms, which consists of many macrophages closely adherent to each other (epithelioid cells) and T-lymphocytes. Some of the macrophages fuse to form multinucleated giant cells. Many of the macrophages contain the infectious agents. The macrophages are highly activated (ie, enlarged and have a large number of lysosomes and increased phagocytic capacity) and have an enhanced capacity to nonspecifically inhibit the growth or kill intracellular microorganisms. Macrophage activation is stimulated by soluble mediators (lymphokines) produced by specifically sensitized T-lymphocytes. The granuloma may undergo necrosis, fibrosis and calcification. At any point, the process may become quiescent, progress locally or disseminate distantly, depending on the balance between host defenses and virulence of the microorganism.

SELECTED READINGS

Gwaltney JM Jr, Moskalski PB, Hendley JO: Hand-to-hand transmission of rhinovirus colds. *Ann Intern Med* 1978;88:463.

Huxley EJ, Viroslav J, Gray WR, Pierce AK: Pharyngeal aspiration in normal adults and patients with depressed consciousness. *Am J Med* 1978;64:564.

Knight V: Viruses as agents of airborne contagion. *Ann NY Acad Sci* 1980;353:147.

Riley RL: Airborne infection. *Am J Med* 1974;57:466.

Tigertt WD, Benenson AS, Gochenen WS: Airborne Q-fever. *Bact Rev* 1961; 25:285.

2 Host Defenses in the Respiratory Tract

Sheila Ann Murphey

The respiratory tract is well provided with a variety of defenses against the noxious agents and elements that abound in our environment. These defense mechanisms are both specific and nonspecific and include mechanical, secretory and phagocytic systems. This discussion will emphasize the ability of the lung to remove, neutralize or kill the broad spectrum of microorganisms that can cause respiratory tract infections. The alterations in host defenses caused by toxins, drugs, underlying disease states and certain respiratory tract infections, which then render the host more susceptible to pulmonary infections, also will be discussed.

AERODYNAMIC DEFENSES

The earliest set of defenses encountered by potentially pathogenic agents entering the respiratory tract by inhalation are the aerodynamic defenses that are intended to filter out or to remove particulate material from the airstream by impaction or sedimentation. The efficiency of the aerodynamic defenses varies with the size and shape of the particles to be removed, their hygroscopic characteristics, their velocity and their portal of entry (nose or mouth). In the nose, the process begins with the filtration of very large particles by the nasal vibrissae. Most particles greater than 10 μm impact on the surfaces of the nasal septum and turbinates, since the convoluted surfaces and narrow passages encourage turbulent airflow. As the airstream then changes direction at the nasopharynx, most of the remaining particles of about 10 μm in size impact on the posterior wall of the pharynx. The nasopharynx and oral fauces are well provided with lymphoid tissue, the adenoids and tonsils, to assist in dealing with these impacted particles, both animate and inanimate.

The airstream entering the upper trachea contains relatively few particles larger than 10 to 15 μm in size. The airway above the vocal cords is narrow and irregular, causing turbulence and forcing both larger and smaller particles onto the mucociliary blanket which lines the tracheobronchial tree. Below the vocal cords, sedimentation, which removes most particles of 5.0 to 0.2 μm, becomes more important than impaction. The airstream velocity slows as it enters the progressive bifurcations of the tracheobronchial tree. Both the number and the angles of the branches are important, since the probability of a particle landing on a bronchial wall is proportional to the cosine of the angle between the parent and the daughter bronchus. Larger particles tend to be removed in the more proximal bronchial tree, while smaller ones may reach the peripheral airways before being deposited onto the mucociliary blanket.

Particles smaller than 0.1 μm are rather randomly deposited throughout the airways by their brownian motion. Inertia and gravitational forces have little effect on such small particles. Their removal in the respiratory tract is thus inefficient and most are exhaled rapidly.

AIRWAY REFLEXES

The airway reflexes are an important adjunct to the aerodynamic defenses of the respiratory tract. The cough is an effective means for removing excessive secretions or foreign materials from the tracheobronchial tree. The person coughing takes a deep inspiration, then begins to exhale against the closed glottis. Intrapleural pressures can thus rise rapidly, to over 100 mm of mercury. As the glottis is suddenly opened, pressures in the trachea and the major bronchi fall rapidly and the bronchial caliber is reduced. The linear airflow velocity increases dramatically, to values approaching 85% of the speed of sound. Secretions lining the walls of the narrowed bronchi protrude into the bronchial lumen where the high airflow velocity propels them into the larger airways.

Bronchoconstriction prevents or reduces penetration of inhaled materials into the distal areas of the respiratory tract. Mucosal edema and the vagally mediated contraction of smooth muscle in the tracheobronchial tree result in narrowed airways with increased airflow resistance. Many physical and immunologic stimuli may initiate bronchoconstriction, including mechanical irritation of the upper airway, inhalation of irritant gases, certain droplet aerosols and certain dusts.

EPITHELIAL ADHERENCE

The oropharynx serves as the portal of entry for all sorts of ingested and inhaled materials and contains a large and complex residual bacterial flora to which new organisms are constantly being introduced. In spite of innumerable opportunities for diversification, however, the general composition of the oropharyngeal flora of normal persons remains fairly constant, especially in the various microenvironments of the mouth.

The ability of the buccal epithelium to preferentially permit adherence of a relatively nonpathogenic bacterial population is an important host defense. Adherence of bacteria to the oropharyngeal squamous epithelial cells results from interaction between the bacterial surface and specific receptors on host cells. Glycoproteins on bacterial cell walls are thought to be responsible for adherence of the "normal" mouth flora. Salivary glycoproteins have been shown to inhibit the adherence of streptococci to buccal epithelial cells. While the exact mechanisms and specificity of bacterial adherence to epithelial cells are not fully understood, changes in the adherence characteristics of buccal epithelial cells have been demonstrated in patients in intensive care units, in postoperative patients, in smokers, and in patients with acute respiratory infections or influenza. Epithelial cells from such patients have been shown to permit increased numbers of gram-negative bacilli to adhere to the cell surface. In postoperative and intensive care unit patients, these changes in adherence are associated with colonization of the oropharynx by gram-negative bacilli. Epithelial cells, which permit binding of increased numbers of gram-negative bacilli, bind fewer streptococci. The binding of gram-negative bacilli is not very species-specific and can be blocked by binding of concanavalin A but not by bovine serum albumin or by phytohemagglutinin. The actual number of binding sites for gram-negative bacilli seems to increase in the oropharynx of the host impaired by acute illness or surgery. The resulting changes in the oropharyngeal flora, and increase in potentially pathogenic gram-negative bacilli, increases the risk of pulmonary infection by these organisms in affected patients.

MUCOCILIARY BARRIERS

From the nasopharynx to the terminal bronchioles, the ciliated respiratory epithelium acts in concert with the goblet cells and mucous gland secretions to provide a very efficient trapping and removal system for particulate and soluble materials and is known as the mucociliary transport system. Each of the pseudostratified ciliated respiratory epithelial cells deploys approximately 200 cilia, 5 μm long and 0.3 μm in diameter. The coordinated movements of the respiratory cilia sweep the overlying mucus blanket towards the oropharynx where the mucus and its entrapped material either then may be swallowed or expectorated.

Ultrastructural studies of the respiratory cilia reveal arrangement of nine pairs of microtubules which surround a central pair of microtubules (Figure 2-1). The smaller of the units in the nine outer microtubule pairs (subunit A) has two short dynein arms which project towards the next outer pair of microtubules. The nine outer microtubule doublets are connected to each other by nexin links. Radial spokes extend from the A subunit of each outer microtubule doublet to the sheath surrounding the central microtubule pair. The nine outer microtubule doublets extend down to a basal plate; the central axial pair does not reach this far. The bending of cilia seems to result from sliding of the outer doublet microtubules using the dynein arms as bridges. Dynein has been shown to have adenosine triphosphate activity and may function analogously to the myosin bridges of muscle. The central microtubules may play a role in coordinating ciliary movement.

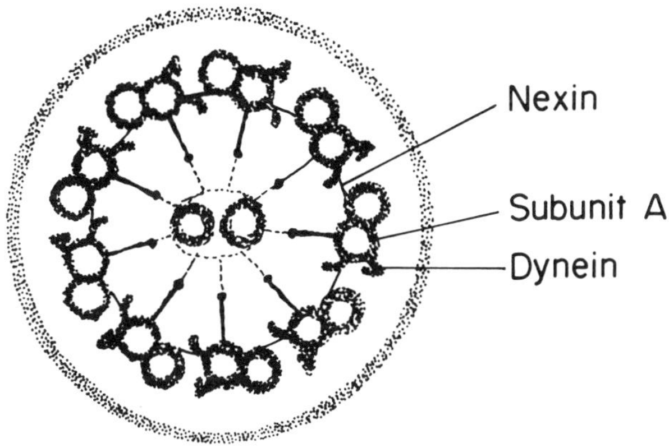

Figure 2-1 A schematic diagram of the cross-section of a cilium.

A variety of congenital ultrastructural abnormalities recently have been described which can render cilia completely immobile or significantly dysfunctional and which thus alter rates of mucociliary clearance. Sturgess et al (1980) have proposed classifying these abnormalities as "ciliary dyskinesis"—Type 1: defective dynein; Type 2: defective radial spokes; and Type 3: microtubule transposition. The Type 1 defect was first described by Elaisson et al in patients with Kartagener's syndrome; individuals with chronic sinobronchial infections without Kartagener's syndrome have been found to have the other cilial defects described.

The mucous blanket is produced by both the goblet cells and the mucous secretory glands. Goblet cells release their mucus by rupture of the cell surface, while the mucous gland secretions are excreted through ciliated ducts onto the surface of the respiratory epithelium.

The mucous blanket actually consists of two functional layers: a 5-μm deep layer of low shear fluid, which behaves as a sol, rests on the epithelial surface and covers the beating cilia. Above this lies a viscous higher shear gel-like layer, 2 μm thick. The tips of the cilia reach the gel layer at the peak of their stroke. The gel layer is impermeable to water and may protect the underlying periciliary fluid level from dehydration. It also serves as a barrier/trap to particles settling on the mucociliary blanket.

Mucus is a complex mucopolysaccharide polymer whose gel structure is dependent on the arrangement of its long glycoprotein mucins linked through hydrogen and disulfide bonds. Water, which comprises 95% of mucus, is organized in part at least by hydrogen bonding in this glycoprotein "skeleton." In the presence of infection or inflammation, tracheobronchial secretions become more viscous and tenacious, interfering with normal mucous flow. This increased viscosity results from several factors, including increased disulfide bonding between the glycoprotein mucins and the addition of deoxyribose nucleoprotein fibrils from disintegrating phagocytic cells which are then incorporated into the mucus gel.

The respiratory epithelium cilia beat ineffectively or not at all unless covered by their mucous blanket, requiring that both components be considered together in studies of mucociliary transport. It is known that cilia beat at 1000 and 1500 cycles per minute in waves that result in a progressive increase in velocity as mucus approaches the upper airway. Linear velocities of mucus transport range from 0.5 to 1 mm per minute in the small airways to as much as 5 to 20 mm in the main bronchi and trachea. Rates are not necessarily uniform at each level—mucosal injury, areas of squamous metaplasia and eddy formation may produce local slowing. Nevertheless, almost all material deposited on the normal mucociliary transport system is removed within 24 hours.

Ciliary movement can be affected by many physical and chemical stimuli. Oxygen is necessary for ciliary motion, although 100% oxygen depresses mucociliary transport. Local levels of calcium, potassium, and hydrogen may affect function, and it has been shown that cardiac glycosides can reverse the ciliary dysfunction caused by hypoxia in an animal model. Cigarette smoke slows ciliary beating and produces incoordination. The physical characteristics of the mucous blanket can result in major alterations in mucociliary transport. When mucous gland hypertrophy occurs, the increased volume of secretions is associated with an increase in mucous viscosity and impaired mucous transport.

ALVEOLAR DEFENSES

Particles ranging from 2 μm to 0.2 μm may escape being deposited onto the mucociliary blanket to reach the pulmonary alveoli. The alveolar walls are lined by two types of epithelial cells. The Type 1 squamous pneumocyte is a large cell thinly stretched over a very large area. Cytoplasmic extensions of the Type 1 pneumocyte may actually reach from one alveolus into another. These cells do not replicate in the alveoli and, because of their large exposed surface area, are susceptible to a wide variety of toxic insults. The Type 2 granular pneumocyte is a smaller, roughly cuboidal cell which is usually found at the alveolar septal junctions. It is recognized by its characteristic lamellar cytoplasmic inclusions that are the storage form of the surfactant which this cell secretes into the alveolar lining fluid.

Once a particle has landed on an alveolar surface, it is likely to be promptly ingested by a pulmonary alveolar macrophage, the resident phagocyte of the lung. The particle will be killed and/or digested by the alveolar macrophage or will leave the alveolus inside the macrophage by one of several routes. Alveolar macrophages and their load of ingested material may travel from the alveolus out of the terminal bronchioles and thence onto the mucociliary transport system or they may migrate through the interstitium into the pulmonary lymphatic channels and on to the pulmonary lymph nodes. Uningested particles may be carried along in the alveolar lining fluid out to the alveolar ducts and the terminal bronchioles or into the pulmonary lymphatic channels that lie close to the terminal bronchioles. Uningested particles in the lymphatic channels may then be ingested by macrophages that have migrated into the lymphatics from the interstitial spaces or perhaps ingested by the lymphatic endothelial cells.

The pulmonary alveolar macrophage is the main defense of the alveolus. The origin of the pulmonary macrophage, like other tissue macrophages, is the bone marrow. From the marrow, circulating monocytes reach the pulmonary interstitium and become a self-replicating population which serves as the source for alveolar macrophages. The alveolar macrophage population is capable of DNA synthesis and production of colony-stimulating factor. Patients receiving chemotherapy for acute leukemia have been shown to have normal numbers of alveolar macrophages in spite of severe peripheral monocytopenia.

Alveolar macrophages vary in size from 15 to 50 μm in diameter; the nucleus-to-cytoplasm ratio averages about 1:3. The cytoplasm contains Golgi bodies, mitchondria, predominantly rough endoplasmic reticulum, free ribosomes, glycogen granules and a wide variety of inclusion bodies resulting from the fusion of the primary lysosomes and the digestive vacuoles. Scanning electron microscopy of alveolar macrophages reveals a very ruffled cell membrane.

The alveolar macrophage is well adapted to its habitat in the pulmonary alveolus and, in spite of its origin from common bone marrow precursor, differs metabolically in several important respects from other tissue macrophages. The resting alveolar macrophage has a much higher rate of oxygen consumption than do peritoneal macrophages or polymorphonuclear leukocytes. During phagocytosis, however, oxygen consumption increases to a lesser extent than in other phagocytic cells. Alveolar macrophages have more mitochondria and more cytochrome oxidase than do peritoneal macrophages. They also have lower levels of the glycolytic pathway enzymes, such as pyruvate kinase and phosphofructokinase, than do their peritoneal counterparts. These differences indicate that the alveolar macrophage, which exists in a relatively aerobic environment (ambient PO_2 approximately 100 mmHg) is dependent primarily on oxidative phosphorylation for its metabolic needs. The peritoneal macrophage, which exists in an environment low in oxygen

(PO_2 approximately 5 mmHg) utilizes anaerobic glycolysis for most of its energy needs.

Ingestion of particles is an active process which requires metabolic energy. The phagocytizing alveolar macrophage consumes oxygen ("the respiratory burst") and relies heavily on oxidative phosphorylation to provide the energy needed for phagocytosis. It also makes some use of anaerobic glycolysis. Incubation in relatively anaerobic conditions (an ambient PO_2 of less than 25 mmHg) will inhibit particle phagocytosis by alveolar macrophages. In normal aerobic conditions, metabolic poisons that block anaerobic glycolysis, such as iodoacetate or sodium fluoride, will also interfere with alveolar macrophage phagocytosis. In contrast to the alveolar macrophage, other phagocytes, such as peritoneal macrophages and polymorphonuclear leukocytes, can sustain phagocytosis for at least the short periods under anaerobic conditions by using anaerobic glycolysis as their sole energy source.

The alveolar macrophage, however, is an adaptable cell. The inhibition of phagocytosis seen in anaerobic conditons is reversible if the cell is soon returned to an aerobic environment. When alveolar macrophages are cultivated in hypoxic conditions for periods of 96 hours, their levels of glycolytic enzymes increase and the activity of the oxidative phosphorylation pathway enzymes decrease, indicating a functional adaption to the hypoxic environment.

The mechanics of ingestion by alveolar macrophages, unlike the energetics, seem to be similar to those of other phagocytic cells. The process has been well described by Stossel (1974). A particle must be recognized by the phagocyte as a candidate for phagocytosis. Coating of particles by certain serum proteins can promote "recognition" if the phagocytic cell has specific surface membrane receptor sites for these proteins or "opsonins." The best-defined opsonins are IgG and the third component of the complement. Alveolar macrophages, like polymorphonuclear leukocytes, monocytes and peritoneal macrophages, have specific surface membrane receptors for the Fc fragment of IgG and for the C_3b fragment of C_3. When alveolar macrophages are "activated," as by administration of Calmette-Guérin bacillus to the donor animal, the number or affinity (or both) of the IgG and the complement receptors on the cells increases. Such activated cells have been shown to ingest more particles than nonactivated cells.

It is not understood how an opsonized particle, coated with IgG and C_3, signals its presence to the phagocytic cell at some distance from it, over what distance such a "signal" can effectively travel, or exactly how the phagocytic cell receives that "signal." It is clear, however, that movement of the phagocytic cell toward the opsonized particle and ingestion of the particle are active processes which require directed movement of the phagocytic cell. The alveolar macrophage, like other phagocytic cells, has a system of contractile proteins which allow movement around and ingestion of particles. These proteins include actin, myosin, actin-binding protein and a cofactor required for activation of the myosin-associated, magnesium-requiring ATP-ase. Stossel has proposed that fibrils of actin polymers form a tangled mesh in cytoplasm. Particle contact or other signals somehow activate the actin-binding protein, which then causes cross-linking of actin into microfilaments and provides a rigid structure for the cytoplasmic gel. Myosin, in the presence of its cofactor, can now cause contraction of the gel and localized distortion and increased fluidity in areas of pseudopod formation. Many details of this process are not yet well understood, including the roles played by microfilaments and microtubules.

Alveolar macrophages will respond with directed movement to chemotactic stimuli. Their pattern of chemotaxis to various stimuli differs from the responses of peritoneal macrophages and monocytes in some respects. Endotoxin-activated serum, whose principal chemotactic factor is C_5a, and lymphocyte-derived chemotactic factor elicit very poor chemotactic responses from alveolar macrophages. On the other hand, bacterial chemotactic factors, small peptides released during bacterial growth, and the N-formylmethionyl peptides will provoke a very good chemotactic response from alveolar macrophages. As in phagocytosis, the metabolic energy for alveolar macrophage chemotaxis is derived from both oxidative phosphorylation and anaerobic glycolysis. Incubation in relatively low oxygen environments inhibits alveolar macrophage chemotaxis. Interestingly, incubation in hyperoxic conditions for several hours also depresses alveolar macrophage chemotaxis without affecting cell viability.

Once the particle to be ingested has been reached and the pseudopodia of the alveolar macrophage have surrounded it to form the phagocytic vacuole, a number of microbicidal mechanisms are brought into action. As the phagosome is forming, granules in its vicinity fuse with the phagosome membrane and discharge their contents into it (degranulation) forming the phagolysosome. The lysosomes of alveolar macrophages contain a variety of materials with antimicrobial activity— lysozyme, cathepsin, hydrolytic enzymes, such as β-glucuronidase, β-galactosidase, and acid phosphotase, aryl-sulfatase and phospholipases. Alveolar macrophages recently have been shown to contain two cationic proteins with a rather broad spectrum of antimicrobial activity in their lysosomes. Alveolar macrophages also produce a variety of neutral proteinases which may have both antimicrobial and less specific digestive functions. These include collagenase, elastase and plasminogen activators.

The antimicrobial materials just mentioned comprise the nonoxygen-dependent microbicidal mechanisms of the alveolar macrophage. The oxygen-dependent microbicidal activity of the alveolar macrophage, although still incompletely understood, probably plays the major role in the killing of many pulmonary pathogens. A variety of stimuli, which have in common interaction with the phagocytic cell surface membrane, can trigger the "respiratory burst" in phagocytic cells. Suitable agents include particles such as opsonized bacteria, unopsonized inanimate materials like latex particles, the plant lectin concanavalin A, and soluble materials such as phorbol myristate acetate, several ionophores and fluoride ions, and the activated fragment of the fifth complement component C_5a. Activation of the respiratory burst, which follows an appropriate stimulus by 30 to 60 seconds, does not require the occurrence of either phagocytosis or degranulation. Activation seems to be an energy-dependent process since it can be blocked when both glycolysis and mitochondrial oxidative phosphorylation are inhibited.

Activation of the respiratory burst initiates a marked increase in oxygen uptake by phagocytic cells. The alveolar macrophage, unlike other phagocytic cells, consumes part of this oxygen in the mitochondrial respiratory chain instead of using most or all of it to form reactive oxygen radicals. Part of the oxygen uptake, however, is utilized in the production of hydrogen peroxide (H_2O_2), superoxide anion (O_2^-) and other reactive oxygen-containing metabolites. The generation of superoxide anion and hydrogen peroxide in alveolar macrophages is very probably catalyzed by the enzyme NADPH oxidase, since alveolar macrophages from a patient with chronic granulomatous disease have been shown to have the same metabolic deficiencies as the polymorphonuclear leukocytes and the monocytes of patients with CGD. In addition to superoxide anion and hydrogen peroxide, alveolar macrophages also have been shown to produce hydroxyl radicals (•OH). Both hydroxyl radicals and superoxide anions are highly reactive intermediate radicals and are probably capable of doing significant oxidative damage to microbial cell membranes. However, their exact contribution to microbial killing by phagocytes remains unclear. Hydrogen peroxide is produced from superoxide anion by the action of superoxide dismutase. In the polymorphonuclear leukocyte, hydrogen peroxide interacts with myeloperoxidase and with halide ions to form a potent in vitro antimicrobial system which iodinates bacterial cell wall components. The clinical significance of the hydrogen peroxide–myeloperoxidase system remains unclear, however, since the polymorphonuclear leukocytes of patients with myeloperoxidase deficiency show impaired killing of *Candida albicans*, but normal killing of many bacteria. Moreover, patients with myeloperoxidase deficiency rarely have difficulty with infections. The alveolar macrophage contains no myeloperoxidase and does not iodinate ingested bacterial particles, although it kills such bacteria promptly. It has been postulated that catalase, which alveolar macrophages do have, can replace myeloperoxidase in the H_2O_2–halide–myeloperoxidase system. However, there is no good evidence to support this postulate, and the relative contributions of the various oxygen-containing reactive intermediates to total microbicidal activity of the alveolar macrophage require further study.

During the ingestion of large numbers of particles, phagocytic cells internalize a substantial amount of their cell surface and eventually can no longer ingest particles. These satiated cells can be shown to have lost many of their surface membrane receptors. New cell surface and surface receptors can be generated, in time, by mononuclear phagocytes such as the alveolar macrophage, but not by the neutrophil. Since, under comparable in vitro conditions, alveolar macrophages migrate more slowly, ingest more slowly and even kill more slowly than neutrophils, it would be possible to overwhelm their microbicidal capacity if a large enough microbial challenge is suddenly presented. It is not surprising, therefore, that the alveolar macrophage can recruit assistance for dealing with such contingencies.

It recently has been shown that the alveolar macrophage can synthesize and release a neutrophil chemotactic factor, a low molecular weight, relatively heat-stable substance. Release of the neutrophil chemotactic factor by alveolar macrophages is stimulated by phagocytosis of bacterial particles, such as *S. aureus* and *S. albus*, or inanimate particles, such as zymosan and Sepharose-4B and by immune complexes. Serum opsonization of the particles by C_3b significantly augments the release of alveolar macrophage neutrophil chemotactic factor compared to phagocytosis of unopsonized particles. Purified C_3b alone can induce release of the neutrophil chemotactic factor. Particles coated with IgG, though not with complement, can also cause alveolar macrophages to produce and release neutrophil chemotactic factor.

The alveolar macrophage functions in the thin layer of fluid lining the alveoli. This fluid medium contains several materials that are important for normal alveolar macrophage function and several that are produced or destroyed by the alveolar macrophages. Surfactant, a major component of the alveolar lining material, is synthesized in the Type II alveolar lining cell. Its major component is dipalmitoyl lecithin. The alveolar macrophage contains lysosomal hydrolytic enzymes that are capable of degrading surfactant. It is not surprising, therefore, that radiolabeling studies have shown that alveolar macrophages ingest and catabolize surfactant and probably play the major role in its clearance. Changes in surfactant composition can thus alter alveolar macrophage function; conversely, changes in alveolar macrophage catabolism of surfactant can lead to alterations in pulmonary function.

Alveolar lining fluid also contains small amounts of phospholipids, neutral lipids and proteins including albumin, transferrin, α1-antitrypsin, immunoglobulins G, A and E, occasionally IgM and small amounts of complement including C_3, C_4, C_5, C_6, C_9, and Factor B of the alternative complement pathway and free IgA secretory component. In addition to all of the above, alveolar lining fluid from certain animal species may contain an as yet undefined substance that enhances alveolar macrophage microbicidal activity for some bacterial species.

Although some of the immunoglobulin present in bronchoalveolar fluid originates in the systemic circulation and reaches the alveoli by transudation from pulmonary capillaries, specific IgG and IgA are locally produced by the pulmonary lymphocytes. Bronchopulmonary lavage has demonstrated the presence of T-lymphocytes, B-lymphocytes, and "null" cells in bronchoalveolar fluid, which comprise a fairly stable resident pulmonary lymphocyte population. This population can be augmented by emigration of systemic lymphocytes into the lung. Local administration of antigen can provoke a local immune response in the respiratory tract. The nature of the response will vary with the antigen, its distribution and the dose. A relatively small dose of antigen administered directly to the respiratory tract may elicit only a pulmonary response, either humoral or cellular or combined. A large dose may evoke a systemic as well as a local immune response when antigen reaches the systemic circulation and lymphoid tissues. Relatively large particles will be preferentially deposited in the upper airway where the local humoral response will be predominantly IgA antibody. Immunoglobulin A can agglutinate microbial particles, which may enhance mucociliary clearance. It can neutralize a variety of respiratory viruses including common pathogens such as influenza, rhinoviruses and respiratory syncytial viruses. It also can reduce or prevent attachment of bacteria to mucosal surfaces and so can prevent colonization as an initial stage in infection.

Antigens that reach the lower respiratory tract will elicit a humoral response which is mostly immunoglobulin G. Immunoglobulin G can perform a number of antimicrobial functions. It opsonizes microbes alone or, together with complement, it neutralizes many viruses and toxins, agglutinates particles and lyses susceptible gram-negative bacilli in the presence of complement. Pulmonary production of IgM and IgE also has been demonstrated, but their role in the pulmonary defenses is not as clear as that of IgG and IgA. IgM is variably present in small amounts in respiratory secretions; although it can fix complement and lyse susceptible gram-negative bacilli and can agglutinate particles, it does not function as an opsonin and may play a very small role in the normal defenses of the lung.

The pulmonary alveolar macrophage plays a significant role in processing antigens that reach the lower levels of the respiratory tract, thus becoming involved in both the humoral and cellular immune responses. The alveolar macrophage is also the effector cell for cell-mediated immune responses in the lung. Immune T-lymphocytes can respond to specific antigen by two methods. One is lymphocyte-mediated cytotoxic T-lymphocyte destruction of cells carrying membrane antigens to which the T-lymphocytes have been sensitized. It is not clear that this reaction occurs in the respiratory tract. The second T-lymphocyte response to the presence of antigen is the release of lymphokines, soluble mediators that evoke macrophage responses. These lymphokines include macrophage migration-inhibitory factor, which is probably identical to macrophage-activating factor, macrophage-aggregation factor, macrophage-fusion factor, chemotactic factor and cytotoxic factor. "Activation" of alveolar macrophages may occur after direct exposure to certain materials, such as endotoxin, or in response to lymphokine production by sensitized T-lymphocytes. The activated macrophage, a larger cell with a larger complement of surface membrane receptors and of hydrolytic enzymes is a more efficient phagocytic cell, now capable of killing certain microbes, such as *M. tuberculosis, L. monocytogenes, T. gondii,* which it is unable to kill in an unactivated state. It also becomes cytotoxic for virus-infected cells.

The multiple defenses of the respiratory tract are designed primarily to deal with airborne microbial invasion of the lung. Infection can easily reach the lung, however, via the bloodstream since the pulmonary capillaries receive almost the entire venous return. Although the defenses of the lung from hematogenous invasion have not been extensively studied, it is relatively easy to envision how the alveolar macrophage is probably responsible for their modulation.

The presence of virulent microbes in sufficient numbers in the pulmonary capillary bed may be accompanied by some or many of the following events: release of endotoxin, release of bacterial cell wall peptides that are chemotactic for phagocytic cells, activation of the alternative complement pathway, formation of antigen–antibody complexes, generation of vasoactive substances and endothelial damage. Alveolar macrophages are present in the pulmonary interstitium as well as in the alveoli and so are readily accessible to the signals listed above, especially if capillary integrity is compromised and soluble mediators or even microbes reach the interstitium. As mentioned above, alveolar macrophages will release neutrophil chemotactic factor when stimulated by the presence of bacteria, especially when the bacteria are opsonized with IgG and C_3b, or when stimulated by the presence of antigen–antibody complexes or C_3b alone. If the alveolar or interstitial concentrations of immunoglobulins or complement are increased because of altered vascular permeability, this may facilitate particle opsonization and add to the effect of alveolar macrophage-derived chemotactic factor in recruiting neutrophils into the lung to deal with the microbial invasion. The altered vascular permeability also may allow microbial antigen to reach systemic as well as pulmonary lymphatic tissue, thus insuring a systemic as well as a local immune response to the inciting pathogen.

Complex and complementary, the various defenses of the respiratory tract can be damaged by a number of environmental, infectious and even pharmacologic agents. Since a number of defense mechanisms may be simultaneously affected by a single agent or disease, details of the pathogenesis of impaired pulmonary defenses remain unclear in many instances. In addition, in vitro studies of isolated segments of the lung defenses, such as in vitro pulmonary alveolar macrophage function, do not always reflect the complex interactions occurring in the lung in vivo.

A typical example is the work done by many investigators on the effects of viral infections on pulmonary antibacterial defenses. In in vivo animal studies, influenza infection impairs pulmonary bactericidal activity against aerosols of *S. aureus.* However, in in vitro assays of alveolar macrophage function, influenza virus infection of the macrophages does not impair their ability to ingest and kill *S. aureus.* Additionally, macrophage chemotaxis has been shown to be impaired in vitro during influenza infection. Murine parainfluenza 1 viral infections will interfere with the in vitro ability of mouse alveolar macrophages to bind *Candida krusei,* but will not affect their ability to kill *S. epidermidis* and *S. aureus.* Murine cytomegalovirus will inhibit the in vitro phagocytosis of *S. aureus* by murine alveolar macrophages. Obviously, the interactions between different viruses and the various aspects of the pulmonary defenses, even the multiple defensive activities of the alveolar macrophage, are complex and still incompletely understood.

Alcoholic intoxication also has a number of effects on the antimicrobial defenses of the lung. In addition to the obvious risk of aspiration of oropharyngeal contents following severe inebriation with altered mental status, chronic alcoholism may alter the adherence characteristics of the buccal epithelium and predispose to oropharyngeal colonization with gram-negative bacilli. Acute intoxication impairs in vivo clearance of bacterial aerosols in experimental animals, but the exact mechanisms by which the lung defenses are impaired have not been studied in detail.

Immunosuppressive therapy, whether using corticosteroid administration alone or in combination with cytotoxic agents results in an increased risk of pulmonary infection and has been shown to have a variety of adverse consequences in the lung. Studies in animal models have shown that glucocorticosteroids can depress in vivo pulmonary clearance of bacterial aerosols. A combined regimen of hydrocortisone and cyclophosphamide will also decrease the numbers of alveolar macrophages that can be recovered by bronchopulmonary lavage (which cortisone alone does not do). In vitro studies of alveolar macrophage phagocytic ability after pretreatment with steroids alone or in combination with cyclophosphamide have shown no impairment of ingestion. Both cortisone and cyclophosphamide have been shown to reduce alveolar macrophage chemotaxis. Additionally, cortisone and cyclophosphamide reduce the amount of chemotactic activity for neutrophils produced by cultures of alveolar macrophages and reduce the biosynthesis of C_2 and C_4 by alveolar macrophages.

Glucocorticosteroids profoundly depress both the number and function of circulating T cells. T-lymphocyte production of lymphokines is required for the "activation" of alveolar macrophages; without activation, alveolar macrophages cannot kill several important opportunistic pathogens such as *Toxoplasma gondii,* mycobacteria, etc. When the effects of steroids and cytotoxic agents on neutrophil numbers and on responsiveness to chemotactic stimuli, such as those generated by alveolar macrophages, are considered, the susceptibility of immunosuppressed patients to pulmonary infection is not surprising.

Patients with congenital or acquired disorders of their immune systems—immunoglobulin deficiencies, abnormalities of cellular immunity, disorders of classic or alternative complement pathway components or defects in neutrophil or monocyte function—are more susceptible to pulmonary infections. Disease states that impair these host defenses, such as neoplasms, cirrhosis, sarcoidosis and renal failure, also increase the risk of pulmonary infection.

Nevertheless, in spite of environment assaults and endogenous deficiencies, the multiple specific and nonspecific defenses of the respiratory tract work remarkably well together in protecting the lung against infection.

SELECTED READINGS

Babior BM: Oxygen-dependent microbial killing by phagocytes. *N Engl J Med* 1978;298:659-668,721-725.

Dauber JH, Daniele RP: Chemotactic activity of guinea pig alveolar macrophage. *Am Rev Resp Dis* 1978;117:673-684.

Elaisson R, Mossberg B, Comner P, et al: The immobile cilia syndrome. A congenital ciliary abnormality as an etiologic factor in chronic airway infections and male sterility. *N Engl J Med* 1977;297:1-6.

Gadek JE, Hunningbake GW, Zimmerman RL, et al: Regulation of the release of alveolar macrophage-derived neutrophil chemotactic factor. *Am Rev Resp Dis* 1980;121:723-733.

Green GM: The J. Burns Amberson Lecture—In defense of the lung. *Am Rev Resp Dis* 1970;102:691-703.

Green GM, Jakab GJ, Low RB, et al: Defense mechanisms of the respiratory membrane. *Am Rev Resp Dis* 1977;115:479-514.

Hocking WG, Golde DW: The pulmonary alveolar macrophage. *N Engl J Med* 1979;301:580-581,639-645.

Johanson WG, Higuchi JH, Chaudhuri TR, et al: Bacterial adherence to epithelial cells in bacillary colonization of the respiratory tract. *Am Rev Resp Dis* 1980;121:55-63.

Kleinerman ES, Daniels CA, Polsson RP, et al: Depression of macrophage accumulation in influenza-infected mice. *Am J Pathol* 1976;85:373–382.

Lauweryns JM, Baert JH: Alveolar clearance and the role of the pulmonary lymphatics. *Am Rev Resp Dis* 1977;115:625–683.

Mills J: Effects of Sendai virus infection on function of cultured mouse alveolar macrophages. *Am Rev Resp Dis* 1979;120:1239–1244.

Newhouse M, Sanchis J, Bienenstock J: Lung defense mechanisms. *N Engl J Med* 1976;295:990–998,1045–1052.

Nugent KM, Pesanti EL: Effect of influenza infection on the phagocytic and bactericidal activities of pulmonary macrophages. *Infect Immun* 1979;26: 651–657.

Patterson-Delafield J, Martinez RJ, Lehrer RI: Microbicidal cationic proteins in rabbit alveolar macrophages: A potential host defense mechanism. *Infect Immun* 1980;30:180–192.

Pennington JE, Harris EA: Influence of immunosuppression on alveolar macrophage chemotactic activities in guinea pigs. *Am Rev Resp Dis* 1981;123: 299–304.

Stanley JD, Pesanti EL: Replication of murine cytomegalovirus in lung macrophages: Effect on phagocytosis of bacteria. *Infect Immun* 1980;29:1152–1159.

Stossel TP: Phagocytosis. *N Engl J Med* 1974;290:717–723,774–780,833–839.

Sturgess JM, Chas J, Turner JA: Transposition of ciliary microtubules: Another cause of impaired ciliary motility. *N Engl J Med* 1980;303:318–322.

3 *Radiographic Manifestations of Pneumonia: An Approach to Differential Diagnosis*

Linda Griska

Radiographs of the chest are important in all patients suspected of having pneumonia. The roentgenogram can confirm clinical findings, establish the extent of disease, and suggest an etiologic organism in many cases. Serial radiographs are of value in following the course of the disease, the development of complications, and the rapidity of clearing.

An abnormal chest x-ray of the type compatible with pneumonia also can be produced by many noninfectious diseases. These include pulmonary emboli, pulmonary edema, alveolar hemorrhage, "shock" lung, and tumors such as alveolar cell carcinoma or metastatic disease. Although radiographic findings may be nonspecific, correlation of these findings with the clinical history, physical examination, laboratory studies, and other investigations will yield a positive diagnosis in the majority of cases.

Occasionally, pneumonia may be present without an abnormal chest x-ray. For example, a severely neutropenic patient may not be able to produce an inflammatory pulmonary infiltrate. Rehydration of the dehydrated patient may make an undetectable infiltrate apparent. Early in the course of many pneumonias the symptoms and signs precede radiographic evidence, and therefore the most common cause for a "negative" chest x-ray may be a matter of timing.

Recognition of several common x-ray patterns can be the basis for construction of a differential diagnosis of pulmonary disease. The following examples illustrate several major radiographic patterns and the disease entities that produce them. Pneumonia is considered in the differential diagnosis of all of the patterns. The salient radiographic features specific for individual organisms will be described.

LOCALIZED ALVEOLAR INFILTRATES

The alveolar patterns are produced by diseases that predominantly involve the air spaces or acini of the lung. The infiltrates appear as fluffy, ill-defined, coalescent opacities. The "air bronchogram" is the radiographic hallmark of this pattern and is due to the presence of air-filled, patent bronchi surrounded by alveoli filled with something other than air, ie, inflammatory exudate in the case of pneumonia. The infiltrates may be homogeneous, or inhomogeneous with zones of aerated lung separating focal areas of infiltrate. The distribution of the infitrates may be segmental, nonsegmental, or lobar. Bronchopneumonia produces segmental involvement because of the mechanism of spread along the bronchial tree; however, the exudate of acute alveolar pneumonia characteristically spreads centrifugally via the pores of Kohn, unimpeded by segmental boundaries, and consequently these infiltrates become nonsegmental in distribution. The alveolar infiltrate thus can become lobar in distribution, and is referred to as lobar consolidation (Figure 3-1). In most instances there is not significant displacement or invasion of the contiguous fissures.

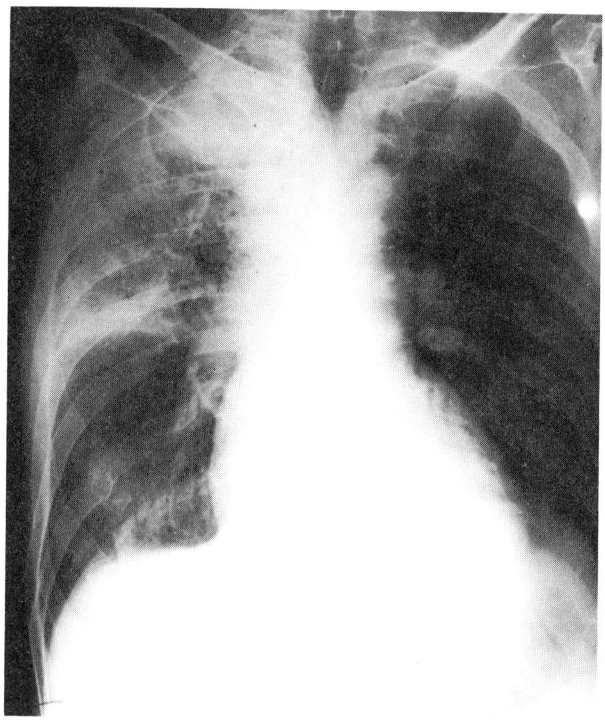

Figure 3-1 The right upper lobe is opacified due to infiltrate. Air bronchograms are present.

Bacterial pneumonia is the classical cause of localized alveolar infiltrates (Table 3-1). Pneumococcal pneumonia is still the major etiology. In untreated or inadequately treated cases, pleural effusion or even empyema may develop, but lung abscess is uncommon. It is unusual for more than one lobe to be involved.

Table 3-1
Localized Alveolar Infiltrates: Common Etiologies

1. Pneumococcal pneumonia—most common.
2. *Klebsiella* pneumonia—lobar enlargement evidenced by bowing or bulging of a fissure favors *Klebsiella* or pneumococcal Type III pneumonia.
3. Staphylococcal pneumonia—pneumatoceles may form.
4. Streptococcal pneumonia—empyema common.
5. Anaerobic pneumonia—favored if posterior segment right upper lobe or superior right lower lobe with cavitation.
6. Tuberculous pneumonia
7. Histoplasmosis—acute pneumonic form.
8. Legionnaire's disease

Acute *Klebsiella pneumoniae* pneumonia shows the same general roentgenographic features as acute pneumococcal pneumonia: homogeneous parenchymal consolidation containing an air bronchogram. Two features that aid its differentiation are: 1) a tendency for the formation of voluminous inflammatory exudate with resultant bulging of fissures and 2) a tendency to abscess and to cavity formation which is rare in acute pneumococcal pneumonia.

Staphylococcus aureus pneumonia produces parenchymal consolidation that is segmental in distribution. The disease most commonly occurs following influenza or in debilitated or immunosuppressed patients. Abscess formation with subsequent communication with the bronchial tree and the appearance of fluid-containing cavities is fairly common, occurring in 25% to 75% of cases. Pyopneumothorax may occur as a complication. In children, a distinctive characteristic is the development of pneumatoceles. These cystic spaces are commonly thin-walled and are thought to result from check valve obstruction of a communication between a peribronchial abscess and the lumen of a bronchus. Many pneumatoceles contain fluid levels. They usually appear during the first week of thc pneumonia and disappear spontaneously, frequently within six weeks. The common method of development of acute staphylococcal pneumonia is by inhalation or aspiration of the organism, but occasionally organisms reach the lung as septic emboli, particularly in intravenous drug abusers or in hospitalized patients with infected intravenous access sites. The x-ray appearance, then, is not of segmental consolidation but one of multiple nodular masses throughout the lungs which may subsequently cavitate.

In most respects, the roentgenographic characteristics of *Streptococcus pyogenes* pneumonia are indistinguishable from those of other causes of acute bacterial pneumonia. The tendency to produce pneumatoceles or pyopneumothorax found in acute staphylococcal pneumonia is absent, and lung abscesses and cavities rarely develop, although empyema is common.

Legionnaire's disease (*Legionella pneumophila* pneumonia) most commonly presents radiographically as an alveolar infiltrate of lobar distribution. Lower lobe involvement is most common, although all lobes have been reported to be involved. Small pleural effusions are present in up to two thirds of cases. Radiographic progression for several days following therapy has been noted, despite clinical response.

Anaerobic infections also produce alveolar infiltrates. Anaerobic infections may result from aspiration of food or gastric secretions in the postoperative state, and in alcoholics, epileptics, comatose patients or those with laryngeal or swallowing disorders. The distribution of pneumonia from aspiration of material contaminated with oral anaerobic microflora reflects gravitational flow, most commonly affecting posterior segments of the right upper lobe or superior segments of the right lower lobe (aspiration in the recumbent position), or basal segments of the lower lobes (aspiration when erect). In the majority of cases, necrosis will occur relatively early and become apparent as single or multiple thick-walled, irregular cavities in dependent lung regions. Empyema is common, and nearly always associated with parenchymal disease.

Reinfection (adult) tuberculosis has a strong predilection for producing alveolar infiltrates in the apical and posterior segments of the upper lobes and the superior segments of the lower lobes. These lesions often are multiple and poorly circumscribed, particularly in the early or exudative phase of the disease. Soft, fluffy, alveolar lesions may coexist with "hard" lesions of fibrotic strands, cavitation and calcification.

Pneumonic consolidation is a fairly common feature in acute histoplasmosis and thus may simulate acute bacterial air space pneumonia. Hilar lymph node enlargement is common, but because it is uncommon in acute bacterial pneumonia, this finding should suggest acute histoplasmosis, especially in endemic areas. Histoplasmosis sometimes is manifested by unilateral or bilateral enlargement of hilar, mediastinal or intrapulmonary lymph nodes, without roentgenographic evidence of parenchymal disease. This form is particularly common in children, in whom it may produce tracheal obstruction. Unlike tuberculosis, primary histoplasmosis rarely gives rise to pleural effusion. Typical punctate splenic calcifications have been reported in up to 50% of cases in some endemic areas.

Pulmonary actinomycosis, nocardiosis, blastomycosis and cryptococcosis may also present as alveolar infiltrates. Actinomycosis involves the lower lobes more commonly than the upper, pleural thickening is common, and the adjacent ribs may show destructive or periosteal changes. Cutaneous sinuses may be formed. X-ray findings in North American blastomycosis are completely nonspecific. The usual pattern is one of acute alveolar pneumonia, most often nonsegmental. The upper lobes are affected more frequently than the lower, in a ratio of 3:2. Cavitation occurs in no more than 15% of cases. Nodules are less common than in histoplasmosis or coccidioidomycosis. Hilar and mediastinal lymph node enlargement and pleural effusion are uncommon. Calcification of parenchymal lesions is rare. Pulmonary involvement occurs in two thirds of cases of nocardiosis and may be segmental, lobar or diffuse. Nocardial infection often occurs in association with pulmonary alveolar proteinosis, and is a common opportunistic pathogen in immunosuppressed patients.

DIFFUSE ALVEOLAR INFILTRATES

The diffuse alveolar pattern has characteristics that aid in its recognition. The infiltrates are soft, fluffy, poorly circumscribed and often confluent. All lobes of both lungs may be involved, although not necessarily to a uniform extent (Figure 3-2). Air bronchograms are noticeable in the consolidated areas. The differential diagnosis of this type of lesion is based on the type of material replacing air in the alveoli, ie, blood, inflammatory exudate, tumor, edema fluid. Alveolar hemorrhage, diffuse pneumonia, pulmonary edema, alveolar proteinosis, and alveolar cell carcinoma can all produce diffuse alveolar infiltrates and be indistinguishable radiographically (Table 3-2).

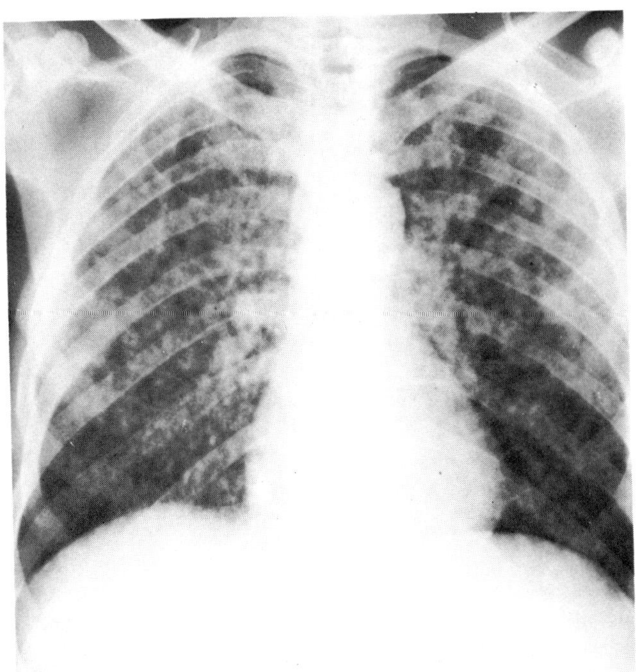

Figure 3-2 Bilateral diffuse alveolar infiltrates are present.

Table 3-2
Diffuse Alveolar Infiltrates: Differential Diagnosis

1. Pneumonia due to *Pneumocystis carinii*, cytomegalovirus, varicella-zoster, *Aspergillus*, etc
2. Pulmonary edema
3. Pulmonary hemorrhage
4. Alveolar proteinosis
5. Alveolar cell carcinoma
6. Shock lung
7. Oxygen toxicity
8. Uremia

Of the pneumonias, *Pneumocystis carinii* infection in the later stages progresses to alveolar consolidation. The radiographic changes are diffuse and may resemble those of pulmonary edema, ie, be more severe centrally than peripherally.

An identical roentgenologic pattern may occur in pneumonia due to cytomegalovirus, and there is no way of distinguishing the two roentgenographically. Terminally, the lungs may be massively consolidated, to the point of almost complete airlessness. The hilar lymph nodes do not enlarge. Pleural effusion is uncommon.

Acute chickenpox (varicella-zoster) pneumonia presents roentgenographically with diffuse, patchy alveolar infiltrates. Hilar lymph node enlargement may be present. Roentgenographic clearing may take months and many patients will have residual scarring. An interesting sequela of chickenpox pneumonia is widespread, tiny calcifications predominantly in the lower lungs. The calcifications are less than 2 to 3 mm in diameter and vary in number. These patients have a remote history of chickenpox during adult life.

Aspergillus sp may give rise to two types of diffuse alveolar lesions: 1) invasive aspergillosis which occurs in immunosuppressed individuals; and 2) allergic aspergillosis which occurs in asthmatics, and the pulmonary lesions (which have a predilection for upper lobes) represent a combination of mucoid impaction and allergic alveolitis. The mycetoma form of aspergillosis is discussed under nodular lesions.

NODULAR LESIONS

Nodular lesions (Figure 3-3) most commonly are due to metastatic tumor. Of the infectious diseases, fungi and mycobacteria produce granulomas that appear radiographically as parenchymal nodules (Table 3-3).

Histoplasmoma is a relatively common form of pulmonary histoplasmosis. It is usually a solitary, sharply circumscribed nodular shadow seldom more than 3 cm in diameter. In most cases, the lesion is in a lower

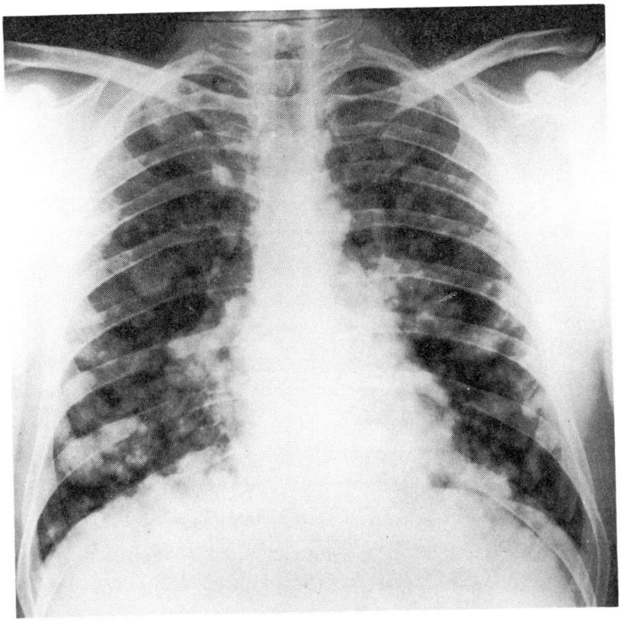

Figure 3-3 Multiple bilateral pulmonary parenchymal nodules.

lobe, often with satellite lesions nearby; many calcify, producing the "target" lesion that is virtually pathognomonic of this disease. Hilar lymph node calcification is common, although node enlargement is unusual. Histoplasmomas seldom exceed four or five in number and often differ considerably in size.

The most common form of pulmonary involvement in cryptococcosis roentgenographically is a fairly well-circumscribed lesion, 2 to 8 cm in diameter. The masses usually are peripheral and a pleural base is often characteristic. Cavitation is relatively uncommon. Hilar and mediastinal lymph node enlargement are unusual, as is pleural effusion. Calcification

Table 3-3
Multiple Nodular Lesions: Differential Diagnosis

1. Metastases
2. Granulomas (eg, histoplasmosis, tuberculosis, blastomycosis, coccidioidomycosis)
3. Hamartomas
4. Arteriovenous malformations
5. Septic emboli with abscess
6. Rheumatoid nodules
7. Wegener's granulomatosis
8. Sarcoidosis
9. Pulmonary infarcts

is rare. Widely disseminated disease rarely may give rise to a miliary or diffuse pattern.

Pulmonary nodules of coccidioidomycosis are not roentgenographically distinguishable from other granulomas. Nodules may excavate to form thin-walled cavities. Cavitation occurs predominantly in the upper lobes and, unlike tuberculosis, it may develop in the anterior segment.

The invariable roentgenographic appearance of a pulmonary fungus ball (usually an aspergilloma) is a solid, rounded mass within a spherical cavity, separated from the wall of the cavity by a crescent-shaped air space. Fluid levels are not seen within the cavities. The intracavity fungus ball occurs more commonly in upper than lower lobes, probably because it so frequently occupies a tuberculous cavity. Most of the cavities are thin walled. The differential diagnosis should include a fragment of tissue in a carcinoma that has undergone necrosis, a mass of necrotic lung tissue in an abscess, a disintegrating hydatid cyst and an intracavitary blood clot.

CAVITARY AND CYSTIC LESIONS

A cavity forms when an area of necrosis develops in the lung parenchyma (Table 3-4). The drainage of liquid necrotic material from the area is replaced by air. The remaining tissue around the periphery of the lesion constitutes the wall. Important differential characteristics of the wall include thickness and a smooth versus irregular contour (Figures 3-4 and 3-5). Cavities may or may not have associated air fluid levels.

Acute cavitating or necrotizing pneumonia is commonly due to *Pseudomonas aeruginosa* or anaerobic bacteria. *Klebsiella pneumoniae*, *Staphylococcus aureus* and *Proteus* sp also may cause necrosis in severely consolidated areas of pneumonia after several days. Cavities in anaero-

Table 3-4
Cavitary and Cystic Lesions: Differential Diagnosis

1. Necrotizing pneumonia with abscess formation—*Pseudomonas* and anaerobes most common
2. Granulomas due to *M. tuberculosis* and fungi
3. Bronchogenic carcinoma
4. Metastatic neoplasm, especially squamous cell neoplasms of head and neck origin
5. Bleb or bulla
6. Cystic bronchiectasis
7. Echinococcal cyst
8. Pulmonary infarcts
9. Pneumatocele—staphylococcal pneumonia in children
10. Rheumatoid granulomas
11. Wegener's granulomatosis

bic pneumonia characteristically are in dependent segments and contain air fluid levels.

A distinctive characteristic of staphylococcal pneumonia in children is the development of pneumatoceles. These cystic spaces are commonly thin walled and are thought to result from ball valve obstruction of a communication between a peribronchial abscess and the lumen of a

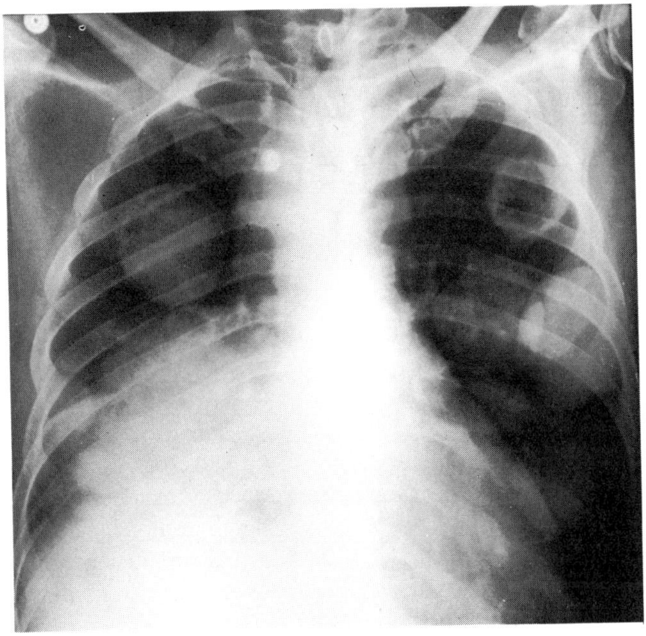

Figure 3-4 Bilateral thick-walled cavitary lesions are present.

Figure 3-5 Bilateral thin-walled cavities are demonstrated by tomography.

bronchus. They usually appear during the first week of pneumonia and disappear spontaneously, within six weeks. In adults, abscess formation in staphylococcal pneumonia is fairly common.

Fungi, mycobacteria and actinomycetes often show necrosis, sometimes after several weeks. The cavities of tuberculosis vary in size and number. The walls of the cavities may be irregular and air fluid levels are rare. The cavities of coccidioidomycosis are typically thin walled.

Pulmonary echinococcal cysts may become cavitary when communication develops with the bronchial tree. Rupture may occur between the pericyst and endocyst, permitting air entry between these layers and producing the appearance of a thin crescent of air around the periphery of the cyst—the "crescent" sign. The second form of bronchial communication occurs directly with the endocyst. After the cyst has ruptured into the bronchial tree, its membrane may float on the fluid within the cyst, giving rise to the classic "water lily" sign.

Necrosis with cavitation may occur in certain rare infections such as pneumonic plague, tularemia, and melioidosis.

DIFFUSE INTERSTITIAL, MICRONODULAR AND MIXED PATTERNS

The interstitial patterns are produced by diseases that preserve the alveolar air space and cause the tissues surrounding the air spaces to increase in volume. The appearance is predominantly an increase in linear or reticulated markings (Figure 3-6) or finely stippled nodules. The differential diagnosis of intersititial disease is extensive (Table 3-5). Of the pneumonias, *Pneumocystis carinii*, viral and mycoplasma pneumonias generally affect the interstitial tissues, whereas bacterial pneumonias more commonly are alveolar. The differential diagnosis of interstitial pattern in immunocompromised patients, for example, includes *Pneumocystis* or cytomegalovirus pneumonia as well as various noninfectious diseases such as lymphangitic metastases, radiation or drug-induced change and chronic pulmonary hemorrhage with resultant hemosiderosis.

The x-ray patterns of mycoplasma and viral pneumonias are commonly indistinguishable. In the early stages, acute interstitial inflammation is apparent as a fine reticular pattern. This is followed by signs of air space consolidation of patchy distribution. In mycoplasma pneumonia, the infiltrates tend to be segmental, predominantly of the lower lobes, hilar lymph node enlargement is rare in adults, and pleural effusion is uncommon.

Primary pneumonia caused by measles (rubeola) virus produces a reticular pattern throughout the lungs, indicating the location of the disease in the interstitium. Hilar lymph node enlargement is usual.

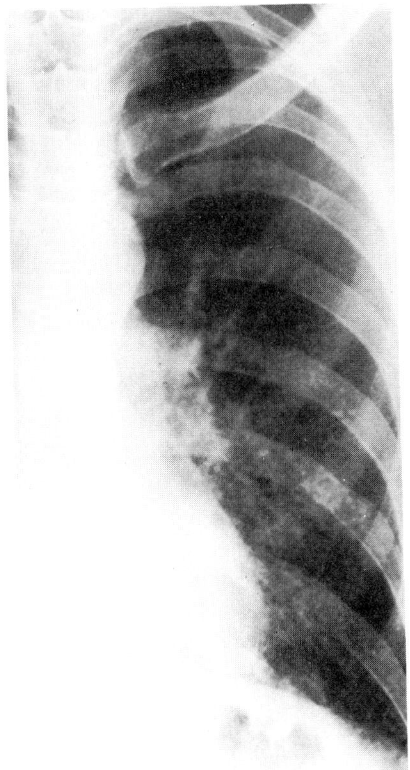

Figure 3-6 The linear reticular appearance is characteristic of interstital disease.

The diffuse micronodular (miliary) pattern is comprised of innumerable small nodules which usually appear to be 3 to 5 mm in diameter (Figure 3-7). Miliary tuberculosis remains the classic example of this pattern (Table 3-6).

Table 3-5
Diffuse Interstitial Disease: Differential Diagnosis

1. Lymphangitic metastases
2. Pneumoconioses
3. Drug hypersensitivity
4. Congestive heart failure
5. Sarcoidosis
6. *Pneumocystis carinii*, viral or mycoplasma pneumonia
7. Collagen vascular disease
8. Tuberous sclerosis
9. Amyloidosis
10. Desquamative interstitial pneumonia

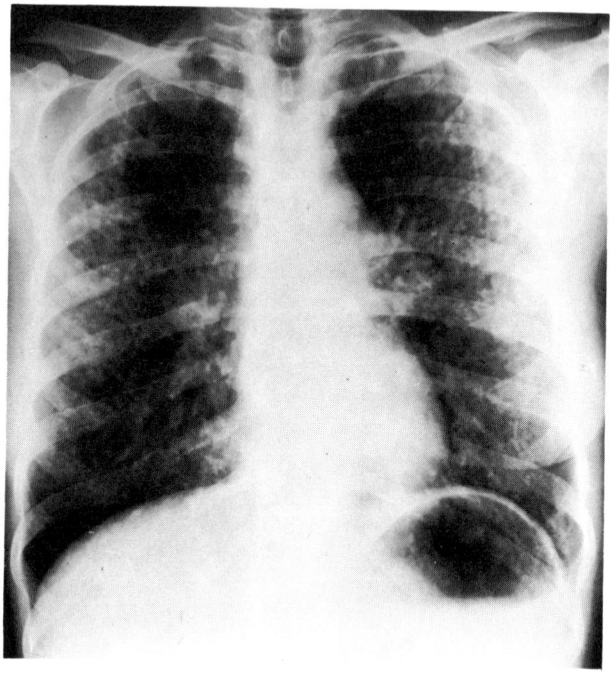

Figure 3-7 This fine micronodular interstitial pattern is miliary.

Frequently, imaging modalities other than plain chest radiographs can be of value to exclude other etiologic possibilities in the differential diagnosis of pneumonia and in the evaluation of complications of pneumonias, such as pleural involvement, necrosis with abscess formation, pneumothorax, fibrosis, or chest wall involvement. Ventilation/perfusion lung scans and, when necessary, pulmonary arteriograms may be obtained to diagnose pulmonary emboli, since both pneumonia and pulmonary emboli can produce similar plain chest roentgenograms. Transthoracic Chiba needle lung biopsies may be performed by the radiologist under fluoroscopic control to obtain tissue from a pulmonary nodule for cytologic and microbiologic analysis. The chest x-ray done with the patient in various tilting positions, such as the cross-table lateral decubitus

Table 3-6
Diffuse Miliary Disease: Differential Diagnosis

1. Tuberculosis
2. Metastatic malignancy
3. Pneumoconiosis
4. Sarcoidosis
5. Alveolar microlithiasis
6. Tuberous sclerosis

Table 3-7
Chest Radiographic Findings in Pneumonia

Organism	Distribution	Other Findings
A. BACTERIA		
Anaerobic organisms	Alveolar pattern. Posterior segments of upper lobes and superior segments of lower lobes.	Abscess formation in most cases; empyema common. Associated with atelectasis approximately 50%. Air-fluid levels common.
Escherichia coli	Alveolar pattern. Nonsegmental. Lower lobes.	Pleural effusion frequent; cavitation uncommon. Affects debilitated patients.
Klebsiella Enterobacter, Serratia	Alveolar pattern. Nonsegemental. Upper lobe predilection.	Tendency to expansion of lung; cavitation common. Air bronchogram usual. Pleural effusion may be present.
Legionella pneumophila	Alveolar pattern. Nonsegmental. All lobes; lower lobes more frequently.	Small pleural effusions common; cavitation unusual.
Mycobacterium tuberculosis (Primary)	Anterior segment of upper lobe or medial segment of middle lobe.	Ipsilateral hilar or paratracheal lymph node enlargement usual in children, but only 50% of adults. Pleural effusion 10% in children, 30% in adults. Cavitation and miliary spread rare. Atelectasis results from either compression from enlarged lymph nodes or endobronchial tuberculosis.
Myobacterium tuberculosis (Postprimary)	Inhomogeneous pattern. Upper lobe predilection, predominantly posterior and apical segments, also superior segment lower lobe.	Cavitation common. Infection may cross interlobar fissures from one lobe to another, but frequently is segmental in distribution.
Proteus	Alveolar pattern. Nonsegmental. Upper lobe predilection.	Abscess formation frequent.
Pseudomonas aeruginosa	Alveolar pattern. Nonsegmental less common than segmental. May be diffuse.	Pleural effusion common; cavitation common.

Table 3-7 (continued)

Organism	Distribution	Other Findings
Staphylococcus aureus	Alveolar pattern. No lobar predilection.	Abscess formation common with or without bronchopleural fistula and pyopneumothorax.
Streptococcus pneumoniae	Alveolar pattern. Nonsegmental. Dependent portions of upper and lower lobes.	Air bronchogram usual; cavitation rare.
Actinomyces israelii *Nocardia* sp	Alveolar pattern. Lower lobe.	Cavitation common; pleural effusion and extension into chest wall usual with or without rib destruction. May transgress interlobar fissures.
Mycoplasma pneumoniae	Lower lobes; interstitial pattern with superimposed inhomogeneous alveolar infiltrates.	Pleural effusion uncommon and lymph node enlargement rare.
B. FUNGI		
Aspergillosis	Alveolar pattern. May produce aspergilloma.	Common presentation is as opportunistic invader.
Blastomycosis	Alveolar pattern. Nonsegmental. Upper lobe predilection.	Cavitation uncommon; pleural effusion and chest wall involvement rare.
Candida albicans	No predilection.	May cavitate.
Coccidioidomycosis	Lower lobe predilection.	Hilar and paratracheal lymph node enlargement may be present. Cavitation common, thin walled.
Cryptococcosis	Lower lobes.	Cavitation uncommon. Lymph node enlargement uncommon. Common presentation as discrete mass.
Histoplasmosis		Hilar lymph node enlargement common. In primary infection, atelectasis or obstructive pneumonitis from compression by enlarged hilar nodes. Cavitation may occur.

Organism	Distribution	Other Findings
C. PARASITES		
Entamoeba histolytica	Alveolar. Nonsegmental. Right lower lobe.	Right pleural effusion very common; cavitation infrequent.
Pneumocystis carinii	Generalized.	Peri-hilar interstitial pneumonitis initially. Massive air space consolidation in terminal stage; pleural effusion very uncommon.
D. VIRUSES		
Influenza Adenoviruses Coxsackie	Interstitial pattern. Predominantly lower lobes.	X-ray pattern indistinguishable within the group and from mycoplasma pneumonia.

*Adapted from Fraser and Pare (1979).

view, is often useful for the recognition of mobile pleural effusions, confirmation of fluid levels, and displacement of opacities, eg, a fungus ball within a cavity. The lordotic view frequently provides relatively unobstructed visualization of disease in the lung apices.

Ultrasound may be utilized for the diagnosis of pleural effusions. Diagnostic and/or therapeutic thoracentesis can be more safely performed under ultrasonic guidance, especially in patients who have loculated pleural effusions. Conventional tomography may be necessary to diagnose and localize pulmonary nodules and to detect early cavitation. Computed tomography can be useful for pleural, bony, and thoracic wall involvement, evaluation of the mediastinum for lymphadenopathy, and also for the detection of calcification in pulmonary nodules.

Chest radiographs can be among the most difficult to interpret, even for an experienced radiologist. However, if the patterns of disease, as discussed, are recognized and the differential diagnoses applied in conjunction with the clinical findings, the correct diagnosis often can be made (Table 3-7).

SELECTED READINGS

Fraser RG, Pare JAP: *Diagnosis of Diseases of the Chest.* Philadelphia, WB Saunders, 1979.

Kirby BD, Pecks H, Meyer RD: Radiographic features of Legionnaire's disease. *Chest* 1979;76:5,562–563.

Lillington GA, Jamplis RW: *A Diagnostic Approach to Chest Diseases.* Baltimore, Williams and Wilkins, 1977.

Reeder MM, Felson B: *Gamuts in Radiology.* Cincinnati, Audiovisual Radiology of Cincinnati, Inc, 1975.

4 *Complications of Pneumonia*

Paul L. Marino

There are numerous complications that may arise as a result of pulmonary infections, ranging from the relatively nonspecific complications seen in many types of infections (eg, dehydration), to more specific complications characteristic of infection with a particular organism (eg, cold agglutinin antibodies produced in *Mycoplasma pneumoniae* infections). Most of these complications can be placed in one of two general categories. The first category includes complications that occur during the acute phase of the infection. These may be evident locally in the thorax or may be systemic. The second category includes the more chronic complications of infection. These latter abnormalities tend to be restricted to the lung parenchyma, and they characteristically persist despite resolution of the acute infection.

ACUTE COMPLICATIONS

Pleural Effusion and Empyema

Classification Pleural effusions are not uncommon in association with acute bacterial pneumonias, occurring in approximately 45% of all cases. The incidence of these "parapneumonic" effusions varies with the causative agent. They more frequently are seen in association with pneumonias caused by gram-negative bacilli (60% of the cases), *Staphylococcus aureus* (50% of the cases), *Streptococcus pneumoniae* (40% to 60% of cases) and anaerobic organisms (35% of cases), but can be seen with virtually any type of bacterial pneumonia. Small effusions also may be seen in up to 20% of cases of viral or *Mycoplasma pneumoniae* pneumonias.

Most parapneumonic effusions are sterile and resolve spontaneously as the pneumonia resolves, but may be associated on occasion with persistent fever. These are called "uncomplicated" parapneumonic effusions, and are characterized by the following: 1) a gram stain that shows no organisms; 2) a negative pleural fluid culture; 3) a pleural fluid pH > 7.20; 4) a pleural fluid LDH < 1000 IU/L. Effusions of this type are more commonly associated with pneumococcal, mycoplasma and viral pneumonias. In contrast, some parapneumonic effusions either are infected, or prone to becoming infected, and these effusions will not resolve without external drainage. These are referred to as "complicated" parapneumonic effusions, and can be identified by any of the following: 1) a gram stain that reveals organisms; 2) a positive pleural fluid culture; 3) a pleural fluid pH < 7.0; 4) a pleural fluid glucose < 40 mg/100 mL; or 5) a pleural fluid LDH > 1000 IU/L. Effusions of this type are more likely to be seen in association with pneumonias caused by anaerobic organisms, *S. aureus*, or gram-negative enteric bacilli.

The differentiation between uncomplicated and complicated parapneumonic effusions cannot be reliably made on the basis of the white blood cell count in the pleural fluid. However, pleural fluid that is grossly purulent in appearance is almost always a complicated (ie, infected) effusion. These purulent effusions are called empyemas, and they signify extension of the pulmonary infection into the pleural space. The route of extension can be a bronchopleural fistula, rupture of a lung abscess into the pleural space, spread via the lymphatics, or hematogenous seeding of the pleura. The most common causes of empyema are gram-negative organisms such as *E. coli* and *Pseudomonas aeruginosa* (cultured in 40% to 60% of cases), *S. aureus* (present in 30% to 50% of the cases) and anaerobic organisms (cultured in 30% to 70% of cases). Empyemas are frequently mixed infections, containing both anaerobic and aerobic organisms. Less common causes of empyema are pneumococci, *M. tuberculosis*, and *Nocardia asteroides*.

Diagnostic approach In any pulmonary infection, the chest x-ray should be carefully examined for the presence of a pleural effusion. If the routine chest x-ray taken in posterior-anterior and lateral positions are suggestive of an effusion, an x-ray taken in the lateral decubitus position should be obtained to differentiate pleural thickening from pleural fluid. Failure of a lateral decubitus film to reveal free-flowing fluid does not rule out a pleural effusion, since empyema fluid frequently is loculated and thus will not flow despite changes in body position. If loculated fluid is suspected, ultrasound examination of the area in question has proven valuable in differentiating pleural thickening from pleural effusion.

If a pleural effusion is demonstrated by the above techniques, the decision to perform a thoracentesis will depend on the individual case. Thoracentesis may be withheld in the following situations: 1) when the pneumonia is caused by an organism that does not commonly result in an empyema (eg, viral pneumonia); 2) when the pneumonia is responding to antimicrobial therapy; or 3) when an effusion is very small, and not increasing in size. On the other hand, thoracentesis should be performed in the following circumstances: 1) when the pneumonia is caused by an organism that is frequently associated with an empyema (eg, *S. aureus*); 2) when the pneumonia and effusion are progressing despite antimicrobial therapy; 3) when an effusion is loculated; or 4) when the causative agent has not been identified by routine methods.

After a thoracentesis is performed, the pleural fluid should be examined for gross appearance, cell count, glucose and LDH concentrations and pH. A gram stain of the fluid should be inspected carefully, and cultures for aerobic organisms, fungi, and acid-fast bacilli should be performed. Special anaerobic culture techniques should be used if anaerobes are suspected, or when the pleural fluid has a foul odor. It is preferable to culture a pleural effusion prior to initiating antibiotic therapy, since cultures obtained during antibiotic therapy may be negative due to suppression (but not eradication) of the causative agent.

Therapy Aspiration of uncomplicated pleural effusions may be associated with a cessation of unexplained fever. Since infection of the pleural space is a closed-space infection, external drainage is required in addition to appropriate antibiotic therapy. This is recommended in all cases when the pleural fluid is grossly purulent, or when the gram stain or culture of the pleural fluid is positive. External drainage is also recommended in complicated parapneumonic effusions when the gram stain and culture are negative, but the pleural fluid pH is less than 7.0.

Closed drainage of the pleural space is accomplished by placing a large bore thoracostomy tube into a dependent region of the fluid accumulation. Multiple tubes may be necessary if the fluid is loculated. The chest tube should be attached to underwater-seal drainage; application of suction to the pleural space is only necessary if there is an associated pneumothorax or bronchopleural fistula. The adequacy of drainage is assessed by the following: 1) clinical signs of infection (ie, fever, WBC count), 2) chest x-rays, and 3) the character and amount of drainage. Successful drainage is characterized by defervescence, radiographic resolution of the pleural effusion, and a decrease in the amount of fluid drained daily. Chest tubes usually can be removed when the fluid is no longer purulent and when the amount of drainage is less than 50 mL/day.

On occasion, closed drainage of the pleural space is not successful in completely eradicating the pleural space infection. This can occur when a large peel forms over the visceral pleura, thus preventing the lung from expanding to eradicate the pleural space, or when multiple loculated pockets of fluid are present. In the former situation, open thoracotomy drainage can be instituted. This procedure consists of resecting a rib segment to create a large opening into the infected space; this opening is kept patent with a large drainage tube, or by creating a pleuro-cutaneous fistula with a flap of skin. Since open drainage exposes the pleural space to atmospheric pressure, it is important to document that the lung will not collapse prior to performing the procedure. An alternative to open drainage is surgical decortication. This involves removal of the thickened peel of visceral pleura, thus allowing the lung to expand and eradicate the pleural space. As this is considered a major surgical procedure, it is reserved for patients who are considered healthy enough to withstand the procedure. Multiple loculations in the pleural space usually are treated by opening the pleural space and manually disrupting the loculations; this procedure can be combined with decortication if deemed necessary.

Prognosis An empyema that is treated with appropriate antibiotics and early chest tube drainage generally responds favorably. However, the mortality from empyema can be high in elderly debilitated patients with chronic underlying disease, or in empyema following thoracic surgery. In these situations, the mortality from empyema may exceed 50% despite appropriate therapy.

Systemic Complications

Complications of pneumonia frequently result from invasion of a particular organ by the offending microorganisms (eg, a meningitis that results from bacteremic seeding of the meninges). However, there are other complications of pneumonia that cannot be directly attributed to dissemination of the causative agent. This section will focus on these latter phenomena.

Fluid and electrolytes Dehydration and hypernatremia can frequently accompany pneumonia, particularly in the elderly. This usually results from an increase in insensible fluid loss secondary to fever, along with poor oral intake of fluids. Therapy in this setting usually consists of fluid infusion to replete intravascular volume and correct the plasma hypertonicity.

Hyponatremia secondary to inappropriate secretion of antidiuretic hormone (ADH) occasionally may be seen in association with various infections involving the lungs. This has been reported in association with bacterial pneumonias (particularly pneumococcal pneumonia and Legionnaires' disease), lung abscess, viral pneumonias and pulmonary tuberculosis. The source of the excess hormone production in these situations is not known, but some feel the hormone is elaborated by the altered lung tissue. The diagnosis of inappropriate ADH is suggested by the appearance of a low serum osmolality in association with a paradoxically high urine osmolality and an elevated urine sodium concentration. Treatment involves restriction of water intake and specific therapy of the underlying lung disorder. The excess ADH production generally subsides as the pulmonary infection resolves.

Hematologic Anemia is commonly seen in chronic infections involving the lung (eg, mycobacterial or fungal diseases). In this situation, the anemia is primarily the result of a defect in the transfer of iron from reticuloendothelial cells in the bone marrow to developing normoblasts. Since there is relatively little iron available for hemoglobin synthesis, the erythrocytes frequently are hypochromic and microcytic, as seen in iron-deficiency anemia. However, iron therapy is of no value in this type of anemia because of the faulty transfer of iron to developing red blood cells. Anemias associated with chronic infection are frequently mild, and subside as the infection resolves.

A decrease in red blood cell survival can be seen in association with certain pneumonias. *Mycoplasma pneumoniae* pneumonia can result in the production of IgM antibodies that agglutinate human red blood cells at 4° C (ie, cold agglutinins of the anti-I variety). Antibodies of this type are produced in approximately 50% of cases of *M. pneumoniae* pneumonia (depending on the severity of the disease) and usually reach peak titers of 1:64 to 1:256 two to three weeks after onset of illness. However, clinically significant hemolysis is not evident until titers exceed 1:512 and therefore hemolysis is not commonly apparent in pneumonia caused by *M. pneumoniae*. In the presence of high antibody titers, hemolysis and stasis of blood in peripheral tissues (ie, hands, feet, nose and ears) may occur when the fever falls or upon exposure to the cold. These complications usually disappear within two to three months.

Cold agglutinins also can be detected in some viral pneumonias (eg, influenza, adenovirus) and in psittacosis, but almost never result in clinically evident hemolysis. Viral pneumonias also may be associated with an autoimmune hemolytic anemia resulting from antibody-induced red blood cell agglutination that does not require cold temperatures (eg, "warm" antibody hemolytic anemia). However, hemolysis in this setting also is usually mild.

Coagulopathies can be evident in certain pulmonary infections. The most common is disseminated intravascular coagulation (DIC), which frequently accompanies gram-negative bacillary bacteremia. DIC also may be seen in pneumonias caused by influenza, herpes simplex, *M. pneumoniae* and *Legionella pneumophila*. Isolated thrombocytopenia has been reported in viral pneumonias, particularly influenza, and is attributed to absorption of the virus to platelets with subsequent platelet lysis.

Hepatic Bacterial pneumonias are commonly associated with mild elevations in liver enzymes without evidence of invasion of the liver by the infectious agent. In this situation, there usually is no significant hepatocellular dysfunction. However, severe bacterial pneumonias (particularly pneumococcal, staphylococcal and gram-negative bacillary pneumonias) can cause intrahepatic cholestasis, manifested by elevated levels of alkaline phosphatase and bilirubin in the blood. Although the etiology of this phenomenon is not clear, the appearance of jaundice in the setting of a bacterial pneumonia can indicate a poor prognosis.

Renal Severe pulmonary infections, like most severe infections, are associated with marked increases in protein catabolism. The resultant load of nitrogenous breakdown products delivered to the kidneys frequently is too great to be completely eliminated in dehydrated patients or those with preexisting renal disease. This produces a progressive azotemia. Because renal function does not actually deteriorate, the serum creatinine concentration fails to rise to the same extent as the blood urea nitrogen. The overall picture is thus one of "prerenal azotemia," and is of little pathologic significance. Legionnaires' disease may be associated with increases in serum BUN and creatinine, but these elevations usually are mild.

Mild degrees of proteinuria (less than 500 mg/day) may be seen with active pulmonary infections. This is a nonspecific finding, and is probably the result of an increase in the glomerular filtration of small plasma proteins that frequently accompanies infection and fever.

CHRONIC COMPLICATIONS

Pulmonary Function

Abnormalities in pulmonary function resulting from acute pneumonia (Chapter 7) usually include a combination of airways obstruction, a decrease in lung compliance, and a decrease in the diffusing capacity for carbon monoxide (D_LCO). These abnormalities commonly result in a decrease in both the arterial PO_2 and the arterial PCO_2. An elevation in arterial PCO_2 above normal levels usually is seen only in the far advanced stages of acute pneumonia.

In bacterial pneumonias, the acute abnormalities in pulmonary function commonly resolve completely when the pneumonia resolves radiographically. On the other hand, abnormalities in pulmonary function (eg, D_LCO) can persist for up to one year after radiographic resolution of severe viral pneumonias. Although most viral pneumonias eventually resolve completely, there is a suggestion that some may progress to chronic interstitial fibrosis.

Chronic Pneumonia

Chronic pneumonia generally is defined as a pulmonary infection that persists clinically and radiographically for more than four to six weeks. The most common infectious causes of chronic pneumonia are mycobacterial and fungal agents. Most bacteria and viruses that cause acute pneumonia do not produce a persistent pulmonary infection. Among the organisms that typically cause acute pneumonia, only anaerobes, *S. aureus*, and gram-negative bacilli, such as *Pseudomonas aeruginosa*, are capable of causing chronic infections. However, this occurs only in debilitated patients with chronic underlying disease. Chronic pneumonia is the subject of another chapter in this book, and will not be covered further in this section (see Chapter 12).

Bronchiectasis

Bronchiectasis is a disorder characterized by irreversible destruction and dilatation of the airways. It may be localized to one lobe, but more commonly involves two or more lobes of the lung. The etiology of bronchiectasis is not clear in many cases, but a history of prior pulmonary infection is obtained in approximately 50% of the cases. The antecedent infection frequently occurs in childhood, and is most commonly a bronchiolitis or pneumonia, particularly pneumonias complicating pertussis or measles. Other commonly cited causes of bronchiectasis include: 1) recurrent infections occurring distal to a site of airways obstruction, such as seen in cystic fibrosis with airways obstruction from thick mucus plugs; 2) acquired hypogammaglobulinemia with recurrent bronchopulmonary infections; 3) pulmonary involvement with *M. tuberculosis*; or 4) necrotizing pneumonias, such as aspiration pneumonitis. Most of the commonly encountered pneumonias in adults do not result in the development of bronchiectasis.

The major problem in bronchiectasis is persistent or recurrent bronchopulmonary infections in involved lung segments. This results primarily from two processes: 1) a tendency for the damaged airways to collapse due to loss of elastic retraction forces; and 2) a defect in mucociliary clearance. Patients commonly have a history of chronic cough associated with the production of copious amounts of purulent or bloody sputum. Chest x-rays may reveal a crowding of markings in specific segments due to loss of volume, and cystic spaces containing air fluid levels can be seen in advanced cases. Definitive diagnosis requires bronchography to demonstrate the dilated airways. Treatment generally consists of appropriate antibiotics to control infection, along with chest percussion and postural drainage to clear secretions from involved segments. Surgical resection of involved lobes is occasionally indicated when the bronchiectasis is restricted to a single lobe and recurrent pneumonia is a major problem. Advances in antimicrobial therapy have resulted in a marked decline in the mortality from bronchiectasis, and adults with this disease frequently reach an advanced age.

SELECTED READINGS

Pleural Effusion and Empyema

Finland M, Barnes MW: Changing ecology of acute bacterial empyema: Occurrence and mortality at Boston City Hospital during 12 selected years from 1935 to 1972. *J Infect Dis* 1978;137:274–291.

Light RW: Management of parapneumonic effusions. *Arch Intern Med* 1981; 141:1339–1341.

Light RW, Girard WM, Jenkinson SG et al: Parapneumonic effusions. *Am J Med* 1980;69:507–512.

Sandiweiss DA, Hanson JC, Gosink BS, et al: Ultrasound in diagnosis, localization, and treatment of loculated pleural empyema. *Ann Intern Med* 1975;82:50–53.

Snider GL, Saleh SS: Empyema of the thorax in adults: Review of 105 cases. *Dis Chest* 1968;54:12–17.

Weese WC, Shindler ER, Smith IM, et al: Empyema of the thorax then and now. *Arch Intern Med* 1973;131:516–520.

Systemic Complications

Davies MG: Pneumonia causing the syndrome of inappropriate secretion of antidiuretic hormone. *Br J Clin Pract* 1977;31:82–84.

Fahrlander H, Huber F, Gloor F: Intrahepatic retention of bile in severe bacterial infections. *Gastroenterology* 1964;47:590–599.

Murray HW, Masur H, Senterfit LS, et al: The protean manifestations of mycoplasma pneumonia infection in adults. *Am J Med* 1975;58:229–242.

Spanos A, Christopher JS: Inappropriate secretion of antidiuretic hormone with chronic chest infections. *Br Med J* 1974;3:785–786.

Yu VL, Kroboth FJ, Shonnard J, et al: Legionnaires' disease: New clinical perspective from a prospective pneumonia study. *Am J Med* 1982;73:357–361.

Pulmonary Function

Berven H: Studies on the cardiopulmonary function in the post-infectious phase of "atypical" pneumonia. *Acta Med Scand* 1962;172(suppl):382–393.

Bocles JS, Ehrenkranz NJ, Marks A: Abnormalities of respiratory function in varicella pneumonia. *Ann Intern Med* 1964;60:183–195.

Winterlauer RH, Ludwig WR, Hammar SP: Clinical course, management, and long-term sequelae of respiratory failure due to influenza viral pneumonia. *Johns Hopkins Med Bull* 1977;141:148–152.

Bronchiectasis

Clark NS: Bronchiectasis in childhood. *Br Med J* 1963;1:80–88.

Kometzko NFJ, Carton RW, Leroy EP: Causes of death in patients with bronchiectasis. *Am Rev Resp Dis* 1969;100:852–858.

Schachter EN, Basta W: Bronchiectasis following heroin overdose. *Chest* 1973;63:363–366.

Suhs RH, Dowling HF, Jackson GG: Hypogammaglobulinemia with chronic bronchitis or bronchiectasis. *Arch Intern Med* 1965;116:29–38.

5 Use of the Clinical Microbiology Laboratory

Matthew E. Levison

The clinical microbiology laboratory often is crucial in the care of patients with pneumonia. If therapy is not to be entirely empiric, the results of sputum, blood or pleural fluid cultures are necessary, not only for accurate diagnosis but also for proper selection of antimicrobial therapy and evaluation of the adequacy of dosing.

COLLECTION OF SPECIMENS FOR MICROBIOLOGIC EXAMINATION

The validity of microbiologic laboratory data depends on the care with which the specimen has been obtained. The most important step in isolating microorganisms from clinical material is proper collection of the specimen to prevent or minimize contamination with the normal microflora.

Within moments after birth, the skin and mucosal surfaces adjacent to the skin (nasopharynx, oropharynx, oral cavity, colon, vagina and anterian third of the urethra) become colonized with bacteria. Each site harbors a characteristic flora which differ from one another in microbial densities and diversity of species. Certain bacteria adhere more frequently to epithelial cells from certain sites. This selective adherence undoubtedly determines in large part the type of indigenous flora on the various surfaces. The flora remains rather stable in spite of almost constant contact with a variety of different organisms from the environment or from other body surfaces. However, under the influence of host and environmental factors, the flora can change. For example, the frequency of finding various Enterobacteriaceae or *P. aeruginosa* as components of the flora of the nasopharynx and oral cavity increases with aging, poor dentition, alcoholism, severe underlying disease, hospitalization, and antibiotic therapy.

Inhaled particles larger than 10 μm are filtered out in the nasal cavity so that a large variety of environmental organisms may be found at this site, but the predominant organisms are *Staphylococcus aureus* and *Staphylococcus epidermidis*. The flora in the nasopharynx includes *S. pneumoniae*, *Neisseria* and *Hemophilus* and in the tonsillar crypts, anaerobes including *Bacteroides*, *Fusobacterium*, *Veillonella* and *Actinomyces*. The gingival crevice has a population of about 10^{11} organisms/g made up of over 200 different species, predominantly obligate anaerobes, including *Bacteroides melaninogenicus*, *B. oralis*, *Actinomyces*, *Fusobacterium*, *Peptostreptococcus*, *Peptococcus*, *Veillonella*, *Borrelia* and *Treponema*, in addition to the facultative anaerobic viridans streptococci. A polymicrobial aggregate also extends out of the gingival crevice onto a glycoprotein layer adherent to the dental surfaces (plaque). The saliva contains about 10^8 organisms/mL which have been washed from the dental plaque and the mucosal surfaces of the oral cavity. The lower respiratory tract (trachea, bronchi and alveoli) normally are not colonized. Bacteria that may be inhaled or aspirated into the lower respiratory tract are removed by the mucociliary barrier and phagocytosis.

The normal microflora may contain organisms capable of producing disease, and their presence in cultures may be diagnostically meaningless if there was a possibility of contamination. Prevention of contamination may be easier for some specimens than others. Specimens from the lower respiratory tract obtained by percutaneous lung aspiration or transtracheal aspiration require only decontamination of the skin with iodine-iodophor or alcohol. However, specimens obtained across heavily contaminated surfaces (expectorated sputum) are routinely contaminated and results of their culture must be interpreted with caution.

BLOOD CULTURE

Although blood cultures are only positive in up to about 30% of patients with bronchogenic pneumonia, culture of the blood is often the most important clinical microbiologic procedure. Bacteremia indicates a highly invasive process and organisms isolated from blood should be assumed to be pathogenic unless they both typically are members of the skin microflora (*S. epidermidis* or *Propionibacterium* sp) and are isolated from only one of several blood cultures. But even these skin organisms can be pathogenic in the proper clinical setting; for example, these organisms are among the most frequent causes of prosthetic cardiac valve endocarditis.

Bacteremia may be transient or continuous. Continuous bacteremia is characteristic of intravascular infection, such as endocarditis in which about 20 to 200 organisms/mL of blood are found at all times unrelated to changes in fever pattern. This number represents the steady state when the rate of clearance is balanced by the rate at which bacteria are entering the circulation. Transient bacteremia is clinically manifested by chills and fever, but because of rapid clearance mechanisms, by the time blood is obtained for culture, bacteremia may no longer be present.

Blood should be obtained from a patient suspected of having transient bacteremia in a different manner than blood from a patient with continuous bacteremia. To detect transient bacteremia, blood should be collected as close as possible to the onset of chills or fever. A relatively large volume of blood should be taken; for example, a minimum of two to three separate blood cultures taken at 15-minute intervals, to increase the sensitivity for detecting low grade bacteremia. In contrast, to detect continuous bacteremia, three to five separate blood cultures should be obtained, each one to two hours or more apart. In patients with intravascular infection, all of the blood cultures obtained in this manner usually are positive.

Blood should be collected before administration of antibiotics. If antibiotics are already being given, blood can be collected 1) in special equipment that contains a resin that removes certain antibiotics, 2) when lowest antibiotic concentration in blood is expected, or 3) the blood specimen can be divided into small aliquots which can each be cultured in relatively large volumes of broth (eg, 5 mL of blood divided into 1 mL portions, each of which are cultured in bottles containing 45 mL of broth *vs* the usual method of placing 5 mL of blood in one bottle containing 45 mL of broth). Usually 10 mL of blood is collected for each blood culture and 5 mL inoculated into one bottle for aerobic incubation and 5 mL into another for anaerobic incubation. Blood cultures should be incubated for two to three weeks to assure detection of some slow-growing pathogens.

SPUTUM CULTURES

Sputum culture and gram stain are the most common techniques used to make a bacteriologic diagnosis in cases of pneumonia. Bacteremia and empyema, diagnostically definitive when found, occur too infrequently to be generally useful. However, sputum culture may fail to yield the etiologic agent. Up to about 50% of the patients with bacteremic pneumococcal pneumonia fail to have pneumococci cultured from their sputum. In addition, in the process of collection by either expectoration or aspiration via an orotracheal catheter, sputum routinely becomes contaminated with oropharyneal secretions. Isolation of pneumococci from contaminated specimens does not permit differentiation of pneumonia from carriage of pneumococci in the nasopharynx. In some patients two or more potential pathogens can be recovered from the sputum. Similarly, both the high incidence of gram-negative bacillary pneumonia and the acquisition of gram-negative bacilli in the pharyngeal flora in hospitalized, seriously ill patients further compound the difficulties in interpreting cultures of sputum in patients with nosocomial pneumonias.

Several methods have been suggested to obtain more reliable data from respiratory secretions. Washing of sputum to remove bacteria that might have originated in upper respiratory secretions, quantitative culture of liquefied sputum and bronchoscopy to obtain lower respiratory secretions for culture may not reliably decrease contamination to acceptable levels, especially for the diagnosis of nosocomial gram-negative bacillary pneumonia.

Although the value of bacteriologic study of sputum remains in serious doubt for the reasons just cited, it is likely that expectorated sputum specimens will continue to be submitted to clinical bacteriology laboratories for culture because of medical contraindications to more aggressive methods such as transtracheal or transthoracic lung aspiration.

Most authorities suggest an objective system for evaluating the quality of lower respiratory tract secretions based on the numbers of leukocytes and squamous epithelial cells on gram-stained smears under 100 × magnification. As confirmed by Murray and Washington (1975), specimens containing fewer than 10 epithelial cells per field are acceptable for culture.

The gross appearance of the specimen is an unreliable indicator of oropharyngeal combination. Further, the presence of variable numbers of alveolar macrophages or leukocytes does not improve the bacteriologic results when substantial numbers of squamous epithelial cells are present. If there are ≥ 10 epithelial cells/100 × field, another sputum should be obtained.

It is important, however, to reserve such a screening technique for sputum bacteriology only. In cases of suspected mycobacterial, fungal, mycoplasmal, or viral respiratory illness, the degree of oropharyngeal contamination is relatively less important. In all of these cases, the procedures used are selective for cultivation of the suspected etiologic agent and are inhibitory to contaminating bacterial flora. In such instances, the presence of leukocytes or alveolar macrophages in a gram-stained smear is indicative of the quality of the specimen.

Culture of early morning, freshly expectorated sputum on three or more occasions, or of expectorated sputum induced by a heated aqueous aerosol of 10% glycerol and 15% sodium chloride, is useful for recovery of mycobacteria and fungi. Gastric washings obtained after induced coughing may increase the yield of mycobacteria. Use of pooled specimens for isolation of mycobacteria, however, because of overgrowth of contaminants are unnecessary and undesirable.

Transtracheal aspiration can be used to obtain material uncontaminated by oropharyngeal secretions. An Intracath set is generally used. The plastic catheter is passed via a needle across the cricothyroid membrane. A syringe with a few milliliters of nonbacteriostatic saline is attached to the catheter, the saline is injected, followed by aspiration of secretions into the syringe. The saline injection often elicits a vigorous coughing reflex. The procedure is carried out rapidly, and care is taken to ensure collection before the vigorous cough expels the catheter into the pharynx. In skilled hands, this procedure has low morbidity, but subcutaneous emphysema, hemoptysis, cardiac arrhythmias, and anxiety are all common sequelae. Paratracheal abscess and death are rarer complications. Thus, this procedure should not be a routine part of the workup for all cases of pneumonia. The procedure should not be done on patients who have blood PO_2 < 50 mmHg, who are coughing vigorously or have a bleeding diathesis, because the risks of transtracheal aspiration outweigh the risk of empiric treatment based upon clinical judgment or obtaining specimens by other means. Thus, inability to obtain sputum is not always an indication for transtracheal aspiration.

Specific indications for transtracheal aspiration include: 1) pneumonias in immunosuppressed hosts in whom rapid diagnosis is critical, 2) suspected tuberculosis in children not yielding organisms by other diagnostic maneuvers, 3) nosocomial aspiration pneumonia in which polymicrobial colonization of the oropharynx makes the etiologic agent uncertain, and 4) progressive pneumonia despite seemingly appropriate antibiotic therapy.

Transtracheal aspiration reliably yields the etiologic agent of bacterial pneumonia provided that there has been no prior treatment with antimicrobial drugs. The frequency of false-negative cultures is reported to be 1% if the specimen is collected before administration of antimicrobial drugs. False-positive cultures are unusual in persons without chronic lower respiratory tract disease, but are commonly encountered among those with chronic bronchitis.

The direct-needle aspiration of a pulmonary infiltrate through the chest wall is an older technique that has been recently revived. In both pediatric and adult patients, it has proven to be relatively safe. By comparison with transtracheal aspiration, lung aspiration more frequently is diagnostic. For example, simultaneous recovery of multiple potential pathogens occurs less frequently from lung aspiration than concurrently performed transtracheal aspirate. With lung aspiration, pneumothorax is the major complication, at times requiring a chest tube. Rare complications include air embolism and hemoptysis. Potentially, empyema could occur.

It seems prudent not to perform lung aspiration on patients with bullous lung disease, patients unable to suspend respiration for four to five seconds, patients with respiratory failure in whom positive pressure respirators may be used, or in patients with a bleeding diathesis. Similar to transtracheal aspiration, lung aspiration is not necessary for the appropriate management of most cases of community-acquired pneumonia. The risks must be balanced against the expected benefits.

Open lung biopsy, although having the potential morbidity and mortality associated with thoracotomy, provides the most information. In some instances, the etiology of pulmonary infections may only be diagnosed by biopsy of the lung. In patients for whom open lung biopsy is a serious risk, transbronchial lung biopsy using a fiberoptic bronchoscopic technique, may provide findings that are diagnostic. Due to the small size of the transbronchial biopsy specimen (1 to 3 mm), however, the findings may not be representative of the overall disease process. If the transbronchial lung biopsy shows only inflammation or fibrosis, when infection is strongly suspected and the need to know the specific diagnosis is crucial, then open lung biopsy should be considered (unless a specific contraindication exists). Transbronchial or open lung biopsy may be necessary to establish the diagnosis of infection due to *Pneumocystis carinii*, *Aspergillus*, or *Legionella pneumophila* in immunocompromised hosts, and it may be helpful in either establishing or confirming infections due to mycobacteria and viruses. Special stains on biopsy material for mycobacteria, *Legionella*, *Pneumocystis* and fungi (eg, Ziehl-Neelson, Dieterle, silver methenamine and PAS), and fluorescent antibody studies for *Legionella* may rapidly disclose the etiology.

AEROBIC BACTERIOLOGY OF LOWER RESPIRATORY SECRETIONS

Specimens from the lower respiratory tract unless otherwise requested, are routinely plated on 1) a nonselective agar for aerobic incubation such as blood agar, 2) a selective medium of facultative gram-negative rods, such as desoxychlolate agar, 3) a selective agar for facultative gram-positive cocci, such as phenylethyl alcohol agar, and 4) a supplemented chocolate agar plate incubated in 5% CO_2 for isolation of *Hemophilus* species. Although adequate to support growth of many lower respiratory pathogens, such procedures because of media, incubation conditions or incubation time may fail to identify more fastidious pathogens. The laboratory should be specifically notified that these fastidious pathogens are suspected so that specimens may be processed appropriately. Organisms requiring special notice include anaerobes, mycobacteria, *Nocardia*, *Chlamydia*, *Mycoplasma*, viruses and fungi.

Pneumococci, after 18 hours of incubation on the surface of blood agar plates, give rise to smooth, glistening colonies from 1 to 2 mm in diameter, except for Type 3, which forms much larger, glistening ("mucoid") colonies that are easily recognizable. As the culture ages, autolytic changes begin in the center of the pneumococcal colony which may collapse, giving it a checker-like appearance. The rate and extent of autolysis are highly variable from strain to strain. Identification of pneumococcal colonies on the surface of blood agar plates is facilitated greatly by the use of low-power magnification (45 ×) provided by a dissecting microscope. The colonies on blood agar are surrounded by a zone of alpha hemolysis which increases in size as the culture ages.

Most sputum specimens will contain viridans streptococci as contaminants from the oral cavity. Under ideal circumstances, it may be possible to differentiate the pneumococcus from viridans streptococci on colonial morphology alone. However, in most cases, except for the highly characteristic colonies of Type 3 pneumococcus, differentiation cannot be made with assurance. Since pneumococci can survive in sputum for long periods of time, delay in arrival of specimens at the microbiology laboratory probably does not account for the fact that pneumococci are not isolated from sputum cultures in 50% of patients with bacteremic pneumococcal pneumonia. The most probable reason is failure of technologists to recognize pneumococcal colonies. Identification of pneumococci in respiratory secretions may be improved with the use of sheep blood agar containing gentamicin; however, duplicate plating on plain sheep blood agar is required. Recognition of pneumococci in sputum cultures also can be enhanced either by placing an optochin disc on the primary culture plate, using the bile test (a drop of 2% bile) on the primary culture plate, anaerobic incubation, or the availability of results from a gram-stained smear to the person who examines the culture.

ANAEROBIC BACTERIOLOGY OF LOWER RESPIRATORY TRACT SECRETIONS

If specimens contain even minute amounts of secretions from the upper respiratory tract and mouth, they should not be eligible for anaerobic cultivation because of contamination from the large populations (10^{11} to 10^{12} microorganism/g) of anaerobes on these mucosal surfaces. Only methods that bypass the upper respiratory tract (ie, transbronchial aspiration, percutaneous lung aspiration) will yield specimens from the lung adequate for anaerobic bacteriology.

Fluid specimens should be collected in a needle and syringe for anaerobic bacteriology. Air can then be expelled from the pus-filled needle and syringe and the needle plugged with a sterile rubber stopper, as would be done for blood gas determinations, to avoid excessive exposure to oxygen. The specimen also can be inoculated into an oxygen-free tube to assure an anaerobic environment while in transport to the laboratory.

Specimens should be cultured anaerobically on enriched solid media, such as Schaedler's agar, as soon as possible after collection. Fortunately, established growth (purulent clinical specimens or colonies on solid medium) of most pathogenic anaerobes tolerate the presence of room air for a fairly long time (eg, eight or more hours). However, not infrequently, a laboratory that may promptly inoculate plates for anaerobic culture will put them into a jar, which is then left open in room air until more cultures arrive to fill the jar before it is finally sealed. Of course, during this waiting period the first batch of plates continue to be exposed to oxygen, thus perhaps altering viability of inoculated organisms. It is desirable to store inoculated media in a holding jar into which a constant flow of deoxygenated CO_2 gas is directed. Once closed, the jar should optimally not be opened for 48 hours. Liquid media, such as thioglycolate broth, should be heated in a boiling water bath for 20 minutes prior to use to remove dissolved oxygen and then cooled. Even when properly reduced, thioglycolate should be supplemented with either 10% ascitic fluid or sterile rabbit serum to improve growth of anaerobes. The inoculated supplemented medium should also be incubated anaerobically. It is not satisfactory merely to seal the tube for incubation in room air. The easiest way to achieve acceptable results is to loosen the cap on the specimen-containing tube of thioglycolate broth and put the tube into an anaerobic jar.

The Gas Pak is a simple, convenient system for obtaining an anaerobic environment. This system consists of a disposable hydrogen-carbon dioxide generator pack easily activated by the addition of water. The hydrogen released from the generation combines with the oxygen in the presence of a palladium catalyst to form water, which condenses on the inner walls of the jar. An oxygen-sensitive indicator is included to detect any failure of the jar.

Only a few anaerobic species commonly cause pulmonary infection. These include *Bacteroides melaninogenicus*, *Fusobacterium nucleatum*, and various *Peptostreptococcus* and *Peptococcus*. Fortunately, the techniques for cultivation and identification of these anaerobic bacteria have been simplified now so that the bacteriology of the major anaerobes encountered clinically can be carried out quite easily in the average laboratory with relatively simple tests, many of them the same type of tests being used for identification of aerobic and facultative bacteria.

A direct microscopic examination of clinical specimens should supplement anaerobic incubation. Anaerobic infections are characteristically polymicrobial and this will be reflected in the gram stain of a properly collected specimen of lower respiratory secretions, ie, the gram stain will show many different types of microorganisms and an abundance of leukocytes. Direct gram stain will not only demonstrate morphologic and staining characteristics but also will indicate the relative proportions of the various microorganisms in the lesion, thus permitting better interpretation of subsequent culture results. The same relative proportions of all types of organisms seen on direct smear should be recovered in culture. If organisms were present on gram stain but the culture is sterile, anaerobic bacterial infection should be suspected.

OTHER DIAGNOSTIC METHODS

The value of gram stains of sputum has been questioned. Contamination of specimens with the large number of aerobic and anaerobic streptococci in the oropharynx may contribute to poor correlation of the gram stain with the etiology of pneumonia. However, a gram stain of a minimally contaminated sputum (< 10 epithelial cells/100× field) may be quite helpful in suggesting the etiology of the pneumonia.

If an organism has a distinctive cellular morphology or staining characteristic, the most readily available, rapid method for laboratory diagnosis of an infection is the microscopic demonstration of the pathogen in a smear of clinical material. For example, gram-stained smears may reveal encapsulated gram-positive diplococci (*Streptococcus pneumoniae*); gram-positive cocci in clusters (*Staphylococcus* sp); coffee-bean shaped, often intracellular gram-negative diplococci (pathogenic *Neisseria*); tiny, gram-negative coccobacilli (*Hemophilus* or *Acinetobacter*); gram-positive cocci in chains (*Streptococcus*); gram-negative rods pointed at both ends (*Fusobacterium*); oval, large budding forms (yeast); or branching, gram-positive filaments (*Nocardia* or *Actinomyces*).

The Kinyoun modification of the Ziehl-Neelsen stain can demonstrate *Mycobacterium*. *Nocardia* sp is usually weakly acid-fast and requires more rapid decolorization or use of a weaker decolorization. *Legionella* are distinctly seen as dark-brown to black pleomorphic rods with the Dieterle silver impregnation stain and also can be identified by direct immunofluorescence. *Pneumocystis* can be identified by the silver methenamine stain. Wet smears when combined with India ink may be used to demonstrate cryptococci or when used with specific anticapsular antibody can identify *S. pneumoniae*, *N. meningitidis* or *H. influenzae*.

Counterimmunoelectrophoresis (CIE) has been used to detect pneumococcal polysaccharide in serum and urine in patients with pneumococcal pneumonia. Although highly specific for the detection of pneumococcal disease CIE in serum and urine, it is not sensitive enough to be useful. Recently, several studies have demonstrated that CIE of sputum appears to be a sensitive and specific test in patients with pneumonia. However, in patients without pneumonia, pneumococcal antigen also can be detected in the sputum of those with chronic bronchitis and a sputum culture positive for pneumococci.

ANTIMICROBIAL SENSITIVITY TESTING

Dilution Methods (Figure 5-1)

Bacterial susceptibility to antimicrobial agents can be measured quantitatively and expressed as the minimum inhibitory concentration (MIC) or minimum bactericidal concentration (MBC) of the agent for the strain tested. These in vitro data can then be related to anticipated chemotherapeutic levels at the site of infection to provide a logical prediction of the effect of therapy.

To perform these tests, serial twofold dilutions in broth of the antimicrobial agent are inoculated with a nonturbid suspension of the organism so that the broth contains 5×10^5 CFU/mL. For most purposes, an

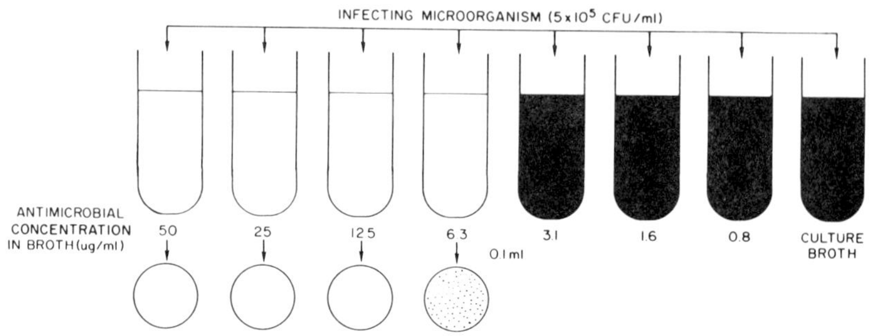

Figure 5-1 Scheme of the broth dilution method. After 18 to 24 hours of incubation, black tubes contain turbid broth and white tubes contain clear broth. Interpretation of results: MIC, 6.3 μg/mL; MBC, 12.5 μg/mL.

antimicrobial concentration of 50 μg/mL is a satisfactory upper limit for routine testing with any antimicrobial agent. Important exceptions are tests of carbenicillin or ticarcillin. Strains of *Pseudomonas aeruginosa* which are inhibited by concentrations of 100 to 125 μg/mL of these two antibiotics are considered susceptible to achievable blood levels. Also, high concentrations will be needed for tests whose results are to be related to urinary concentrations of agents excreted by the kidney.

The mixture consisting of microorganisms, nutrient medium, and antimicrobial agent is then incubated at 37°C for 18 to 24 hours. The minimal concentration of antibiotic that has prevented visible growth (turbidity to the naked eye) is defined as the minimal inhibitory concentration (MIC). Determination of bactericidal levels by transfer of organisms from clear tubes to solid media can then be done. To assess bactericidal activity, 0.1 mL is removed from each clear tube and subcultured onto agar plates. If a $\geq$ 99.9% kill has occurred, the initial inoculum of 5×10^5 CFU/mL will have been reduced to $\leq 5 \times 10^2$ CFU/mL (ie, $\leq$ 50 colonies on the subculture plate). The minimal concentration of antibiotic that has caused a 99.9% kill is defined as the minimal bactericidal concentration (MBC). Results of inhibitory action are available in 48 to 72 hours and bactericidal action, 24 hours later.

The MIC and MBC should be done in a standardized fashion, because variations in culture media, incubation period, and size of inoculum can affect the results. The inoculum size is particularly important when dealing with certain antibiotics and bacteria. For example, when testing the sensitivity of penicillinase-producing staphylococci to penicillin G, the minimal inhibitory concentration can be appreciably lowered by merely lowering the inoculum from 10^5 to 10^3.

The broth dilution test has been the standard method in most infectious diseases research laboratories when quantitative bacterial sensitivities are desired. However, dilution tests have not been used for routine susceptibility testing in most clinical laboratories because of their expense and time until the recent development of microdilution methods.

These miniaturized variants of the broth dilution procedure, commercially available for testing aerobic, facultative and recently anaerobic bacteria, have the serial dilutions of several antimicrobial agents prepared in microtiter trays. In one form, trays are available frozen from regional production centers throughout the United States and Canada. Trays received must be maintained in the frozen state (−20°C or lower) until used. In another form, the dilutions of the antimicrobial agent are lyophilized. This product has the advantage of simpler storage conditions and a somewhat longer shelf-life. Both have been found to produce results comparable to the macrobroth dilution method.

The dosage of the antimicrobial agent should yield a peak concentration in tissues substantially higher than the MIC. To assure attaining these tissue concentrations, blood levels that are three- to fivefold higher than the MIC have been suggested, but it must be realized that such recommendations have been made without well-controlled laboratory–clinical correlative studies. However, if the MIC is the same or higher than achievable blood levels, the organism should be considered resistant to the agent, except for testing of urinary pathogens when the MIC should be correlated to achievable urinary levels. If the MIC is lower than achievable blood levels, but levels anticipated at the site of infection (eg, cerebrospinal fluid) are considerably below blood levels, the organism may well be clinically resistant. Other reasons for discrepancy between the results of the in vitro assay and clinical response are shown in Table 5-1.

Disc Diffusion Method

The disc agar diffusion method is the most frequently performed assay for the in vitro response of bacteria to antimicrobial agents. This method has been standardized, is relatively simple to perform and interpret, results are accurate and reproducible, and it does not require the use of expensive or complex equipment.

Agar plates are streaked over the entire surface with a standardized inoculum of bacteria to be tested. Within 15 minutes discs impregnated with the antimicrobial agent are applied to the surface of the inoculated plates. The number of discs that can be placed on a single plate is limited to 12 or 13 on a 150-mm plate. When a disc is applied to the inoculated surface of the agar medium, the discs absorb water from the agar, thus dissolving the antimicrobial agent, which then diffuses through the adjacent agar. Within 15 minutes after the discs are applied, the plates are incubated at 35°C in air. Any longer delay before incubation will allow excess diffusion of the antimicrobial agent before bacterial growth has started. In the incubator, after an initial lag phase, bacterial growth

Table 5-1
Lack of Prediciton of In Vivo Outcome By In Vitro Assay for Antimicrobial Sensitivity

In Vitro Results	In Vivo Response	Reasons
Resistance	Response	1) Self-limited disease 2) Higher than anticipated drug concentration at the site of infection 3) Microbial density at the site of infection lower than that used in the in vitro assay 4) Use of synergistic drug combinations
Sensitive	No response	1) Poor host defenses 2) Lower than anticipated drug concentration at the site of infection; inappropriate dose, route, rate of administration; secluded focus of infection; local drug inactivation 3) Microbial density at the site of infection higher than that used in the in vitro assay 4) Use of antagonistic combinations

begins and proceeds at a logarithmic rate. The position of inhibitory zone is established early, when actively proliferating bacterial cells are inhibited in those regions of the medium around the disc where the concentration of the drug equals or exceeds the MIC for the organism being tested.

After 18 hours of incubation, the plates are examined, and the diameters of the zones of inhibition are measured to the nearest millimeter. The size of the resulting zone of inhibition is related to the susceptibility of the bacteria, the rate of growth of the bacteria, the number of bacteria inoculated on the surface of the plate, the amount of drug in the disc, the diffusion characteristics of the drug in agar, the depth and viscosity of the agar and incubation conditions. When testing is restricted to only rapidly growing bacterial pathogens (eg, Enterobacteriaceae, *Pseudomonas aeruginosa* and *S. aureus*) and when those factors related to the drug, the inoculum size, the agar medium, and the timing of inoculation, disc placement and incubation are standardized, the diameter of the inhibitory zone is very reproducible. When performed in the standardized fashion, the results of the disc sensitivity testing can be interpreted by referring to a table that correlates the zones of inhibition with breakpoints of MIC values of resistant or susceptible strains (see Table 5-2). An intermediate category between the two MIC breakpoints includes

Table 5-2
Zone Diameter Interpretive Standards and Approximate Minimal Inhibitory Concentration (MIC) Correlates for Selected Antimicrobial Agents

Antimicrobial Agent	Disk Content	Zone Diameter (Nearest Whole mm)		Approximate MIC Correlates*
		Resistant	*Susceptible*	*Susceptible*
Amikacin	30 μg	≤ 14	≥ 17	≤ 16 μg/mL
Ampicillin when testing gram-negative enteric organisms and enterococci	10μg	≤ 11	≥ 14	≤ 8 μg/mL
Ampicillin when testing staphylococci and penicillin G-susceptible organisms	10μg	≤ 20	≥ 29	≤ 0.2 μg/mL
Ampicillin when testing *Hemophilus* sp	10μg	≤ 19	≥ 20	≤ 2.0 μg/mL
Carbenicillin when testing *Proteus* sp and *Escherichia coli*	100μg	≤ 17	≥ 23	≤ 16 μg/mL
Carbenicillin when testing *Pseudomonas aeruginosa*	100μg	≤ 13	≥ 17	≤ 125 μg/mL
Cefamandole	30μg	≤ 14	≥ 18	≤ 10 μg/mL
Cefoxitin	30μg	≤ 14	≥ 18	≤ 10 μg/mL
Cephalothin	30μg	≤ 14	≥ 18	≤ 10 μg/mL
Chloramphenicol	30μg	≤ 12	≥ 18	≤ 12.5 μg/mL
Clindamycin	2μg	≤ 14	≥ 17	≤ 1 μg/mL
Erythromycin	15μg	≤ 13	≥ 18	≤ 2 μg/mL
Gentamicin	10μg	≤ 12	≥ 15	≤ 4 μg/mL
Methicillin when testing staphylococci	5μg	≤ 9	≥ 14	≤ 3 μg/mL
Penicillin G when testing staphylococci	10 U	≤ 20	≥ 29	≤ 0.1 μg/mL
Penicillin G when testing other microorganisms	10 U	≤ 11	≥ 22	≤ 1.5 μg/mL
Sulfonamides	250 or 300μg	≤ 12	≥ 17	≤ 100 μg/mL
Tetracycline	30μg	≤ 14	≥ 19	≤ 4 μg/mL
Trimethoprim-sulfamethoxazole	1.25/23.75μg	≤ 10	≥ 16	≤ 2/38 μg/mL
Tobramycin	10μg	≤ 12	≥ 15	≤ 4 μg/mL
Vancomycin	30μg	≤ 9	≥ 12	≤ 5 μg/mL

*Only MIC breakpoints of susceptible strains are given in this table. For MIC breakpoints of resistant strains, see Lennette et al, 1980, p 464.

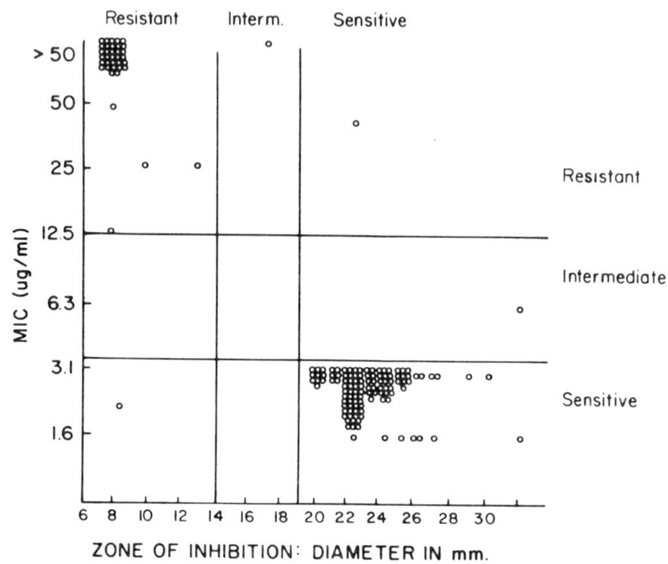

Figure 5-2 Schematic scattergram depicting the inverse relationship between MIC determined by the broth dilution technique and zone diameters determined by the disc diffusion technique. Interpretive MIC and zone size breakpoints are also shown. Only a few major interpretive discrepancies occur; ie, susceptible by one method, but resistant with the other method.

strains only moderately susceptible. These MIC breakpoints which define resistant and susceptible categories for each drug are based on blood levels usually expected with frequently used dose schedules, or urine levels in the case of nitrofurantoin or nalidixic acid.

The correlation of zone diameters with MIC values are derived from studies performed on a large number of strains of a particular microbial species. Because of differences in diffusion in agar, these correlations must be done separately for each drug. Scattergrams are prepared by plotting the MIC value ($\log_2$ scale) against the corresponding zone diameter (arithmetic scale) for each strain tested (Figure 5-2). The scattergram may distinguish between two distinct bacterial populations—a sensitive one and a resistant one—with relatively few organisms of intermediate sensitivity. This bimodal distribution defines the range of zone sizes for the resistant and sensitive populations. In such a scattergram, strains exhibiting large inhibitory zones have low minimum inhibitory concentrations, and those exhibiting small zones, high minimal inhibitory concentrations. Some organisms are characterized by a unimodal distribution indicating that they are either entirely sensitive or resistant.

Organisms resistant by the usual criteria nevertheless may be inhibited by higher levels of antimicrobial agents which can be attained either in the blood by use of larger than usual doses of a relatively nontoxic agent, or at sites of infection where the agent may be concentrated. For example, concentration of certain antibiotics by the kidney may result in urinary levels many times higher than the levels considered in developing breakpoints for systemic infections. In such situations, urinary pathogens that are resistant to certain agents by disc testing might be treated successfully by agents that are concentrated in the urine.

Because the gaseous atmosphere, the media and the duration of incubation necessary for incubation of anaerobes differ from conditions used routinely in the Bauer-Kirby test for aerobes and facultative anaerobes, the interpretation for the Bauer-Kirby test cannot be applied to anaerobes. At the present time, the vast majority of clinically significant anaerobes have reasonably predictable susceptibilities to antimicrobial agents. Thus, antimicrobial therapy for anaerobic infection usually is based on current patterns of susceptibility using agar or broth dilution techniques that have been performed periodically in research laboratories on large numbers of clinical isolates and reported in the literature.

TIME-KILL CURVE

The efficacy of an antibiotic in certain infections is thought to correlate with the rate and completeness of its bactericidal activity: The faster the rate and the more complete the kill, the greater will be the in vivo efficacy. Rapid and complete bactericidal activity is desirable in patients who have systemic defects in host defense mechanisms (eg, agranulocytosis), or who have infection at anatomic sites with defective defenses (eg, the vegetation in endocarditis or the cerebrospinal fluid).

The rate and completeness of the bactericidal action of animicrobial agents alone or in combination may be assessed in vitro by determining the number of surviving organisms at various times after exposure to the agent under controlled laboratory conditions (so-called time-kill studies). Time-kill studies are done in flasks of liquid media which initially contain an inoculum of 10^6 CFU/mL of the microorganism and either no antibiotic (control broth) or broth containing the appropriate concentration of antibiotic or combination of antibiotics.

Combinations of antimicrobial agents often are used in the treatment of serious infections in an attempt to increase therapeutic effect. The interaction can be considered synergistic when the effect observed with the combination is greater than the effect observed with the sum of the effects of the two drugs alone. The interaction can be considered additive or indifferent when the combined effect is equal to the sum of the effects of the two drugs alone or equal to that of the most active drug in the combination. The interaction can be considered antagonistic when the combined effect is less than that of the most active drug alone.

ASSAY FOR ANTIBACTERIAL ACTIVITY IN SERUM

Measurement in vitro of serum bactericidal activity during antibiotic therapy has been suggested as a guideline to therapy (Figure 5-3). The patient's serum is serially diluted in twofold steps with broth or antibiotic-free serum and inoculated with the organism that has been isolated from the patient. The most frequently used inoculum size is 10^5 to 10^6 CFU/mL. To assess bactericidal activity after 18 to 24 hours of incubation, 0.1 mL is then removed from each tube and subcultured onto agar plates. If a $\geq$ 99.9% kill has occurred, the initial inoculum of 5×10^5 CFU/mL will have been reduced to $\leq 5 \times 10^2$ CFU/mL (ie, $\geq$ 50 colonies on the subculture plate). The serum bactericidal activity is defined as the maximal dilution of serum that will result in at least a 99.9% kill (1000-fold reduction) of the inoculum after 18 to 24 hours of incubation. The serum itself in a 1:2 dilution may exhibit antibacterial activity, especially against gram-negative rods, so that only dilutions greater than 1:2 are significant. The use of serum as the diluent is suggested to assay activity of antibiotics that are highly serum protein bound, ie, cefazolin, nafcillin, oxacillin. There are no good data of the precise interpretation of the results, although peak serum bactericidal activity of at least 1:8 dilution is required for survival of rabbits with experimental streptococcal endocarditis. In this model, trough activity has been shown not to be essential.

In man, serum usually is assayed when peak activity is anticipated, ie, end of an IV infusion or one to two hours after IM injection. Although there have been recommendations to attempt to achieve significant serum bactericidal activity at both peak and trough (just before next

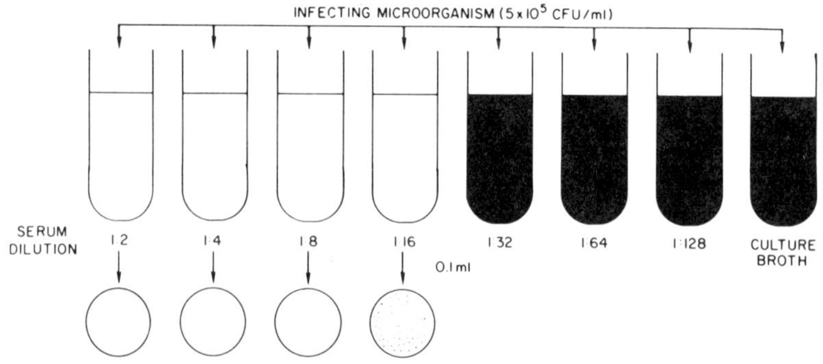

Figure 5-3 Schema of the serum dilution test for bactericidal activity in patients with infective endocarditis. After 18 to 24 hours of incubation, black tubes contain serum in which the organism has grown abundantly and the white tubes contain serum of unchanged turbidity. Interpretation of results: bactericidal at 1:8 dilution.

dose), with some antibiotics such as the aminoglycosides, this may only encourage the development of toxicity without evidence of benefit.

Although most laboratories only consider a 99.9% kill in 18 to 24 hours significant, this rate of bactericidal action has been set more or less arbitrarily. There is no evidence to date that proves that other endpoints, such as 98% or 99% kill in 18 to 24 hours, are inferior to the one requiring 99.9% killing for prediction of a satisfactory clinical response. A form of resistance, called tolerance, recently has been described in which 99.9% kill occurs at 48 or more hours but not after 18 to 24 hours of incubation. The clinical significance of this delayed bactericidal activity is unknown as yet, but is currently under investigation.

Because of the problems with standardization of methods (inoculum size, medium, diluent, incubation conditions, duration of incubation), lack of quality control, arbitrary endpoint (ie, 99.9% kill of a 10^6 CFU/mL inoculum in 18 to 24 hours), and lack of confirmation of clinical efficacy, no firm recommendations can be given for specific indications or interpretation of results. Most authorities recommend that chemotherapy is to be adjusted to attain high serum bactericidal activity (in at least a 1:8 dilution) to create a sufficient concentration gradient to achieve bactericidal activity at the site of infection for clinical situations in which host defense mechanisms do not function optimally. Treatment for bacterial endocarditis is the most widely accepted indication for measurement of serum bactericidal activity. These tests in serum also may be indicated for the treatment of osteomyelitis and serious infections in patients with agranulocytosis and in CSF for treatment of meningitis.

DETERMINATION OF CONCENTRATIONS OF ANTIMICROBIAL AGENTS IN BODY FLUIDS

The primary indications for determination of serum concentrations of antimicrobial agents are: 1) determination of the adequacy of dosing, and 2) avoidance of drug toxicity. There is no justification or need for routine measurement of agents, such as penicillins and cephalosporins, which may be safely given in large doses that result in blood levels greatly in excess of MICs and MBCs. Exceptions include: 1) infection with organisms having a relatively high MIC, especially in patients with impaired host defenses, to assure adequacy of dosing; or 2) use of a β-lactam antibiotic in a patient with impaired drug elimination, when even these usually innocuous agents may result in toxicity due to excessive serum levels. The aminoglycosides are the usual agents for which assays are indicated because of their narrow therapeutic range and the possibility of severe damage to renal and auditory function when excessively high serum levels occur. The aminoglycosides have variable dose/blood level relationships even in patients with normal renal function. In renal failure their elimination is significantly altered, and dosing must be adjusted based on measurements of serum levels. In addition, in patients on combined therapy, aminoglycosides can be inactivated in vivo by penicillins, such as carbenicillin or ticarcillin, resulting in a biologically inactive compound. This effect is most pronounced when blood levels of the β-lactam are high and sustained, as in the presence of renal failure. This might result in an unexpectedly short half-life and low blood levels of the aminoglycoside. In addition, if the β-lactam were to be discontinued in these patients on combined therapy, the subsequent "overshoot" of the aminoglycoside blood level could result in ototoxicity and nephrotoxicity.

To determine concentrations of antimicrobial agents in clinical specimens, several different methods are used. The microbiologic assay is probably still the most commonly used method, but immunologic and physicochemical methods are also available. None of these three basic methods are clearly superior to another. The microbiologic assay is least costly, but requires trained microbiology personnel and takes six or more hours to obtain results. If the patient is receiving multiple antimicrobial agents, the microbiologic assay will measure total antimicrobial activity of the serum due to all the antimicrobial agents to which the assay organism is sensitive. Special procedures must be done to nullify agents not to be measured. For example, the β-lactams in a specimen can be destoyed by β-lactamase and aminoglycosides can be removed by cellulose phosphate. However, the activity of other agents such as vancomycin, rifampin, tetracycline, clindamycin and chloramphenicol is difficult to remove. Multiresistant assay organisms can be used in such situations, but the laboratory is then required to have a number of these multiresistant strains readily available. An agent whose elimination from the body is delayed, even if given to the patient up to several days prior to obtaining the specimen, may interfere with the microbiologic assay of another subsequently administered agent. For these reasons, all of the antimicrobial medications that have been recently used to treat the patient should be known to the personnel performing the microbiologic assay.

The radioimmunoassay and enzyme immunoassay are rapid and specific for the agent to be measured, but are only available for aminoglycosides and are more expensive than the bioassay to perform. High pressure liquid chromatography (HPLC) is also specific for the agent to be tested, is rapid and can be used to measure almost all antimicrobial agents, but the equipment is expensive and requires experienced personnel.

SELECTED READINGS

Barrett-Conner E: The non-value of sputum culture in the diagnosis of bacterial pneumonia. *Am Rev Respir Dis* 1971;103:845–848.

Davidson D, Tempest B, Palmer DL: Bacteriologic diagnosis of acute pneumonia. Comparison of sputum, transtracheal aspirates, and lung aspirates. *JAMA* 1976;235:158–163.

Lennette EH, Balows A, Hausler WH Jr, et al: Manual of Clinical Microbiology, ed 3. Washington, DC, American Society of Microbiology, 1980.

Murray PR, Washington JA: Microscopic and bacteriologic analysis of sputum. *Mayo Clin Proc* 1975;50:339–344.

6 *Use of Antimicrobial Agents*

Matthew E. Levison

The outcome of life-threatening infection frequently depends on the early institution of appropriate antimicrobial therapy. Appropriate use of an antimicrobial agent requires a microbiologic diagnosis (either tentative or proven), and knowledge of the spectrum of activity of various antimicrobial agents, the concentrations required to inhibit or kill most susceptible strains, and the pharmacology of these agents.

SIGNIFICANCE OF BACTERIOSTATIC VERSUS BACTERICIDAL ACTIVITY

Agents may be divided into those that are bacteriostatic and those that are bactericidal. Bacteriostatic agents have a minimal bactericidal concentration (MBC) that is much higher than the minimal inhibitory concentration (MIC); whereas, bactericidal agents have an MBC approximately equal to the MIC. The MBC is defined by convention as the minimal concentration that reduces a microbial population of about 10^5 to 10^2 or less organisms/mL, a 99.9% or more kill, after overnight incubation in vitro, and the MIC is defined as the minimal concentration that prevents development of visible turbidity after overnight incubation of a clear microbial suspension of 10^5 organisms/mL. Bactericidal action is expected from the penicillins, cephalosporins, aminoglycosides and vancomycin; whereas, erythromycin, tetracyclines, chloramphenicol, clindamycin, lincomycin, and sulfonamides generally are bacteriostatic. However, this division is not strict as bactericidal agents may be bacteriostatic against certain microorganisms and vice versa. For example, chloramphenicol is bactericidal against pneumococci, *H. influenzae* and meningococci, and penicillin has poor bactericidal activity against enterococci.

Bacteriostatic agents require normal body defense mechanisms to clear the infection. If the defenses are inadequate, infection treated with bacteriostatic agents may relapse once therapy is stopped. Infections in which host defense mechanisms seem to be at least partially lacking either at the local site, or systemically, require treatment with bactericidal agents. High cure rates in these situations may depend to a large extent on total elimination of the pathogen by a bactericidal antimicrobial agent. Examples include meningitis in which the cerebrospinal fluid lacks complement activity, endocarditis in which the vegetation lacks infiltration with granulocytes, and infection in patients with severe granulocytopenia ($\leq$ 500 polymorphonuclear granulocytes/mm^3).

Treatment of endocarditis with erythromycin, clindamycin, tetracycline or chloramphenicol usually will be unsuccessful. Similarly, treatment of enterococcal endocarditis with penicillin alone usually will not be successful unless an aminoglycoside is added to result in a bactericidal effect. Treatment of meningitis due to *H. influenzae*, meningococci or pneumococci with chloramphenicol which is bactericidal against these organisms will result in high cure rates. However, the cure rate for meningitis due to *E. coli*, against which chloramphenicol is only bacteriostatic, is low when treated with this antibiotic. In addition, the cure rate in *S. aureus* pneumonia or bacteremia treated with bacteriostatic agents is low; much better results are achieved with penicillins, cephalosporins or vancomycin. The leukopenic patient with serious gram-negative bacillary infection also seems to fare better with bactericidal therapy such as penicillins, cephalosporins and/or aminoglycosides.

In other infections, however, there seems to be no advantage of bactericidal over bacteriostatic agents (eg, pneumococcal pneumonia, urinary tract infection).

EMPIRIC THERAPY

To avoid delay in institution of antimicrobial therapy, seriously ill patients usually require therapy before confirmation of the specific microbiologic cause and before the antimicrobial susceptibility of the pathogen is known. Such treatment should be directed at the organisms that would *most likely* cause the patient's illness, with antimicrobial agents that are *most likely* to be active against the suspected pathogens. To achieve maximum benefit, agents should be chosen that would be active against the highest percentage of strains at the lowest concentration and that have the lowest toxicity. For example, in a hospitalized patient with agranulocytosis and a sudden onset of chills and fever, infection due to *Pseudomonas aeruginosa* or Enterobacteriaceae is highly probable. If it is known that gentamicin or tobramycin inhibit only 90% of these organisms at this particular hospital, whereas amikacin inhibits 99%, then amikacin should be chosen. Amikacin, although in general less potent than gentamicin or tobramycin, is less toxic on a mg/kg body weight basis and can be used in higher doses to achieve higher serum levels in vivo to compensate for its lesser potency. At times, when organisms are equally sensitive to all three aminoglycosides, the degree to which serum levels will exceed the minimal levels necessary for a therapeutic effect will be greater for amikacin than for the two other aminoglycosides after usual dosing regimens.

Because one agent may not have a wide enough spectrum against all the potential pathogens in a given clinical situation, therapy with a combination of agents may have to be initiated. In addition to the use of combinations of antimicrobial agents in empiric regimens to increase the spectrum of activity, combinations also are frequently required in mixed infections.

Combination therapy also is used in the anticipation that the bacterial densities may fall more rapidly, inhibitory activity may occur at significantly lower concentrations of each agent, and emergence of resistant mutants may occur less frequently than if the agents were used alone. Combination therapy in empiric regimens may be simplified to the single most effective and least toxic agent when antimicrobial sensitivities become known. However, granulocytopenia and immunocompromised patients may benefit by continuance of combined therapy with several agents to which the isolated pathogen is susceptible.

SYNERGISM AND ANTAGONISM– COMBINATION THERAPY

When antimicrobial agents are used in combination, certain in vitro observations can be made. There may be more rapid or more complete bactericidal activity (called *synergism*); there may be no change in bactericidal activity (called *indifference*); or there may be less bactericidal activity (called *antagonism*) than would occur when agents were used alone.

Synergism occurs mainly when two bactericidal agents are combined, indifference when bacteriostatic agents are combined and antagonism when a bacteriostatic agent is combined with a bactericidal agent. However, these interactions are not totally predictable and in vitro testing is necessary to determine the true interaction.

Antagonism and synergism have been shown clinically to be of significance in very few situations. These are all examples of infections in which sterilization of the site of infection depends primarily on the antimicrobial agent. For example, pneumococcal meningitis treated with penicillin plus a tetracycline (a bacteriostatic agent) has a higher mortality rate than when treated with penicillin alone (a bactericidal agent). In the experimental animal with endocarditis, a bacteriostatic agent combined with a bactericidal agent is antagonistic. Synergism occurs in enterococcal endocarditis when an aminoglycoside is added to penicillin; without addition of an aminoglycoside, the relapse rate is very high. It is likely that synergism is also important in the leukopenic patient with serious *P. aeruginosa* infection treated with an aminoglycoside (eg, tobramycin) plus a penicillin (eg, ticarcillin) in whom better results are achieved with combination therapy.

ACTIVITY OF AGENT AT SITE OF INFECTION

In a patient with serious infection, it is important to locate the primary source of the infection, for results of therapy will not be satisfactory unless the antimicrobial agent is present in effective concentrations at this site. Many tissues, such as lung, are well perfused and tissue levels of antimicrobial agents are similar to blood levels. However, relatively large doses of an antimicrobial may be necessary to achieve high-spiking blood levels, and thus assure adequate penetration into more poorly perfused tissues or otherwise less accessible sites (necrotic tissues, abscesses, cerebrospinal fluid).

For example, many agents pass through the blood-brain barrier poorly and attain low cerebrospinal fluid concentrations as compared to serum concentrations (eg, penicillins), although higher concentrations usually are achieved in the presence of meningeal inflammation. Therefore, high doses of penicillins are required in meningitis. Some agents, such as chloramphenicol, sulfonamides and rifampin, achieve adequate cerebrospinal fluid levels with the usual doses. Clindamycin and the so-called first and second generation cephalosporins are not satisfactory agents in the treatment of central nervous system infection, since such diffusion is unpredictable. The vegetation of endocarditis also is probably an area where penetration of some antimicrobials is impaired; therefore, large doses are required to assure adequate diffusion into the infected vegetation. In contrast, urinary levels of most antibiotics are very high in patients with normal renal function. Most agents penetrate well into inflamed joints and other body cavities, excluding the cerebrospinal fluid. Therefore, there is no advantage in instilling agents into body cavities such as the pleural, peritoneal and joint spaces.

Local conditions at the site of infection may compromise the activity of the antimicrobial agent. For example, the activity of many agents may be lessened against dense microbial populations: large microbial populations may be more likely to harbor a few resistant mutants than sparse populations; this resistant subpopulation may subsequently emerge as the predominant organism during therapy. Furthermore, dense populations may produce a greater amount of an enzyme capable of destroying the agent locally. Aminoglycosides and erythromycin are much less active at an acid pH (as in an abscess or infected body fluid) or the usual pH of urine; sulfonamides are relatively inactive in abscesses because of the presence of large concentrations of para-aminobenzoic acid; and abscesses are anaerobic and aminoglycosides are not active against anaerobically metabolizing bacteria. For these reasons, drainage of pus and removal of foreign bodies are essential for effective therapy.

Since many pneumonias are a mixture of purulent tracheobronchitis plus parenchymal infection, the height, timing and duration of peak antibiotic levels in bronchial secretions may be important. The alveolar and interstitial fluid concentrations of antimicrobial agents closely approximate serum levels. However, levels in bronchial secretions may be considerably below serum levels. Simple passive diffusion along a concentration gradient appears to be the method for transport of most antibiotics between blood and bronchial secretions. In this case, higher serum levels achieved by an intravenous bolus should be accompanied by higher bronchial levels. Penetration of certain drugs into bronchial secretions also may be favored by the bronchial inflammation (eg, ampicillin, cephalexin, clindamycin).

Local intrabronchial antibiotic might persist after the antibiotic has been cleared from serum. Reabsorption or respiratory cleansing mechanisms, such as mucociliary movement and coughing, may be important in clearing antibiotics from the bronchial lumen. Intrabronchial metabolism of an antibiotic also could occur.

The clinical significance of poor diffusion of drug into bronchial secretions may vary with the pathogen. Those relatively resistant organisms (*P. aeruginosa*) may persist in bronchial secretions during therapy although cleared from the lung, while relatively sensitive organisms (pneumococci) may be cleared from both bronchial secretions and lungs.

CHEMOPROPHYLAXIS

Antimicrobial agents can be used to prevent the development of infection. To accomplish this, the antimicrobial agent is administered to obtain blood and tissue levels at the time of exposure to the infectious agent(s). For example, to prevent wound infections following surgery, since exposure occurs during the surgical procedure, antimicrobial drugs should be administered either intramuscularly about one hour prior to surgery or intravenously at the start of surgery. Prophylactic antibiotics are not recommended for clean operations in which a foreign body is not implanted since the expected rate of infection is less than 1% to 5%. Prophylaxis is indicated for: 1) operations in which a critical foreign body is implanted, eg, prosthetic cardiac valve, arterial graft or a prosthetic joint; 2) contaminated surgery, eg, biliary tract surgery in patients likely to have bactobilia (those over 70 years of age, or those who have common duct stones or are jaundiced), vaginal hysterectomy, or surgery on an unprepared bowel; or 3) dirty surgery, eg, surgery in the presence of pus, perforated viscus, or traumatic wound.

Chemoprophylaxis also is recommended for patients at risk of developing infective endocarditis in those situations most likely to be associated with transient bacteremia, such as dental procedures associated with gingival bleeding, bronchoscopy, tonsillectomy, adenoidectomy or other oropharyngeal surgery, instrumentation or surgery of the genitourinary tract and surgery on the lower intestinal tract. Antimicrobial agents should be given at a time that results in maximal blood levels during the period of anticipated bacteremia.

In other situations, exposure to the infectious agents may be unpredictable and require continuous prophylaxis, such as oral penicillin to prevent recurrent pneumococcal infection in patients with multiple myeloma or benzathine penicillin to prevent recurrent rheumatic fever following streptococcal infection.

Antimicrobial agents also can be used to treat an early or asymptomatic phase of an infection to prevent the development of symptoms. Examples include chemoprophylaxis of: 1) active tuberculosis in high-risk tuberculin-positive individuals; 2) intra-abdominal or wound infection following surgery for a ruptured appendix or perforated colon; 3) meningococcal infection in close household contacts of a patient with this disease; or 4) *P. carinii* pneumonia in leukemic children.

Situations in which prophylactic antibiotics have been shown to be ineffective include the prevention of pneumonia in comatose patients with penicillin and streptomycin or in congestive heart failure patients with chloramphenicol; prevention of tracheal colonization by pathogenic organisms with broad-spectrum antibiotics; prevention of bacterial complications of viral respiratory infections; and prevention of acute exacerbations of asthma with penicillin V.

Whenever chemoprophylaxis is used, drug toxicity must be weighed against the risk of infection. Chemoprophylaxis is used in situations in which the risk of development of infection exceeds the potential toxicity of the antimicrobial agent or in which development of infection would result in significant morbidity and mortality, although the risk is low (eg, prosthetic valve endocarditis).

EXCRETION OR INACTIVATION OF THE ANTIMICROBIAL AGENT

The rate of excretion or inactivation of an agent will determine the duration of activity in serum and at other sites. The rate of elimination determines in part the peak serum concentration when the antimicrobial agent is relatively slowly absorbed (ie, when administered by oral, intramuscular or slow intravenous routes).

Most antimicrobial agents are excreted by the kidneys. These agents include most penicillins, cephalosporins, aminoglycosides, tetracyclines, vancomycin and polymyxins. Many penicillins and cephalosporins are excreted by renal tubular secretion as well as by glomerular filtration; probenecid has a marked effect in reducing the rate of excretion of these drugs by blocking tubular secretion. The aminoglycosides, most tetracyclines, vancomycin, sulfonamides and polymyxins are excreted mainly by glomerular filtration. Erythromycin, lincomycin, clindamycin, rifampin and nafcillin (a penicillin) are excreted mainly in the bile. Doxycycline is excreted mainly by the intestinal tract into the stool. Some agents are inactivated by the liver prior to excretion; cephalothin and certain other cephalosporins (cephapirin, cefotaxime) are deacetylated, chloramphenicol is conjugated by glucuronyl transferase and isoniazid is acetylated in the liver. The rate of acetylation of isoniazid is genetically determined (ie, rapid or slow acetylators).

MAINTENANCE DOSING IN PATIENTS WITH IMPAIRED ELIMINATION

Repeating the administration of the usual dose at the usual dosing interval in patients with abnormally prolonged elimination will lead to accumulation. To prevent toxic accumulation of the drug, either the maintenance dose can be reduced, the dosing interval can be increased, or both can be done in proportion to the reduction in drug elimination. With impaired renal function, it is essential to modify dosage regimens of aminoglycosides, vancomycin, polymyxins, tetracyclines (other than doxycycline), sulfonamides and flucytosine. When large doses of penicillins or cephalosporins are being used, it is also prudent to lower the dosage. With severe impairment of liver function, it may be necessary to decrease doses of the following: erythromycin, lincomycin, clindamycin, chloramphenicol and nafcillin.

Dosage schedules for patients with impaired renal function usually can be adjusted satisfactorily. Indices of renal function (such as serum creatinine) provide an estimate of the necessary adjustment. Formulas, graphs, nomographs, and computer programs have been devised for adjustment of dosage schedules for individual drugs, including the aminoglycoside antibiotics.

Adjustment of dosage schedules for patients with impaired hepatic function is difficult, since hepatic drug elimination is not consistently correlated with any of the routine hepatic function tests.

Adjustment of dosage schedules on the basis of pharmacokinetic principles, whether estimated by rule of thumb or by computer, is necessarily only an approximation; final adjustment must be made by measurement of drug concentrations in serum.

ROUTE OF ADMINISTRATION

Peak serum levels will be higher and attained more rapidly with rapid intravenous injection than with the other routes of administration. When the absorption from the site of drug administration is slow relative to rate of elimination (eg, slow intravenous, intramuscular or oral administration), the height of the peak serum concentration will be lessened, and the time to peak and duration of levels will be lengthened (Figure 6-1). Oral and even intramuscular administration cannot

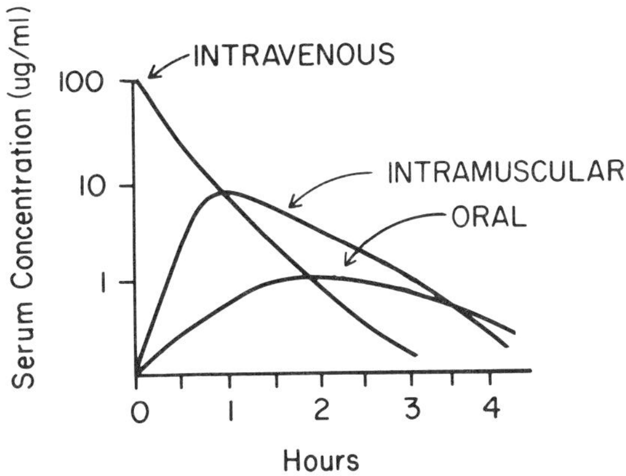

Figure 6-1 Semilog plot of the serum concentrations of an antimicrobial agent after IV, IM, and oral administration.

guarantee rapid and complete access of a drug to the systemic circulation. This would require the drug to be injected directly into the vascular system. Therefore, therapy by the oral or even intramuscular route is considered only in less serious infections, which will not be too adversely affected by slow or erratic absorption, and in infections caused by very sensitive organisms, because blood and tissue levels usually will be lower following oral rather than parenteral administration. An exception would be infection in the urinary tract that can be treated with an oral agent that is concentrated in the urine. It is most prudent to give oral agents in the fasting state (preferably one to two hours before meals), but an agent like ketoconazole is better absorbed when given with meals. Some agents are not absorbed orally (eg, aminoglycosides, vancomycin) or are destroyed by gastric acid (eg, methicillin). For systemic infections, these agents must be given by injection. Some agents are absorbed as well orally as by intravenous injection (eg, chloramphenicol).

The route of administration frequently limits the size of the dose. Large doses that usually are used to treat infections at relatively inaccessible sites or infections due to relatively insensitive organisms usually require intravenous administration because of intestinal intolerance with these doses when given orally or excessive volume with these doses when given intramuscularly. The intravenous route also may be preferred over intramuscular administration with patients in shock or in critically ill patients requiring rapid attainment of therapeutic levels. In addition, absorption from intramuscular injection sites may be impaired in diabetics. Some agents are too painful to use intramuscularly and must be given intravenously when parenteral administration is required (eg, large doses of penicillin G, tetracycline or erythromycin). Intramuscular administration is also avoided in patients with a bleeding diathesis.

PHARMACOKINETICS

Pharmacokinetics is the quantitative study of the time course of disposition (the absorption, distribution, metabolism and excretion) of drugs in the body. The optimal size, route and frequency of individual doses, the need for and the appropriate size of loading doses, and the time course of accumulation in the body during repeated administration are functions of the pharmacokinetics of a drug.

Because of the relative ease of measurement, pharmacokinetics usually are described in terms of blood levels. However, it is important to remember that the therapeutic effects require effective drug concentrations at sites of infection. It is thought that these local concentrations of antimicrobial agents should be equal at least to the minimal concentrations that can inhibit the growth of the microorganism in vitro (MIC). Furthermore, the minimal concentrations that can kill the microorganisms in vitro (MBC) are thought to be required at those sites of infection where host defenses are impaired. Because of the arbitrary characteristics of the in vitro testing system with regard to the medium, incubation conditions, duration of incubation, inoculum size, in vitro results may not adequately predict the in vivo situation. Therefore, the in vivo concentrations optimally should exceed the MIC or MBC. The extent by which the in vivo levels at the site of infection exceed the MIC or MBC and for how long is not well defined, but probably depends on the organisms, the stage of the infection (eg, bacterial densities and rate of growth), and local factors at the site of infection that diminish either the activity of the agent or adequacy of host defenses.

Pharmacokinetic models view the body as a homogeneous pool or compartment, or a series of compartments into which a drug is distributed and from which it is eliminated. The fate of many antimicrobial agents is described by the two-compartment model: a central compartment of small apparent volume and a peripheral compartment of larger apparent volume. Drugs distribute rapidly throughout the central compartment, which consists of the serum or blood volume together with the extracellular fluid of highly perfused tissues such as the heart, lungs, liver, kidneys, and endocrine glands. The peripheral compartment is formed by less perfused tissues, such as muscle, skin, and body fat into which drugs enter more slowly. In addition to tissue perfusion, distribution of drug between serum and tissues is also determined by protein binding, diffusibility, lipid solubility, molecular size, pK value, tissue binding, and active transport.

Rapid intravenous injection is the simplest method of drug administration for pharmacokinetic analysis. When administered in this manner, all of the drug is initially found in the central compartment. The concentration in the central compartment immediately after injection is equal to

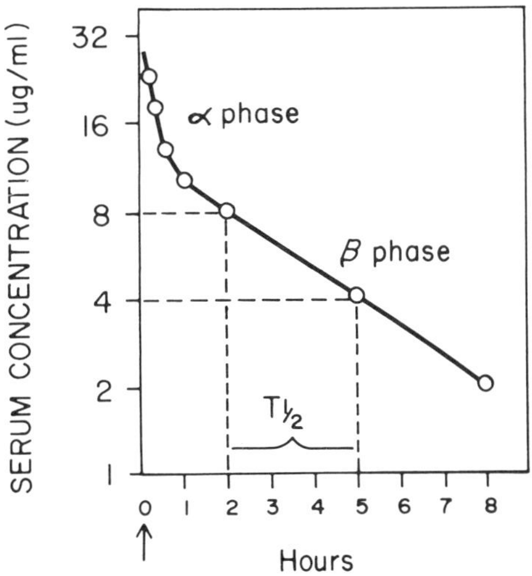

Figure 6-2 Schematic graph of serum concentrations plotted on the logarithmic scale versus time after a single IV bolus of an antimicrobial agent as predicted by a two-compartment model. Calculation of serum half-life (T½) from the slope of the curve during the elimination, or β phase is shown.

the dose divided by the volume of the central compartment. Changes in dose will result in a proportional change in height of this peak concentration.

A plot of the logarithm of serum concentration versus time yields a curve with two distinct linear components (Figure 6-2). The initial rapid fall in concentration, called the "alpha" or "distribution" phase, mainly represents the relatively rapid process of drug distribution from central to peripheral compartments.

Once distribution is complete, the curve enters the relatively slow "beta" or "elimination" phase, during which drug disappearance is determined mainly by irreversible elimination due to metabolism and renal or biliary excretion.

The total apparent volume of distribution (V_d) is defined as the volume in which the drug is distributed after absorption and distribution are complete. A large V_d implies wide distribution or extensive tissue uptake or both. A small V_d indicates that distribution is limited and tissue uptake is not extensive. Volume of distribution is expressed as volume per unit body weight. Drug dosage should be suitably adjusted for abnormally lean or obese individuals and for those who are markedly dehydrated or edematous, with appropriate regard for whether the drug is distributed in fat or in the extracellular fluid compartment. For a drug distributed in extracellular fluid, if the volume of distribution is expanded (eg, by ascites), unexpectedly low serum levels will be attained unless the dose is increased. Drugs (eg, the aminoglycosides) that are not distributed in adipose tissue will have a volume of distribution proportional to lean body weight. As obese body weight increases, failure to base aminoglycoside dose upon lean body weight could result in serum levels significantly in excess of the desired level. Dosage for aminoglycosides should be based on lean weight plus 50% of the adipose weight (actual body weight–lean body weight) to prevent development of potentially toxic serum levels in obese patients.

The rate of elimination can be described by the elimination half-life ($T\frac{1}{2}$), which is the time it takes for the serum concentration to fall 50% (or for 50% of the drug present in the body to be eliminated). A short $T\frac{1}{2}$ indicates rapid elimination (see Figure 6-2).

Total clearance of a drug is another index of drug elimination from the central compartment. Metabolism, excretion by the kidney, exhalation by the lungs, and fecal excretion are the usual methods of drug elimination that determine clearance. Clearance of a drug is inversely proportional to $T\frac{1}{2}$ and directly proportional to the V_d.

When a drug is excreted by the kidney, its renal clearance can be calculated by division of the rate of urinary excretion of the drug by the serum concentration. Alternatively, one can multiply total drug clearance by the fraction of the administered dose that appears unchanged in the urine. Total clearance less renal clearance equals the extent of clearance by nonrenal mechanisms.

MODES OF ADMINISTRATION

Continuous Intravenous Infusion

On occasion, antimicrobial agents are given by continuous intravenous infusion; for example, aqueous crystalline penicillin G can be given as 10 to 20 million units per day by a continuous intravenous infusion to treat pneumococcal or meningococcal meningitis or streptococcal endocarditis. The pharmacokinetics of a constant rate infusion (Figure 6-3) reveals the serum concentration gradually rises to reach a plateau. The time required to achieve the plateau serum concentration depends only on the $T\frac{1}{2}$. About 95% of the plateau serum concentration is attained after four to five half-lives. The magnitude of the plateau serum concentration depends on the infusion rate, $T\frac{1}{2}$ and V_d. The plateau serum concentration will be heightened by increasing the infusion rate or, among drugs administered in the same manner, the drug having a relatively longer $T\frac{1}{2}$, a smaller V_d, or a lower total body clearance will have the higher plateau concentration.

For example, in normal adults the $T\frac{1}{2}$ of penicillin G is about one-half hour and plateau penicillin levels would be expected after two hours of infusion. If 5 million units of penicillin G is administered by continuous infusion over a six-hour period, a plateau serum level is 12 to 20

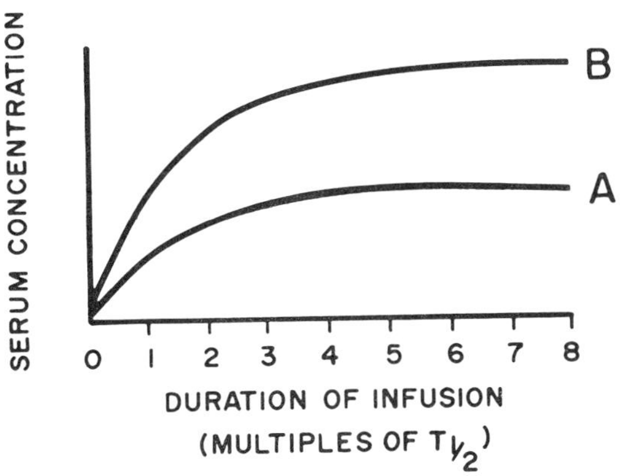

Figure 6-3 Schematic graph of serum concentrations versus time during IV infusion at a constant rate (A) and at twice that rate (B).

μg per mL. Plateau serum levels are stable if a constant infusion pump is used. However, if the infusion is given by an ordinary intravenous drip, large serum level fluctuations occur, despite close supervision of the infusions. Because therapeutic serum concentration may not be achieved initially by continuous intravenous infusion, in emergency treatment of serious infections, such as meningitis, an initial rapid injection of penicillin G should be given intravenously to achieve a high level of penicillin quickly, and this can then be followed by continuous penicillin infusion. Continuous infusion was once considered preferable because of rapid excretion of penicillin, but many clinicians now prefer rapid intermittent intravenous infusions of high concentration penicillin solutions via a secondary intravenous bottle.

Intermittent Dosing (Figure 6-4)

Continuous infusion therapy attempts to maintain a constant serum concentration of the drug above the MIC for the pathogen. Experimental studies on dosing intervals, in the late 1940s and early 1950s by Eagle et al, showed clearly that the concentration of antibiotic need not continuously exceed the MIC for the organism. In fact, most antimicrobial agents are now given intermittently. This mode of administration results in a high peak concentration of drug in serum which then falls at regular intervals to levels below the MIC for the pathogen.

Of importance is the fact that after the concentration has fallen below effective levels, the surviving bacteria do not immediately recover from the toxic effects of the drug. The term *postantibiotic effect* refers to a period of variable duration after complete removal of the drug when there is no growth of the target organism. The postantibiotic effect has

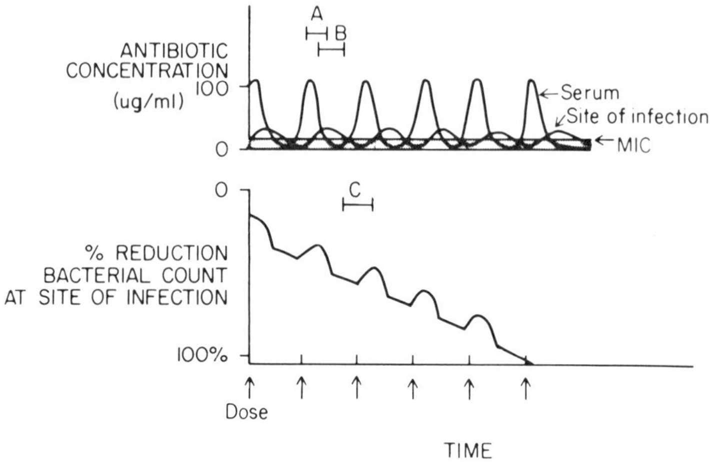

Figure 6-4 The effect of repeated administration of a bactericidal antibiotic on the bacterial population at the site of infection. A—The period that serum levels are above the MIC. B—The period that levels of the antibiotic at the site of infection are above the MIC. C—The period after levels of antibiotic at the site of infections are below the MIC, ie, the postantibiotic effect.

now been documented for many organism-antibiotic combinations. During the drug-free period following exposure to an antibiotic, the damaged but still viable organisms may be more susceptible to phagocytosis and intracellular killing, and continue to die under the impact of the body's defense mechanisms.

The fact that the number of bacteria remains stable or continues to fall for a considerable period after the drug concentration is below the MIC, makes possible discontinuous drug administration. Eventually, however, the organisms do recover from the toxic effects of the drug and resume multiplication. The longer the interval between doses, the greater is the degree to which remultiplication during the drug-free period counteracts the effect of the preceding dose.

The degree to which the drug-free interval can be prolonged without seriously compromising the therapeutic effect depends on a number of factors: 1) the danger is obviously greater with a rapidly multiplying organism than with a slowly multiplying organism (eg, *Mycobacterium tuberculosis* which has an in vitro generation time of several days versus *E. coli* which has a generation time of 20 minutes); 2) the concentration of the drug to which the organisms have been exposed and the duration of the exposure affect the time required for the bacteria to recover; 3) some species recover from the toxic effects more slowly than others; 4) the smaller the number of organisms that survive the preceding dose the less harm is done by regrowth for several generations. If the bacterial population in the infected host had been reduced from 10^9 to 10 organisms, several hours would elapse before their remultiplication became of clinical significance. However, if the number of bacteria had been reduced only from 10^9 to 10^7 organisms, regrowth for even a few generations could have a serious effect on the evolution of the infection.

During the recovery phase, the metabolically inactive bacteria are least susceptible to β-lactam and aminoglycoside antibiotics; but when the surviving organisms ("persisters") begin to grow again, they regain their previous sensitivity to these drugs, so that a little regrowth may be beneficial for the action of certain antimicrobial agents.

Discontinuous drug administration also results in spiking high peak concentrations in the serum. The height of the peak concentration determines the degree of tissue penetration. In an area of chronic inflammation with walled-off foci of infection, which only slowly equilibrates with the serum and surrounding tissue fluids, relatively high serum concentrations may be necessary to assure the presence of an effective concentration at the foci of infection. Although peak concentrations are achieved more slowly in tissue than in serum, concentrations may remain high in tissues longer than in the serum and may persist in tissues even after the drug is no longer detectable in the serum.

Similar to continuous infusion, when single doses are given at a specified dosage interval, drug accumulation may occur. After each dose, the serum concentration reaches a maximum, at which point the rate the drug leaves the central compartment exceeds the rate at which it enters from the absorption site. During the rest of the dosage interval, the serum concentration falls to a minimum value. If not all of the agent is eliminated before the next dose is given, the drug will accumulate, giving progressively higher serum levels until a steady state eventually is reached at which time the amount of drug eliminated per dosage interval equals the amount of drug administered. Steady-state serum concentrations are attained in about four to five T½ and are high when doses are large or frequent, when drug elimination is slow, or when the apparent volume of distribution is small. Since the drug is almost totally eliminated in four T½, accumulation will not occur if the dosage interval is four to five T½.

Dosage interval is selected primarily by consideration of the fluctuations in drug concentration that can be tolerated without excessive toxicity or loss of efficacy. In addition, consideration is given to patient convenience and compliance. For example, the penicillins in aqueous solution are often administered at intervals much greater than their T½ because a satisfactory effect can be achieved without toxicity despite the large fluctuations in serum levels, and because the schedule is convenient for the patient. Indeed, most antimicrobial agents are administered approximately every four or more T½ (Table 6-1).

A few antimicrobial agents traditionally are given at intervals less than the time required for total elimination. The dosing interval for vancomycin, tetracyclines, trimethoprim-sulfamethoxazole and amphotericin is approximately equal to the T½ (Figure 6-5A). Plateau levels of vancomycin and tetracycline would be achieved at 24 hours (4 × T½), trimethroprim-sulfamethoxazole at two to three days and amphotericin at four days. When clinically indicated, a "loading" dose (Figure 6-5B), larger than the subsequent maintenance dose may be recommended at times in an attempt to achieve prompt therapeutic levels. However, load-

Table 6-1
Relation of Recommended Dosing Intervals to Serum T½ for Antimicrobial Therapy in Patients with Normal Renal Function

Antimicrobial Agent	Serum T½ (Hours)	Recommended Dosage Interval (Hours)
Penicillin G	0.5	4
Nafcillin	0.5	4
Cephalothin	0.5	4
Cefotaxime	1.0	4
Ampicillin	1.5	4-6
Carbenicillin	1.5	4
Chloramphenicol	2.5	6
Clindamycin	2.0	6-8
Cefazolin	2.0	8
Moxalactam	2.0	8
Gentamicin	2.0	8
Tobramycin	2.0	8
Amikacin	2.0	12
Vancomycin	6.0	6-12
Tetracycline	6.0	6
Trimethoprim-Sulfamethoxazole	16/10	12
Amphotericin	24	24

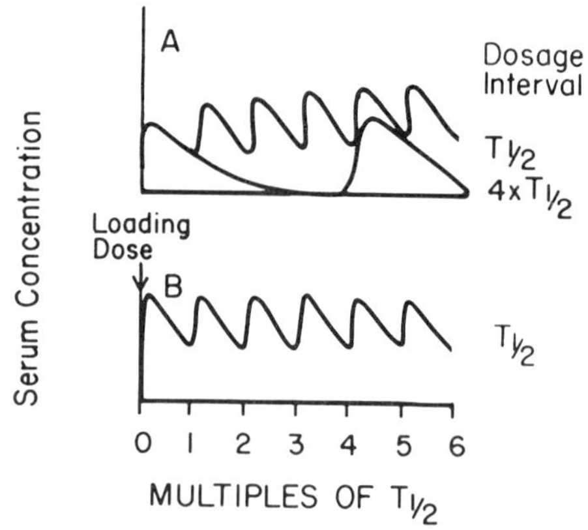

Figure 6-5 Schematic graph of the effect on serum concentrations of varying the dosage interval during repeated administration. A—without loading dose; B—with loading dose.

ing doses for these antimicrobial agents usually are not required since the serum levels after the initial dose usually are therapeutic and subsequent plateau levels are not any more toxic when these agents are given by the recommended fixed dosage schedules.

MONITORING DRUG CONCENTRATIONS

Determination of serum or tissue levels of antimicrobial agents may be useful to indicate therapeutic or toxic effects in the following situations: 1) dosing patients with uncertain or changing drug elimination; 2) adjusting the dosage of an antimicrobial agent that has a small difference between the optimal therapeutic level and the minimal toxic level; or 3) when treating an organism with a relatively high MIC. Collection of serum at peak concentrations allows determination of the maximum antimicrobial activity of the patient's serum. Trough measurements reveal the duration of activity. Peak serum levels occur about one to two hours after IM or oral administration. Peak serum levels also occur immediately at the end of an IV infusion, prior to completion of the distribution phase. Such levels collected prior to completion of distribution should not be used to calculate elimination half-life. Instead, two levels during the elimination phase, about two hours apart, are the minimum number of points needed to ascertain the elimination half-life of an antimicrobial agent (see Figure 6-2). For aminoglycosides, the first level obtained one hour after an IM injection or one-half hour after the end of a 30-minute IV infusion should be about 4 to 8 μg/mL for gentamicin and 15 to 25 μg/mL for amikacin; the second level obtained immediately before the next dose should be $\leq$ 2 μg/mL for gentamicin and tobramycin, and $\leq$ 5 μg/mL for amikacin. These levels are done on about the third and fifth day of therapy. A progressive rise in trough levels for these antibiotics would indicate a rising T½ and, because they are eliminated by glomerular filtration, deterioration in renal function.

Similarly, the antimicrobial activity of serial dilutions of the patient's serum during therapy may be tested in vitro against the organism that is infecting the patient. The maximum serum bactericidal dilution is related to the serum concentration of a bactericidal agent in the following way: the serum concentration of the antimicrobial agent divided by the MIC (equivalent to the MBC for a bactericidal agent) approximates the maximum dilution of serum that exhibits bactericidal activity (Figure 6-6). This relationship is, of course, subject to great variation since each series of dilutions has an inherent error of $\pm$ one dilution. If the half-life of the antibiotic being used is short, if the dosing interval is greater than four to six half-lives, or if the organism is relatively insensitive, the activity at the trough level may be zero, yet peak concentrations may be adequate (Figure 6-6).

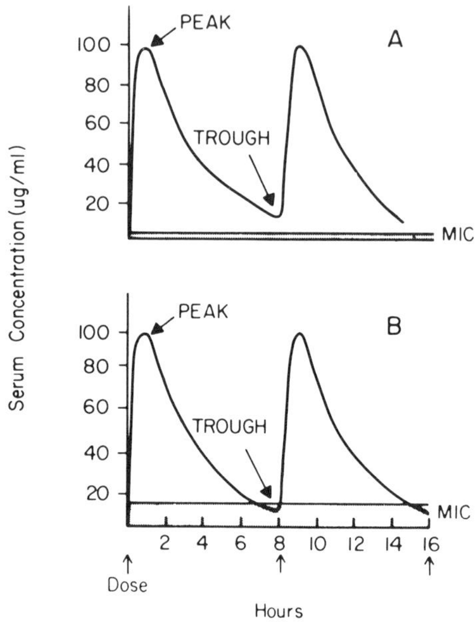

Figure 6-6 Schematic graph of serum concentrations of a bactericidal antibiotic. A—MIC = 3.1 μg/mL. Peak serum bactericidal activity should be 1:32 (peak serum concentration of 100 μg/mL ÷ MIC of 3.1 μg/mL), and trough activity of 1:4 (trough concentration of 12 μg/mL ÷ MIC of 3.1 μg/mL). B—MIC = 12.5 μg/mL. Peak serum bactericidal activity should be 1:8 (peak serum concentration of 100 ÷ MIC of 12.5), trough activity of < 1:2 (trough concentration of 12 ÷ MIC of 12.5).

DURATION OF THERAPY

The recommendations for duration of therapy of most infections are based on empiric observations of optimal response and minimal risk of relapse. The majority of infections are treated for seven to 14 days. Unnecessary prolongation of therapy may increase risks of drug toxicity or supra-infection. Symptomatic group A streptococcal infections should be treated for ten days in an attempt to prevent rheumatic fever. Infective endocarditis and serious staphylococcal infections usually require at least four weeks of treatment. With suppuration (lung abscess, liver abscess, etc) and osteomyelitis, longer therapy usually is needed. Mycobacterial and deep fungal disease may require a year or more of therapy.

TOXICITY OF ANTIMICROBIAL AGENTS

All drugs have side effects. The side effects may be local (eg, pain or phlebitis at the site of administration), allergic (eg, rash, hepatitis, serum sickness-like reaction or anaphylaxis), metabolic (eg, sodium loading, hypokalemic alkalosis from carbenicillin) or organ toxicity (eg, nephrotoxicity from aminoglycosides). Allergic reactions are not dose related, whereas metabolic and organ toxicity occur most frequently following use of excessive dosage, or in patients with impaired drug elimination and with prior disease in the target organ of drug toxicity. Clindamycin and many other antibiotics have caused pseudomembranous colitis due to colonic overgrowth of enterotoxin-producing *Clostridium difficile*.

Toxicity may be related to the patient's age, renal function, pregnancy or interaction with concurrently administered drugs. For example, nephrotoxic and ototoxic agents, such as the aminoglycosides, are more likely to cause toxicity in cachetic elderly patients who have an age-related reduction in renal function. The serum creatinine concentration may be lower than would be expected for that degree of renal impairment because of a reduced muscle mass. If the serum creatinine is used as the index of renal function in these patients to guide dosing of aminoglycoside antibiotics, excessively large doses may be given. The creatinine clearance, which is not dependent on muscle mass, would be a more reliable index of renal function in this situation. Tetracycline can cause damage to the teeth in the fetus when used in pregnancy or in the child before 8 years of age. Sulfonamides can cause kernicterus in the newborn by displacement of bilirubin from serum albumin, and chloramphenicol can cause the lethal "gray baby syndrome" in the newborn.

ANTIMICROBIAL THERAPY OF PULMONARY INFECTIONS

The antimicrobial therapy of various pulmonary infections discussed in this book is given in Table 6-2. The dosages given in the table are for adults with normal renal function unless otherwise specified.

Failure of Therapy with Antimicrobial Agents

The failure of seemingly appropriate antibiotic therapy to produce a satisfactory clinical response is fairly common and may relate to several factors.

Delay of therapy If initiation of therapy is delayed, eventually a point of no return is reached in the course of serious infections beyond which therapy is not effective. This is true even in infections with organisms that are highly susceptible to antibiotics (eg, pneumococcal pneumonia). It is, therefore, important to start therapy promptly in the seriously ill patient.

Incorrect diagnosis A patient who does not have an infection or has a viral infection cannot be expected to respond to antimicrobial therapy. Diagnostic errors may also result from attributing pathogenicity

Table 6-2
Antimicrobial Therapy of Pulmonary Infections

Antimicrobial Agent	Indication	Daily Dose*	Interval	Route	Duration	Toxicity or Comments
Adenine arabinoside (Vira-A)	Herpes simplex	15 mg/kg	qd	IV	10d	
Amantadine (Symmetrel)	(1) Prevention of influenza A infection prior to development of protective antibodies following vaccination or when vaccination is contraindicated	200 mg	q12h	po	(1) ≤ 90d	Depression, psychosis, CHF, orthostatic hypotension, urinary retention
	(2) Therapy of early influenza A infection				(2) Until 1-2d after disappearance of symptoms	
Aminoglycosides						
Amikacin (Amikin)	Serious infection due to Enterobacteriaceae or *P. aeruginosa*	15 mg/kg	q8-12h	IM, IV	2-3w	Nephrotoxicity, ototoxicity
Gentamicin (Garamycin)		5 mg/kg	q8h	IM, IV	2-3w	
Tobramycin (Nebcin)		5 mg/kg	q8h	IM, IV	2-3w	
Streptomycin (Streptomycin)	(1) Plague	(1) 30 mg/kg	q12h	IM	10d	Ototoxicity
	(2) Tularemia	(2) 15 mg/kg	q12h	IM	10d	
	(3) Tuberculosis (with INH)	(3) 15 mg/kg, then 15 mg/kg	qd, then 2-3 × w	IM IM	2-3m, then ≤ 18m	
Amphotericin (Fungizone)	Aspergillosis, cryptococcosis, candidiasis, histoplasmosis, mucormycosis coccidioidomycosis	0.3-0.7 mg/kg	qd (alternate d at higher dose)	IV (6h infusion)	≥ 6w	Fever, phlebitis, nephrotoxicity anemia, hypokalemia
Antimony sodium gluconate (Pentostam)	Kala-azar	6 mL	qd	IV	6d in India 30d in Africa	Available from CDC (404-329-3670)
Bithionol (Actamer, Biton)	Paragonimiasis	30-50 mg/kg	alternate d	po	14 doses	Available from CDC (404-329-3670)

Cephalosporins						
Cephalothin (Keflin)	(1) Infection due to susceptible Enterobacteriaceae	(1) 4-12g	q4-6h	IV	2-3 w	Phlebitis, hypersensitivity
Cephapirin (Cefadyl)	(2) *S. aureus*	(2) 4-12g	q4-6h	IV	4-6 w	
Cephradine (Velocef)	(3) *S. pyogenes*	(3) 2g	q6h	IM, IV	2w	
	(4) *S. pneumoniae*	(4) 2g	q6h	IM, IV	2w	
Cefazolin (Kefzol, Ancef)	(1)-(4)	1.5-6g	q8h	IM, IV	2-6w	
Cefamandole (Mandol)	(1)-(4) and *H. influenzae*	2-12g	q4-6h	IM, IV	2-6w	
Cefoxitin (Mefoxin)	(1)-(4) *H. influenzae* and *B. fragilis*	2-12g	q4-6h	IM, IV	2-6w	
Cefotaxime (Claforan)	(1)-(4) *H. influenzae* (*B. fragilis, P. aeruginosa* variable)	2-12g	q4-6h	IM, IV	2-6w	
Cefoperazone (Cefobid)	(1)-(4) *H. influenzae* (*B. fragilis, P. aeruginosa* variable)	3-6g	q8h	IM, IV	2-6w	Phlebitis, hypersensitivity, ↑ prothrombin time
Moxalactam (Moxam)	(1)-(4) *H. influenzae* (*B. fragilis, P. aeruginosa variable*)	3-6g	q8h	IM, IV	2-6w	Phlebitis, hypersensitivity, ↑ prothrombin time
Chloramphenicol (Chloromycetin)	(1) Susceptible Enterobacteriaceae (2) *H. influenza* (3) Anaerobic infection (4) *Rickettsia* (5) *Chlamydia*	50 mg/kg	q6h	po, IV	2-3w	Reversible bone marrow depression, aplastic anemia, gastrointestinal reactions, neurotoxic reactions, hypersensitivity, gray syndrome in neonates
Clindamycin (Cleocin)	(1) Anaerobic pneumonitis (2) Anaerobic lung abscess	0.9-2.4g or 0.9g	q6-8h q8h	IM, IV po	(1) 10d (2) 2m	Diarrhea, colitis
Cotrimoxazole (Bactrim, Septra) Trimethoprim (TMP) + Sulfamethoxazole (SMX)	(1) Pneumocystosis	(1) 20 mg/kg TMP-100 mg/kg SMX	q6h	IV, po	14d	Blood dyscrasias Hypersensitivity
	(2) Susceptible Enterobacteriaceae or *H. influenzae*	(2) 320 mg TMP-1600 mg SMX	q12h	IV, po	14d	

Table 6-2 (continued)

Antimicrobial Agent	Indication	Daily Dose*	Interval	Route	Duration	Toxicity or Comments
Diethylcarbamazine	Filariasis	6 mg/kg	TID	po	14d	
Diiodohydroxyquin	Amebiasis – to eliminate cyst excretion in stool	1950 mg	TID	po	21d	
Erythromycin (E-mycin, EES, Erythrocin, Ethril, Bristamycin, Pediamycin, Wyamycin, Robimycin)	(1) *S. pneumoniae* (2) *S. pyogenes* (3) *Mycoplasma* (4) Legionnellosis (5) *Bordetella* (6) *Chlamydia trachomatis*	(1) 1-2g (2) 1-2g (3) 1-2g (4) 2-4g (5) 2g (6) 40 mg/kg	q6h q6h q6h q6h q6h q6h	po, IV po, IV po, IV po, IV po IV	10d 10d 10d 14d 14d 10d	(6) Pediatric dose
Flucytosine (Ancobon)	Cryptococcosis (with amphotericin)	50-150 mg/kg	q6h	po	6w	Bone marrow depression, diarrhea, elevated liver enzymes
Isoniazid	Tuberculosis (with rifampin, streptomycin or ethambutol)	300 mg	qd	po, IM	9-18m	Neurotoxic reactions, hepatitis, anemia, hypersensitivity
Mebendazole (Vermox)	Hookworm, ascaris	200 mg	q12h	po	3d	Embryotoxic and teratogenic in rats; contraindicated in pregnancy
Metronidazole (Flagyl)	(1) Anaerobic infection (not optimal as single agent)	(1) 15 mg/kg, then 30 mg/kg	1st dose, then q6h	IV, po	2-3w	Gastrointestinal reactions, metallic

Metronidazole (continued)	(2) Amebiasis (with diiodohydroxyquin)	(2) 2250 mg	q8h	IV, po	10d	taste, antibuse-like effect, carcinogenic in rodents, mutagenic in bacteria
Niridazole	Schistosomiasis	25 mg/kg	BID	po	5-7d	Except in hepatosplenic schistosomiasis
Penicillins						
Crystalline Pencillin G	(1) Anaerobic pneumonitis	(1) 6-20 million units (mU)	q4-6h	IV	10-14d	Hypersensitivity
	(2) Anaerobic lung abscess	(2) 6-20 mU	q4-6h	IV	10-14d	(2) Oral therapy should be continued 2-3 m
	(3) *Actinomyces*	(3) 20 mU	q6h	IV	4-6w	(3) Oral therapy should be continued 6-8 m
	(4) Anthrax	(4) 20 mU	q6h	IV	7-10d	
	(5) *S. pneumonice*	(5) 2-20 mU	q4-6h	IV	7-10d	
Procaine Penicillin G	*S. pneumoniae* *S. pyogenes*	1.2 mU	q12h	IM	7-10d	
Phenoxymethyl Penicillin V	(1) Anaerobic lung abscess	(1) 2g	q6h	po	2-3m	
	(2) *Actinomyces*	(2) 2g	q6h	po	6-8m	
	(3) *S. pneumoniae*	(3) 1-2g	q6h	po	7-10d	
Oxacillin (Prostaphlin)	*S. aureus* infection	4-12g	q4-6h	IM, IV	4-6w	
Methicillin (Staphcillin)	*S. aureus* infection	4-12g	q4-6h	IM, IV	4-6w	Nephritis, neutropenia
Nafcillin (Nafcil, Unipen)	*S. aureus* infection	4-12g	q4-6h	IM, IV	4-6w	Neutropenia
Ampicillin	Susceptible Enterobacteriaceae or *H. influenzae*	4-12g	q4-6h	IM, IV	2-3w	
Carbenicillin (Pyopen)	Susceptible Enterobacteriaceae, *P. aeruginosa, H. influenzae, B. fragilis*	30g	q4h	IV	2-3w	
Mezlocillin (Mezlin)		18g	q4h	IV	2-3w	
Ticarcillin (Ticar)		18g	q4h	IV	2-3w	
Piperacillin (Pipracil)		18g	q4h	IV	2-3w	
Azlocillin (Azlin)		18g	q4h	IV	2-3w	

Table 6-2 (continued)

Antimicrobial Agent	Indication	Daily Dose*	Interval	Route	Duration	Toxicity or Comments
Pentamidine	Pneumocystosis	4 mg/kg	qd	IM	14d	Obtainable from the CDC
Pyrimethamine	Toxoplasmosis (life- or sight-threatening) (use with sulfadiazine and folinic acid)	50 mg, then 25 mg	qd qd	po po	3d 1m	
Rifampin (Rifadin)	(1) *S. aureus* infection (use with either antistaphylococcal penicillin, cephalosporin or vancomycin)	(1) 600 mg	qd	po	4-6w	
	(2) Tuberculosis (with INH)	(2) 600 mg	qd	po	≥ 9m	
	(3) Legionellosis (with erythromycin)	(3) 600 mg	qd	po	2w	
Sulfisoxazole or Sulfadiazine	(1) Nocardiosis	(1) 6-12g	q6h	IV, then po	2-3w, then ≥ 12m	
	(2) Toxoplasmosis	(2) 75-100 mg/kg	q6h		1m	
Thiabendazole	(1) Strongyloidiasis	(1) 50 mg/kg	q12h	po	3d	
	(2) *Toxocara* (visceral larva migrans)	(2) 50 mg/kg	q12h	po	1-2w	
	(3) *Ancylostoma braziliense* (cutaneous larva migrans)	(3) 25 mg/kg	q24h	po	2d	
Tetracycline	(1) *Actinomyces*	(1) 2g	q6h	po	6-8m	
	(2) Plague	(2) 2g	q6h	IV	7-10d	
	(3) Tularemia	(3) 2g	q6h	IV	7-10d	
Vancomycin	*S. aureus* infection	2g	q6h	IV	4-6w	

*Doses are for adults with normal renal function unless otherwise specified. The package inserts should be consulted for current or more complete manufacturer's recommendations on dosage, indications and adverse reactions.

to noninvasive commensals isolated from contaminated specimens or environmental organisms accidentally inoculated into cultures. Recently, epidemics of "pseudobacteremia" and "pseudo"-urinary tract infection have been reported due to *Pseudomonas cepacia* that had contaminated iodine-iodophor solutions or chlorhexidine solutions used to cleanse the body surfaces prior to obtaining cultures.

Normal variation in clinical course Impatience for a dramatic clinical improvement may result in needless switches of antimicrobial agents. For example, adequately treated acute pneumococcal pneumonia or pyelonephritis commonly may take three to four days before marked improvement is evident, although improvement usually occurs sooner.

Failure to deliver the agent to the site of infection in therapeutic concentrations Patients may fail to comply with prescribed oral therapy. Errors can be made in filling prescriptions. In addition, errors can occur in carrying out prescribed drug schedules on busy hospital wards. This requires review with the patient, pharmacist or nurse when faced with seeming antibiotic failures.

The dose may not be appropriate for the site of infection. Dosage guidelines in package inserts may be inadequate to achieve effective levels in relatively inaccessible tissues, such as the central nervous tissue, abscesses, endocarditic vegetations, or bone. These infections generally require maximal dosage. Several drugs, such as nalidixic acid, nitrofurantoin and cephaloglycin, are limited to use in lower urinary tract infections because of failure to achieve adequate blood or tissue levels.

The route of administration may be inappropriate. Intravenous therapy is required for patients in shock. Absorption of orally administered drug may be impaired by food in the stomach, other oral medications or diseases associated with malabsorption.

The interval between doses may be too long because relatively rapid elimination of the drug allows regrowth of the pathogen at the site of infection.

Adverse conditions at the site of infection Antimicrobial agents will not work well in an area of necrosis, foreign body or pus. For example, aminoglycosides are not very active in anaerobic conditions or at an acid pH, as in infected body fluids, pus or acid urine. Penicillin will not kill bacteria that are not multiplying (eg, as in pus). In addition, antibiotic may be destroyed locally by enzymes (eg, β-lactamase) produced by dense microbial populations or in mixed infections. In the presence of obstruction (eg, in the biliary or urinary tract) effective antimicrobial levels may not be achieved in bile or urine. For these reasons, pus must be drained and necrotic tissue debrided, foreign bodies removed, and obstruction relieved.

Complicating febrile illness Seeming antibiotic failure can be due to phlebitis at the site of intravenous lines, abscesses at sites of intramuscular administration or venous thrombophlebitis in the legs and pulmonary emboli in a bedridden patient.

Microbial resistance An antimicrobial agent will not be effective when the organism is resistant. This can occur from unrecognized pathogens (eg, treatment of an intra-abdominal abscess containing aerobes and anaerobes with antibiotics active only against the aerobes). Resistance may be present and not recognized unless special tests are used (eg, incubation at reduced temperatures for detection of resistance to methicillin among *S. aureus*). Resistance can develop in the original pathogen as the patient is being treated, or suprainfection with a new resistant organism can occur. Administration of high doses of antimicrobial agents usually results in some qualitative alterations in the patient's microbial flora. This is commonly manifested by colonization with one or more organisms, usually antibiotic resistant gram-negative bacilli or fungi. Occasionally, an invasive suprainfection of clinical significance may occur due to these microorganisms. Distinguishing colonization from suprainfection may be difficult. Suprainfection usually is manifest by a worsening clinical course, often after an initial improvement, the appearance of new findings on physical examination or new radiologic and microbiologic findings, and absence of other factors predisposing to drug failure.

Apparent failure related to drug fever Fever due to the antimicrobial agent itself may develop after initial response and is most likely to occur with penicillins, cephalosporins, vancomycin and amphotericin B. When this is the case, the patient often seems to be clinically improving despite the fever. If a search fails to disclose other causes for fever outlined above, drug fever may be present, especially if eosinophilia or skin rash has developed. Drug fever, however, may occur in their absence. If the drug is critical, it should be continued despite the fever. If the drug is not critical, discontinuation with or without substitution of another agent generally results in defervescence in two to three days.

SELECTED READINGS

Barza M, Weinstein L: Penetration of antibiotics into fibrin loci in vivo. I. Comparison of penetration of ampicillin into fibrin clots, abscesses and interstitial fluid. *J Infect Dis* 1974;129:59–65.

Barza M, Samuelson T, Weinstein L: Penetration of antibiotics into fibrin loci in vivo. II. Comparison of nine antibiotics: Effect of dose and degree of protin binding. *J Infect Dis* 1974;129:66–72.

Barza M, Brusch J, Bergeron MG, et al: Penetration of antibiotics into fibrin loci in vivo. III. Intermittent vs. continuous infusion and the effect of probenecid. *J Infect Dis* 1974;129:73–78.

Eagle H, Fleischman R, Musselman AD: Effect of schedule of administration on the therapeutic efficacy of penicillin. Importance of the aggregate time penicillin remains at effectively bactericidal levels. *Am J Med* 1950;9:280–299.

Eagle H: Experimental approach to the problem of treatment failure with penicillin. I. Group A streptococcal infection in mice. *Am J Med* 1952;13:389–399.

Greenblatt DJ, Koch-Weser J: Drug therapy. Clinical pharmacokinetics. *N Engl J Med* 1975;293:702–705, 964–970.

7 *Pulmonary Function Defects in Lower Respiratory Tract Infection*

Paul E. Epstein

The effects of pneumonia on lung function are more complicated than they first appear. Since efficient gas exchange depends on the intimate contact of inspired air with perfusing blood, any process that blocks this contact damages the efficiency of lung function. In fact, patients who have roentgenographically demonstrable pneumonias are commonly noted to be dyspneic and hypoxic. Certainly, a major cause of these findings is the presence of inflammatory cells and fibrinous exudate filling the alveoli. However, the careful observer becomes suspicious of such a simplistic explanation when he recognizes that air hunger is often greater than one would expect from the radiographic extent of the pneumonia.

ABNORMALITIES OF VENTILATION

In the normal lung, a localized decrease in ventilation produces a concomitant decrease in local perfusion. It is well recognized that hypoxemia is a powerful pulmonary artery vasoconstrictor. Local alveolar hypoxia, due to diminished ventilation, is capable of producing localized pulmonary vascular spasm with a resultant decrease in blood flow through the poorly ventilated area of the lung. Conversely, lung segments that are poorly perfused frequently are shown to have decreased ventilation. It has been suggested that the mechanism responsible for this latter observation is that poorly perfused segments receive less carbon dioxide-laden venous blood; the resultant alveolar hypocapnia produces bronchoconstriction localized to the poorly perfused area of lung. Of these two effects, abnormalities of ventilation appear to be more powerful in producing a matching blood flow than are decreases in perfusion in producing localized hypoventilation. Ventilation/perfusion lung scans take advantage of these differences in distinguishing between pulmonary embolism and pneumonia. Pneumonia is frequently recognized on lung scans as showing matching ventilation/perfusion abnormalities, while pulmonary embolism shows a perfusion defect without a matching ventilation defect.

Clearly, this logic is an oversimplification of the true pathophysiology of pneumonia. If perfusion followed ventilation precisely, then the effects of pneumonia on arterial blood gases would be no greater than that observed when a similar volume of lung tissue is removed at surgery. In fact, hypoxia does not occur even when a whole lung is removed from an otherwise normal person. On the other hand, a moderate-sized unilateral pneumonia can cause a major decrease in arterial oxygenation.

CAUSES OF HYPOXEMIA

From a physiologic standpoint, hypoxemia can be caused by only four mechanisms: hypoventilation, ventilation/perfusion abnormalities, diffusion abnormalities, or shunts. The hypoxemia noted in patients with pneumonia can be partially reversed by breathing supplemental oxygen. Usually, however, even when the patient breathes an inspired fractional concentration of oxygen of 100% (FIO_2 of 1.0), a degree of hypoxemia remains. Hypoventilation is not a feature of uncomplicated pneumonia and therefore is not responsible for the observed hypoxemia. The hypoxemia of both ventilation/perfusion abnormalities and diffusion abnormalities will be reversed entirely by administration of oxygen. Diffusion abnormalities must be widespread and severe in order to cause arterial hypoxemia and are unlikely to be involved in the hypoxemia of pneumonia. The hypoxemia caused by a shunt mechanism will not be corrected by oxygen administration because the shunted blood never flows through areas of lung where oxygen is available for exchange. The fact that exogenous oxygen administration only partially relieves the hypoxemia of pneumonias indicates that the hypoxemia is produced by more than one physiologic mechanism. In all probability both intrapulmonary shunts and ventilation/perfusion abnormalities contribute to the blood gas abnormalities seen in pneumonia.

CHARACTERISTICS OF LOWER RESPIRATORY TRACT INFECTIONS

Obviously, the specific type of infective organism and the clinical circumstances surrounding invasion of the lung has an important effect on the exact method of disease production. Nonetheless, most lower respiratory tract infections share a number of common characteristics. To a greater or lesser extent each of the types of pneumonia involve the bronchi or bronchioles, the alveoli, the interstitium, the pulmonary vasculature and the pleura. Both hypoxemia and sepsis may have wide-ranging effects on other organs. Any of these effects may be exaggerated in the individual who has preexisting pulmonary disease. For instance, patients with chronic obstructive pulmonary disease are not only more likely to develop pneumonia but also respond to the infection in qualitatively and quantitatively different ways than the normal individual. Pulmonary function studies performed on patients in the acute phase of pneumonia have shown that the vital capacity is reduced to a level lower than would be expected considering the volume of lung involved by the infection. Two possible mechanisms include a change in the compliance of the lung and pleural pain that limits the movement of the chest wall.

Studies of the viscoelasticity of the lung have shown that pulmonary compliance is substantially reduced in patients with pneumonia. Pressure-volume measurements in the normal lung show a linear relationship between distending pressure and the change in volume up to a level of about 2 L. Therefore, even when there is consolidation of one whole lung, no significant change in compliance should be observed within the usual bounds of tidal breathing. Surprisingly, actual measurements on patients with pneumonia have shown that elastic resistance in the acute phase of the illness is frequently at least double the value recorded on the same patients following recovery. The reasons for this change are not absolutely clear, but may be due to vascular engorgement or interstitial edema in areas of lung that are not clinically involved in the infection.

The change in pulmonary viscoelasticity appears to be roughly proportional to the observed respiratory rate. A poorly understood control mechanism has been recognized to regulate work of breathing to the most efficient level. As a result, even though the lung becomes generally less compliant in pneumonia, the work of breathing rises only slightly. This occurs because the tidal volume decreases while the rate of respiration increases. This is the same type of breathing pattern seen in patients with pulmonary fibrosis.

Chest pain, caused by pleural irritation, also plays an important role in setting the respiratory pattern in patients with pneumonia. Lobar pneumonias ordinarily extend out to the pleural surface and frequently cause pleural irritation. Although viral pneumonias are less consistently pleural based, the viral process itself frequently involves the pleura and may produce pain on breathing. Bronchopneumonias, in general, are less likely to cause this problem but, on occasion, may abut the pleura and cause pain. No matter what the type of pneumonia, however, the patient with this complication frequently has a rapid, shallow breathing pattern like the one just described as being due to changes in viscoelasticity. The effects of these mechanisms can be separated by treating the pleural pain with analgesics such as codeine or meperidine. The shallow, rapid breathing pattern due to pleural pain will ordinarily revert to normal and the patient will be less likely to tire and require mechanical assistance to breathing. Adequate pain relief in pneumonia is particularly important in patients with chronic obstructive pulmonary disease (COPD). These patients cannot easily tolerate a rapid respiratory rate since COPD is characterized by frequency dependence of compliance. This means that the work of breathing increases markedly as respiratory rate increases, leading to exhaustion and progressive hypoventilation. It is prudent to initiate pain therapy in patients with COPD with small does of an easily reversible narcotic. Adequacy of ventilation must be monitored with arterial blood gas analysis, paying particular attention to changes in PCO_2 and pH. The dose of analgesic should be increased slowly until adequate pain relief is achieved without depressing ventilatory drive.

Lung volumes may also be affected by pleural effusions caused by the inflammatory process. Small parapneumonic effusions are of little functional significance and are of importance only in their differentiation from empyemas. Large effusions, however, may affect pulmonary function in two ways. First, the effusion is a space-occupying process within a relatively fixed thoracic volume; its presence must, therefore, decrease all measured lung volumes. Second, the weight of a large effusion sitting on a diaphragm flattens the muscle and may even change the configuration from convex upward to convex downward. When the muscle is everted, diaphragmatic contraction may have the paradoxical effect of decreasing the intrathoracic volume. At the very least, inspiratory efforts will be unable to achieve the negative intrapleural pressure that is normally produced by a similar level of exertion. Therefore, the work required to maintain adequate ventilation rises. For these reasons, removal of even relatively small amounts of pleural fluid in a dyspneic patient with massive effusion produces an unexpectedly large symptomatic relief. It should be remembered that for every liter of fluid removed at thoracentesis more than a kilogram of downward pressure is removed from the diaphragm. Although improvement in symptoms may be excellent, the change in fluid level seen roentgenographically frequently is rather small. This finding simply demonstrates that the depressed diaphragm rises before the upper fluid meniscus falls. Recent studies by Brown et al (1978) have shown that the symptomatic improvement is substantially greater than the improvement in pulmonary mechanics. Removal of 1 L of fluid generally produces substantial symptomatic relief without exposing the patient to the unnecessary risks of major fluid shifts and hypovolemic hypotension. "Tapping the pleura dry" may be visually satisfying to the physician, but generally is unnecessary and may be of greater danger than help to the patient. If, however, the fluid is an empyema, it becomes mandatory to evacuate the pleural space completely in order to avoid loculation of the fluid and permanent trapping of the lung by fibrous tissue.

Purulent secretions are cleared from the alveoli largely through the tracheobronchial tree by way of coughing, although there is some resorption of fluid through the interstitium and some clearance via the mucociliary elevator. As secretions are being cleared through the bronchi there is partial blockage of the bronchial lumens. Airway resistance rises markedly with minor changes in luminal diameter. In fact, resistance to air flow varies inversely with the fourth power of the bronchial radius. As a result of changes in airway resistance, an altered pattern of airflow is produced and ventilation/perfusion relationships are altered. If these secretions are not cleared promptly, hypoxemia is the usual consequence. Hypoxemia itself can drive respiration to a more rapid rate. The ability to fill alveoli with air during a given time span depends on the numerical product of pulmonary compliance and airway resistance. Ordinarily, compliance changes relatively slowly when compared to the rapid changes that can occur in airway resistance. Therefore, if two different areas of lung having equal compliance are served by bronchi, one of which is patent and one of which is partially blocked by secretions, airflow in a given inspiratory cycle will be greater to the unobstructed area. As respiratory rate increases, turbulence in the partially obstructed bronchus increases. Since turbulence also increases flow resistance, ventilation to the partially obstructed area actually decreases when the rate of breathing increases.

Viral lower respiratory tract infections have a deleterious effect on the mucociliary system in that cough, inflammation and edema in the bronchial submucosa produces detachment of ciliated epithelial cells. Sheets of desquamated bronchial epithelial cells, known as Creola bodies, can be identified in expectorated sputum. These bodies are not specific for viral pneumonia since they are also found in secretions from patients with asthma and chronic bronchitis. As a result of this desquamative process, the efficiency of the mucociliary system is diminished in lower respiratory tract infections.

Body position is important in determining the degree of hypoxia produced by unilateral pneumonia. Since the pattern of blood flow and ventilation within the lung are largely determined by gravity in the normal individual, certain generalizations can be made about changes that occur when alveoli become filled with fluid and cellular debris. Normally, in the standing or sitting position, the greatest percentage of blood flow per unit volume of lung goes to the most dependent portion of the lung. Conversely, the smallest amount of blood flow per unit volume of tissue goes to the apices. This occurs because hydrostatic pressure exerts the greatest distending force on vessels at the lung bases and provides the greatest driving force for blood through the distended vessels. With each increment of height from the lung base there is a corresponding decrement of hydrostatic pressure.

Similarly, if the lung can be visualized as being suspended by a suction cup from the extreme apex of the chest. The alveoli at the top of the lung are distended not only by the negative intrapleural pressure but also by the weight of the lung tissue suspended beneath them. In the resting position of ventilation (functional residual capacity), these apical alveoli are already nearly completely distended and therefore receiving very little extra ventilation during tidal breathing. On the other hand, the alveoli at the extreme base of the lung are distended only by intrapleural pressure since no weighty lung tissue is suspended beneath them to drag them open. These basal alveoli have much greater potential for expansion during tidal breathing than the alveoli at the apex. Since ventilation and perfusion are both greatest at the lung base, gas exchange in that area is also proportionately greater than in any other portion of the lung.

The same gravitational effects occur in the recumbent position; the most dependent portion of lung receives the greatest share of both ventilation and perfusion. In the patient with unilateral pneumonia, hypoxia is made substantially worse by lying the patient on his side with the diseased lung in the down position. In this circumstance the infected alveoli in the down lung will be unable to ventilate efficiently while blood flow to the down lung will continue to be maximized by gravity. This produces ventilation/perfusion abnormalities and results in hypoxia. Oxygenation can be improved by putting the good lung in the down position.

When pneumonia results from aspiration of gastric contents, the effects of hydrochloric acid on the pulmonary parenchyma becomes an important pathogenic factor. Infective fluid entering the lungs with a pH below 2.4 produces a chemical burn of both the bronchial mucosa and the alveolar walls. Tracheobronchial secretions are very effective buffers of the acid and ordinarily bring the pH of the aspirated fluid up to at least 7.0 within 10 minutes. However, during that period of time there is damage both to the mucociliary system and to the alveolar lining cells. Type 1 pneumocytes, which normally form a thin epithelial barrier between the alveolar lumen and interstitium, become vacuolated and rounded before they die and are removed. Type 2 pneumocytes are also susceptible to damage by hydrochloric acid. These cells ordinarily have two functions: surfactant production and regeneration of Type 1 cells. Surfactant production is disrupted by acid damage to the Type 2 pneumocytes and this results in progressive atelectasis in the affected portions of the lung.

The inflammatory effects of gastric acid aspiration extend into the pulmonary capillary bed where endothelial cell damage loosens the intercellular junctions and permits leakage of plasma and formed elements into the interstitium and then into the alveoli.

Although infection is not a primary event in gastric acid aspiration, the processes described above provide favorable culture conditions for microbial agents and damage the self-cleansing mechanisms of the lung. If particulate matter is aspirated along with the acid, obstruction of bronchi may occur and potentiate the damage.

ADULT RESPIRATORY DISTRESS SYNDROME

The adult respiratory distress syndrome (ARDS), which was first recognized as pulmonary decompensation following nonthoracic trauma, recently has been associated with several types of pneumonia. Most prominent among the pulmonary infections leading to ARDS are various viral pneumonias, although several types of bacterial pneumonias also have been implicated.

Both qualitatively and quantitatively, ARDS produces different effects on pulmonary function than does pneumonia alone. From a morphologic standpoint, the changes are most similar to those described above for disease caused by aspiration of gastric acid. ARDS is, in fact, a common accompaniment of acid aspiration as well as microbial invasion. The most striking anatomic changes in ARDS are noted in the pulmonary parenchymal epithelium. The alveolar surface is denuded of epithelial covering, and proteinaceous fluid along with cellular elements fill the alveolar spaces. Hyaline membranes, reminiscent of the respiratory distress syndrome of newborn infants, cover the alveolar walls. The basement membrane and the interstitium become porous to fluid and large protein molecules; massive edema occurs with the onset of ARDS. In addition to fluid and protein accumulation, cellular elements of the blood are seen escaping from the capillaries into the interstitium. The basement membrane on the capillary side of the interstitium is mildly edematous but appears relatively normal. The most surprising anatomical finding in ARDS is the relative normality of the capillary endothelium. Considering the magnitude of fluid shifts across the alveolar capillary membrane in ARDS, one would expect to see gross disruption of the endothelial lining. This generally is not the case. Endothelial cells are somewhat more vacuolated than normal and there is focal cytoplasmic swelling. Endocytotic activity in the endothelial cells is greatly increased and may account for some of the fluid transport that obviously occurs in ARDS. However, there are few areas denuded of capillary lining cells, and fibrin clots usually plug these injured areas effectively. In addition, cell junctions appear to be relatively intact.

These curious findings, confirmed by many investigators present an anomalous situation that is as yet unexplained. The huge fluid shifts seen in ARDS must be due to alteration of both the capillary and the alveolar lining. Yet, when examined at autopsy, capillary endothelium is only mildly disturbed. One theory to explain this situation is that the capillary leak occurs early in the course of the disease and that the endothelial damage is repaired rapidly. Alveolar lining cells (Type 1 pneumocytes), however, are regenerated slowly from differentiation of Type 2 pneumocytes and may not keep pace with capillary repair.

The diagnosis of ARDS complicating pulmonary infection depends on the rapid deterioration of oxygenation accompanied by signs of diffuse, noncardiogenic pulmonary edema. Specifically, the patient develops tachypnea and hypoxemia that is refractory to oxygen administration. Foamy secretions are expectorated, and auscultation of the chest reveals bilateral rales. The roentgenogram shows diffuse, fluffy alveolar infiltrates, but characteristically, the heart size is normal. An important feature that differentiates cardiogenic from noncardiogenic pulmonary edema is the pulmonary capillary wedge pressure that is normal or low in patients with ARDS and elevated in patients with cardiogenic pulmonary edema.

Functional abnormalities follow directly from the anatomic derangements seen in ARDS. Since surfactant production is damaged by loss of Type 2 pneumocytes, microatelectasis occurs and produces hypoxia by widespread shunting of blood through vessels serving the closed alveoli. Fluid, protein and cellular leakage into alveoli causes both shunting and ventilation/perfusion mismatching, worsening the hypoxemia. Alveoli that fill with foreign material decrease the space available for air and the functional residual capacity (FRC) is thus diminished. The FRC, which normally provides a reservoir of oxygen to buffer minor changes in respiratory pattern, is no longer as effective in this task. This results in a relative instability of blood oxygenation. Meanwhile, interstitial edema produces induration of the normally compliant lung tissue leading to alteration of pressure/volume relationships and increasing the work of breathing. Thus, as the oxygen cost of breathing is rising, the ability of the lungs to supply oxygen to the blood falls dramatically.

Adequate management of the infectious process that caused ARDS is not necessarily effective in controlling the train of events described above. Special techniques of respiratory therapy and fluid management will be detailed in Chapter 8.

SELECTED READINGS

Agostini E: Mechanics of pleural space. *Physiol Rev* 1972;52:57.

Awe WC, Fletcher WS, Jacob SW: The pathophysiology of aspiration pneumonitis. *Surgery* 1966;60:232.

Bachofen M, Bachofen H, Weibel E: Lung edema in the adult respiratory distress syndrome, in Fishman A, Renkin E (eds): *Pulmonary Edema.* Baltimore, Williams and Wilkins, 1979.

Brown NE, Zamel N, Eberman E: Changes in pulmonary mechanics and gas exchange following thoracentesis. *Chest* 1978;74:540.

Colp CR, Park SS, Williams MH: Pulmonary function studies in pneumonia. *Am Rev Resp Dis* 1962;85:808.

Epstein RL: Constituents of sputum: A simple method. *Ann Intern Med* 1972;77:259.

Herzog H, Staub H, Richterich R: Gas-analytical studies in severe pneumonia. *Lancet* 1959;1:593.

Hurewitz A, Bergofsky EH: Adult respiratory distress syndrome. *Med Clin North Am* 1981;65:33.

Marshal R, Christie RV: The visco-elastic properties of the lung in acute pneumonia. *Clin Sci* 1954;13:403–408.

Remolina C, Khan AV, Santiago TV, et al: Positional hypoxemia in unilateral lung disease. *NEJF* 1981;304:523.

Sibbald WJ, et al: Clinical correlates of the spectrum of lung microvascular injury in human noncardiac edema. *Crit Care Med* 1983;11(2):70.

8 *Respiratory Care in Pneumonia*

Paul E. Epstein

This chapter deals with various aspects of the respiratory care of patients with pneumonia, exclusive of antimicrobial therapy. It should be emphasized at the outset that the proper selection and administration of antimicrobial therapy is the single most important aspect of care in patients with pneumonia. The necessity for specialized respiratory care requiring hospitalization in any given individual depends on the severity of hypoxemia. Most young, previously healthy individuals with radiographic infiltrates involving one lobe of the lung do not require hospitalization for treatment. Factors favoring hospitalization include advanced age, coexistent pulmonary or cardiac disease, severe dyspnea, dehydration, cyanosis, delirium and multilobar infection.

NONINVASIVE METHODS OF OXYGENATION

Adequate oxygenation frequently is a problem in patients with pneumonia, since hypoxemia (or at least a widened alveolar-arterial oxygen gradient) is a constant companion of pulmonary infection. Arterial blood gas analysis should be performed whenever the patient is dyspneic or cyanotic in order to plan for appropriate therapeutic intervention. Supplemental oxygen should be administered when the arterial oxyhemoglobin saturation falls below 90%. Arterial blood gas analysis should be repeated 20 to 30 minutes after initiation of oxygen administration to assure an adequate improvement in blood gases. At a normal arterial pH, 90% saturation is reached at approximately a PO_2 of 60 mmHg. Below that level, the saturation falls rapidly with small decrements in PO_2, and minor physiologic deterioration can lead to major decreases in oxygen content of the blood. Two noninvasive methods of oxygen administration have gained wide acceptance; oxygen masks and nasal prongs.

Oxygen masks can maintain inspired oxygen concentration between 21% and 90% without resorting to endotracheal intubation. The actual inspired oxygen level depends not only on the fractional concentration of oxygen reaching the mask, but also on the rate of gas flow to the mask and the patient's peak inspiratory flow rate. For example, peak inspiratory flow in a person breathing at a normal rate may reach 15 L/min at some point during the respiratory cycle. If the oxygen mask being used delivers 100% oxygen at 5 L/min, at the instant of peak inspiratory flow the patient entrains twice as much room air as oxygen. As a result, even on a constant flow of oxygen, the actual inspired oxygen concentration may vary widely, depending upon the patient's respiratory pattern. These variations can be eliminated by providing very high gas flow through a loose fitting mask. Venturi masks provide such high flows, with deliberate entrainment of a fixed percentage of room air to achieve a predetermined inspired oxygen concentration. Very high and stable inspired oxygen levels can be obtained by combining high flow masks with a reservoir bag that collects oxygen flow during expiration and supplements oxygen volume during peak inspiratory flow.

The major problems with oxygen masks are that they are uncomfortable to wear and must be removed during meals. Nasal prongs generally are more comfortable and can be worn throughout the day. However, they cannot be used to achieve as high an inspired oxygen level as is possible with a mask. Studies have been performed that demonstrate effective oxygenation by nasal prongs even in mouth breathers.

Oxygen Dosage

Oxygen, like other drugs, should be administered in the proper dosage. Overvigorous administration of oxygen can be harmful to the patient with previously normal lungs as well as to the patients with obstructive lung disease. For reasons that are still unclear, some patients with chronic obstructive pulmonary disease (COPD) become insensitive to carbon dioxide as a respiratory stimulant. These patients maintain ventilation as a result of the hypoxic drive to breathe. When supplemental oxygen is administered in a dose that elevates the arterial PO_2 above the stimulatory level, minute ventilation falls until a hypoxic level is reestablished. In the patient with COPD who develops pneumonia, arterial PO_2 falls. An important question for the physician to answer is how much should the arterial PO_2 be raised in a patient with severe COPD who, under the best of circumstances, maintains hypoxic arterial blood gases. If previous determinations of arterial blood gases have been made when the patient was not affected by pneumonia, the premorbid level of PO_2 should be reestablished by supplemental oxygen therapy. If no previous arterial blood gases are available, controlled, low-flow oxygen should be given to raise the arterial PO_2 to 60 mmHg.

In no case is it acceptable to permit hypoxia to reach dangerously low levels out of fear that respiration will be suppressed by supplemental oxygen therapy. If respiratory drive is suppressed, it will occur in relation to the concentration of oxygen administered. For example, if the inspired oxygen concentration is raised from 21% to 24% using a Venturi mask, the initial rise in alveolar PO_2 will be 22 mmHg. If the initial arterial blood gases were PO_2 35 mmHg, PCO_2 60 mmHg, pH 7.32, the result would be to raise the PO_2 to 57 mmHg. Assuming the worst possible situation, the respiration might be suppressed back to (but no lower than) a PO_2 of 35 mmHg. If the respiratory quotient is 0.8, the greatest possible rise in PCO_2 would be 22 × 0.8, or 17.6 mmHg. This would elevate the arterial PCO_2 to 77.6 mmHg. While this rise in PCO_2 would not be helpful, neither would it cause dangerous acidosis or CO_2 narcosis. In fact, the worst case as outlined above rarely occurs. More commonly, the rise in arterial PO_2 will be more modest and the suppression of ventilation will be small, if it occurs at all. Nonetheless, the potential benefits far outweigh the potential risks in such a stiuation. Relatively stable equilibrium points will be achieved within 20 to 30 minutes after changing the inspired oxygen concentration, and arterial blood gas analysis should be performed at that interval after each change in oxygen therapy.

Oxygen Toxicity

The concept of controlled oxygen therapy is also important when patients with pneumonia require high levels of oxygen supplementation in order to achieve an acceptable arterial PO_2. Oxygen toxicity has been recognized as a clinical entity since 1897. It first became a common clinical problem when premature infants developed retrolental fibroplasia after being treated with oxygen in the neonatal period. Over the past 15 years, the focus of clinical oxygen toxicity has shifted to the adult lung, as more efficient methods of oxygen delivery have been devised for treatment of patients with acute pulmonary disease. The biochemistry of oxygen toxicity has been described in several publications and is beyond the scope of this chapter. Suffice it to say here that various enzyme activities are disrupted by high levels of oxygen. Many careful studies have shown that the alveolar PO_2, rather than the arterial PO_2, is the major determinant of pulmonary oxygen toxicity. As a result, the physician must be mindful of the inspired PO_2 as well as the results achieved in maintaining acceptable arterial blood gases.

Although there is no universal agreement on the exact level at which oxygen supplementation leads to histological change in the pulmonary parenchyma, most investigators agree that clinically important effects do not occur below an inspired oxygen level of 50% to 60%. Above those levels, the patient is likely to experience some deleterious effects of prolonged oxygen administration. The higher the inspired oxygen level, the more rapid is the onset of oxygen toxicity. Although there is variable susceptibility among individuals to the effects of oxygen, most patients exposed to an inspired oxygen level of 100% (at 1 atmosphere pressure) begin to have histologic changes in the pulmonary parenchyma within 12 to 24 hours after initiation of therapy. Within 24 to 48 hours, clinical problems assert themselves and often consist of retrosternal burning discomfort and increasing cough. Shortly thereafter, absorption atelectasis occurs and the arterial PO_2 begins to fall due to shunting of blood through unventilated areas of lung. Hypoxia that is refractory to therapy occurs within several days and, unless the inspired oxygen level can be reduced, the patient will die of respiratory failure.

Histologically, the toxic effects of oxygen are expressed in two phases. The first phase is an exudative process that results from destruction of Type 1 alveolar epithelial pneumocytes and damage to capillary endothelial cells. Marked interstitial edema occurs as proteinaceous fluid and cellular elements escape from the damaged capillaries. Hyaline membranes line the alveolar surfaces. If the oxygen administration is continued at high concentration, a proliferative phase, characterized by interstitial fibrosis, will supervene. The histologic changes are virtually identical to those seen in adult respiratory distress syndrome.

It should be remembered that patients with pneumonia are commonly hypoxic because of intrapulmonary shunting and that major escalation of inspired oxygen levels may produce only minor changes in arterial oxygen content. In view of the danger of oxygen toxicity, care should be taken to balance the potential benefits of a specific rise in arterial PO_2 against the danger of pulmonary damage.

The only clinically useful means of treating pulmonary oxygen toxicity is by reducing the inspired oxygen level. Even a relatively brief diminution of inspired oxygen levels is thought to be helpful in that tolerance to the toxic effects of oxygen is occasionally induced by transient lowering of inspired oxygen levels. The goal of inducing tolerance to oxygen is of real and practical importance even though it is frequently impossible to take steps necessary to achieve it without producing dangerous hypoxemia.

Despite the recognized danger of oxygen toxicity, short-term (less than 12 hours) exposure to 100% oxygen (at 1 atm) is not hazardous to the patient without carbon dioxide retention. Therefore, there should be no hesitation to administer high levels of oxygen for brief periods when a patient with pneumonia is in an unstable condition or is being transported between medical facilities.

TECHNIQUES TO IMPROVE CLEARANCE OF SECRETIONS

There is no universal agreement on the usefulness of other respiratory therapy maneuvers in the treatment of patients with pneumonia. However, various techniques are widely used to improve the clearance of secretions from the tracheobronchial tree. They generally fall into the categories of humidification, aerosol therapy and chest physiotherapy.

Humidification

Mucociliary clearance in the tracheobronchial tree is most efficient in a humid atmosphere. Many studies have shown that drying of the tracheal mucus surface retards the flow of pulmonary secretions toward the glottis. Humidification of inspired gas ordinarily occurs in the upper airways, particularly during nasal breathing. This process consists of adding molecular (as opposed to particulate) water to the inspired gas by means of evaporation from the nasal mucosal surface until 100% saturation is achieved. Efficiency of the system is taxed during pneumonia by the devlopment of fever and by the tendency toward mouth breathing as a response to dyspnea. Since saturation of the inspired air is a function of temperature, elevation of body temperature leads to increased evaporation from the mucosal surface. If the efficient nasal baffling produced by the turbinates is bypassed by mouth breathing, humidification must take place in the trachea. This increase in evaporation from the trachea causes excessive drying and produces a deterioration in mucociliary clearance. For these reasons, it is appropriate to treat patients suffering from pneumonia with heated gas humidifiers, usually delivered by face mask.

Aerosol Therapy

An aerosol is defined as a suspension of particulate matter in gas. Strictly speaking, the particles may be either solid or liquid, but for purposes of respiratory therapy the particles are nearly always liquid. Aerosol treatments are classified as either bland or medicated depending upon the nature of the particles suspended in the inhaled gas. If the particles are made of water or saline, the aerosol is considered bland. Medicated aerosols contain bronchodilators, mucolytic agents or steroids. Aerosolized particle deposition within the tracheobronchial tree depends on both the particle size and the velocity of airflow during inspiration. Particles larger than 5μm in diameter are likely to be deposited in the upper airways. Similarly, rapid shallow respiration, as might occur in patients with acute pneumonia, increases turbulence and promotes upper airway deposition of particles. The particles deposited in the upper airways woud not be expected to have any significant effect on the clearance of pneumonia, since the infection occurs in the peripheral areas of the lung. Even when bland aerosols contain particles smaller than 5 μm in diameter that are deposited in the peripheral airways, there has been no convincing evidence that there is effective augmentation of mucus transport.

Medicated aerosols are useful under specific circumstances. Few physicians would dispute the effectiveness of aerosolized bronchodilators in the treatment of bronchospasm that interferes with mucus clearance. There is considerably more doubt about the routine use of bronchodilators when no wheezing is detected. Aerosolized mucolytic agents, such as acetyl cysteine, are irritating to the bronchi and frequently cause diffuse bronchospasm. Consequently, their use is probably not warranted in the treatment of pneumonia, except when mucus plugging of bronchi with resultant atelectasis can be demonstrated roentgenographically.

Chest Physiotherapy

Postural drainage and chest physiotherapy, consisting of chest clapping and vibration, has been shown to be effective in removing secretions from the bronchi in patients with chronic obstructive pulmonary disease. Even though there is significantly more sputum removed from those receiving postural drainage and chest physiotherapy than from untreated controls, no measurable improvement in pulmonary function or arterial blood gases can be detected.

When these techniques are applied to patients with uncomplicated pneumonia, the results have been impressive only for their ineffectiveness. In one randomized prospective study of 54 patients with pneumonia (Graham and Bradley, 1978) the administration of racemic epinephrine aerosol, postural drainage and chest physiotherapy every four hours along with antibiotics was compared to antibiotic administration alone. There was no detectable difference between the test group and the control group with respect to resolution of fever, length of hospital stay, rate of clearing of x-ray film or mortality. The implication of the study is that the respiratory therapy maneuvers that are commonly applied in the treatment of patients with pneumonia are ineffective, expensive and potentially harmful. It should be remembered, however, that this series dealt with patients who had uncomplicated pneumonias. As such, there is no reason to suspect that these particular patients had defective bronchial clearance mechanisms. It is conceivable that the same therapeutic measures, when applied to patients with pneumonia complicated by chronic bronchitis, would be helpful in resolving the alveolar process. Active debate on this subject is likely to continue for many years, since well-controlled studies with chronic obstructive pulmonary disease are difficult to design and conduct.

INVASIVE METHODS OF OXYGENATION

Endotracheal Intubation

Endotracheal intubation in patients with pneumonia usually is performed for purposes of mechanical ventilation or occasionally for management of secretions in the patients with altered ability to cough. Other reasons for intubation, particularly in the obtunded patient, include the assurance of a patent airway and the prevention of aspiration of foreign material into the lungs. Although each patient must be evaluated individually for the necessity for intubation and mechanical ventilation, certain guidelines may be used in the decision-making process. Deterioration of arterial blood gas status is probably the most compelling reason to initiate invasive respiratory procedures. If the arterial PO_2 cannot be maintained at a level of 60 mmHg or greater on an inspired oxygen level of less than 60%, intubation and mechanical ventilation should be considered in order to decrease the oxygen cost of breathing. Similarly, a rising arterial PCO_2 should alert the physician to the onset of respiratory fatigue and impending exhaustion. Measurement of the alveolar/arterial oxygen difference is of limited usefulness in patients with pneumonia since a right to left shunt is to be expected in this setting. Vital capacity measurements are easily performed at the bedside and can help predict the need for intubation and mechanical ventilation. An inability to achieve a vital capacity of at least 12 to 15 mL/kg of body weight suggests that coughing will be ineffective and secretions will collect in the lower respiratory tract. Measurements of maximum inspiratory and maximum expiratory pressures help evaluate the patient's ability to perform respiratory work, but should not be used as a primary decision-making tool. It is difficult to perform more sophisticated tests of pulmonary function in very ill patients and, from a practical standpoint, it is unlikely that they will help in decision making.

Most of the modern endotracheal tubes are made of pliable plastic materials that assume the shape of the trachea when exposed to body temperature. Soft, high volume, low pressure cuffs allow relatively long-term retention of the tube before the threat of tracheal damage requires tracheostomy. It is generally accepted that these tubes may be left in place for about two weeks before tracheostomy is performed. Nasotracheal tubes are more easily tolerated by the patient than are orotracheal tubes. In addition, use of a nasotracheal tube allows for firmer fixation of the device into correct position and affords better protection against kinking or closure by compression. The larger diameter of the orotracheal tube, on the other hand, permits easier access for suctioning or bronchoscopy, should that procedure become necessary. While the tube is in place, erosion of the mucosa may occur over several days and hemoptysis is commonly observed. If this sign is ignored, the tube may perforate the trachea and erode into the innominate artery, causing death by exsanguination. Clearly, the onset of hemoptysis should be carefully evaluated by bronchoscopy and either the tip of the tube should be moved or a tracheostomy should be performed.

If a nasotracheal tube has been inserted, the resultant mucosal inflammation may interfere with normal paranasal sinus drainage and produce severe sinusitis. After an endotracheal tube has been removed, formation of scar tissue occasionally produces tracheal stenosis. This complication usually is seen in prolonged intubations, but may rarely occur following very short periods of assisted ventilation. The problem ordinarily declares itself as intractable, progressive dyspnea several months to two years following extubation.

Subglottic stenosis by scar tissue formation is seen at operation or autopsy. The diagnosis of this complication can be made by pulmonary function testing. A flow volume loop demonstrating truncation of the expiratory phase of maximum effort is highly suggestive of upper airway obstruction; peak expiratory flow is diminished and the flow rate remains stable throughout a large portion of the vital capacity maneuver. The inspiratory curve as seen on the flow volume loop is the mirror image of the expiratory phase in patients with fixed upper airway obstruction.

Mechanical Ventilation

Mechanical ventilation performed on patients with pneumonia follows the same general principles observed in respiratory failure of other etiologies. The primary goals of therapy are to maintain adequate oxygenation and to provide sufficient alveolar ventilation to stabilize the arterial PCO_2. Ordinarily, oxygenation is more problematical than is ventilation. If arterial PO_2 cannot be raised to at least 60 mmHg while breathing at an oxygen level of 60% or less, the physician should be prepared to institute positive end expiratory pressure breathing (PEEP). The purpose of this maneuver is to enlarge the functional residual capacity as a means of reopening alveoli that have become atelectatic as a result of the disease process. PEEP therapy improves oxygenation by reestablishing ventilation to perfused alveoli and by decreasing the right-to-left shunt fraction of cardiac output. In the setting of pneumonia, PEEP works best in diffuse lung disease as might be encountered in viral or *Pneumocystis carinii* infections. Use of PEEP in localized infections, such as lobar pneumonia, frequently causes deterioration of arterial blood gases. This evidently occurs because alveoli in the unaffected areas of lung are more susceptible to stretching by the application of positive pressure than are those filled with fiuid and cellular debris. The more normal alveoli are thus able to transmit pressure more effectively to the pulmonary capillary walls, causing decreased blood flow through the normal areas of the lung. Pulmonary blood flow is then diverted to the abnormal alveoli that are not being ventilated. This causes an increase in shunt fraction and a decrease in arterial oxygen level.

Other complications of PEEP include the depression of cardiac output by decreasing venous return to the heart and the production of pressure-related damage to the lungs. This latter complication is known as pulmonary barotrauma. The injuries caused by barotrauma are pneumothorax and pneumomediastinum, both of which are more common at high PEEP pressures than at low pressures.

Keeping these complications in mind, it is wise to use PEEP only up to the level necessary to maintain adequate oxygenation. Ordinarily this goal can be reached by applying end expiratory pressure between 5 and 15 cm H_2O. On rare occasions, higher levels of PEEP have been used successfully.

Therapy of ARDS

Some patients with pneumonia develop the adult respiratory distress syndrome (ARDS) as a result of their infection. The onset of this syndrome can be recognized by the development of refractory hypoxemia accompanied by diffuse, bilateral pulmonary edema in the face of normal pulmonary capillary wedge pressure measurements. Therapy of ARDS is, in large part, an extension of the principles already discussed. PEEP has been particularly useful in the management of the hypoxemia of ARDS. Great care must be taken not to allow PEEP pressures to decrease oxygen delivery to the tissues by depressing cardiac output. Even if arterial PO_2 levels rise as a result of better ventilation/perfusion ratios, a decrease in cardiac output caused by diminishing venous return may lead to worsening tissue hypoxia. Measurements of mixed venous PO_2 have been used effectively in the evaluation of oxygen delivery and are helpful in following the results of therapeutic intervention. This requires insertion of a balloon-tipped, flow-directed catheter (eg, Swan-Ganz catheter) into the pulmonary artery, a procedure that has become routine in the management of critically ill patients.

Another advantage of having a pulmonary artery catheter in place is that fluid balance can be closely monitored by following pumonary capillary wedge pressure. This is particularly important in patients with ARDS because pulmonary capillary permeability is much greater than normal. The major determinants of fluid movement, according to Starling's law, are capillary permeability, colloid osmotic pressure and hydrostatic pressure. Since plasma colloid osmotic pressure is relatively stable (despite the fact that it might be low in patients with ARDS), small changes in hydrostatic pressure across the pulmonary capillary bed can produce major fluid shifts from the intravascular space into the alveoli. These shifts can be minimized by keeping the pulmonary capillary wedge pressure low as long as left ventricular filling pressure is not compromised. While the patient with a normal myocardium will do best at a wedge pressure of 16 mmHg, sepsis itself may compromise myocardial contractility. Therefore, in these very ill patients cardiac output should be monitored using a thermodilution catheter. Diuretics are commonly used to effect this volume control and help manage the ARDS.

Intravenous infusion of albumin has not been helpful in raising the plasma colloid osmotic pressure, since leakage of plasma proteins into the alveoli may actually compound the fluid clearance problems. Steroid therapy in ARDS, while widely used, is of unproven benefit. The data thus far presented is not strong enough either to support or to condemn the use of steroids in this situation.

Membrane Oxygenation

At one time, it was thought that the respiratory failure of overwhelming pneumonia might be managed effectively by providing long-term gas exchange by means of a membrane oxygenator. This heart-lung machine has the advantage over bubble oxygenators of allowing no direct contact between the gas phase and the liquid phase (blood). As a result, there is very little erythrocyte damage caused by the machine, and patients can be oxygenated for periods measured in weeks while the lungs are nonfunctional. Unfortunately, such severely damaged lungs are unable to recover sufficiently to allow long-term survival. A large multicenter trial by Zapol et al (1979) failed to show that the membrane oxygenation was more effective than conventional therapy in improving mortality from acute respiratory failure.

SELECTED READINGS

Campbell EJM: The Burns Amberson Lecture, The management of acute respiratory failure in chronic bronchitis and emphysema. *Am Rev Respir Dis* 1967; 96:626.

Clark JM: The toxicity of oxygen. *Am Rev Respir Dis* 1974;110:40.

Deneke SM, Fanburg BL: Normobaric oxygen toxicity of the lung. *N Engl J Med* 1980;303:78.

Goldstein RS, Young J, Rebuck AS: Effect of breathing pattern on oxygen concentration received from standard face masks. *Lancet* 1982;8309(2):1188.

Graham, WG, Bradley DA: Efficacy of chest physiotherapy and intermittent positive-pressure breathing in the resolution of pneumonia. *N Engl J Med* 1978;299:624.

Haugaard N: Cellular mechanisms of oxygen toxicity. *Physiol Rev* 1968;48:311.

Henley DC, Hutchinson DCS, Donald KW: Behavior of apparatus for oxygen administration. *Br Med J* 1963;2:1081.

Hurewitz A, Bergofsky EH: Adult respiratory distress syndrome: Physiologic basis of treatment. *Med Clin North Am* 1981;65:33.

Mulfoefer JC, Holford FD, Kerghley JFH: The effect of oxygen administration on mixed venous oxygenation in chronic obstructive lung disease. *Chest* 1974;66:122.

Proceedings of the Conference on the Scientific Basis of Respiratory Therapy. *Am Rev Respir Dis* 1974;110(Part 2):1–204.

Weisman IM, Rinaldo, JE, Rogers RM: Positive end-expiratory pressure in adult respiratory failure. *N Engl J Med* 1982;307:1381.

Zapol W, Snider M, et al: Extracorporeal membrane oxygenation in severe acute respiratory failure. *JAMA* 1979;242:193.

9 *Strategies in the Approach to Treatment of Pneumonia*

Elias Abrutyn

For clinicians, detection of pneumonia likely to be infectious in origin is not difficult, but determination of the causative agent is often difficult indeed. This difficulty arises in part because the number of causative agents is large. The difficulty also arises because the clinical findings associated with many of these agents are similar. Moreover, the procedures that can be applied to make a definitive diagnosis (transtracheal aspiration, lung biopsy, etc) are used only infrequently, because they are invasive. Blood cultures, a less invasive test used frequently, may permit a definitive diagnosis, but they are often negative. Pleural and pericardial fluid cultures, if positive, may also permit definitive diagnosis, but involvement of these serosal membranes sufficient to permit definitive diagnosis is infrequent.

As a consequence, the practitioner usually is forced to rely on a combination of clinical-epidemiologic data, supported by the demonstration and/or isolation of the putative agent from sputum. However, there are difficulties with these. Clinical-epidemiologic data is often nonspecific since most agents cause similar signs and symptoms and sputum, the source for demonstration or isolation of the putative etiologic agent, is likely to be contaminated with organisms that colonize the upper respiratory tract and are unrelated to the primary pathologic process. The latter observation forces clinicians to consider whether a given organism, either seen on sputum gram stain or isolated from sputum, is causative or merely a contaminant.

Despite the absence of specificity in clinical information and the potential for attributing the cause of infection to a contaminant, this combination is the only information available for most patients with pneumonia, since definitive diagnostic procedures are rarely performed. The goal of this chapter, therefore, is to describe an approach for integrating the commonly available clinical, epidemiologic, and laboratory data, permitting a presumptive etiologic diagnosis and initial therapy when the patient is first evaluated and before the results of cultures are known. This process is important, even when definitive tests are to be performed, because it guides choice of initial therapy before the tests are done and the results are known. It is also important because it helps determine which studies should be performed on specimens from those procedures.

The approach to be outlined requires the information obtained from a *complete* history and *thorough* physical examination as well as the results of chest x-rays and gram stain of sputum (if obtainable). This information represents the minimum data that must be available when the clinician first approaches the question of appropriate therapy. In collecting these data, particular emphasis should be placed on an accurate history regarding pets, occupation, hobbies, travel, and recent contact with others having an infectious disease, as this information may suggest specific etiologies that need to be considered.

INITIAL EXAMINATION: DOES THE PATIENT HAVE PNEUMONIA?

One should first be certain that a patient with symptoms suggestive of a lower respiratory tract infection indeed has pneumonia and not some other respiratory tract problem. To that end, evidence is sought demonstrating involvement of the lung parenchyma. The evidence supporting parenchymal involvement includes physical findings (rales, dullness, or other signs) or the appearance of an infiltrate on chest x-ray in an area of lung not known to be similarly involved before and not explicable by any other disease process. Occasionally, patients with pneumonia have normal chest x-rays at the first evaluation, developing an infiltrate during the first 24 hours or so of observation. In such cases, some physical findings suggestive of pneumonia are frequently present, even if the x-ray appears normal. Examples include early pneumococcal pneumonia, metastatic pneumonia in bacteremic patients, and pneumonia in neutropenic patients not able to mount an inflammatory response. A clue to such a process may be tachypnea and an otherwise unexplained depression in blood oxygen tension. The absence of physical or chest x-ray findings in a patient with symptoms consistent with pneumonia should suggest a process that may mimic pneumonia such as tracheobronchitis. Certain noninfectious diseases involving the lung (immunologic, neoplastic, pulmonary embolus, etc) may also mimic pneumonia and require differentiation.

After determining that pneumonia is present, it is useful to define whether it is acute or chronic and, in each instance, whether the host is normal or immunosuppressed. The latter term describes patients with a malignancy who may have depressed host defenses and those receiving cytotoxic, radiation, or steroid therapy. What follows is an approach to the usual case, the normal host with an acute pneumonia. Details regarding other subsets may be found elsewhere in this volume.

THE ACUTE PNEUMONIAS: SIGNIFICANCE OF SPUTUM PRODUCTION

The patient with an acute pneumonia, that is pneumonia of recent onset, may present with fever, chills, malaise, weakness, dyspnea, chest pain, or other symptoms in any combination. These symptoms are common to most cases of pneumonia and are nonspecific. Although they serve to lead the clinician to suspect the presence of pneumonia, they are of relatively little value in defining the cause.

In addition to these symptoms, the patient with pneumonia usually has a cough. Cough may be accompanied by sputum production ("productive cough"), or it may be associated with little or no sputum production ("dry" or "flu-like" cough). Pneumonias associated with a productive cough are likely to be of bacterial origin, whereas those with a dry or flu-like cough are likely to be produced by a different set of agents. The latter group of agents has been referred to in clinical terminology as the group producing the atypical pneumonia syndrome or as "nonbacterial" pneumonias, the term being placed in quotes because some causes of atypical pneumonia are indeed bacteria. The terms "bacterial" and "nonbacterial" pneumonia may thus be used to refer to a specific type of organism in a microbiologic sense. But, as sometimes used by clinicians, they may be used to denote pneumonias with or without sputum production, respectively, each with a different set of etiologies. The terms "typical" and "atypical" pneumonia are used similarly. The distinction between sputum- and nonsputum-producing pneumonias is of value in denoting etiology and represents a useful point of departure for differentiating the cause of pneumonia in a given case (see Chapter 10 and 11).

THE ACUTE PNEUMONIAS: EVALUATION OF THE SPUTUM BY GRAM STAIN

Having assessed the magnitude of sputum production, the next step in every patient is examination of the sputum gram stain, if sputum can be obtained. Conceptually, this involves three steps: 1) evaluation of the adequacy of the specimen, followed by 2) evaluation of the quantity of polymorphonuclear leukocytes (PMNs) and organisms, and 3) evaluation of the kind and number of the organisms present, particularly the predominant type. The results permit one to determine whether the process is inflammatory in nature and hence consistent with infection, and often provides an indication of etiology in cases likely to be bacterial in origin.

Assuming proper staining technique, the adequacy of the specimen is judged on the basis of whether squamous epithelial cells and alveolar macrophages are present or absent. Specimens containing large quantities of squamous epithelial cells (the cells lining the mucosa of the upper respiratory tract) are considered inadequate, because these cells indicate sampling of the upper respiratory tract rather than lower tract where the pneumonia is occurring. On the other hand, the absence of significant quantities of epithelial cells and/or the presence of alveolar macrophages is considered to mean that the specimen is representative of lower respiratory tract secretions and hence is suitable for examination. Inadequate specimens should be discarded and another sample must be examined.

Next, the number of PMNs and bacteria are assessed. In simplistic fashion and for purposes of developing a useful construct, one may consider that there may be few or many PMNs and few or many bacteria, leaving aside for a moment the morphologic appearance of the organism(s) present. As shown in Figure 9-1, stratification of each variable (PMNs and bacteria) into two categories (few or many) leads overall to a total of four combinations that possibly may be found. However, it should be appreciated that this scheme applies not only to sputum, but to any specimen evaluated with the gram stain. As shown, a given specimen must show one of the following patterns: 1) few PMNs and few bacteria; 2) few PMNs and many bacteria; 3) many PMNs and few bacteria; and 4) many PMNs and many bacteria.

The significance of each of these patterns can be approached by understanding the meaning of each variable (PMNs and bacteria). The presence of PMNs in sputum, or any other specimen for that matter, indicates that an inflammatory process is present. Accordingly, infection as one cause of inflammation would be expected to evoke an inflammatory response in the lung, which is then reflected in the sputum by the presence of PMNs, a major host defense against infection. PMNs should be present with infection, but they may be also present in the absence of infection, if an inflammatory process other than infection is occurring in the lungs or airways. Conversely, the absence of PMNs indicates the absence of inflammation and, by inference, the absence of infection. In such cases, a noninflammatory cause for a pulmonary infiltrate should be sought such as congestive heart failure. In brief, the presence of PMNs

		Bacteria: Few	Bacteria: Many
PMNs	Few		
	Many		

Figure 9-1 Scheme for classifying the sputum gram stain.

denotes the presence of inflammation, one cause of which is infection. PMNs should be found when infection is present and their absence should initiate a search for a noninfectious, noninflammatory cause of disease.

Of those specimens containing many PMNs, some have few bacteria and others many bacteria. PMNs, as stated, indicate inflammation; this, coupled with the simultaneous presence of many bacteria, permits the inference that a bacterial infection is the stimulus evoking the inflammatory response. The gram stain then that is consistent with bacterial infection is the one showing many PMNs and bacteria, especially if alveolar macrophages are also present. The second possibility, many PMNs and few bacteria, is consistent with either an inflammatory process of a noninfectious nature, or more pertinent to the topic under discussion, an infectious process caused by agents either poorly or not at all visible on gram stain. This pattern may be seen in those infections classified as associated with a dry or flu-like cough, the atypical or nonbacterial pneumonias.

Both of the remaining patterns, few PMNs–few bacteria and few PMNs–many bacteria, indicate the absence of inflammation and hence, the absence of infection. The former pattern may be seen, for example, in patients with pulmonary edema. The latter pattern might be found in patients who are colonized, but not infected, such as post-tracheostomy patients whose tracheobronchial tree is colonized with *Pseudomonas aeruginosa*.

The final step in examination of sputum gram stains is evaluation of the morphologic appearance of the organism(s) in the sputum and determination of the predominant type. In smears showing many PMNs and many bacteria, the predominant organism is considered the likely cause of the pneumonia.

In brief, a construct to aid in interpretation of gram stains and in diagnosis of the cause of an infection has been presented. Patients with acute pneumonia and sputum production are likely to have gram smears showing many PMNs and many bacteria; those with a dry cough should have smears showing many PMNs and few bacteria, if sputum is obtainable. It is important to appreciate the situations when application of this scheme may not be helpful: 1) diagnosis of pneumonia behind an obstruction; 2) diagnosis in neutropenic patients not able to mount an inflammatory response; 3) diagnosis in patients with chronic bronchitis whose sputum often shows PMNs and organisms related to persistent inflammation of broncheal mucosa; and 4) in patients who have received antibiotic therapy likely to alter the kind and number of organisms in the sputum. It should also be appreciated that the utility of the gram stain in diagnosis of pneumonia has been questioned, but despite less than optimal sensitivity and specificity, its use continues to be recommended by many. With that caveat in mind, the decision to treat or not to treat a particular patient should not rest on the results of the gram stain alone, but rather on the likely diagnosis given all the clinical as well as laboratory findings. Thus, therapy for a particular infection should always be begun if the weight of evidence suggests that a treatable cause of pneumonia is present, even if this conclusion is not supported by the gram stain.

To summarize the approach thus far, we 1) determine whether or not the patient has pneumonia and 2) stratify those with pneumonia into those with and without sputum production, indicating in clinical parlance a typical bacterial pneumonia or an atypical pneumonia syndrome, respectively. Then, the sputum is examined: many PMNs and many bacteria are the likely findings in those with sputum production and many PMNs and few bacteria are likely in those with a dry cough, if sputum is at all obtainable. Finally, in patients with apparent bacterial pneumonia, the morphologic appearance of the organism(s) present is evaluated, and the predominant type, indicating the likely etiology is determined.

BACTERIAL PNEUMONIAS

One of the following is likely to be seen in sputum smears of patients with bacterial pneumonia: gram-positive cocci, gram-negative rods, gram-negative diplococci, or mixed gram-positive and gram-negative organisms.

Gram-Positive Cocci

The gram-positive cocci causing bacterial pneumonia include *Streptococcus pneumoniae* (lancet-shaped diplococci), *Staphylococcus aureus* (cocci in clusters or tetrads), and *S. pyogenes* (cocci in chains). Whereas these organisms are easily recognized when grown in laboratory media, they are sometimes difficult to distinguish in direct smears of material from patients such as sputum. Often, however, clinical information may be helpful in diagnosis. (The clinical and epidemiologic findings that should be sought in supporting these diagnoses may be found in Chapter 10.)

Therapeutically, penicillin is the drug of choice for pneumococcal and streptococcal pneumonia. A penicillinase-resistant penicillin is preferred, but a first generation cephalosporin (cefazolin, cephalothin, or other) may be used as initial therapy for possible staphylococcal pneumonia pending culture and sensitivity tests. Doses and alternatives for the penicillin allergic patient or for the patient with a methicillin-resistant *Staphylococcus* may be found in the chapters about these organisms. When the likely etiologic diagnosis for a pneumonia caused by a gram-positive coccus is unclear, the group may be adequately covered with a penicillinase-resistant penicillin or a cephalosporin as detailed for the *Staphylococcus*, while awaiting results of laboratory tests. However, vancomycin should be given if methicillin-resistant *S. aureus* is suspected.

Gram-Negative Rods

Pneumonia caused by one of the Enterobacteriacae (*Escherichia coli*, *Klebsiella pneumoniae*, *Proteus* sp, etc) or *P. aeruginosa* is uncommon, but in certain situations the risk is increased. Gram-negative rod pneumonia is often hospital-associated (nosocomial) and must always be considered in hospitalized patients developing pneumonia. Chronic and severe illness, pulmonary disease, prior antibiotic therapy, and endotracheal intubation are examples of factors that promote colonization of the nasopharynx, with gram-negative rods increasing the risk of pneumonia with these agents after aspiration. Pneumonia after use of contaminated respirator equipment occurs, and it is a rare complication of bacteremia (*P. aeruginosa* pneumonia in a burn patient). Alcoholism is prominent in those with community-acquired gram-negative pneumonia. Again, the features characterizing pneumonias caused by these agents should be sought elsewhere in this volume.

Given the diversity of organisms causing gram-negative pneumonia, the inability to reliably identify specific organisms on gram smear, and the high associated mortality, broad and antimicrobial coverage is recommended. Among the regimens that can be employed pending culture and sensitivity reports, we prefer: 1) a third generation cephalosporin (cefotaxime, moxalactam, cefoperazone, etc) plus an aminoglycoside, although some specialists might not include the latter drug, or 2) an antipseudomonal penicillin, such as piperacillin, plus an aminoglycoside. The former regimen is preferred when *Klebsiella* infection seems likely, the latter when *P. aeruginosa* is likely. In selecting specific antimicrobics, the susceptibilities of organisms in each institution must be considered. After the infecting organism is identified and susceptibilities determined, consideration should be given to stopping the aminoglycoside and to employing other less expensive β-lactam antibiotics, if cure can be achieved with a less toxic, less expensive regimen. *P. aeruginosa* infection, however, always requires combined therapy.

Gram-Negative Diplococci and Hemophilus influenzae

The causes of pneumonia showing gram-negative diplococci in sputum include *Neisseria meningitidis*, *Acinetobacter calcoaceticus*, and *Branhamella catarrhalis*. For the purposes of discussion, *H. influenzae* has been included in this group, recognizing that it is described as a tiny gram-negative rod; however, inclusion in this group seems justified as it may appear in sputum as a diplococcus.

A regimen that may be used as initial therapy pending culture results is ampicillin plus gentamicin. Ampicillin has activity against *H. influenzae* and *N. meningitidis*, and gentamicin has activity against *Acinetobacter*. If disease caused by penicillinase producing *H. influenzae* is prevalent, then another regimen should be employed. The third generation cephalosporins have in vitro activity against penicillinase-producing and nonpenicillinase-producing *H. influenzae*, *N. meningitidis*, some *Acinetobacter* isolates, and possibly *B. catarrhalis*. One of these cephalosporins, combined with gentamicin, should provide excellent coverage.

Mixed Gram-Positive and Gram-Negative Organisms

In the absence of chronic bronchitis, the occurrence of mixed gram-positive and gram-negative organisms on gram stain in relatively equal proportions is highly suggestive of infection after aspiration of oropharyngeal secretions. This type of smear is found in patients with lung abscess or necrotizing anaerobic pneumonitis. The pleomorphic appearance of organisms on gram smear is an excellent clue to these diseases. The presence of foul-smelling sputum reflecting involvement of anaerobes, particularly in those with abscess or necrotizing pneumonia, may be helpful. Clinically, the patient may be acutely or chronically ill, and may have an underlying disease that alters central nervous system function such as epilepsy, alcoholism, or drug addiction. Other clues to aspiration include pneumonia in patients with poor gag reflex, or in patients with esophageal diseases such as achalasia or tracheoesophageal fistula.

Therapy for aspiration pneumonia depends in part on the material that has been aspirated. Patients with aspiration of inert nontoxic materials (water, saline, blood, etc) and gastric or other acid at low pH generally are followed carefully without antimicrobial therapy until evidence of infection is found (new or higher fever, new infiltrates appearing 36 to 48 hours after aspiration, purulent sputum, and a consistent gram stain).

Aspiration of oropharyngeal secretions is often followed by a pneumonia with clinical features resembling the other bacterial pneumonias, later complications include necrotizing pneumonitis, lung abscess, or empyema. Therapy for the early pneumonias is indicated when evidence of infection is present and the choice of drug depends in part on the setting in which the aspiration occurred. Community-acquired disease may be treated with penicillin or clindamycin; some data suggests clindamycin may be superior. In hospital-acquired disease, *S. aureus*, the aerobic gram-negative rods, and *P. aeruginosa* are often implicated and therapeutic regimens designed to cover these possibilities may be necessary, if a specific etiologic diagnosis cannot be made.

Other

The previous discussion describes an approach helpful in the vast majority of bacterial pneumonias, yet occasionally other important causes of bacterial pneumonia in the United States require consideration. Fortunately, exposure and/or contact in the history is often helpful in indicating the need to consider these diagnoses. *Pasturella multocida*, a small gram-negative rod, is acquired from infected animals, such as dogs or cats, from bites or scratches, and causes pulmonary abscesses as a result of bacteremic spread. *Yersinia pestis* (the plague bacillus), also a tiny gram-negative rod, is acquired after exposure to infected rodents (rats or prairie dogs in the southeast United States) or their fleas; human-to-human transmission via aersol occurs and is devastating. *Francisella tularensis*, the agent of tularemia is associated with exposure to infected animals (rabbits, muskrats, and others), bites from infected fleas, deerflys, and mosquitoes, or, rarely, ingestion of contaminated meats. Finally, there are descriptions of other etiologies, but these appear uncommon; Fick and Reynolds (1983) have provided a useful tabulation of such agents.

ATYPICAL OR NONBACTERIAL PNEUMONIA

Treatable causes of atypical pneumonia (cough with little or no sputum production) include infection with *Mycoplasma pneumoniae*; *Legionella pneumophila* or related organisms; *Coxiella burnetii*, the agent of Q fever; and *Chlamydia psittaci*, the agent of ornithosis, also called psittacosis. *Mycoplasma* and *Legionella* infection appear common, but the others are rare. In adults, other common causes of atypical pneumonia include influenza A virus, influenza B virus, and adenovirus.

The practical considerations regarding therapy for this group of pneumonias may be summarized as follows. Tetracycline, effective against the agents of Q fever and psittacosis, should be administered if the history is appropriate and the clinical illness is compatible with this diagnosis. Tetracycline is also effective for *Mycoplasma* infections. In the absence of a history suggesting either Q fever or psittacosis, administration of erythromycin should be considered because it is effective against two of the common causes of this syndrome, *Mycoplasma* and *Legionella* infection, neither of which can be diagnosed rapidly with methods available today. If an illness caused by influenza A virus is suspected, amantadine may be given.

CHRONIC PNEUMONIA

The diagnostic considerations in patients with chronic pneumonia (pneumonia with a protracted clinical course) include mycobacterial, fungal, and nocardial infection, as well as actinomycosis. The course associated with anaerobic infection such as lung abscess, also may be protracted, but the diagnosis usually is apparent. Useful clues to the diagnosis of chronic pneumonias may be obtained from the history (eg, exposure to tuberculosis or travel to an area endemic for a particular fungus) and from chest film (eg, apical-posterior infiltrates in tuberculosis). The sputum examination is also of value, but techniques other than the gram stain may be required (acid-fast stain for mycobacteria, modified acid-fast stain for nocardial, etc). The approach to diagnosis and treatment of these illnesses may be found in other chapters of this book.

PNEUMONIA IN THE IMMUNOSUPPRESSED HOST

Pneumonia in the immunosuppressed host is a challenging, perplexing problem. The etiologic considerations in these patients includes not only the organisms already discussed in this chapter, but also several microbes that rarely produce disease in hosts with normal defenses. Examples of these "opportunistic" pathogens include *Pneumocystic carnii*, *Toxoplasma gondii*, cytomegalovirus, several species of fungi (*Aspergillus*, *Candida*, and the *Zygomycetes*) and others. Additional complexity derives from the fact that simultaneous infection with more than one organism occurs.

The initial approach to diagnosis of pneumonia in immunosuppressed host should be the same as that described for normal hosts. However, in the presence of neutropenia the value of the gram stain as a diagnostic aid often is severely reduced. Moreover, many of the agents causing disease in this group cannot be diagnosed with this technique. In light of the range of etiologic agents causing disease and the difficulties in diagnosis, the need for invasive procedures is enhanced. The major initial decisions, therefore, revolve around assessing the need for invasive procedures (fiberoptic bronchoscopy with or without transbronchial biopsy, transthoracic biopsy, or open lung biopsy) and the scope of antimicrobial coverage.

Occasionally, it is apparent that the patient has a viral illness requiring symptomatic therapy only. Antibiotics, with their attendant potential toxicities, should not be administered. The decision should be made whether withdrawal of immunosuppressive therapy is required to boost host defenses or whether continued therapy is important for treatment of the underlying disease. In some cases, it is clear that the patient has a treatable bacterial infection. Under such circumstances, treatment of the likely pathogen without invasive testing is appropriate. Most frequently, the diagnosis after initial evaluation is in doubt and invasive procedures are considered. Some patients in this latter group are given broad antimicrobial coverage, invasive procedures being undertaken only if the patient fails to respond after an appropriate interval and the diagnosis remains in doubt. In others, such procedures are performed immediately with or without antimicrobial coverage. It should be appreciated that the decision for invasive procedures depends not only on the need for an etiologic diagnosis, but also the ability of the patient to tolerate the test.

It should be clear that the management of such patients involves complexities not encountered in normal patients with pneumonia. The decisions regarding an appropriate antimicrobial regimen for a particular patient and the timing and sequencing of invasive procedures tax the skills of the most experienced clinicians. Additional discussion about these points can be found in the other chapters about infection in immunocompromised host, but those without experience in this area are best advised to seek expert help when confronted by such patients.

SELECTED READINGS

Bartlett JG: Aspiration pneumonia. *Clin Notes Resp Dis* 1980; Spring issue:3–8.

Basiliere JL, Bistrong HW, Spence WF: Streptococcal pneumonia: Recent outbreaks in military recruit populations. *Am J Med* 1968;44:580–589.

Bayer AS, Chow AW, Anthony BF, et al: Serious infections in adults due to Group B streptococci: Clinical and serotypic characterization. *Am J Med* 1976;61:498–503.

DiPoala JA: Prognosis of pneumonia: Sputum culture and gram stain. *NY State J Med* 1977;77(8):1259–1262.

Fick RB, Reynolds HY: Changing spectrum of pneumonia—News media creation or clinical reality. *Am J Med* 1983;74:1–8.

Goodhart GL, Abrutyn E, Watson R, et al: Community-acquired Acinetobacter calcoaceticus var anitratus pneumonia. *JAMA* 1977;238:1516–1518.

Irwin RS, Woelk WK, Coudon WL III: Primary meningococcal pneumonia. *Ann Intern Med* 1975;82:493–498.

Johnson JE III: Acute pulmonary infection, in Cluff LR, Johnson JE (eds): *Clinical Concepts of Infectious Diseases*, ed 2. Baltimore, Williams and Wilkins, 1978, pp 236–250.

Kohler RB, Zimmerman SE, Wilson M, et al: Rapid radioimmunoassay diagnosis of Legionnaires' disease: Detection and partial characterization of urinary antigen. *Ann Intern Med* 1981;94:601–605.

Lerner MA: The gram negative bacillary pneumonias. *DM* 1980;22(2):1–56.

Levison ME, Mangura CT, Lorber B, et al: Penicillin versus clindamycin for the treatment of anaerobic lung abscess. *Ann Intern Med* 1983;98:466–471.

McKinney, RM, Porschen RK, Edelstein PH, et al: Legionella longbeachae species nova, another etiologic agent of human pneumonia. *Ann Intern Med* 1981;94:739–743.

Murray HW: Antimicrobial therapy in pulmonary aspiration. *Am J Med* 1979; 66:188–190.

Pennington JE: An empiric approach to pneumonia. *Med Times* 1977;105:36–43.

Pierce AK and Sanford JP: Aerobic gram negative bacillary pneumonias. *Am Rev Resp Dis* 1974;110:647–658.

Rein MF, Gwaltney JM Jr, O'Brien WM, et al: Accuracy of gram's stain in identifying pneumococci in sputum. *JAMA* 1978;239:2671–2673.

Shulman JA, Schlossberg D: *Handbook for Differential Diagnosis of Infectious Diseases*. New York, Appleton Century-Crofts, 1980, pp 134–149.

Sickles EA, Greene WH, Wiernik PH: Clinical presentation of infection in granulocytopenic patients. *Arch Intern Med* 1975;135:715–719.

White RJ: Chemotherapy of pneumonias. *J R Coll Physicians Lond* 1979; 13:21–22.

10 *Typical Pneumonia Syndrome*

Oksana M. Korzeniowski

Since a large number of infectious agents can produce pneumonia, one can arrive at a more rapid microbiologic diagnosis if the pathogens are grouped as causes of one of several, relatively distinct syndromes. On the basis of clinical presentation, pneumonias can be classified either as "typical" or "atypical". In typical bacterial pneumonia, respiratory symptoms predominate, the onset is sudden and purulent sputum is produced copiously. In contrast, atypical pneumonia is characterized by an illness in which constitutional symptoms and extrapulmonary manifestations predominate over the respiratory features and sputum production is scanty. Atypical pneumonia will be discussed in a separate chapter.

Several other clinical syndromes can be described to facilitate a microbiologic diagnosis. For example, when the typical pneumonia syndrome is acquired in the community, the pathogens include *Streptococcus pneumoniae*, *Hemophilus influenzae*, *Staphylococcus aureus*, *Streptococcus pyogenes*, or rarely, *Klebsiella pneumoniae*. When acquired in the hospital or occurring in compromised patients, the organisms which include *S. aureus*, *Pseudomonas aeruginosa*, enteric gram-negative organisms and fungi, reflect the more resistant flora encountered in an environment constantly exposed to high concentrations of antibiotics. Nosocomial pneumonias and pneumonia in compromised patients are discussed in Chapters 15, 17 and 18, respectively.

Another common pneumonia syndrome occurs in patients who have underlying conditions that cause dysphagia or unconsciousness and that result in aspiration of mouth contents. An indolent pneumonia which frequently cavitates to produce large abscesses results from such insults. The infection usually is polymicrobial and the organisms implicated in these infections usually are anaerobic streptococci, fusobacteria and *Bacteroides* sp, especially *B. melaninogenicus*. Patients who aspirate within hospital or institutional environments and have undergone colonization of their nasopharynx with hospital flora, may develop aspiration pneumonia complicated by the presence of *S. aureus* and resistant enteric bacilli. This type of pneumonia will be further discussed in Chapter 16.

ETIOLOGY AND EPIDEMIOLOGY

The typical pneumonia syndrome usually is the result of bronchogenic spread of the pathogen and may occur as a suprainfection in patients rendered susceptible by a previous viral infection of the upper or lower respiratory tract. There is no age-specific predisposition, although the incidence of infection increases with advancing age. Infants are also more susceptible. Most patients are adults above the fifth decade who have some underlying chronic obstructive pulmonary disease (COPD), cardiovascular or other chronic disease.

Of the few organisms commonly implicated in community-acquired typical pneumonia syndrome (Table 10-1), by far the most common pathogen is the pneumococcus. This is due to a high endemic carriage rate of this organism in the nasopharynx, existence of multiple virulent strains, no development of cross-immunity to heterologous strains, and susceptibility of patients at all age ranges. Outbreaks of pneumococcal pneumonia can occur following large outbreaks of influenzal illness. Patients with inadequate opsonizing antibody levels (ie, those with splenectomy or multiple myeloma) are particularly susceptible to recurrent attacks of a particularly virulent form of bacteremic pneumococcal infection.

Table 10-1
Typical Bacterial Pneumonia Etiologic Agents

Community Acquired
Common
S. pneumoniae
H. influenzae
S. aureus
Uncommon
K. pneumoniae
S. pyogenes
P. aeruginosa
N. meningitidis
Rare
Y. pestis
P. pseudomallei
Acinetobacter

H. influenzae type B, previously thought to cause pneumonia mainly in children under the age of 5, is gaining prominence as the organism responsible for severe bacteremic pneumonia in alcoholics and patients with COPD, as well as in previously healthy patients. In addition, patients with COPD frequently are carriers of nontypable strains of *H. influenzae*. These strains had been thought to cause a less severe abacteremic form of pneumonia. Recent data, however, suggest that bacteremia and metastatic infection also occur frequently as a consequence of pulmonary infection with these strains.

Klebsiella pneumoniae is the only enteric gram-negative organism implicated with any frequency in community-acquired infections. Again, the elderly, alcoholics and individuals with chronic obstructive pulmonary disease are particularly susceptible.

In the past, pneumonia caused by *S. aureus* was uncommon in adults except in those convalescent from a recent influenzal lower respiratory tract infection or in individuals with cystic fibrosis. However, the recent increased community abuse of parenteral drugs has resulted in a large group of individuals with *S. aureus* bacteremia/endocarditis and resultant metastatic pulmonary infection.

With the advent of highly effective antibiotic therapy for pharyngitis and impetigo, *Streptococcus pyogenes* has become an uncommon cause of pneumonia. Outbreaks of this infection are still occasionally encountered in individuals rendered susceptible by previous influenzal infection.

Although many other organisms may cause community-acquired pulmonary infection, their frequency is quite rare and susceptibility is dependent on either a severe compromise in pulmonary defenses (ie, *Pseudomonas* pneumonia in patients with cystic fibrosis) or unlucky exposure to a rare pathogen; for example, plague pneumonia among those exposed to an infected rat population or *Neisseria meningitidis* pneumonia in military recruits.

CLINICAL FEATURES

A general symptom complex is applicable to all typical bacterial pneumonias. The onset is usually acute. Systemic complaints of malaise are usually present; however, pulmonary symptoms predominate. Dyspnea, chest discomfort, pleuritic pain, or chest "splinting" associated with a cough productive of purulent or blood-tinged sputum are prominent features. Clinical signs include fever, tachycardia, tachypnea. Labored breathing, cyanosis and confusion are noted in advanced cases. Physical examination early in the illness may reveal only fine crepitant rales over the involved portion of the lung. Progression to lobar involvement is accompanied by signs of consolidation, eg, dullness to percussion, vocal fremitus, whispered pectoriloquy and bronchial breathing. Extension of the pneumonia to pleural surfaces can be accompanied by pleural effusions. Physical signs of pleural involvement include pleural friction rubs, dullness to percussion, decreased breath sounds and egophony. If necrosis of the lung leads to the development of large cavities, cavernous or amphoric breathing may be heard directly over the cavitary lesion. Pneumonias located in the lower lobe regions may cause inflammation of the diaphragmatic surface. Referral of pain to the abdominal region in association with diaphragmatic splinting may clinically mimic an acute intra-abdominal process and lead to a false diagnosis of peritonitis or acute cholecystitis.

RADIOLOGIC FEATURES

The classic radiographic features of an advanced typical bacterial pneumonia consist of dense lobar consolidation. The infection may involve one or more lobes and be either unilateral or bilateral. A pleural effusion may be present. Since the introduction of effective antimicrobial therapy, such a classic presentation has become uncommon. The chest x-ray most frequently now shows a localized bronchopneumonic pattern, which is almost never diagnostic and, in fact, may be indistinguishable from infections caused by nonbacterial pathogens. In patients with rapid onset of infection and clinical signs of severe dehydration, no infiltrates may be detectable even in the face of prominent clinical findings.

Certain radiographic features, when present, may be of diagnostic aid. Upper lobar consolidation with a bowing of the fissure ("bulging fissure sign") suggests *Klebsiella* pneumonia. Multiple bilateral nodular infiltrates with central cavitation suggest infection due to *S. aureus*. *S. aureus* pneumonia, particularly in children, results in ill-defined thin-walled cavities ("pneumatoceles"), bronchopleural fistulas and empyema. Cavitation is unusual in pneumococcal pneumonia due to serotypes other than Type 3. Diffuse patchy bronchopneumonia that progresses to microabscesses which may coalesce into large abscesses is most suggestive of *Pseudomonas* infection, although necrosis of lung parenchyma may occur with other gram-negative organisms such as *Klebsiella*, *Proteus*, and *E. coli*.

LABORATORY FEATURES

The most useful maneuver for the initial diagnosis of typical bacterial pneumonias is a gram stain examination of the sputum. Most patients with bacterial pneumonia produce copious amounts of purulent or mucopurulent sputum. Exceptions are patients with severe dehydration, patients with obstructive lesions, obtunded patients who cannot cooperate and patients who are too weak to mount an effective cough. Gross examination of the sputum is rarely helpful, since even pneumonia due to pneumococci or *Klebsiella* infrequently cause production of a "classic" sputum. More useful diagnostically is the odor of sputum which usually is feculent in lung necrosis due to anaerobic bacteria.

Microscopic examination of expectorated sputum should reveal numerous polymorphonuclear leukocytes, occasional alveolar macrophages and many bacteria. The presence of large numbers of squamous epithelial cells suggests contamination of the specimen with saliva, and thus the sample cannot be used for diagnostic evaluation. The gram stain morphology of the organisms can be of significant diagnostic aid (Table 10-2). Microscopic differentiation of the gram-positive cocci can be

Table 10-2
Differential Features of Common Bacterial Pathogens

Bacterial Pathogens	Susceptibility	Clinical Features	Associated Sites of Infection	Sputum Gram Stain
S. pneumoniae	All ages Splenectomy Chronic lymphatic leukemia Multiple myeloma Sickle cell anemia Postinfluenza COPD, smokers	Rusty sputum Single shaking chill Bacteremia 25–50% Pleural effusions	Arthritis Meningitis Endocarditis Sinusitis	Encapsulated lancet-shaped gram-positive diplococci or short chains Quellung reaction positive
H. influenzae	Young children < 5 years of age COPD Alcohol abusers Postinfluenza	Pleural effusion common Bacteremia	Otitis Sinusitis Meningitis Epiglottitis Facial infection	Small gram-negative pleomorphic encapsulated bacillus (Group B) Occasionally disease caused by nontypable strains
S. aureus	Metastatic infection in parenteral drug abusers or patients with infected intravenous catheters Postinfluenza Cystic fibrosis Inhospital aspiration	Pleuritic chest pain Multiple thin walled abscesses ("pneumatoceles") Cardiac murmurs	Endocarditis Cerebritis Metastatic abscesses Skin furuncles	Gram-positive cocci in clusters

Table 10-2 *(continued)*

Bacterial Pathogens	Susceptibility	Clinical Features	Associated Sites of Infection	Sputum Gram Stain
S. pyogenes	Postinfluenza COPD	Pleural effusion or empyema (up to 90%) Bacteremia 12%	Tonsillitis Mediastinitis	Gram-positive cocci in chains Quellung reaction negative
K. pneumoniae	Alcohol abusers COPD Neonates Nosocomial	"Currant jelly" sputum Bulging fissure Lung necrosis	–	Large gram-negative rod with capsule
P. aeruginosa	Neutropenic Intubated Respiratory therapy ICU-Burn unit Cystic fibrosis	Green sputum Fulminant course Necrotizing with multiple small and large abscesses	Skin lesions (ecthyma gangrenosum)	Gram-negative rod (encapsulated in patients with cystic fibrosis)
Enteric bacilli	Same as *P. aeruginosa*	Variable	–	Gram-negative rod

enhanced with the use of pneumococcal anticapsular antibody (Quellung reaction). Speciation of gram-negative organisms is not feasible microscopically and must be done by cultivation of sputum.

Blood cultures, if positive, provide a more specific bacteriologic diagnosis, although they are frequently negative even in patients with systemic toxicity. Similarly, positive cultures of pleural effusions, when present, are specific for the etiology of the underlying pneumonia.

Most patients with typical bacterial pneumonia mount a leukocytosis with predominance of early forms of polymorphonuclear leukocytes. Exceptions can be found among patients who are very young or very old, debilitated individuals and those with overwhelming infections.

DIAGNOSIS

A preliminary diagnosis of bacterial pneumonia that allows institution of antimicrobial therapy can be made on the basis of the clinical setting, the physical findings and the gram stain morphology of the sputum. Diagnostic precision can be enhanced by gram stain examination of any other available fluids, eg, pleural fluid, aspirates of skin lesions.

Because of the similarity in pulmonary manifestation among the bacterial pneumonias, clinical differentiation of etiologic agents is dependent primarily on nonpulmonary sites of involvement and on historical clues (Table 10-2). In community-acquired infections, a history of a single shaking chill, production of rusty sputum, and statistical odds favor the diagnosis of pneumococcal infection. Evidence of splenectomy or a generalized disease process, such as sickle cell disease, myeloma or chronic lymphocytic leukemia (CLL), should suggest the possibility of pneumococcal or *H. influenzae* pneumonia. The association of meningitis with pneumonia is also most likely due to either the pneumococcus or *H. influenzae*, since both organisms show a high predilection for involving the central nervous system. The presence of sinusitis or purulent otitis might provide additional clues to these two organisms. A dusky facial rash or epiglottitis may indicate *H. influenzae* infection.

Patients who relapse in the convalescent phase of a viral respiratory illness are liable to have postinfluenzal bacterial pneumonia, at times life-threatening, caused by the pneumococcus, *H. influenzae*, *S. aureus* or group A streptococcus (*S. pyogenes*). The concomitant presence of tonsillitis or a large pleural effusion favors *S. pyogenes* as the causative organism. A rapidly progressive, highly toxic pulmonary infection in an alcoholic who is producing copious mucoid bloody ("currant jelly") sputum is consistent with a *Klebsiella* pneumonia. Signs of consolidation might be localized to the upper lobes. Patients with cystic fibrosis are particularly susceptible to pneumonias caused by *S. aureus* and *P. aeruginosa*, both because of impaired mucociliary function of the tracheobronchial tree and because of frequent exposure to antibiotics that suppress the more sensitive organisms usually responsible for community-acquired pneumonias.

Parenteral drug abusers who are susceptible to the common community-acquired pneumonias are also at particular risk of developing pneumonia as a result of aspiration while intoxicated or as a result of hematogenous dissemination of organisms from sites of intravenous drug injection. Onset of metastatic pneumonia is abrupt, but the clinical presentation may mimic an acute pulmonary embolus with fever, severe respiratory distress and pleuritic chest pain. Cough and production of purulent sputum may not occur early in the course of illness. Pulmonary findings usually are bilateral, and insufficiency murmurs originating in the tricuspid, mitral or aortic valves may be present as a result of concomitant cardiac valve involvement with infective endocarditis. The most common cause of metastatic pulmonary infection in this population is *S. aureus*, although infections with gram-negative organisms such as *Serratia*, *Proteus* and *Pseudomonas* have occurred.

Definitive diagnosis resides in identification of the etiologic agent by culture from sputum, blood or pleural fluid. If sputum samples are unavailable or inadequate, more invasive procedures might be indicated when definitive bacteriologic results are imperative, ie, in immunocompromised hosts or in patients unresponsive to initial empiric therapy. Transtracheal aspiration yields uncontaminated bronchial secretions, but it is contraindicated in uncooperative patients, hypoxic patients and individuals with coagulopathies. Fiberoptic bronchoscopy might yield an adequate sputum sample, but results must be interpreted with caution since oropharyngeal contamination also occurs with this technique. Thus, with this technique anaerobic cultures are completely invalid, but a single organism isolated on confluent aerobic growth is most likely to be the offending pathogen. The diagnostic yields of percutaneous, transbronchial or open lung biopsy are quite high, but these procedures are rarely indicated in the normal host with an acute pneumonia.

THERAPY

Both the choice of antimicrobial agent(s) and the route of administration should be determined by the provisional diagnosis and by the severity of illness of the patient (Table 10-3). Young, healthy individuals with a localized infiltrate and minimal toxicity ("walking pneumonia") might respond adequately to oral antipneumococcal therapy with penicillin or erythromycin. Older (or younger) individuals with more severe respiratory compromise or with underlying illnesses require hospitalization, hydration, oxygenation, vigorous pulmonary toilet and intravenous administration of antimicrobial agents.

Table 10-3
Typical Bacterial Pneumonia Therapy

Etiology	Empiric Therapy
S. pneumoniae	Penicillin or erythromycin
H. influenzae	Ampicillin (for nonpenicillinase-producing strains), cefamandole, cefotaxime, or moxalactam
S. aureus	Penicillinase-resistant penicillin, cephalosporin (1st generation) or vancomycin
S. pyogenes	Penicillin or cephalosporin
K. pneumoniae	Moxalactam, cefotaxime, or cephalorsporin plus aminoglycoside

Clinical response to therapy generally is prompt with pneumococcal pneumonia, although resolution of x-ray abnormalities may be delayed. *H. influenzae*, *S. pyogenes*, *S. aureus* and the enteric gram-negative organisms respond more slowly with a prolonged convalescence. Intravenous therapy should be continued for a minimum of 10 to 14 days or longer depending on the clinical resolution of the infection.

Patients at high risk for pneumococcal pneumonia or its complications (ie, splenectomized patients, those with underlying pulmonary and cardiovascular disease, the elderly) should be immunized with the polyvalent pneumococcal vaccine and yearly with influenza vaccine. (See Chapter 20.)

SELECTED READINGS

Berkmen YM: Uncommon acute bacterial pneumonias. *Semin Roentgenol* 1980; 15:17–24.

Bruton JL, Eidelman D, Aberman AA: Diagnosis and treatment of pneumonia. *Comprehensive Therapy* 1982;8(9):8–18.

Fisk RB Jr, Reynolds HY: Changing spectrum of pneumonia—News media creation or clinical reality? *Am J Med* 1983;74:1–8.

Genereux GP, Stilwell GA: The acute bacterial pneumonias. *Semin Roentgenol* 1980;15:9–16.

George WL, Finegold SM: Bacterial infection of the lung. *Chest* 1982;81:502–507.

Lerner AM: The gram-negative bacillary pneumonias. *DM* November 1980:1–56.

Lerner AM, Jankauskas K: The classic bacterial pneumonias. *DM* February 1975.

McHenry MC: The infectious pneumonias. *Hosp Prac* 1980;12:41–52.

Meyer RD, Edelstein PH, Kirby BD, et al: Legionnaires disease: Unusual clinical and laboratory features. *Ann Intern Med* 1980;93:240.

Ort S, Ryan JL, Barden G, et al: Pneumococcal pneumonia in hospitalized patients. Clinical and radiologic presentations. *JAMA* 1983;249:214–218.

11 *Atypical Pneumonia Syndrome*

Jerome Boscia
Oksana M. Korzeniowski

The atypical pneumonia syndrome may result from infection by *Mycoplasma*, *Chlamydia*, *Rickettsia*, other bacteria viruses or fungi. Differentiation among the common causes of atypical pneumonia is based on a combination of epidemiologic, clinical, radiologic and laboratory findings. This provides a presumptive diagnosis which then allows institution of empiric antimicrobial therapy. Definitive diagnosis of atypical pneumonia usually is made retrospectively by serologic tests.

ETIOLOGY AND EPIDEMIOLOGY

The pathogens causing the atypical pneumonia syndrome are listed in Table 11-1. The most common pathogen of atypical pneumonia is *Mycoplasma pneumoniae*. This organism may rank second to *Streptococcus pneumoniae* among all the infectious causes of pneumonia in adults in the United States. Other relatively common causes of atypical pneumonia are influenza viruses and *Legionella pneumophila*. All the other pathogens listed in Table 11-1 are either uncommon causes of pneumonia in adults or their consideration as a causative agent depends on documentation of exposure of the patient to an unusual source of infection.

Table 11-1
The Pathogens of the Atypical Pneumonias

Bacteria
Legionella pneumophila (Legionnaires' disease) and legionella-like organisms
Francisella tularensis (tularemia)
Bacillus anthracis (anthrax)
Mycoplasma pneumoniae
Chlamydia psittaci (psittacosis)
*Chlamydia trachomatis**
Coxiella burnetii (Q fever)
Viruses
Influenza, adenovirus, parainfluenza*, respiratory syncytial virus*
Fungi
Histoplasma capsulatum (histoplasmosis)
Coccidioides immitis (coccidioidomycosis)

*These pathogens mainly cause pneumonia in the pediatric age group and will be discussed in subsequent chapters.

The epidemiologic features of the atypical pneumonias are compared in Table 11-2. The incubation periods, seasonality and age susceptibility of patients usually are of limited diagnostic value. For instance, young adults during their second and third decades of life are more likely to have *Mycoplasma pneumoniae*, whereas viral pneumonias occur in individuals who become ill during outbreaks of respiratory infections in the winter months. Person-to-person transmission of disease occurs commonly only with *Mycoplasma* and viral pneumonias. *Mycoplasma* pneumonia is a slowly spreading respiratory illness (due to a prolonged incubation period and respiratory carriage of the organism) within closed populations (eg, families, dormitory students, military recruits.) Influenza viruses cause disease in epidemic patterns, while adenoviruses are rare causes of pneumonia except under crowded environmental conditions such as those encountered by military recruits. The elderly and individuals with chronic underlying cardiorespiratory diseases are particularly susceptible to Legionnaires' disease and influenza pneumonia.

The most reliable differential epidemiologic feature of the atypical pneumonias is an elicited exposure to infected animals or environmental sources. Legionnaires' bacilli have been isolated from water and soil, and pneumonias due to these organisms have occurred among individuals exposed to aerosols generated by water-cooling towers, heat-exchange units, and excavation sites. Contact with infected psittacine birds and pigeons is a prerequisite for the development of psittacosis. This disease is seen among birdfanciers, pet store owners or bird breeders. Q fever can occur among ranchers or slaughterhouse workers who come in contact with infected sheep or cattle or infected animal tissues. Tularemia is seen in hunters or other outdoorsmen having contact with infected rabbits or ticks. Anthrax can occur in those having contact with infected goat hair, skin, or wool. Histoplasmosis occurs from inhalation of spores from soil fertilized with chicken and bat droppings. Environmental exposure to the spores of coccidioidomycosis occurs in the San Joaquin Valley and other areas of southern California, southern Arizona, New Mexico, and southwest Texas.

CLINICAL, RADIOGRAPHIC AND LABORATORY FEATURES

The "typical" bacterial pneumonias are characterized by an illness of abrupt onset with high fever, cough productive of purulent sputum, dyspnea, pleuritic chest pain, and signs of pulmonary consolidation on physical examination. In contrast, the "atypical" pneumonias are usually a more insidious illness with fever, nonproductive cough and prominent constitutional symptoms (severe headache, malaise, myalgias.) Physical

Table 11-2
Comparative Epidemiologic Features of the Atypical Pneumonias

Atypical pneumonias	Incubation Period (days)	Seasonality	Patient Age	Exposure to Infected Animal or Sources	Person-to-Person Transmissions	Underlying Chronic Diseases
Mycoplasma pneumonia	14–21	Year round	Adolescents and young adults	–	+	–
Legionnaires' disease	2–10	Year round (summer peak)	Adult	Cooling towers, condensers, excavation sites	–	+
Psittacosis	7–14	Year round	Adult	Psittacine birds, pigeons, turkeys, pet shops, zoos	–	–
Q fever	14–28	Year round	Adult	Cattle, sheep, goats, contaminated milk	–	–
Tularemia	1–14	Year round	Adult	Rabbits, ticks	–	–
Anthrax	1–5	Year round	Adult	Goat hair/skin, wool, bonemeal fertilizer	–	–
Viral pneumonia	1–3	Winter	All	–	+	+
Histoplasmosis	3–21	Year round	All	Chickens, bats, river valleys	–	–
Coccidioidomycosis	7–28	Year round	All	California, southwest USA	–	–

examination at most discloses rales and rhonchi. Signs of pulmonary consolidation are rarely present.

Although there is considerable overlap in the manifestations of the atypical pneumonias, some distinctive clinical, radiographic and laboratory features that aid in their differentiation are presented in Table 11-3. Bullous myringitis (one or more serous fluid-filled blebs, often sagging in appearance, that may cover most of the surface of the tympanic membrane) may accompany pneumonia caused by *Mycoplasma pneumoniae*. Cold agglutinin antibodies that cross-react with the specific adult red blood cell antigen I develop in about 50% of patients with *M. pneumoniae* infections during the second to third week of illness. In patients with high titers of cold agglutinins, clinically significant hemolytic anemia may occur. Gastrointestinal disturbances, hematuria, and mental confusion in the absence of inflammatory changes in the CSF are prominent features in Legionnaires' disease. Splenomegaly, epistaxis, and Horder's spots (a scant evanescent macular rash on the face resembling the rose spots of typhoid fever) suggest psittacosis. Liver involvement is common in Q fever, but its clinical manifestations are variable. In one series of 180 patients with Q fever, 5% had jaundice, 11% hepatomegaly, and 7% liver tenderness. In some patients with Q fever, clinical evidence of hepatitis may predominate over that of pneumonitis. Culture-negative infective endocarditis rarely complicates the course of Q fever. A cutaneous ulcer and regional lymphadenopathy may be present with tularemic pneumonia. Substernal or precordial chest pain are common complaints with tularemia, anthrax, histoplasmosis and coccidioidomycosis. Although anthrax presents initially as an atypical pneumonia, it rapidly becomes a devastating respiratory illness which usually results in death within 24 hours despite treatment. Hemorrhagic meningitis may complicate anthrax in less than 5% of patients. Erythema nodosum and skin rashes may be seen, especially in adult women, with acute coccidioidomycosis.

Radiographically, the atypical pneumonias appear as interstitial or patchy bronchopneumonic infiltrates, although consolidation may develop in later stages of illness. The radiographic findings in Legionnaires' disease are particularly variable. Patchy infiltrates may progress to dense, even nodular, bilateral involvement. Exudative pleural effusions are occasionally present in *Mycoplasma* pneumonia, Legionnaires' disease, tularemia, anthrax, and coccidioidomycosis. The pleural effusions of tularemia may be bloody. Bilateral hilar adenopathy is seen with tularemia, anthrax and the pneumonias of fungal origin.

A mild leukocytosis develops in most of the atypical pneumonias, except for those of viral etiology and in psittacosis in which leukopenia may occur. If sputum is available, the gram stain reveals mononuclear or polymorphonuclear leukocytes, but no predominant organism is seen.

Table 11-3
Distinctive Clinical, Radiographic, and Laboratory Features of the Atypical Pneumonias

Atypical Pneumonias	Clinical Features	Radiographic Features	Laboratory Features
Mycoplasma pneumonia	Upper respiratory tract symptoms Bullous myringitis Hemolytic anemia Myocarditis Meningoencephalitis	Occasional pleural effusion	Cold hemagglutinins
Legionnaire's disease	Relative bradycardia Abdominal pain Vomiting and diarrhea Hematuria Mental confusion	Occasional pleural effusion	Abnormal liver and renal function tests Increased CPK
Psittacosis	Relative bradycardia Epistaxis Horder's spots Splenomegaly	–	Normal or low leukocyte count
Q fever	Relative bradycardia Tender hepatomegaly Endocarditis	–	Abnormal liver function tests
Tularemia	Substernal chest pain Relative bradycardia	Bilateral hilar adenopathy common Occasional bloody pleural effusion	Normal or low leukocyte count
Anthrax	Precordial discomfort Hemorrhagic meningitis	Mediastinal adenopathy common Occasional pleural effusion	–
Viral pneumonia	Upper respiratory tract symptoms	–	
Histoplasmosis	Erythema nodosum Substernal discomfort	Bilateral hilar adenopathy common	–
Coccidioidomycosis	Chest pain Erythema nodosum	Bilateral hilar adenopathy common Occasional pleural effusion	–

Routine sputum cultures reveal normal respiratory flora, except with anthrax, in which case the organism is easily recovered. In an appropriate clinical setting, detection of abnormalities in liver and renal function tests and an elevated CPK should suggest the diagnosis of Legionnaires' disease. Laboratory studies indicating the presence of hepatitis occur in one third of patients with Q fever.

DIAGNOSIS

Direct isolation of the offending pathogen from the respiratory secretions, pleural fluid, blood or tissue of a patient with atypical pneumonia usually requires specialized and sometimes hazardous culture techniques not available in routine laboratories. However, with appropriate and careful culture techniques, it is possible to recover any of the organisms known to cause atypical pneumonia. Except for Legionnaires' disease, microscopic demonstration of the organism in sputum is unusual. Therefore, biopsy of tissues such as the lung is necessary for histologic confirmation. *Legionella pneumophila*, however, has been demonstrated in sputum and pleural fluid with Dieterle silver stain and direct fluorescent antibody staining. Recently developed techniques can detect the *Legionella* antigen in urine. Skin tests for histoplasmosis and coccidioidomycosis have limited value as diagnostic tools and are most useful for defining endemic areas of disease. However, in an appropriate clinical setting, the documented conversion of a negative skin test may be considered diagnostic. The histoplasmin skin test should be used with caution since it causes seroconversion and therefore may be a source of further diagnostic confusion. Definitive diagnosis of an atypical pneumonia is frequently made retrospectively through employment of serologic tests. A fourfold or greater rise in antibody titer between acute and convalescent sera is confirmatory of an acute infection. The results, however, are usually unavailable early in the course of the illness when therapy is most beneficial. Therefore, a presumptive diagnosis must be made in order to institute empiric therapy. By combining the key clinical, epidemiologic, radiographic and laboratory features of a particular illness, diagnostic specificity is enhanced and a more rational choice of antimicrobial therapy may be made.

THERAPY

The empiric antimicrobial therapy based on a presumptive clinical diagnosis is listed in Table 11-4. If no clues exist to suspect psittacosis, Q fever, tularemia or anthrax, erythromycin should be employed as the most appropriate antimicrobial agent, since it is effective against *Mycoplasma* pneumonia and Legionnaires' disease, the two most common

Table 11-4
Empiric Antimicrobial Therapy for the Atypical Pneumonias

Pneumonia	Antimicrobial Agent
Mycoplasma pneumonia	Erythromycin or tetracycline
Leionnaires' disease	Erythromycin (+ rifampin if severe or nonresponsive)
Psittacosis	Tetracycline
Q fever	Tetracycline
Tularemia	Streptomycin
Anthrax	Penicillin (the addition of streptomycin may be synergistic)
Influenza A	Amantadine
Histoplasmosis or Coccidioidomycosis	Amphotericin B or ketoconazole (only in severe or progressive disease)

atypical pneumonias. In severe or nonresponsive cases, rifampin could be added to the regimen since it shows in vitro synergistic activity with erythromycin against *Legionella pneumophila*. Amantadine is effective for the prophylaxis and early treatment of uncomplicated influenza A, but its efficacy is still unproven for pneumonia. Treatment of pulmonary histoplasmosis or coccidioidomycosis depends on documentation of severe or progressive disease. Standard therapy resides in administration of intravenous amphotericin B; however, oral ketoconazole is emerging as a less toxic and possibly equally effective alternative agent.

SELECTED READINGS

Brachman PS, Kaufmann AF, Dalldorf FG: Industrial inhalation anthrax. *Bact Rev* 1966;30:646.

Cunha BA, Quintiliani R: The atypical pneumonias: A diagnostic and therapeutic approach. *Postgrad Med* 1979;66:95.

Davis GS, Winn WC, Beatty HN: Legionnaires' disease: Infections caused by *Legionella pneumophila* and legionella-like organisms. *Clin Chest Med* 1981;2:145.

Derrick EH: The course of infection with *Coxiella burnetii*. *Med J Aust* 1973;1: 1051–1057.

Levine DP, Lerner AM: The clinical spectrum of *Mycoplasma pneumoniae* infections. *Med Clin North Am* 1978;62:961.

McHenry MC: The infectious pneumonias. *Hosp Pract* December 1980:41.

Miller RP, Bates JH: Pleuropulmonary tularemia: A review of 29 patients. *Am Rev Resp Dis* 1969;99:31.

Mufson MA, Zollar LM: Nonbacterial respiratory infections. *DM* November 1975.

Murray HW, Tuazon C: Atypical pneumonias. *Med Clin North Am* 1980;64:507.

Schaffner W, Drutz DJ, Duncan GW, et al: The clinical spectrum of endemic psittacosis. *Arch Intern Med* 1967;119:433.

Swartz MN: Clinical aspects of Legionnaires' disease. *Ann Intern Med* 1979; 90:492.

12 *Chronic Pneumonias*

Jaime Carrizosa
William B. McNamee, Jr.

The pulmonary infections that evolve gradually over a period of weeks to months are caused by numerous microorganisms (Table 12-1). The lung may be the only organ involved or be part of a multisystem illness. Symptoms tend to be highly variable in accordance with the diverse nature of the infectious agents. Usually, constitutional and pulmonary symptoms predominate. However, occasionally extrapulmonary manifestations lead the patient to seek help.

Table 12-1
Organisms that Cause Chronic Pneumonia

Bacteria
Actinomyces israelii
Nocardia asteroides
Pseudomonas pseudomallei
Mixed anaerobic oral flora
Mycobacteria
Mycobacterium tuberculosis
Mycobacterium kansasii
Mycobacterium avium-intracellurare
Fungi
Blastomyces dermatitidis
Coccidioides immitis
Histoplasma capsulatum
Paracoccidioides brasiliensis
Crytococcus neoformans
Sporothrix schenkii
Protozoa
Entamoeba histolytica
Helminths
Paragonimus westermani
Echinococcus granulosus

Although this chapter will discuss only the infectious causes of chronic pneumonia and an approach to their diagnosis, it must be kept in mind that numerous noninfectious processes give rise to a similar syndrome (Table 12-2). The diagnostic approach must consider all the noninfectious as well as infectious causes.

Table 12-2
Noninfectious Diseases

Sarcoidosis
Malignancy
Primary
Metastatic
Vasculitis
Collagen vascular disease
Wegener's granulomatosis
Hypersensitivity—Churg-Straus allergic granulomatosis
Goodpasture's syndrome
Radiation pneumonitis
Drug-induced pneumonitis
Extrinsic allergic alveolitis
Desquamative interstitial pneumonia syndrome
PIE syndromes (Pulmonary infiltrate with eosinophilia)
Eosinophilic granuloma
Alveolar proteinosis

ETIOLOGY

Among the bacterial causes, actinomycosis and mixed anaerobic pleuropulmonary disease are quite similar. The organisms responsible for both these pneumonias are part of the normal oral flora, and infection arises following aspiration of these organisms. Both give rise to necrotizing pneumonias that generally remain confined to the lung. Nocardiosis, despite closely resembling actinomycosis in its pulmonary manifestations, has a pathogenesis and presentation more similar to the disseminated fungal infections or tuberculosis. As with these latter microorganisms, *Nocardia* is acquired exogenously via inhalation. The primary infection is in the lung, but widespread dissemination may lead to numerous sites of extrapulmonary disease which frequently dominate the clinical picture, as may happen in fungal infections and tuberculosis. Melioidosis, similar to nocardiosis, may be acquired in nature via inhalation. A subacute or chronic illness may follow reactivation of infection in lung, bone, skin, lymph nodes, spleen or other site of metastatic infection. The chronic pulmonary form of melioidosis mimics tuberculosis. Other bacteria, such as *S. aureus*, one of the Enterobacteriaceae, especially *Klebsiella pneumoniae* or *P. aeruginosa*, generally give rise to acute pneumonia, but may cause chronic necrotizing pneumonia, usually in the impaired or debilitated host.

Tuberculosis is the only form of chronic pneumonia in which man is the only reservoir and transmission depends on person-to-person spread. In adults, tuberculosis is almost always due to endogenous reactivation. Extrapulmonary manifestations are quite common, as primary infection generally includes widespread hematogenous dissemination. In contrast, atypical mycobacteriosis is acquired in nature. Infection usually is confined to the lungs, except in compromised patients, and pulmonary infection with these atypical mycobacteria is most commonly seen in patients with underlying lung disease.

North American blastomycosis, South American blastomycosis (paracoccidioidomycosis), coccidioidomycosis and cryptococcosis frequently cause disseminated infection similar to that seen in nocardiosis or tuberculosis. Histoplasmosis occasionally disseminates, but more commonly causes chronic cavitary disease limited to the lung. This type of histoplasmosis usually is seen in patients with chronic obstructive lung disease with repeated exposure to *Histoplasma capsulatum*. Their altered pulmonary clearance mechanisms favors the development of local infection, with tissue necrosis leading to chronic cavitary disease. *Coccidioides immitis* and *Sporothrix schenkii* also give rise to chronic cavitary lung disease. In the infections caused by these fungi, the cavities evolve from the primary pneumonic infiltrate and often occur in patients with no underlying lung disease.

Protozoa and worms are infrequent causes of chronic pneumonia in this country but may be acquired abroad. Only *Entamoeba histolytica* is endemic in some areas of the United States. *E. histolytica* presents as a pleural effusion or lung abscess, both of which arise from contiguous spread from a subphrenic infection. *Paragonimus westermani* is the lung fluke. Man acquires the infection by ingesting raw infected shellfish. The worm migrates through the intestinal wall and subsequently through the diaphragm to the lung causing chronic nodular or cavitary disease that mimics tuberculosis. *Paragonimus* pulmonary disease is now being seen in the United States among refugees from Cambodia. Echinococcosis, caused by the tapeworm, *Echinococcus granulosus* or *multilocularis*, is prevalent in sheepherding countries. This infection is acquired by eating material contaminated with feces of sheep dogs. The intestinal infection is hematogenously disseminated to liver and lung, causing gradually enlarging lung cavities associated with episodes of chest pain, wheezing and even hemoptysis.

Early diagnosis of chronic pneumonias requires careful attention to certain clinical and epidemiologic features (Table 12-3).

Epidemiologic Aspects

The most useful epidemiologic characteristics relate to 1) endemic areas of infection, and 2) the host factors that increase the susceptibility to infection. Table 12-3 shows the endemic areas for each organism causing chronic pneumonia. Many of these diseases cannot be acquired within the United States. Melioidosis, S.A. blastomycosis, echinococcosis and paragonimiasis all belong to this group and their diagnosis requires a

Table 12-3
Clues to the Diagnosis of Chronic Pneumonia

Disease	Location	Source/Mode Spread	Predisposing Underlying Conditions	Extrapulmonary Manifestations	Characteristic Chest X-ray
Actinomycosis	Worldwide	Normal oral flora/ Aspiration	None	Rib destruction Cutaneous sinuses	Mass lesion or dense infiltrate, cavitation, spread to pleura and chest wall
Nocardiosis	Worldwide	Soil decaying vegetable matter/ Inhalation	Defect cell-mediated immunity; High dose corticosteroid therapy; Alveolar proteinosis Chronic granulomatous disease of childhood	Brain abscess Skin and subcutaneous abscess	Confluent bronchopneumonia; cavitation Pleural and chest wall involvement
Melioidosis	Between 20° N and 20° S latitudes in S.E. Asia	Soil, stagnant water/ Inhalation	None	Skin and subcutaneous abscess Lymphadenitis	Nodular infiltrates in upper lobes Cavitation
Mixed anaerobic pleuropulmonary disease	Worldwide	Normal oral flora/ Aspiration	Alcoholism Neurologic disease Esophageal disorder Seizure disorder Recent general anesthesia	Brain abscess	Dependent lung segments, single or multiple cavities with surrounding infiltrate; frequent air fluid level; frequent pleural involvement
Tuberculosis	Worldwide	Person-to-person	Alcoholism Silicosis Gastrectomy	Meningitis, osteomyelitis Lymphadenitis Infiltration of liver and bone marrow	Multiple thick-walled cavities with surrounding infiltrate in upper lobe, often bilateral

Tuberculosis (continued)	Worldwide	Person-to-person	Defective cell-mediated immunity Diabetes mellitus Corticosteroid therapy	Pericarditis Genitourinary involvement Addison's disease	
M. kansasii	Worldwide, but especially Texas, Louisiana, Chicago	Unknown	Chronic obstructive pulmonary disease (COPD) Silicosis		Indistinguishable from tuberculosis; pleural involvement rare
M. avium-intracellulare	S.E. United States	Soil	COPD Silicosis Defective cell-mediated immunity	Rare except in immunocompromised hosts	See above
North American blastomycosis	S.E. and Mid-Atlantic United States Great Lakes region, Manitoba, Africa	Soil Domestic animals	None	Skin, bone and genitourinary tract	Fibronodular, interstitial or alveolar infiltrates, often segmental or lobar
Coccidioidomycosis	S.W. United States, parts Central America	Soil	Greater tendency to disseminate in dark-skinned people or pregnant females	Skin, bone or meninges	Thin-walled, solitary cavities, segmental, alveolar infiltrate with hilar adenopathy
Histoplasmosis	Ohio and Mississippi valleys; endemic foci in 31 states	Soil contaminated with large amount of bird or bat excreta	Extremes of life for disseminated disease; emphysema for chronic cavitary histoplasmosis	Oral mucosal ulcerations, hepatosplenomegaly; infiltration of bone marrow, Addison's disease, mediastinitis	Thick-walled, expanding cavities, interstitial or pathy, nodular infiltrates with hilar adenopathy

Table 12-3 (continued)

Disease	Location	Source/Mode Spread	Predisposing Underlying Conditions	Extrapulmonary Manifestations	Characteristic Chest X-ray
Cryptococcosis	Worldwide	Soil contaminated with bird droppings	Defects in cell-mediated immunity; corticosteroid therapy; lymphoproliferative disorders; alcoholism, diabetes mellitus	Meninges, skin, occasionally bone	Nodular dense infiltrates in lower lobes; cavitation rare
South American blastomycosis	South and Central America	Soil	None	Skin, oral mucosa, lymph nodes	Bilateral alveolar infiltrates in lower lobes; often interstitial infiltrates
Sporotrichosis	Worldwide	Vegetable matter	None		Upper lobe, thin-walled cavities, unilateral
Paragonimiasis	Far East Asia, India, Africa Central and South America	Consumption of raw or pickled fresh water crustacea	None	Rarely abdominal or central nervous system involvement	Cavity often with patchy infiltrates, pleural effusion
Echinococcosis	Greece, Lebanon and other sheep and cattle raising areas	Ingestion of material contaminated with dog feces	None	Hepatic cysts	Rounded, nodular lesions
Amebiasis	Worldwide, primarily underdeveloped countries	Fecal-oral contamination	Male homosexuals	Intestinal amebiasis Hepatic abscess	Infiltrative or cavitary lesion in right lower lobe often with right pleural effusion

history of travel to one of these endemic areas. The travel history must be meticulous because exposure need not be great and latent periods may be as long as two to three decades for certain infections, including melioidosis and S.A. blastomycosis.

Coccidioides immitis, *Histoplasma capsulatum*, *Blastomyces dermatitidis* and the atypical mycobacteria all have endemic areas within the United States. Overlapping of endemic areas is common, except for coccidioidomycosis, and this somewhat limits diagnostic usefulness of a travel history. Likewise, transmission of disease by fomites from endemic areas also lessens the value of utilizing endemic areas in diagnosis. However, despite these limitations, travel history often provides a valuable clue for diagnosis.

Occupational history, hobbies and personal habits are important in acquiring certain infections. Coccidioidomycosis is associated with people doing any type of excavation work, such as archeologists or construction workers, in endemic areas. *H. capsulatum* shows striking association with fowl or bat excreta. Histoplasmosis may follow exposure to soil contaminated with bird excreta during excavation work, bridge painting or barn cleaning. Exposure may also occur while spelunking in bat-infested caves. Melioidosis has occurred in helicopter crewmen in Vietnam due to aerosolization of dust by the propeller. Sporotrichosis represents an occupational hazard for gardeners and vegetable produce handlers, while echinococcosis shows increased frequency in those tending sheep or cattle in endemic areas. Finally, eating habits may be important; paragonimiasis can only be acquired by eating raw seafood from endemic areas.

Certain groups appear more susceptible to particular infections. Dark-skinned people show an increased tendency to develop disseminated or chronic pulmonary forms of coccidioidomycosis. Likewise, women acquiring infection during pregnancy show a similar tendency. White males tend to develop chronic cavitary histoplasmosis even when the statistics are adjusted for their increased incidence of underlying emphysema. The patient age occasionally is helpful. For example, the acute form of disseminated histoplasmosis is a disease of infants, in addition to immunosuppressed adults. Adults otherwise are more likely to have a more chronic form of disseminated disease.

The detection of underlying disease frequently aids in diagnosis, as certain infections show striking association with certain conditions. This is particularly apparent in the immunocompromised host. Nocardiosis, cryptococcosis and mycobacterial disease are associated with defects in cell-mediated immunity. These defects may be drug-induced (eg, corticosteroids or other immunosuppressive medication) or related to the underlying disease (eg, lymphoproliferative malignancies). Other mycotic infections, including histoplasmosis, blastomycosis and coccidioidomycosis have been reported as opportunistic infections, presumably as a result of endogenous reactivation in immunocompromised patients.

Nocardiosis is found with increased frequency in patients with alveolar proteinosis. Silicosis has long been recognized as a risk factor for mycobacterial disease. Preexisting chronic lung disease is a prerequisite for development of chronic pulmonary histoplasmosis and appears important in the development of atypical mycobacterial disease, especially of the *M. avium-intracellulare* type. Conditions associated with aspiration, such as alcoholism, seizure disorder, recent anesthesia, neurologic and esophageal disturbances, are commonly contributory in the development of anaerobic lung abscess.

CLINICAL SYNDROME

Constitutional and chronic pulmonary symptoms often dominate the presentation in many of these diseases. Low grade fever, anorexia, weight loss as well as productive cough, hemoptysis, chest pain and dyspnea are common no matter what the microbial etiology. These symptoms help little to distinguish among diagnostic possibilities, except a putrid odor of the breath and sputum is characteristic for anaerobic lung abscess. However, many of these illnesses present in a disseminated form and each one of these syndromes will have characteristic extrapulmonary manifestations. Involvement of one or several extrapulmonary sites will narrow diagnostic possibilities as discussed below.

Skin

Cutaneous lesions are frequently present in disseminated N.A. blastomycosis and coccidioidomycosis in which they may be the presenting complaint. These lesions are characteristically verrucose or ulcerative. They frequently are multiple and usually involve exposed areas, especially the face. Skin lesions are less common but still important in nocardiosis, cryptococcosis and S.A. blastomycosis. In nocardiosis, skin lesions occur in up to 30% of cases and usually consist of nodular, ulcerative lesions or subcutaneous abscesses. In cryptococcosis, skin lesions are seen in approximately 10% of cases, and usually consist of shallow, initially painless ulcers on the scalp or face.

Mucosa

Oral ulcerations are the characteristic manifestation of the chronic form of disseminated histoplasmosis. Over 50% of these cases present with oral ulcerations. The ulcer may be painless or painful and may involve any portion of the oropharynx or larynx. North and South American blastomycosis, coccidioidomycosis and tuberculosis all occasionally have oral lesions, and in blastomycosis these typically are contiguous with cutaneous lesions and often involve the underlying alveolar bone.

Central Nervous System

Chronic pneumonias often may present with involvement of brain or meninges. Coccidioidomycosis, cryptococcosis and tuberculosis all characteristically involve the meninges. In coccidioidomycosis, meningitis is frequently the initial manifestation of the disseminated form of disease and usually develops within six months of the primary infection. Unlike cryptococcal meningitis, a pulmonary infiltrate is still evident in many patients presenting with meningeal coccidioidomycosis. Brain abscess is seen in up to 25% of the cases of pulmonary nocardiosis and is also associated with anaerobic lung abscess.

Bone

N.A. blastomycosis, coccidioidomycosis and tuberculosis frequently involve bone. The vertebrae are the most common sites of infection, although the skull and long bones are also common sites. Blastomycosis and tuberculosis usually involve the disc space, while in coccidioidomycosis prominent destruction of the vertebrae is common. Cryptococcosis occasionally gives rise to osteolytic lesions.

Genitourinary System

Involvement of the prostate, epididymus and testes is seen in up to 20% of the cases of N.A. blastomycosis and presents as recurrent bouts of epididymitis, sometimes with the development of scrotal ulcer. Tuberculosis involves both the upper and lower genitourinary tract. Asymptomatic renal disease with positive urine cultures is seen in cryptococcosis.

Other Metastatic Sites

Involvement of the liver, spleen, adrenal glands, and the gastrointestinal tract are occasionally seen in both tuberculosis and histoplasmosis.

LABORATORY

Routine laboratory studies will manifest only nonspecific abnormalities in the majority of cases. Abnormalities such as normocytic, normochromic anemia, thrombocytosis, elevated erythrocyte sedimentation rate and polyclonal gammopathy are common. Leukopenia or pancytopenia would suggest the disseminated forms of tuberculosis or histoplasmosis due to their extensive involvement of the reticuloendothelial cells of the bone marrow. Likewise, both tuberculosis and histoplasmosis characteristically involve the hepatic reticulo-endothelial system, leading to abnormal liver function studies, usually characterized by an elevated serum alkaline phosphatase. Eosinophilia, when associated with chronic pneumonia, should suggest one of the parasitic etiologies (eg, paragonimiasis, echinococcosis), although most such cases in the United States will be noninfectious in nature.

Involvement of the genitourinary tract, common in disseminated tuberculosis and N.A. blastomycosis, often gives rise to an abnormal urine sediment. Sterile pyuria or hematuria may be a clue to their diagnosis. Electrolyte disturbances are uncommon with the chronic pneumonias except for hyponatremia. Adrenal insufficiency, manifest by volume depletion, hyponatremia and hyperkalemia, may be a consequence of tuberculosis or histoplasmosis of the adrenal gland. Inappropriate secretion of ADH or the reset osmostat syndrome are other causes frequently associated with intrathoracic diseases, particularly tuberculosis.

RADIOGRAPHIC FINDINGS

The chest x-ray often provides an important clue in diagnosis. However, seldom will the x-ray pattern be unique or pathognomonic for any disease. More often, the x-ray will suggest a group of diseases that typically produce such a picture and thereby help to narrow the differential diagnosis. Great caution must be exercised when using the chest radiograph in this way, as most of these infections are capable of producing the entire spectrum of radiographic appearances.

Cavitary lesions are characteristic of the mycobacterial diseases, melioidosis, sporotrichosis, the chronic forms of histoplasmosis and coccidioidomycosis, and chronic necrotizing pneumonia due to the mixed anaerobic bacteria or Enterobacteriaceae. The majority of cavities found in tuberculosis, histoplasmosis, coccidioidomycosis and sporotrichosis are unilateral and located in the upper lobes. Those infections due to aspiration, whether a solitary lung abscess or multiple cavities secondary to necrotizing pneumonia, usually are located in dependent areas, ie, posterior segments of upper lobes or superior segments of lower lobes. Bilateral distribution suggests mycobacteral disease, although even mycobacterial disease is more frequently unilateral. A prominent, infiltrate surrounding the cavity suggests tuberculosis, bacterial lung abscess or melioidosis. The finding of an air-fluid level strongly favors anaerobic lung abscess but may occur in other diseases. The cavities of chronic histoplasmosis are classically thick walled ($>$ 3 mm) and often show gradual enlargement with time. Chronic pulmonary coccidioidomycosis, although occasionally mimicing tuberculosis with multiple apical cavities, more often present with a solitary thin-walled cavity. Paragonimiasis, when radiographically apparent, gives rise to a pulmonary cavity, while echinococcosis more often gives rise to an irregular mass occasionally with some air within. Also, nocardiosis and actinomycosis, which initially show consolidated or mass-like lesions, tend to cavitate eventually.

The parenchymal infiltrates found in the chronic pneumonias range from interstitial, fibronodular or miliary to dense alveolar consolidation. Parenchymal infiltrates without cavitation usually characterize N.A. blastomycosis, S.A. blastomycosis and cryptococcosis as well as the early stages of nocardiosis and actinomycosis. N.A. blastomycosis produces the entire spectrum of infiltrates with no one pattern significantly more common. S.A. blastomycosis classically gives rise to bilateral, symmetrical alveolar infiltrates most commonly in the lower lobes. Cryptococcosis and actinomycosis most often present with dense nodular infiltrates resembling tumor, while nocardiosis usually becomes manifest as a segmental bronchopneumonia with or without cavitation.

The propensity for pleural involvement is characteristic for certain pathogens. *Nocardia asteroides* and *Actinomyces israelii* both typically extend to involve the pleura with development of empyema. Additionally, these infections also frequently invade the chest wall, leading to bony destruction or cutaneous sinus tracts. Anaerobic bacterial pneumonia also may result in empyema. Tuberculosis is the only mycobacterial disease with frequent pleural involvement. Among the parasites, *Entamoeba histolytica* and *Paragonimiasis westermani* both are frequently accompanied by pleural effusion secondary to pleural involvement during migration from a subdiaphragmatic site.

APPROACH TO THE PATIENT WITH CHRONIC PNEUMONIA

The workup of the patient with chronic pneumonia will depend greatly on the most likely diagnostic possibilities. Many diseases will be excluded by careful consideration of the epidemiologic, clinical and laboratory data. The evaluation of each patient must be individualized based on these data. Five basic diagnostic modalities often aide in diagnosis: 1) smears and cultures of sputum, 2) smears and cultures from extrapulmonary sites, 3) skin testing, 4) serologic testing, and 5) invasive diagnostic methods. The usefulness of each of these methods will vary depending on the pathogen.

Each evaluation should begin with an examination of the sputum. A gram stain, acid fast stain and wet mount all may be helpful depending on the circumstance. The gram stain is likely to be helpful in demonstrating bacteria in pneumonias due to *Pseudomonas pseudomallei*, aspiration pneumonia and the unusual cases of chronic pneumonia due to one of the Enterobacteriaceae. The routine acid fast or fluorochrome stains are useful in demonstrating mycobacteria. A modified version of the acid fast stain (substituting sulfuric for hydrochloric acid in the decolorizer) may be useful in staining the partially acid fast *Nocardia* species. Wet mounts using NaOH or KOH to dissolve concentrated sputum specimens may be useful in the hands of an experienced observer. The NaOH preparation of sputum is useful in demonstrating the operculated eggs of *Paragonimus westermani.* The 10% KOH preparation of sputum is useful in eliminating debris when looking for fungal elements. An India ink preparation or Giemsa stain of sputum may demonstrate *Cryptcoccus neoformans* or *Histoplasma capsulatum*, respectively.

Sputum cultures often provide the diagnosis in chronic pneumonia, although the yield varies significantly depending on the pathogen. Of the organisms causing chronic pneumonia, *Pseudomonas pseudomallei* and Enterobacteriaceae can be recovered on routine bacteriologic culture of expectorated sputum. To culture *Actinomyces* or the anaerobic pathogens causing putrid lung abscess, because the pathogens are anaerobic and part of the normal oral flora, special techniques are required to avoid oropharyngeal contamination and to incubate the specimen anaerobically. Transtracheal aspiration or direct percutaneous aspiration will provide suitable specimens for such cultures. *Nocardia asteroides*, despite being capable of growth aerobically on routine media, is rarely recovered on routine sputum culture because of its slow rate of growth. This organism usually requires at least three to five days for macroscopic colony formation. Since sputum cultures are routinely discarded after 24 to 48 hours, the laboratory must be notified to prolong the incubation period when *Nocardia* is suspected. This may increase the yield; however, overgrowth with normal sputum saprophytes will still limit recovery. *Nocardia* also grow well on Sabouraud and Lowenstein-Jensen agars and thus may be recovered in cultures for mycobacteria or fungi.

The mycobacteria uniformly grow well on artificial media, although their slow rate of growth (four to six weeks) often delays diagnosis. When acid-fast stained smears of sputum are negative and when multiple, appropriate cultures of well-collected specimens are negative, mycobacterial disease is unlikely. Alternatively, great care must be given when interpreting positive sputum cultures particularly when *M. avium-intracellulare* is isolated, as it frequently may represent colonization without tissue invasion.

The yield of sputum cultures in fungal disease will vary with the organism. In the chronic forms of coccidioidomycosis, and N.A. and S.A. blastomycosis, 70% to 100% of confirmed cases yield positive cultures when multiple specimens are collected. In sporotrichosis, despite limited experience, the yield appears comparable. The yield in histoplasmosis is generally lower, with great variability depending on the stage of the disease. In the early stages of histoplasmosis, characterized by an interstitial infiltrate, only 30% have positive sputum cultures, while in later stages when thick-walled cavities exist, the yield increases to 70%. In cryptococcosis, sputum culture generally has a poor yield, with less than 50% of proven cases having positive cultures.

Sources other than sputum may be valuable in diagnosis. In nocardiosis, actinomycosis and anaerobic pulmonary disease, pleural fluid when present offers a readily accessible specimen for examination. Skin lesions either arising via direct spread through the chest wall or secondary to disseminated fungal or nocardial disease provide aspirates or scrapings appropriate for smear and culture. Likewise, the oropharyngeal mucosal and cerebrospinal or synovial fluid all may provide diagnostic material when clinical involvement is found. When genitourinary symptoms exist, urine and prostatic secretions may yield *M. tuberculosis* or *B. dermatitidis*, while *C. neoformans* and *C. immitis* may be recovered in urine despite absence of genitourinary symptoms. Examination of stool may be helpful in amebiasis.

Skin testing appears to be of limited value, contributing significantly only in the diagnosis of tuberculosis. For all skin testing, a positive reaction only indicates past exposure. The tuberculin antigen (purified protein derivative [PPD]) is available in first, intermediate and second strengths, which contain 1, 5 and 250 Todd units, respectively. Occasional false-positive reactions (related to previous sensitization with nontuberculous mycobacteria) and false-negative reactions (related to improperly placed or outdated antigen) occur. However, when a patient has a negative intermediate and second strength PPD in the presence of reactivity to one or more other concurrently placed skin test antigens, such as mumps, *Candida*, streptokinase-streptodornase, tuberculosis is highly unlikely.

Skin test antigens also are available for *C. immitis*, *H. capsulatum* and *B. dermatitidis*. None of these are of much clinical usefulness. The blastomycin skin test shows a high false-negative rate plus considerable cross-reactivity with histoplasmin. The histoplasmin skin test has good sensitivity, but is of little value because at any time, 50% to 60% of the population in an endemic area will be positive. Furthermore, its use will elevate the histoplasmin serologic reaction in histoplasmin-sensitized patients if the mycelial phase antigen is used. Two skin test antigens for *Coccidioides immitis* are available; coccidioidin and spherulin. Skin reactivity to these antigens usually correlates well with controlled disease and is considered a good prognostic sign for recovery. Patients with a chronic, progressive form of coccidioidomycosis generally lack skin test reactivity.

Serology may provide valuable adjunctive information, but rarely is it sufficient for diagnosis. Due to the prolonged nature of the illnesses prior to presentation and diagnosis, only rarely can significant changes in serologic titers be shown. Few serologic tests are available for the diagnosis of bacterial or mycobacterial diseases. The exceptions are melioidosis, for which there are sensitive and specific serologic tests of hemagglutination and complement fixation activity, and *Nocardia*, for which a relatively sensitive, although nonspecific, complement fixation test has been developed. Serology plays a larger role in the diagnosis of the fungal and parasitic diseases. Complement fixation titers are usually elevated in the chronic forms of coccidioidomycosis, histoplasmosis and S.A. blastomycosis. For coccidioidomycosis, the appearance of this antibody in significant titer (≥ 1:16) usually indicates disseminated disease. For N.A. blastomycosis, the complement fixation test is widely available, but is falsely negative in approximately 50% of patients. For sporotrichosis, agglutination tests are available which offer good sensitivity and specificity, and for aspergillosis, an immunodiffusion test is available. Over 95% of patients with disseminated infection with meningeal involvement will have a positive test for cryptococcal antigen by latex agglutination in the cerebrospinal fluid and serum. It appears much less useful in localized pulmonary disease.

For the parasitic diseases, serology often is the key to diagnosis. For echinococcosis, indirect hemagglutination has proven reliable when hepatic disease is present; however, sensitivity is poor when only pulmonary disease is present. An indirect hemagglutination test also is used to diagnose amebiasis. Eightly-seven percent to 100% of patients with parenchymal involvement will have a significant titer; however, care must be taken as 10% of asymptomatic intestinal carriers may manifest significant titers. For paragonimiasis, a complement fixation test is available and often useful.

When the diagnosis cannot be established by the routine smears, cultures or serology, use of invasive methods need be considered. As previously mentioned, transtracheal aspiration may be helpful in the diagnosis of actinomycosis or putrid lung abscess. In the disseminated diseases, extrapulmonary sites often provide easily accessible sites for biopsy. Bone marrow or liver biopsy frequently are useful when the diagnosis of disseminated tuberculosis or histoplasmosis are being entertained. Biopsy of cutaneous, osseous or genitourinary lesions, when present, may be useful to diagnose N.A. blastomycosis, tuberculosis or coccidioidomycosis. When obtaining biopsy specimens, the importance of obtaining appropriate cultures as well as special stains cannot be overemphasized. Mycobacterial as well as fungal culture should be obtained on all such specimens. In addition to the routine stains, special stains to demonstrate fungi (silver methenamine, periodic acid-Schiff, mucicarmine), mycobacteria (acid fast or fluorochrome) and bacteria (Brown-Brenn) should be included.

When no extrapulmonary sites are easily accessible, lung biopsy is often necessary. Generally, fiberoptic bronchoscopy with washings, brushings and transbronchial biopsy is widely available and is the favored approach. Transbronchial biopsy is an attractive method because of the extremely low incidence of serious morbidity, although the small sample of lung obtained limits diagnosis by this method. When transbronchial biopsy is unsuccessful or the lesion does not lend itself to transbronchial biopsy, open lung biopsy may be necessary.

TREATMENT

Treatment in most cases of chronic pneumonia should be reserved until diagnosis is firmly established. Because of the wide variety of diagnoses (infectious and noninfectious), the generally indolent course and considerable toxicity of many of the therapeutic agents, empiric therapy generally is not indicated. Exceptions do exist, however. In the patient with a condition known to predispose to aspiration and with characteristic putrid sputum, treatment with penicillin or clindamycin certainly is reasonable without bacteriologic confirmation. Likewise, when a high clinical suspicion for tuberculosis exists, antituberculous therapy while awaiting results of cultures is indicated.

Specific antibiotic therapy exists for each of the bacterial pneumonias. Until recently, amphotericin B was the only treatment for fungal disease. However, the recent development of the antifungal imidazoles, particularly ketoconazole, may provide a possible alternative treatment. Some of these diseases respond poorly to medical therapy. Treatment of chronic pneumonia generally is prolonged and relapses are not uncommon.

SELECTED READINGS

Adams EB, MacLeod INN: Invasive amebiasis II amebic liver abscess and its complications. *Medicine* 1977;56:325.

Cameron EW: The treatment of pleuropulmonary amebiasis with metronidazole. *Chest* 1978;73:647–650.

Causey WA, Sieger B: Systemic nocardiosis caused by *Nocardia brasiliensis*. *Am Rev Resp Dis* 1974;109:134.

Drutz D, Catanzaro A: State of the art. Coccidioidomycosis. *Am Rev Resp Dis* 1978;117(3):559 Part I, 117(4):727 Part II.

Everett ED, Nelson R: Pulmonary melioidosis: Observations in 39 cases. *Am Rev Respir Dis* 1975;112:331.

Limson BM, Romansky MJ, Shea, JG: An evaluation of twenty-two patients with acute and chronic pulmonary infection with Friedlander's bacillus. *Ann Intern Med* 1956;44:1070–1081.

Lynch PJ, Voorhees JJ, Harrell ER: Systemic sporotrichosis. *Ann Intern Med* 1970;73:23.

Palmer DL, Harvey RL, Wheeler JK: Diagnostic and therapeutic considerations in *Nocardia Asteroides* infection. *Medicine* 1974;53:391.

Pierce AK, Sanford JP: Aerobic gram-negative bacillary pneumonias. *Amer Rev Resp Dis* 1974;110:647.

Sarosi GA, Parker JD, Doto IL, Tosh FE: Chronic pulmonary coccidioidomycosis. *N Engl J Med* 1970;283:325.

Smith AG, et al: Chronic pulmonary sporotrichosis. *Am J Clin Path* 1970;54:401.

Tellis CJ, Putnam JS: Pulmonary disease caused by nontuberculosis mycobacteria. *Med Clin N Amer* 1980;64:433–446.
Tillotson JR, Lerner AM: Characteristics of nonbacteremic pseudomonas pneumonia. *Ann Intern Med* 1968;68:295–307.
Wilson JF, et al: A clinical trial of mebendazole in the treatment of alveolar hydatid disease. *Am Rev Respir Dis* 1978;118:747–757.
Wilson JR, et al: Alveolar hydatid disease. A review of clinical features of 33 indigenous cases of echinococcus multiclocularis infection in Alaskan eskimos. *Am J Trop Med Hyg* 1980;29:1340–1355.

13 *Recurrent Pneumonia*

Elias Abrutyn

Patients with multiple, separate, discrete episodes of pneumonia suffer from recurrent pneumonia. Recurrent pneumonia is to be distinguished from relapsing pneumonia in which patients have more than one bout of clinical disease related to but a single episode of infection. At times, it is difficult to distinguish relapse of a previous infection from onset of a new infection. In general, relapse is suggested when the interval between clinical episodes is brief, but exceptions occur. An understanding of the natural history of the infection in question may also be helpful.

INCIDENCE

The precise incidence of recurrent pneumonia is unknown. Although single case studies are frequent, there is a paucity of systematic studies. The available data, however, suggests that patients with recurrent pneumonia are common. For example, in a retrospective study, Winterbauer et al found 429 persons older than 14 years of age who were hospitalized with acute infectious pneumonia over an 11-year period (January 1957 through December 1967). Of these, 306 had two episodes and 116 had three or more episodes of pneumonia. In that study, recurrent pneumonia was defined as two or more episodes of acute nontuberculous infectious pneumonia, with the interval between episodes exceeding one month; the time criteria served to exclude patients with pneumonia in relapse. Among a subset of 158 patients whose course could be followed, 47 had five or more episodes of pneumonia. They also reviewed several older studies of pneumonia from the preantibiotic era, which included a total of 15,000 patients with lobar pneumonia; the rate of recurrence ranged from 13.6% to 22%. More recent studies also indicate that patients with multiple separate episodes of pneumonia are common.

In 1966, Kjellman reported on studies performed on 14 children with asthma and recurrent pneumonia who were found among the 125 asthmatic children on the register of the department of pediatrics. In a more recent study, Oseasohn, Skipper, and Tempest maintained surveillance for pneumonia in a Navajo community over a two-year period (November 1971 through October 1973). They found that 14.5% of patients $\leq$ 15 years old and 7.6% of those > 15 years old had multiple episodes of pneumonia. Finally, in 1981, Beard, Maxwell, and Thong reported on studies performed on 119 children referred over three years for evaluation of recurrent upper and lower respiratory complaints; 38 had two or more bouts of pneumonia, and the remainder had repeated upper respiratory tract infections. In that study, patients with recurrent pneumonia from an obvious cause or immunodeficiency syndrome were excluded.

PATHOPHYSIOLOGY

Pneumonia, as stated many times in this book, develops as a result of aspiration or inhalation of contaminated materials, or as a secondary infection complicating bacteremia. Moreover, the risk of developing pneumonia is enhanced in patients whose systemic or local defenses are compromised. Conceptually, the conditions predisposing to pneumonia in general would similarly predispose to recurrent pneumonia, if the condition is present either intermittently or persistently. It follows that a localized abnormality predisposing to pneumonia should be sought in patients when the same area of lung is recurrently involved, and a more generalized predilection should be considered when several different areas are recurrently involved, but exceptions occur.

ETIOLOGY

Table 13-1 modified from Dauber and Fogerty (1980) presents a list of disorders associated with recurrent pneumonia by system. At the outset, it should be appreciated that statistical evidence rigorously associating some of the disorders with recurrent pneumonia is lacking. Inclusion, however, seems warranted on the basis of their appearance in lists of associated illnesses in patients with pneumonia, as a result of studies of the natural history of the disorder in question, or clinical experience. Review of the various disorders and the approach to their diagnosis will help define the various procedures and tests that may be required in evaluating patients with recurrent pneumonia.

RESPIRATORY DISORDERS

A variety of congenital, hereditary, and acquired disorders of the respiratory tract are associated with recurrent pneumonia.

Bronchial obstruction is a feature common to many of these conditions, and should be considered in the differential diagnosis of patients with recurrent pneumonia. Obstruction may be intralumenal (eg, from aspirated foreign body), intramural (eg, from congenital bronchial stenosis, bronchogenic carcinoma, or bronchial adenoma), or it may be due

Table 13-1
Selected Disorders Associated with Recurrent Pneumonia*

Respiratory	Neurologic
Asthma	Seizures
Bronchial adenoma	
Bronchiectasis	Substance Abuse
Bronchogenic carcinoma	Alcoholism
Bronchogenic cyst	Drug abuse
Bronchial stenosis	
Cystic fibrosis	Immune Deficiency
Chronic bronchitis	Antibody deficiency
Chronic obstructive pulmonary disease	Complement deficiency
Kartagener's syndrome	Cell-mediated immunity deficiency
Pulmonary sequestration	Mixed disorders
	Phagocyte disorders
Cardiac	Quantitative
Congestive heart failure	Qualitative
Gastrointestinal	Miscellaneous
Tracheoesophageal fistula	Diabetes mellitus
Diseases of striated muscle	Renal failure
Disease of nervous system	Sickle cell anemia
Motor disorders	
Collagen-vascular diseases	
Gastroesophageal reflux	
Diverticulum	

*Modified from Dauber and Fogarty (1980).

to compression from an extrabronchial mass (eg, from hilar lymph nodes). Obstruction promotes the development of pneumonia by inhibiting operation of normal clearance mechanisms. Thus, secretions may pool and become secondarily infected; if aspiration occurs, pneumonia may develop. When obstruction is present, recurrences may occur in the anatomic area served by the compromised bronchus.

The *right middle lobe syndrome* is one special instance of recurrent localized infection. In that disorder, infection is associated with right middle lobe atelectasis. This propensity to atelectasis has been attributed to compression of the right middle lobe bronchus from enlarged peribronchial lymph nodes, to impaired collateral ventilation, and to anatomic factors. Repeated episodes of infection and atelectasis may be followed by bronchiectasis and/or chronic fibrosis of the right middle lobe.

The history of repeated recurrences of pneumonia in the same anatomic area is a clue suggesting obstruction. The history may also reveal evidence of the possibility of foreign body aspiration, symptoms suggestive of bronchogenic carcinoma, or symptoms of carcinoid syndrome (flushing, diarrhea, etc) in the rare instance of mediator-producing bronchial adenoma. Signs of obstruction, such as localized wheezing or unilateral loss of chest volume, may be present on physical examination. During the acute episode of pneumonia, the chest film shows a pulmonary infiltrate as expected, but it may also show additional abnormalities suggesting obstruction such as a mass or enlarged hilar nodes. Chest films taken between episodes may be particularly useful in revealing important abnormalities not detectable during the acute episode, but abnormalities may be present and the chest film nevertheless can be normal. The presence and cause of obstruction are best defined by flexible fiberoptic bronchoscopy, and this procedure should be considered when obstruction is a likely cause of recurrent pneumonia.

Bronchiectasis is an anatomic abnormality of the bronchial tree in which there is abnormal dilatation due to a weakness or destruction of the structural components. In this pathological condition, as in obstructing lesions, there is abnormal pooling of secretions, secondary infection, and aspiration leading to pneumonia. Bronchiectasis may be congenital, may follow necrotizing pulmonary infection (*Staphylococcus aureus*, measles, pertussis, influenza, or tuberculosis), or may follow destruction of the bronchial wall after aspiration of gastric acid; it also is associated with cystic fibrosis and occurs in other conditions. The lesions in bronchiectasis may be diffuse or localized, and those in the dependent lower regions of the lungs (due to, for example, pertussis or measles) are more likely to be associated with symptoms than those in the better drained upper regions (due to prior tuberculosis).

The interval between the primary inciting event and pneumonia may be long. Some patients with bronchiectasis are symptomatic (cough, sputum production, etc) almost all of the time, but others suffer infrequently. The chest film may be helpful, but the test of choice for diagnosis is bronchography (a radiographic procedure employing contrast material that permits visualization of the bronchial tree). Transient bronchiectasis may be found in association with several types of acute pulmonary infections. Therefore, bronchography following an acute pulmonary infection should be delayed to avoid detecting transient abnormalities. Most patients with bronchiectasis respond well to therapy with antibiotics and maneuvers promoting adequate drainage; surgery may be of particular value in localized disease, if conservative management fails.

Studies of patients with *chronic obstructive pulmonary disease* and/or *chronic bronchitis* suggest that such patients are susceptible to recurrent pulmonary infections, perhaps because of abnormal clearance mechanisms. In chronic bronchitis, the tracheobronchial secretions become secondarily infected with *Streptococcus pneumoniae* and *Hemophilus influenzae*. These bacteria are easily visualized on gram stain of sputum and may be cultured easily, if appropriate techniques are used.

They should be considered in the differential diagnosis of pneumonia in these patients.

Studies of patients with *asthma*, another common clinical condition, similarly indicate that such patients are susceptible to repeated pulmonary infection.

Cystic fibrosis is a genetic disease involving the lungs, pancreas, and mucous glands of the gastrointestinal tract; transmission is autosomal recessive. Disease is commonly detected in childhood, but occasional cases are first detected in adults. The diagnosis is made by use of the sweat test which shows high sodium chloride concentration. Clinically, bronchitis, emphysema, and recurrent pneumonia occur and *Pseudomonas aeruginosa* (especially a mucoid variant) is a common pathogen in patients with this disorder.

Another genetic disorder predisposing to pneumonia is *Kartagener's syndrome*. It is a rare autosomal recessive disorder characterized by recurrent sinusitis, otitis media, and pulmonary infection plus situs inversus; affected males may be impotent. Structural and functional abnormalities of spermatozoa and the cilia of the respiratory tract epithelium have been described and neutrophil migration is depressed. Relatives with infection but without situs inversus have been identified and the names "immotile cilia syndrome" and "ciliary dyskinesis" have therefore been suggested as alternative designations for this syndrome.

Pulmonary sequestration is a developmental abnormality associated with recurrent pneumonia in which a portion of lung is partially separated from the normal bronchial tree. It may (intralobar) or may not (extralobar) have a pleural investment from normal lung, but in both cases the blood supply is from aberrant vessels. Arteriography is the test of choice, although abnormalities suggesting the diagnosis may be seen on chest x-ray or tomograms of the chest. Surgical excision may be required.

Cysts may be formed during development or they may be acquired. They occur in a variety of locations, and those that communicate directly with a bronchus are prone to infection.

CARDIAC DISORDERS

Congestive heart failure was prominent among illnesses associated with recurrent pneumonia in one series and is often found as an associated illness in studies of patients with pneumonia. Whether congestive heart failure per se is a risk factor for recurrent pneumonia is unclear, but both conditions occur in many patients.

GASTROINTESTINAL DISORDERS

The feature common to gastrointestinal disorders that is associated with recurrent pneumonia is the propensity for recurrent aspiration. Disorders of the swallowing mechanism and esophageal diseases in particular need to be considered, including developmental abnormalities, diseases of striated muscle, diseases of motor function, collagen-vascular disorders, and others.

Tracheoesophageal (TE) fistula may arise as a developmental defect or as an acquired disease from a process such as trauma, tumor, or infection in the area adjacent to both organs. Some anatomic types are manifest shortly after birth and are easily detected. The least common type is characterized by a short patent connection between esophagus and trachea and may first become apparent in adult life. Clinically, patients complain of cough during meals when liquids (more commonly) or solids pass from the esophagus through the connection and enter the trachea, stimulating the cough reflex and predisposing the pneumonia. The diagnosis may be made by cine-esophagogram, but endoscopic examination of the esophagus and/or trachea may be necessary. Methylene blue is occasionally used in diagnosis (swallowed methylene blue may traverse the abnormal connection and turn the respiratory secretions blue). Surgery is curative. Other malformations, such as *congenital esophageal stenosis*, predispose to pneumonia, but they are rare and become manifest early in life.

Swallowing requires coordinated contraction of a series of muscles (tongue, pharynx, upper esophageal sphincter, and the proximal esophagus). *Diseases affecting these striated muscles* would also likely be associated with recurrent aspiration; examples include myasthenia gravis, myotonic dystrophica, dermatomyositis, and oculopharyngeal dystrophy. *Diseases of the central and peripheral nervous system* affecting the nerves controlling the muscles involved in swallowing may also be associated with aspiration; examples include cerebrovascular accidents, polio, amyotrophic lateral sclerosis, multiple sclerosis, and Huntington's chorea. It is unlikely that patients with these disorders will have recurrent pneumonia as their mode of presentation, but rather recurrent pneumonia complicates advanced disease. Treatment of the acute episode of aspiration usually is successful, but the key to adequate management is prevention. A depressed gag reflex is an easily detectable clinical finding indicating the need for preventive measures. Permanent tracheostomy, feeding gastrostomy, or cricopharyngeal myotomy are occasionally required for management.

Achalasia, a motor disorder of the esophagus, is characterized by 1) a failure in coordinated peristalsis and 2) a failure of the lower esophageal sphincter to relax normally. Dysphagia is common, but heartburn is rare. Regurgitation without bile or acid shortly after meals is common. The esophagus dilates in long-standing disease and halitosis from putrefaction in the pooled materials occurs. Routine chest x-ray may show an abnormal esophagus and occasionally an air-fluid level. Barium examination is used in diagnosis. Mechanical dilatation or surgery are used in management.

Scleroderma, a collagen-vascular disease, affects the skin and several other organs. When the esophagus is involved, motility may be sufficiently disturbed to promote aspiration.

Zenker's diverticulum is an outpouching of the posterior nasopharynx which becomes interposed between the esophagus and spine causing dysphagia. Repeated filling and emptying occurs predisposing to aspiration. Barium studies are useful in diagnosis and surgery in management.

Gastroesophageal reflux, if severe, may similarly predispose to aspiration and pulmonary infection. Aspirated gastric acid may damage the lung and cause pulmonary infiltrates without infection being present, but secondary infection in damaged areas occurs.

NEUROLOGIC DISORDERS

As in the gastrointestinal disorders predisposing to pneumonia, repeated aspiration is a common feature. A list of neurologic disorders affecting swallowing esophageal function was detailed previously. Nervous system diseases, not affecting esophageal function but also associated with recurrent pneumonia, include those associated with depressed consciousness, such as seizures, and those described previously which impair the gag reflex. The best approach to management is application of appropriate methods to prevent aspiration.

SUBSTANCE ABUSE

Patients with drug abuse or alcoholism are also prone to aspirate during episodes of severe central nervous system depression or in association with withdrawal seizures. Diagnosis is not difficult, but complete abstinence from the abused substance, the best preventive measure, is often difficult to achieve.

IMMUNE DEFICIENCY STATES

Defects in the immune system are uncommon causes of recurrent pneumonia, but such defects are important to recognize, because therapy is often helpful. Components of the immune system include: 1) B cells (lymphocytes that mature into antibody-producing plasma cells), 2) T cells (lymphocytes that modulate B cell function and release soluble substances called lymphokines that mediate cellular immunity), 3) complement (circulating serum proteins important in host defense and inflammation and that together with antibody comprise the humoral immune system), and 4) phagocytic cells.

ANTIBODY DEFICIENCY SYNDROMES

The B cell system is important in defense of bacterial infection, especially due to *Staphylococcus aureus*, streptococci, and *H. influenzae*. Defects may be suspected if repeated infection with these organisms occurs, and in disorders with depressed antibody production, otitis media, sinusitis, and pulmonary infection are common.

Congenital X-linked hypogammaglobulinemia is the prototype antibody-deficiency syndrome. The disease becomes manifest early in life after maternal antibody has been metabolized. The affected males suffer from recurrent infections with pyogenic organisms, including pneumonia. Bronchiectasis and pulmonary insufficiency are common. Diagnostically, one finds low to absent immunoglobulin levels, absent B cells in peripheral blood, and intact cellular immunity. Replacement therapy with gammaglobulin injections is helpful.

Common variable hypogammaglobulinemia, the most common functional antibody deficiency in adults, resembles the previous disease. However, this disorder affects both males and females; it can present at any age, but often does so in the third decade of life. The nature of the defect is unclear. In addition to recurrent pulmonary infections, malabsorption and autoimmune-like phenomena (pernicious anemia, hemolytic anemia, rheumatoid arthritis, and others) occur. Lymphadenopathy and splenomegaly may be present. Bronchiectasis is a late complication and the incidence of malignancy is increased. Total immunoglobulin levels are low, but B cell enumeration and T cell responses are variable. As in the previous disorder, replacement therapy with gammaglobulin is helpful.

Selective IgA deficiency is the most common antibody deficiency syndrome occurring in approximately one in 600 persons; however, most persons with this deficiency are asymptomatic. Sinopulmonary infections are common when infections occur, but only occasional patients have recurrent pneumonia. It is unclear at this time what factors cause the occurrence of infection in IgA-deficient persons. Gastrointestinal disease, allergy, and autoimmune phenomena are common. In contrast to the previous disorders, gammaglobulin and blood products should be avoided, because IgA-deficient persons make anti-IgA antibody after exposure to materials containing IgA, establishing the conditions for anaphylaxis. Treatment requires aggressive use of antibiotics for established bacterial infections.

Selective deficiency in IgM and IgG subclasses in varying combinations have been described. Repeated pulmonary infections occur, but these disorders are rare. Patients deficient in IgG and IgA, but with high IgM levels (immunodeficiency with hyper-IgM), may also have recurrent pulmonary infections. Recurrent pulmonary infection may also occur in secondary immunoglobulin deficiency states such as that associated with multiple myeloma or nephrosis.

CELLULAR-IMMUNE DEFICIENCY

The cellular immune system (T cell) is important in defense against viruses, fungi, and some intracellular pathogens (eg, *Mycobacterium tuberculosis*). Defects can be primary or they may be secondary to some other cause. Primary defects are common in children and secondary defects (Hodgkin's disease and other malignancies, steroid therapy, malnutrition, etc) common in adults. Clues suggesting the presence of T cell defects include 1) the occurrence of systemic illness following vaccination with live virus vaccine or BCG, 2) the occurrence of severe or complicated illness with common viral infection, or 3) resistance of oral or mucocutaneous *Candida* infection to respond to therapy.

Representative disorders include *congenital thymic dysplasia* (absent thyroid and parathyroid glands, hypocalemic tetany, cardiac disease, and characteristic facies) and *chronic mucocutaneous candidiasis*. They become manifest early in life. Recurrent bacterial pneumonia is not a prominent feature. Discussion of another disorder, *acquired immune deficiency* (AIDS), and pneumonia may be found in Chapter 17.

MIXED ANTIBODY AND CELLULAR DEFICIENCY

Patients with combined defects in B and T cell function are highly susceptible to infection with broad range of infectious agents including those considered "opportunistic pathogens." Onset is commonly early in life. Representative disorders include ataxia telangiectasia (cerebellar ataxia, oculocutaneous telangiectasis, recurrent sinopulmonary infections, and selective IgA deficiency in 40%) and Wiskott-Aldrich syndrome (eczema, thrombocytopenia, and recurrent pulmonary infections).

COMPLEMENT DEFICIENCY SYNDROMES

In general, deficiency in the early components of the classic pathway (C_1, C_4, C_2) is associated with a lupus erythematosis-like syndrome and deficiency in the late components with recurrent disseminated neisserial infection. Deficiency in C_2 alone, although common, is not generally associated with recurrent pneumonia, but C_2 deficient patients also deficient in Factor B (a component of the alternate pathway), may have repeated pulmonary infection. Patients with C_3 deficiency (decreased production or increased catabolism) or C_5 dysfunction or deficiency are also prone to repeated infection, but these disorders are rare. Patients with sickle cell disease have repeated and/or severe infections. Abnormalities in the function of the alternate pathway of complement activation as well as the RES have been described in these patients; the precise defect, however, is unknown.

PHAGOCYTE DISORDERS

Both quantitative and qualitative defects in phagocyte function have been described. Quantitative disorders may be hereditary (infantile genetic agranulocytosis, benign familial granulocytopenia, and cyclic neutropenia) or acquired. The most commonly encountered disorder is an acquired neutropenia secondary to drugs, in particular, cytotoxic chemotherapy. The risk of infection increases as the granulocyte count falls and the likelihood of infection is high when the neutrophil counts fall below $500/mm^3$.

Qualitative defects associated with recurrent pneumonia include Chediak-Higashi syndrome and chronic granulomatous disease of childhood. Chediak-Higashi syndrome is an autosomal recessive disorder characterized by oculocutaneous albinism, photophobia, and rotary nystagmus. Giant granules seen in many cell types, including neutrophils, are a marker of disease. The abilities of neutrophils to move towards a stimulus (chemotaxis) and to kill (bactericidal activity) are impaired. An accelerated phase resembling lymphoma or leukemia with lymphadenopathy, splenomegaly, and pancytopenia occurs in some patients. Death in childhood is common.

Chronic granulomatous disease is a sex-linked or autosomal recessive disorder. Recurrent infections with *S. aureus* and some aerobic gram-negative rods are common, but infection with catalase-negative organisms (pneumococcus, streptococcus, *H. influenzae*) are rare. The burst in oxidative metabolism that is associated with phagocytosis is defective in these patients. Lymphadenopathy, splenomegaly, and hepatomegaly are common. Pathologic examination of affected tissues shows noncaseating granuloma. The failure in oxidative metabolism is used as the basis of a test used in screening, the NBT test; neutrophils from patients fail to reduce nitroblue tetrazolium dye from yellow to blue. Treatment with ascorbic acid has been of value in some.

Defects in the ability for directed movement (chemotaxis), such as is seen in hyper-IgE syndrome (Job's syndrome), similarly predispose to recurrent bacterial infection and skin problems, including eczema, cold abscesses, and recurrent infection, may be seen. A high IgE level may suggest the hyper-IgE syndrome.

The workup of a patient with possible immunodeficiency may require extensive testing in a specialized laboratory. However, before such testing, the previously described historical clues should be used to define which immunologic functions require evaluation and the readily available tests useful in screening should be performed to determine whether additional specialized evaluation is necessary. The immunology laboratory should be used judiciously; Asherton and Webster (1980) stated that such testing is "unlikely to offer help in the management of most children with recurrent respiratory infections."

The following readily available tests are useful in screening for disorders of immune function. Disorders in antibody-mediated immunity may be assessed by quantitating immunoglobulin levels; by measuring isohemagglutinin titers; and by determining the antibody response after immunization (live virus vaccines should be avoided). Cellular immunity may be assessed using the white blood cell count and differential to measure total lymphocyte count and by evaluating the delayed hypersensitivity response to skin test antigens (*Candida*, trichophyton, mumps, and others). Complement activity may be evaluated by measuring total hemolytic complement (CH_{50}); tests for levels of the specific complement components, C_3 and C_4, are also readily available. Neutrophil function can be assessed with a white blood cell count and differential to measure total neutrophil count and with the NBT test.

MISCELLANEOUS

Diabetes mellitus and renal failure have been considered risk factors for recurrent pneumonia. As in congestive heart failure, conclusive evidence incriminating these disorders as risk factors per se is lacking. Sickle cell anemia has been discussed under complement disorders.

PERSPECTIVE

The previous discussion has focused on several disorders (some rare, some common) that have been associated with recurrent pneumonia. When faced with a patient with recurrent pneumonia, some notion of the relative frequency with which the various disorders occur would be useful. Winterbauer et al performed such a study in 1969 at Johns Hopkins Hospital. Table 13-2, modified from that report, details the illnesses found in 158 patients who had 612 episodes of pneumonia. In interpreting the table, it should be remembered that the study was retrospective, and patients were not evaluated in a standard fashion. Moreover, controls without recurrent pneumonia were not included, so one cannot determine which of the various disorders were significantly associated with recurrent pneumonia; in other words, this table only describes the illnesses found in a large group of patients with recurrent pneumonia.

Accepting these caveats, the following may be said: 1) thoracic and extrathoracic disorders appeared equally frequent, 2) patients without an

Table 13-2
Illness Associated with Recurrent Pneumonia*

Associated Disease	Number
Thoracic	
Chronic obstructive airway disease	46
Congestive heart failure	28
Bronchiectasis	23
History of pulmonary tuberculosis	13
Asthma	12
Previous pulmonary resection	11
Kyphoscoliosis	7
Organization of healing pneumonia	6
Postoperative complication	4
Bronchogenic carcinoma	2
Bronchogenic cyst	1
Silicosis	1
Extrathoracic	
Alcoholism	63
Diabetes mellitus	20
Chronic sinusitis	14
Chronic lymphocytic leukemia	4
Prostatic carcinoma	3
Multiple myeloma	2
Pharyngeal carcinoma	1
Epilepsy	6
Cerebrovascular accident	2
Sickle cell disease	3
Pernicious anemia and neutropenia	1
Aplastic anemia	1
Systemic steroid therapy	6
Systemic lupus erythematosis	3
Hypogammaglobulinemia	2
Primary biliary cirrhosis	1
No Associated Illness	11

*158 patients with 612 infections. Modified from Winterbauer et al (1969).

associated illness were rare, and 3) certain illnesses (bronchogenic carcinoma, multiple myeloma, chronic lymphocytic leukemia, and hypogammaglobulinemia) were uncommon. Importantly, they found that most associated illnesses were apparent before or at the time of hospitalization for the first pneumonia and that the vast majority of associated illnesses could be identified with a history, a physical examination, and a few simple laboratory tests. Other useful points emerging from that study include the observations that the extent of pneumonia and its localization did not depend on the site of the associated illness (thoracic or extrathoracic); that among patients with recurrent (three or more) pneumonia in the same anatomic area, localized lesions were often but not invariably present; and that patients with definite localized disease did not always have pneumonia restricted to that area. Finally, the case fatality ratio (two to six deaths per 100 episodes) was low and was in part related to the extent and frequency of penumonia.

GUIDELINES FOR EVALUATION

From the previous discussion, it should be readily apparent that some disorders associated with recurrent pneumonia are readily identified, but others require invasive or specialized testing and help from a specialist. Given the wide range and large number of diagnostic possibilities, it is also apparent that no rigid battery of tests can be defined for routine application in all patients and that a workup designed to evaluate all possible causes would not be cost-beneficial or wise. Rather, the best strategy is that the history and physical should be used to define the likely diagnostic possibilities, and the possibilities emerging from those procedures should be used to define the subsequent evaluation. In that way, needless and expensive tests can be avoided.

SELECTED READINGS

Allen JC: The diabetic as a compromised host, in Allen JC (ed): *Infection and the Compromised Host: Clinical Correlation and Therapeutic Approaches*. Baltimore, Williams and Wilkins, 1981, pp 229–270.

Ammann AJ, Fudenberg HH: Immunodeficiency diseases, in Stites DP, Stobo JD, Fudenberg HH, et al (eds): *Basic and Clinical Immunology*, ed 2. Los Altos, CA, Lange Medical Publications, 1982, pp 395–429.

Agnello V: Complement deficiency states. *Medicine* 1978;57:1–23.

Asherton GL, Webster ADB: *Diagnosis and Treatment of Immunodeficiency Diseases*. Oxford, Blackwell Scientific Publications, 1980.

Beard LJ, Maxwell GM, Thong YH: Immunocompetence of children with recurrent respiratory infections. *Arch Dis Child* 1981;56:101–105.

Chipps BE, Talamo RC, Winkelstein JA: IgA deficiency, recurrent pneumonias, and bronchiectasis. *Chest* 1978;73:519–526.

Dauber JH, Fogarty CM: Immunodeficiency states and recurrent respiratory tract infections, in Fishmann AP (ed): *Pulmonary Diseases and Disorders*, vol 2. New York, McGraw-Hill, 1980, pp 997–1009.

Dines DE: Etiologic considerations in recurrent pneumonia. *GP* 1967;36:96–105.

Goldstein IM: *Complement in Infectious Diseases*. A Scope Publication, The Upjohn Company, 1980.

Harrell J III: Middle lobe syndrome, in Bordow RA, Stool EW, Moser KM (eds): *Manual of Clinical Problems in Pulmonary Medicine with Annotated Key References*. Boston, Little Brown, 1980, pp 75–77.

Hong R: Immunodeficiency, in Rose NA, Friedman H (eds): *Manual of Clinical Immunology*, ed 2. Washington, DC, American Society of Microbiology, 1980, pp 833–849.

Hosking CS, Fitzgerald MG, Shelton MJ: The immunologic investigation of children with recurrent infection. *Aust Pediatr J* 1977;13(suppl):1–107.

Jomsson MS, McCormick JR, Gilles CG, et al: Kartagener's syndrome with motile spermatozoa. *N Engl J Med* 1983;307:1131–1133.

Kjellman B: Bronchial asthma and recurrent pneumonia in children. Clinical evaluation of 14 children. *Acta Pediatr Scand* 1967;56:651–659.

Malech HL: Abnormal neutrophil migration in Kartagener's syndrome, in Gallin JL (moderator): Disorders of phagocyte chemotaxis. *Ann Intern Med* 1980;92:520–538.

Murray JF: Bronchiectasis and broncholithiasis, in Petersdorf RG, Adams RD, Braunwald E, et al (eds): *Harrison's Principles of Internal Medicine*, ed 10. New York, McGraw-Hill, 1983, pp 1539–1542.

Nerenberg L, Crain L: Pulmonary sequestration. *West J Med* 1980;130:371–374.

Oseasohn R, Skipper BE, Tempest B: Pneumonia in a Navajo community: A two-year experience. *Am Rev Resp Dis* 1978;117:1003–1009.

Palmer D: Alcoholism, infection, and immunity, in Allen JC (ed): *Infection and the Compromised Host: Clinical Correlations and Therapeutic Approaches*. Baltimore, Williams and Wilkins, 1981, pp 121–156.

Pope CE III: The esophagus: Anatomy and developmental abnormalities, in Sleisenger MH, Fordtran JS (eds): *Gastrointestinal Disease, Pathophysiology, Diagnosis, and Management*, vol 1, ed 2. Philadelphia, WB Saunders, 1978, pp 495–503.

Pope CE III: The esophagus: Motor disorders, in Sleisenger MH, Fordtran JS (eds): *Gastrointestinal Disease, Pathophysiology, Diagnosis, and Management*, vol 1, ed 2. Philadelphia, WB Saunders, 1978, pp 513–540.

Van der Weide M, Haasbeck F, Hohmann FR, et al: Two patients with recurrent pneumonia in one lung. *Acta Med Scand* 1980;207:331–335.

Winterbauer RH, Bedon GA, Ball WC Jr: Recurrent pneumonia. Predisposing illness and clinical patterns in 158 patients. *Ann Intern Med* 1969;70: 689–700.

14 *Pneumonias of the Newborn Period and Infancy*

Stephen Baumgart
Alan R. Spitzer
Richard A. Polin

The causes of pneumonia occurring in pediatric patients vary according to the age of the patient. Group B streptococcus (GBS), some gram-negative enteric bacilli and *Staphylococcus aureus* are responsible for bacterial pneumonia in the newborn. GBS pneumonia presents within the first day of life. The clinical and radiographic pattern may simulate respiratory distress syndrome, but shock and apnea are more common in group B streptococcus. *S. aureus*, phage type 80/81, caused severe disease in newborn infants in epidemic proportions in the 1950s, but with the disappearance of this virulent strain, *S. aureus* infection is no longer the major problem it was before. Pneumonia due to gram-negative enteric bacilli occurs in the newborn with altered host defenses.

Pneumonia in the neonate also may result from congenital infection or infection acquired during delivery caused by *Treponema pallidum, Toxoplasma gondii*, rubella, cytomegalovirus and herpes simplex. From 2 weeks to 6 months of age, *Chlamydia trachomatis* is an important cause of afebrile pneumonia. From 2 months until 5 years of age, respiratory viruses are the most common causes of pneumonia. Respiratory syncytial virus is the leading cause, followed by parainfluenza virus type 3, of pneumonia in this age group. Other respiratory viruses include adenoviruses, influenza, echoviruses, and coxsackie viruses A and B. *S. pneumoniae* and *H. influenzae* type B cause bacterial pneumonia in children 6 months to 5 years of age. In children 5 years of age or older, *S. pneumoniae* and *Mycoplasma pneumoniae* are the major causes of pneumonia. *H. influenzae*, although it occurs in this age group, is relatively infrequent.

P. aeruginosa can cause a fatal necrotizing bronchopneumonia in children with cystic fibrosis. *Pneumocystis carinii* can cause pneumonia in debilitated, malnourished premature infants between 2 and 6 months of age and infants under 1 year of age with primary immunodeficiency disorders. Certain organisms, including *Pneumosystis carinii, S. aureus*, gram-negative enteric bacilii, *Nocardia*, fungi, cytomegalovirus and the herpes simplex viruses, cause pneumonia in those who have altered defense mechanisms, such as children being treated with cytotoxic and immunosuppressive drugs for malignancy, collagen-vascular disease or organ transplantation. Influenza virus may become a dominant cause during periods of epidemic spread and adenovirus may cause severe, progressive necrotizing bronchiolitis and pneumonia. Secondary pneumonia due to *S. pneumonia, S. aureus, H. influenzae* or group A streptococci may complicate measles, varicella or influenza.

The purpose of this chapter will be to discuss the epidemiology, clinical presentation, pathology, laboratory diagnosis and therapy of pneumonias commonly occurring during early infancy.

CATEGORIES OF PNEUMONIA

Respiratory distress is the most frequent indication for referral to an intensive care nursery. Lower respiratory tract infections account for a major portion of pulmonary disease during the neonatal period (first 28 days of life) and are an important cause of neonatal mortality and morbidity.

Four categories of pneumonia may be identified in the neonate based on the time of acquisition and age of presentation. Pneumonias that are acquired in utero and are transmitted hematogenously from mother to infant have been termed transplacental pneumonias or "TORCH" infections. TORCH is an acronym that stands for the organisms most frequently responsible for transplacentally acqired infections: *To*xoplasmosis, *Treponema pallidum, R*ubella, *C*ytomegalovirus, and *H*erpes simplex virus. However, other pathogens may also be acquired transplacentally (*Mycobacterium tuberculosis*, varicella-zoster virus, enteroviruses, hepatitis virus, etc). Pneumonias due to the TORCH pathogens may be distinguished by their frequent association with other systemic signs, ie, hepatosplenomegaly, encephalitis, nephritis, osteomyelitis, and rashes.

The second category of pneumonias are the congenital or intrauterine, which occur primarily in stillborn infants or infants dying within 24 hours of birth. These pneumonias can be diagnosed histopathologically by the presence of inflammatory cells in alveoli, often mixed with vernix and squamous cells. Round cells are frequently found in the interstitial spaces between small bronchioles and in the intraalveolar septa. Bacteria are not generally seen in these lung specimens and most cultures are negative. The characteristic findings of bacterial pneumonia (pleurisy, fibrinous exudate, etc) are frequently lacking. Fetal hypoxia and/or birth asphyxia are assumed to be the major factors responsible for these congenital or intrauterine pneumonias. In most cases, bacterial infection is not involved or plays only a minor role.

The third and most common category of neonatal pneumonias are those acquired during labor and delivery. These pneumonias are transmitted to the infant by upward spread of bacteria from the maternal genital tract into the amniotic cavity. The fetus aspirates or inhales the infected amniotic fluid prior to birth. Pathogens responsible for these pneumonias are those which colonize the maternal genital tract (group B streptococcus, *Escherichia coli, Klebsiella*). These infections are fulminant and are frequently associated with signs of cardiovascular instability. Almost one-half the infants suffering bacterial pneumonia succumb to their disease.

The last category of pneumonias are those acquired after birth. These pneumonias may present at variable times during the first month of life and are caused by viral (respiratory syncytial virus, influenza virus, adenovirus), chlamydial or bacterial agents (*Staphylococcus aureus* and coliforms) acquired at delivery, in the nursery or at home. Clinically and radiographically, they resemble the pneumonias of older children and adults, and are frequently bronchopneumonic or interstitial in type.

The pathogens reviewed in this chapter will be chlamydial pneumonia and cytomegalovirus and herpes simplex type 2 viral pneumonias. GBS pneumonia in the neonate is described in Chapter 22.

VIRAL PNEUMONIA IN THE NEONATAL-PERINATAL PERIOD

Viruses represent important, yet frequently undiagnosed agents capable of causing pneumonia in the perinatal and neonatal periods. The high cost of screening for viral infections and the relative lack of effective antiviral chemotherapy have discouraged physicians from vigorously pursuing a specific viral diagnosis when confronted by the neonate with pneumonia. Precise figures as to the frequency of viral pneumonia in the newborn are therefore lacking. The viruses that cause pneumonia in this age group fall into two major categories: those viruses capable of producing congenital infections, (ie, cytomegalovirus, herpes virus and rubella); and those viruses acquired postnatally.

PNEUMONIA CAUSED BY VIRUSES THAT PRODUCE CONGENITAL INFECTION

Cytomegalovirus (CMV)

Epidemiology At the present time, man is believed to be the sole reservoir for cytomegalovirus, with direct or indirect person-to-person contact being the sole pathway for transmission. Oropharyngeal secretions, urine, breast milk, blood, vaginal secretions and seminal fluid have been identified as sources of infection. CMV can be isolated from approximately 3% of pregnant women at term in the United States. The incidence may be higher in other populations. Viral shedding from the cervix may persist for months to years in infected women. Therefore, a substantial reservoir for CMV exists in the general population.

Between 0.5% and 2.5% of newborn infants are infected in utero with CMV. Presumably, many more will acquire the virus during the perinatal period from maternal cervical secretions or ingestion of infected breast milk. By school age, approximately 40% to 60% of children have detectable antibody indicative of prior infection.

The majority of congenitally infected infants are completely asymptomatic at birth, with only 10% showing any signs of the disease in the neonatal period. Typical signs of symptomatic congenital infection include: growth retardation, hepatosplenomegaly, jaundice, thrombocytopenia, purpura, chorioretinitis, microphthalmia, microcephaly, hydrocephalus, deafness, cerebral calcifications and pneumonitis. Those children who are asymptomatic in early life may develop effects later on, in particular, progressive auditory damage and pneumonia. Such "late effects" appear in approximately 10% of congenitally infected infants.

Several recent reports have examined the role of acquired cytomegalovirus infection within the neonatal intensive care unit. Ballard et al (1979) have reported that 16 of 51 infants hospitalized for more than 28 days acquired cytomegalovirus as manifested by viral excretion in the urine or nasopharynx. These authors speculated that CMV infection was acquired from whole blood transfusions received in the nursery. Fourteen infants demonstrated respiratory symptoms of tachypnea and retractions, which were accompanied by hepatosplenomegaly, a "septic" appearance (usually gray pallor), and lymphocytosis. Ventilatory assistance was instituted in all of these cases. The illness lasted approximately two weeks. Three infected infants died and autopsies revealed widespread viral seeding.

Pneumonitis of CMV Pulmonary manifestations of congenital CMV infection usually are overshadowed by the more devastating extrapulmonary manifestations. Infected infants, however, may have extensive alveolar and interstital pulmonary infiltrates. Chest roentgenogram appearance is relatively nonspecific and typically consists of a diffuse interstitial pattern (Figure 14-1). Although infants may have respiratory symptoms shortly after birth, nonspecific signs such as lethargy, poor feeding, apnea, tachypnea and cyanosis are more commonly seen. Lung secretions from infants with CMV pneumonia may be thick and tenacious, leading to extensive atelectasis. Respiratory support may be necessary during the acute phase of the disease and intubation is also helpful in permitting better tracheobronchial toilet in the young infant. The duration of respiratory disease may be from days to weeks.

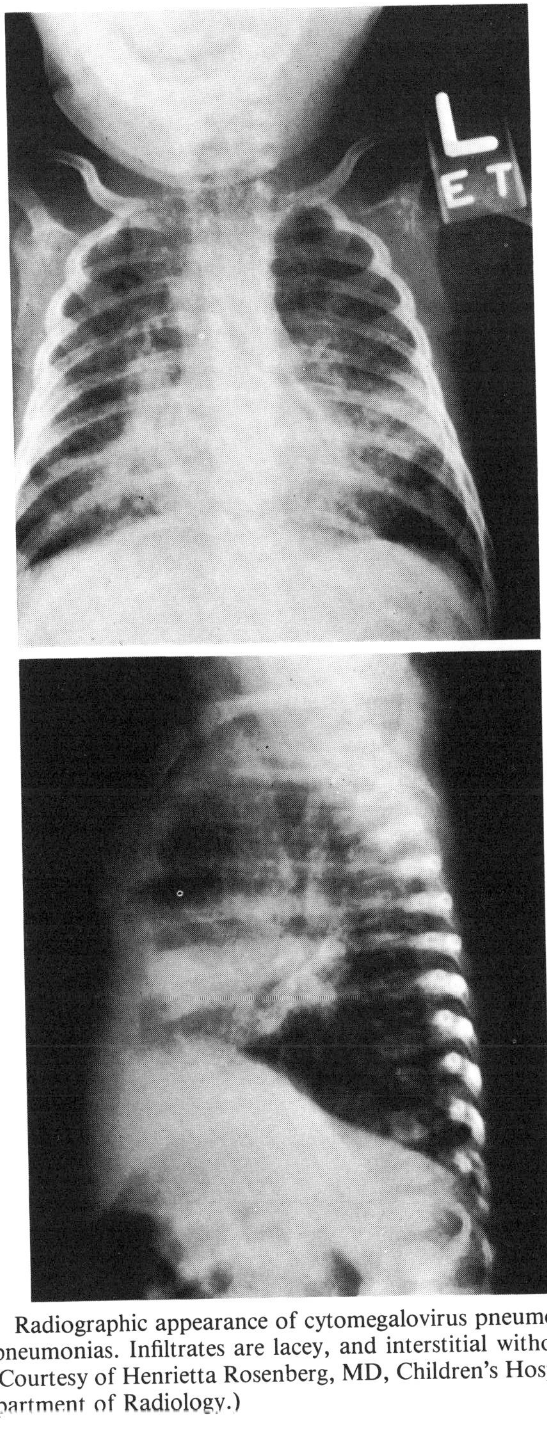

Figure 14-1 Radiographic appearance of cytomegalovirus pneumonia is similar to all viral pneumonias. Infiltrates are lacey, and interstitial without focal consolidation. (Courtesy of Henrietta Rosenberg, MD, Children's Hospital of Philadelphia, Department of Radiology.)

Diagnosis and therapy of CMV Diagnosis of CMV should be confirmed by isolation of virus from urine or tracheobronchial secretions. Depending on the amount of virus present, diagnosis can usually be made after a few days following inoculation of excreta into tissue cultures. Serologic methods that demonstrate viral antibody in serum or secretions can also be used to confirm the diagnosis. Elevated umbilical cord or infant blood IgM that is specific for CMV denotes intrauterine infection and is helpful in screening symptomatic infants.

Treatment of cytomegalovirus in the newborn is primarily preventive. No effective anti-CMV agents presently exist. It is not possible to determine severity of fetal infection prenatally, although maternal infection during pregnancy can be diagnosed by either viral isolation in the urine or complement fixation by antibody in the serum. Active infection, particularly in the first trimester of pregnancy may therefore present the clinician with a difficult management decision regarding termination of pregnancy. Breast milk transmission poses a risk to the premature infant and milk should be screened if used in the intensive care nursery. To date, no serious sequelae from feeding term infants breast milk infected with CMV have been documented.

Acquisition of CMV infection from transfusion of infected blood products has resulted in some advocates advising that blood products given to premature infants be screened for CMV antibody. An alternate approach might be to transfuse the premature infant with only washed, frozen red blood cells, since it is believed that CMV in blood is carried within the white blood cells.

Herpes Virus

Epidemiology Herpes simplex virus (HSV) is a common cause of sexually transmitted disease in the United States (see Chapter 46). The genital tract of the mother represents the source of HSV (usually HSV-2) in most instances of neonatal HSV infection. The majority of maternal infections are asymptomatic. Only 36% of pregnant women with cytologically proven herpetic infections have clinically recognizable lesions. If symptoms are present, they usually consist of vesicular lesions in the cervix, vagina or perineum. Redness, swelling and tenderness may be present, accompanied by local lymphadenopathy. Lesions often ulcerate and may persist in shedding virus for one to three weeks, following which re-epithelialization occurs and viral shedding stops. Following such primary infections, it is believed that the virus travels up sensory nerves, entering a latency period in sensory ganglia. Reactivation may occur at a later time, with lesions reappearing in previously involved areas.

Although infection during pregnancy is in the range of 1%, the rate is significantly less near term, ranging from one in 250 to one in 1000 pregnancies. Transplacental infection may occur, although it is believed to be uncommon. Most often, infection of the newborn infant occurs around the time of birth, either from ascending infection in the mother with premature rupture of membranes, or as the child comes in contact with genital lesions during passage through the birth canal. In addition to rupture of membranes, active primary lesions and premature delivery appear to enhance the rate of neonatal infection. Approximately 120 cases of neonatal herpes virus infection are reported annually in the United States, far less than the predicted rate. Either many cases in neonates are asymptomatic and unrecognized, or other as yet undetermined factors serve to reduce the risk of infection in infants born to affected mothers.

Clinical syndromes The spectrum of findings in the newborn with herpes infection is variable, ranging from asymptomatic to severe overwhelming viremia. The incubation period is typically six to 12 days. The signs of infection most commonly demonstrated include vesicular rash, temperature instability, lethargy, cyanosis, vomiting, jaundice, apnea and respiratory distress. Approximately two thirds of affected infants have severe generalized symptoms with or without central nervous system involvement; in the remaining one third of symptomatic children, infection is localized to skin, eye, oral mucosa or central nervous system. Central nervous system disease may be manifested by irritability, seizures, apnea, bulging fontanelle, opisthotonus, decerebrate posturing or coma. Chorioretinitis, more typically observed in congenital infection with CMV or toxoplasmosis, also may be seen.

Respiratory distress is commonly noted in symptomatic patients and is manifested by tachypnea, retraction, cyanosis and diffusely decreased breath sounds. Radiologically, these babies have a diffuse, nonspecific pattern of interstitial pneumonia and, rarely, patchy infiltrates. Lung involvement frequently necessitates support with oxygen and mechanical ventilation. Prognosis with extensive disease is poor, with a mortality rate of 80% to 90%. Those survivors in whom central nervous system involvement is present have a 60% incidence of severe neurologic sequelae.

Diagnosis and therapy Diagnosis of herpes virus infection is confirmed by viral isolation from lesions in mother or infant, or viral isolation from buccal mucosa, eye, cerebrospinal fluid, or blood buffy coat. In some cases in which the virus appears to be confined to the central nervous system, brain biopsy may be required to confirm a diagnosis of HSV cerebritis. During acute neonatal disease, serologic studies usually are not helpful, since antibody titers to HSV may not rise until several weeks after the onset of infection. Immunofluorescent techniques to quantitate HSV-specific IgM antibodies are available and may be used to measure HSV antibody in convalescent sera to confirm diagnosis.

At present, treatment of symptomatic herpes virus remains primarily supportive, although recent studies suggest that adenine arabinoside (Ara-A) will reduce mortality in babies with disseminated or localized central nervous system disease. The recommended dose of Ara-A is 15 mg per kilogram per day administered by continuous infusion over 12 hours each day for 10 days. Infants with localized disease respond more favorably to therapy than those with disseminated disease, but some infants in both categories demonstrate progression of symptoms. Neurologic impairment in treated babies appears to be reduced by Ara-A.

Prevention of HSV infection is still of critical importance. The mother with active lesions at parturition should be delivered by Caesarean section, preferably within four hours after rupture of membranes. The use of immunoglobulin administered to newborn infants remains controversial, although animal studies support the idea that administered antibody may protect against neonatal disease.

Other Congenital Infections Producing Pneumonitis

Congenital rubella and varicella may also be prenatally acquired and produce a pneumonitis. In both of these infections, pneumonia plays a relatively minor role in the overall symptomatology. Respiratory symptoms and radiographs are nonspecific and appear similar to those seen in the two viruses (cytomegalovirus and HSV) described in detail above.

Postnatally Acquired Viral Pneumonia

Pneumonias caused by viral agents other than those acquired congenitally are occasionally seen in the infant less than 2 months of age. In all cases, exposure to adults or older children who are nasopharyngeal carriers of the organism involved is essential for infection of the infant. Viruses commonly implicated in postnatally acquired pneumonias include respiratory syncytial virus (RSV), parainfluenza viruses, adenoviruses, influenza viruses, and enteroviruses. Late fall to early spring is the season during which these infections most frequently occur.

In infants less than 2 months of age RSV infection rarely produces a bronchiolitic syndrome. More frequently, they display nonspecific findings including hypothermia or hyperthermia, coryza, cough, congestion, anorexia or vomiting and apnea. In infants with RSV and adenovirus infections, apnea may be the most important finding. Tachypnea (respiratory rate greater than 60/min), tachycardia (heart rate greater than 140 beats/min), nasal flaring, retractions, and cyanosis can also be seen. Physical examination may reveal fine rales, diminished air entry, and evidence of pleural effusion. Exanthems may also accompany infection and are typically maculopapular, erythematous eruptions that last for two to three days.

Radiologic findings are variable but most commonly consistent of perihilar infiltrates, or patchy atelectasis. Lobar consolidation is uncommon. Hyperaeration may occur in some infants because of air trapping.

Diagnosis is primarily made by physical and radiologic evaluation.

Leukocyte counts are variable and nonspecific. Rapid slide diagnosis by immunofluorescence for RSV and influenza may be helpful in some cases. Serologic diagnosis is rarely helpful or necessary, and viral isolation techniques do not often influence diagnosis or treatment during the acute phase of the illness. Consequently, the expense for these studies, except during epidemics, usually is not warranted.

Treatment is supportive in nature. Antipyretics, parenteral fluid therapy, and oxygen may be useful in severe cases. For the infant with apnea and bradycardia, careful monitoring in the hospital with ventilatory support may be required.

CHLAMYDIA PNEUMONIA IN INFANCY

Chlamydia trachomatis infection occurs most commonly in adult males, manifested as nongonococcal urethritis. Urethral cultures of 30% to 58% of men with symptomatic urethritis are reported to be positive for *C. trachomatis* and negative for gonococci. Female contacts of this population have a reported incidence of culture positive infection from 21% to 31%. Of these women, 12% to 31% are asymptomatic. These figures have established *C. trachomatis* as the most commonly occurring, venereally transmitted genital infection.

In 1942, Thygerson and Stone first established the association between maternal cervicitis with *Chlamydia trachomatis* and a sterile infant conjunctivitis termed inclusion blennorrhea. Iodinophilic inclusion bodies were demonstrated in epithelial cells scraped from the eyelids of affected infants. Since then, various incidence figures have been reported for the prevalence of *Chlamydia* colonization of the cervix during pregnancy. Early incidence reports of *Chlamydia* infections during pregnancy ranged from 0.8 to 0.34 per 100 live births and were based on cytologic evidence from cervical scrapings. More recently, Hammerschlag et al (1979) reported prospective data on 322 urban women. Culture-positive cervical swabs occurred in 2% of this population. However, 47% of women were cervical secretion antibody-positive and 73% were serum antibody-positive for recent *Chlamydia* infection, suggesting a higher incidence than the 2% culture isolation rate. Other authors have subsequently reported a somewhat higher rate of culture-positive infection ranging from 8.8% to 18%.

Twenty-one percent to 66% of infants born to mothers who are culture-positive for *Chlamydia* during pregnancy will become colonized with *Chlamydia* in the conjunctiva or nasopharynx (Table 14-1). Of these infants one-quarter to one-half will develop symptomatic conjunctivitis or pneumonia. The incidence of *Chlamydia* pneumonia following nasopharyngeal colonization is estimated to range from 3% to 17%. Hammerschlag et al have estimated that if 5% of all pregnant women are

Table 14-1
Follow-up of Infants Born to Chlamydia Culture-Positive Mothers

Study	No. Women Followed During Pregnancy	No. Cervical Cultures Positive (%)	Fraction Of Infants Followed Subsequently Culture Positive (%)	No. Infants with Symptomatic Infection, Pneumonia and Conjunctivitis (%)	No. Infants with Pneumonia (%)
Hammerschlag 1979	322	6 (2)	4/6 (66)	3/6 (50)	1/6 (17)
Frommel 1979	340	30 (8.8)	8/18 (55)	8/18 (55)	2/18 (11)
Heggie 1981	1327	240 (18)	27/95 (28)	23/95 (24)	3/95 (3.1)

colonized by *Chlamydia* and if 10% of infants born from these pregnancies contract pneumonitis, then 15,000 cases of *Chlamydia* pneumonia would occur in the United States each year. The conclusion drawn from these statistics is that *Chlamydia* pneumonia may be the most prevalent "nonbacterial" lower respiratory tract infection in early infancy beyond the immediate neonatal period.

The first report of infant pneumonia attributed to *Chlamydia trachomatis* infection was published in 1975 by Schacter et al. Since this initial report, evidence for the etiologic role of *Chlamydia* in infant pneumonia has accumulated rapidly. The pneumonia syndrome (Table 14-2) is characterized by an indolent onset of respiratory symptoms in infants 2 to 3 weeks of age. Symptoms progress slowly over one to two weeks to an afebrile pneumonitis characterized by a harsh, dry, repetitive cough, similar to pertussis but without paroxysms. The most common age range for diagnosis is between 3 and 11 weeks. Physical exam commonly reveals tachypnea and fine abundant rales generalized over both right and left lung fields. Pardoxically, breath sounds are clear and wheezing is usually absent. Chest roentgenography (Figure 14-2) reveals symmetrical hyperexpansion with diffuse interstitial and patchy alveolar infiltrates. No lobar consolidation is seen, and only occasional pleural reactions occur. Arterial blood gases frequently show mild to moderate hypoxemia and normocapnea. Peripheral white blood cell counts generally manifest an absolute eosinophilia, greater than 400 cells per mm^3. Determinations of serum immunoglobulins characteristically reveal IgG levels greater than 500 mg/dL, IgM greater than 110 mg/dL and IgA greater than 30 mg/dL. The course of *Chlamydia* pneumonia is protracted (two to three weeks). Cough, and radiographic abnormalities may persist more than a month.

The prevalence of *Chlamydia* pneumonia in early infancy has been determined prospectively by culturing infants with lower respiratory tract infections for pathologic bacteria, viruses and other types of

Table 14-2
Chlamydia Pneumonia: Clinical Syndrome

1. History of cough, congestion for 1 to 2 weeks. Onset of symptoms at 2 to 3 weeks of age. Diagnosis of pneumonia presenting at 3 to 11 weeks.
2. Absence of fever, malaise. Mild respiratory distress with tachypnea. Rales with clear air entry, absence of wheezing or air trapping.
3. Chest roentgenogram with hyperinflation, patchy, diffuse alveolar infiltrates. No lobar consolidation.
4. Mild hypoxemia.
5. Eosinophilia $>$ 400 cell/mm^3. IgG $\geq$ 500, IgM $\geq$ 110, IgA $\geq$ 30 mg/dL.
6. Protracted course of 2 to 3 weeks. Abnormal radiography $\geq$ one month.

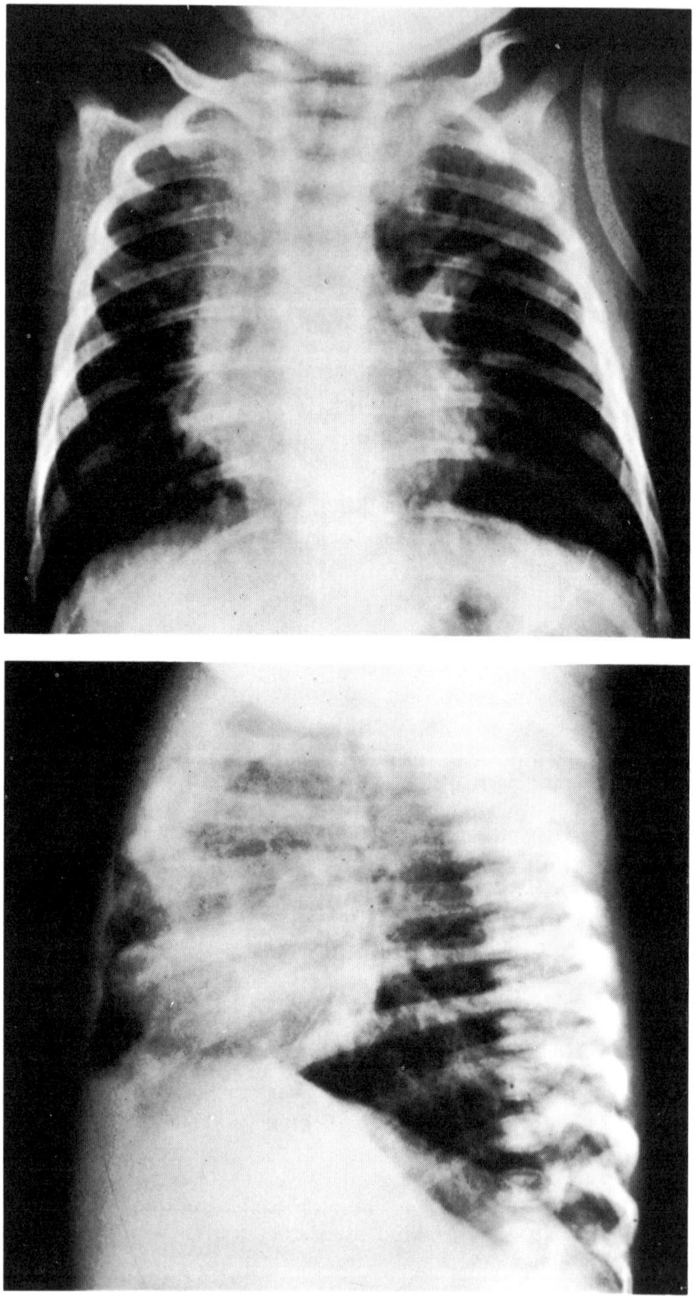

Figure 14-2 Radiographic appearance of *Chlamydia* pneumonia. Hyperinflation of both lung fields with diffuse, patchy alveolar infiltrates. There is no lobar consolidation. (Courtesy of Henrietta Rosenberg, MD, Children's Hospital of Philadelphia, Department of Radiology.)

organisms. Twenty-five percent to 90% of infants presenting with afebrile pneumonia at less than 6 months of age are nasopharyngeal or tracheal culture-positive for *Chlamydia.* A relatively high incidence of coinfection (26% to 50%) with viral and other pathogens has been reported. The most common virus isolated is cytomegalovirus, although coinfections with adenoviruses, rhinoviruses, respiratory syncytial virus and enteroviruses have been described. Stagno et al (1981) found that approximately one half of infant pneumonias that were culture-positive for *Chlamydia* were accompanied by coinfection with cytomegalovirus, *Ureaplasma urealyticum* and/or *Pneumocystis carinii.* Cytomegalovirus, *Chlamydia* and *Ureaplasma* are all acquired venereally, and multiple infections tend to occur in the youngest infants.

Treatment of Chlamydia Pneumonia

Information regarding the treatment of *Chlamydia* pneumonia is sparse. Harrison's study evaluated the use of systemic sulfonamide therapy versus other antibiotics (usually penicillin or ampicillin) retrospectively. *Chlamydia* shedding was eliminated in six of six sulfonamide-treated infants, and in only three of five infants treated with antibiotics ineffective against *Chlamydia* in cell culture. Three infants receiving no therapy continued to shed *Chlamydia* throughout the clinical course of the pneumonia.

Beem et al (1979) reported the only prospective evaluation of antibiotic therapy. In addition to supportive therapy (oxygen, parenteral fluid hydration, and chest physiotherapy), 32 infants received either no antibiotic, sulfisoxazole (150 mg/kg/day), or erythromycin (40 mg/kg/day). Infants managed without chemotherapy continued to shed *Chlamydia* for 10 to 60 days. *Chlamydia* were eradicated by erythromycin on day one in some cases, and in all cases by day six. Sulfisoxazole was also effective in eradicating *C. trachomatis* by day six of therapy. Clinical improvement noted by physical exam occurred by the end of one week in all instances in which antibiotics were administered.

These data suggest that treatment of *Chlamydia* pneumonia in infancy with erythromycin or sulfonamide is beneficial in eradicating organisms from the nasopharynx and in promoting clinical improvement. Since coinfection with *Chlamydia* and *Ureaplasma urealyticum* is possible, erythromycin should be considered the agent of choice until definitive therapeutic trials are conducted.

SELECTED READINGS

Viral Pneumonias

Adams HG, Benson EA, Alexander ER, et al: Genital herpetic infection in men and women: Clinical course and effect of topical application of adenine arabinoside. *J Infect Dis* 1976;133(suppl):A151.

Ballard RA, Drew WL, Hufnagle KG, et al: Acquired cytomegalovirus infection in preterm infants. *Am J Dis Child* 1979;133:482.

Baublis JV, Whitley RJ, Ch'ien LT, et al: Treatment of cytomegalovirus infection in infants and adults, in Pavan-Langston D, Buchanan RA (eds): *Adenine Arabinoside: An Antiviral Agent.* New York, Raven Press, 1975, pp 247–260.

Berkovich S, Taranko L: Acute respiratory illness in the premature nursery associated with respiratory syncytial virus infections. *Pediatrics* 1964;34:753.

Bruhn FW, Mokrohisky ST, McIntosh K: Apnea associated with respiratory syncytial virus infection in young infants. *J. Pediatr* 1977;40:382.

Cheeseman SH, Hrisch MS, Keller EW, et al: Fatal neonatal pneumonia caused by echovirus type 9. *Am J Dis Child* 1977;131:1169.

Glezen WP, Denny FW: Epidemiology of acute lower respiratory disease in children. *N Engl J Med* 1973;288:498.

Hayes K, Danks DM, Gibas H, et al: Cytomegalovirus in human milk. *N Engl J Med* 1972;28:177.

Jacobs JW, Peacock DB, Corner BD, et al: Respiratory syncytial and other viruses associated with respiratory disease in infants. *Lancet* 1971;1:871.

Lang DJ, Ebert PA, Rodgers BM, et al: Reduction of postperfusion cytomegalovirus infections following the use of leukocyte depleted blood. *Transfusion* 1977;17:391.

Miller DR, Hanshaw JB, O'Leary DS, et al: Fatal disseminated herpes simplex virus infection and hemorrhage in the neonate. *J Pediatr* 1970;76:409.

Lake AM, Lauer BA, Clark JC, et al: Enterovirus infections in neonates. *J Pediatr* 1976;89:787.

Light IJ: Postnatal acquisition of herpes simplex by the newborn infant. A review of the literature. *Pediatrics* 1979;63:480.

Monif GRG, Egan EA, Held B, et al: The correlation of maternal cytomegalovirus infection during varying stages in gestation with neonatal involvement. *J Pediatr* 1972;80:17.

Mufson MA, Krause HE, Mocega HE, et al: Viruses, *Mycoplasma pneumoniae,* and bacteria associated with lower respiratory tract disease among infants. *Am J Epidemiol* 1970;91:192.

Nahmias AJ, Josey WE, Naib ZM, et al: Perinatal risk associated with maternal genital herpes simplex infection. *Am J Obstet Gynecol* 1971;110:825.

Nahmias AJ, Roizman B: Herpes simples viruses. *N Engl J Med* 1973;289:667, 719, 781.

Nahmias AJ, Visintine AM:Perinatal herpes simplex virus infection, in Remington JS, Klein JO (eds): *Congenital and Perinatal Infection.* Philadelphia, WB Saunders, 1974, p 156.

Spector SA, Schmidt K, Ticknor W, et al: Cytomegaloviruria in older children in intensive care nurseries. *J Pediatr* 1979;95:444.

Stagno S, Reynolds DW, Pass RF, et al: Breast milk and the risk of cytomegalovirus infection. *N Engl J Med* 1980;19:1973.

Starr JG, Bart RD, Gold E: Inapparent congenital cytomegalovirus infection. *N Engl J Med* 1970;282:1075.

Torphy DE, Ray CG, McAlister R, et al: Herpes simplex virus infection in infants: A spectrum of disease. *J Pediatr* 1970;76:405.

Whitley RJ, Brasfield D, Reynolds DW, et al: Protracted pneumonitis in young infants associated with perinatally acquired cytomegaloviral infection. *J Pediatr* 1976;89:16.

Whitley RJ, Nahmias AJ, Soong SJ, et al: Vidaratine therapy of neonatal herpes simplex virus infection. *Pediatrics* 1980;66:495.

Whitley RJ, Nahmias AJ, Visintine AM, et al: The natural history of herpes simplex virus infections of mothers and newborn. *Pediatrics* 1980;66:489.

Whitley RJ, Soong SJ, Dolin R, et al: Adenine arabinoside therapy of biopsy-proved herpes simplex encephalitis. *N Engl J Med* 1977;297:289.

Yeager AS: Transfusion acquired cytomegalovirus infection in newborn infants. *Am J Dis Child* 1974;128:478.

Yeager AS, Grumet FC, Hafleigh, EB, et al: Prevention of transfusion acquired cytomegalovirus infections in newborn infants. *J Pediatr* 1981;98:281.

Chlamydia Pneumonia

Beem MO, Saxon EM: Respiratory tract colonization and a distinctive pneumonia syndrome in infants infected with *Chlamydia trachomatis. N Engl J Med* 1977;296;306.

Beem MO, Saxon EM, Tipple MA: Treatment of Chlamydia pneumonia in infancy. *Pediatrics* 1979;63:198.

Frommell GT, Rothenberg R, Wong San-pin, et al: Chlamydial infection of mothers and their infants. *J Pediatr* 1979;95:28.

Hammerschlag MR: Chlamydial pneumonia in infants. *N Engl J Med* 1978; 298:1083.

Hammerschlag MR, Anderka M, Semine DZ, et al: Prospective study of maternal and infantile infection with *Chlamydia trachomatis. Pediatrics* 1979; 64:142.

Harrison HR, English MG, Lee CK, et al: *Chlamydia trachomatis* infant pneumonitis. *N Engl J Med* 1978;298:702.

Heggie AD, Lumincao GG, Stuart LA, et al: *Chlamydia trachomatis* infection in mothers and infants. *Am J Dis Child* 1981;135:507.

Paavonen J: Chlamydia infections. *Med Biol* 1979;57:135.

Schacter J, Lun L, Gooding CA, Ostler B: Pneumonitis following inclusion blennorrhea. *J Pediatr* 1975;87:799.

Stagno S, Brasfield DM, Brown MB, et al: Infant pneumonitis associated with cytomegalovirus, chlamydia, pneumocystis and ureaplasma: A prospective study. *Pediatrics* 1981;68:322.

Tipple MA, Beem MO, Saxon EM: Clinical characteristics of the afebrile pneumonia associated with *Chlamydia trachomatis* infection in infants less than six months of age. *Pediatrics* 1979;63:192.

Wang EP, Grayston JT, Alexander ER, et al: Simplified microimmuno-fluorescence test with trachoma-lymphogranuloma venereum (*Chlamydia trachomatis*) antigens for use as a screening test for antibody. *J Clin Microbiol* 1975;1:250.

15 *Nosocomial Respiratory Tract Infections*

Jerome Santoro

DEFINITION

Uniform criteria for the diagnosis of nosocomial lower respiratory tract infections have not been used in the many studies published on this topic. Thus, the true incidence of hospital-acquired pneumonia is not precisely known. The Hospital Infections Branch of the Centers for Disease Control (CDC) criteria are most frequently employed in practice to define nosocomial pulmonary infection. In adults without pulmonary infection on admission there must be onset of purulent sputum no sooner than 48 hours after admission to the hospital or, in those with pneumonia on admission, recrudescence of sputum production and fever and at least one of the following criteria: 1) infiltrate on chest x-ray or physical findings of pneumonia when x-rays are unavailable, or 2) cough, fever, and pleuritic chest pain. In children a diagnosis is made even in the absence of purulent sputum provided that the latter two criteria are met. A diagnosis of pneumonia by the attending physician is also accepted even when the criteria are incompletely fulfilled. Suprainfection is considered to be present when a new pathogen is isolated from the bronchial secretions and the patient deteriorates either clinically or radiographically.

The CDC definitions are imprecise and their use results in overdiagnosis. For instance, a patient with a previous pneumonia may become colonized with *Serratia marcescens* in the hospital and develop new infiltrates due to congestive heart failure or a pulmonary infarction. Someone doing hospital infection surveillance who is not directly caring for the patient might feel that the individual has suprainfection because the criteria are fulfilled. In spite of these shortcomings, the CDC criteria are probably adequate for routine data collection, surveillance, and comparison purposes. When scientifically studying nosocomial respiratory tract infection, more strict criteria (such as those of Johanson et al, 1972) may be more suitable. These criteria are: 1) the appearance of a new infiltrate on x-ray, 2) fever, 3) elevated white blood cell count, and 4) purulent pulmonary secretions. The presence of three of four criteria qualifies as probable infection, while if four are met, the diagnosis of respiratory infection is considered definite.

INCIDENCE, MORBIDITY, AND MORTALITY

Nosocomial infections of the respiratory tract have been reported to occur in a 0.5% to 5% of hospitalized patients, the real figure probably being much closer to 0.5%. These infections account for 10% to 15% of all hospital-acquired infections and rank third behind urinary tract infection and wound infection in order of frequency. However, pulmonary infections account for the greatest number of deaths due to nosocomial infection, and about one half of patients who acquire pneumonia in the hospital die. It has been estimated anywhere from 20,000 to over 100,000 patients die each year from nosocomial respiratory tract infection, and these statistics have been remarkably constant over the last several years.

The acquisition of pneumonia in the hospital is most prevalent among patients on the medical and surgical services, whereas patients on other hospital services tend to have a much lower prevalence rate. Hospital-acquired pneumonia is especially common among terminally ill patients and frequently is the cause of their demise. Many patients who do not die from nosocomial pneumonia most certainly have prolonged hospital stays and, therefore, a huge expenditure of additional health care dollars must result, not to mention the added morbidity to the patient.

PATHOGENESIS

The ways in which bacteria may reach the lung include: 1) hematogeneous spread, 2) bacteria suspended in inhaled gas, 3) by aspiration of pharyngeal contents. Once the organisms reach the alveoli, the efficacy of the host's pulmonary antibacterial defense mechanisms will determine whether or not pneumonia results.

Hematogenous Spread

Although sites of infection distant from the lung can cause bacteremia and subsequent pneumonia, this mode of infection is probably the least common of those mentioned above. However, remote septic foci (eg, intra-abdominal infections) can affect the lung indirectly. For example, patients with intra-abdominal sepsis seem to be predisposed to adult respiratory distress syndrome. Also, dogs that are given peritonitis seem to have impaired clearing of inhaled bacterial aerosols when compared to uninfected control animals. Thus, the presence of infection remote from the lung may be an important predisposition to the development of nosocomial pulmonary infection.

Suspensions in Inhaled Gas

Hospital-acquired gram-negative bacillary pneumonia associated with contaminated nebulizer equipment has long been recognized. In fact, epidemics of pneumonia due to *Klebsiella pneumoniae*, *Pseudomonas aeruginosa*, and *Serratia marcescens* have been traced to these devices. Nebulizers moisten the inhaled gas with aerosols of small particles called droplet nuclei (1.0 to 2.0 μm) which are then able to reach the terminal bronchioles of the tracheobronchial tree. When aerosol reservoirs become contaminated with bacteria, the organisms become suspended in the aerosol as particles and can reach the alveoli. Routine cleaning of nebulizers with acetic acid has been shown to reduce the number of outbreaks of gram-negative rod necrotizing pneumonia within certain hospitals. Humidifiers also moisten inhaled gas, but in contrast to nebulizers, they do not produce small particle aerosols. Therefore, humidifiers probably play a much lesser role in the development of nosocomial respiratory tract infection. The awareness of the potential role of respiratory assistance devices in the production of nosocomial respiratory infections has led to efforts of prevention. A review by Cross and Roup (1981) of the acquisition of nosocomial pneumonia related to respiratory assistance devices showed that respiratory equipment is now rarely a direct cause of hospital-associated pneumonia.

Coughs and sneezes may also generate small particle aerosols capable of reaching the distal parts of the tracheobronchial tree, and exhaled gas from patients on ventilators has been shown to contain gram-negative bacilli. However, except for aerosols produced by patients with tuberculosis, the overall density of bacteria in hospital air that results from these potential sources of infection is usually too low to make these important mechanisms in the production of nosocomial pulmonary bacterial infection. Viruses on the other hand, such as influenza, can spread from person to person through hospitals by droplet nuclei just as they do in the community.

Colonization of the Oropharynx and Aspiration of Pharyngeal Contents

Although the term *aspiration pneumonia* carries a certain connotation, in a sense most pneumonias, whether they be hospital or community-acquired, are due to aspiraton of oropharyngeal contents. Studies have shown that many healthy people aspirate in their sleep. It is reasonable to assume that ill hospitalized patients, especially those who are sedated or have neurologic disease, aspirate even more frequently.

Obviously, healthy individuals do not develop pneumonia when aspiration takes place, whereas hospitalized patients do with appreciable frequency. The reason for this might be related in part to depression of pulmonary defense mechanisms and in part to the phenomenon of pharyngeal colonization with gram-negative bacilli that occurs in the hospital. Pharyngeal cultures from normal, nonhospitalized individuals are rarely positive for aerobic gram-negative bacilli (about 2%). Even when normal individuals are exposed to massive inocula of gram-negative bacilli, colonization of the throat does not take place. However, alcoholics and diabetics have been shown to harbor these organisms more commonly. Johanson and colleagues (1969) noted that hospitalized patients acquired gram-negative bacilli among their pharyngeal flora. Although pneumonia does not invariably develop in individuals who become colonized, it occurs far more frequently in this setting. In the study of Johanson et al for instance, 25% of colonized patients developed pneumonitis as compared to only 3% of those patients who were not colonized. Colonization, and therefore pneumonia, occurred more frequently among more severely ill patients. In fact, about 20% of these individuals were colonized upon admission to the hospital. Colonization may occur as frequently as 75% in this group as compared to 30% to 40% of patients overall.

Although colonization often occurs without antimicrobial therapy, the prevalence is increased when antibiotics are instituted, especially among intensive care unit patients. Other studies have confirmed these findings but suggested an important role for ventilators, nasogastric and endotracheal tubes, and the like. Thus, the bulk of evidence suggests the major determinant of pharyngeal colonization with gram-negative bacilli and a greater risk for subsequent nosocomial pneumonia is severe debility and underlying disease with impairment of the host pharyngeal clearance mechanisms. Antibiotic therapy, nasogastric tubes and ventilatory support devices seem to play adjunctive roles in further impairing pharyngeal clearance mechanisms and thereby facilitating gram-negative rod overgrowth.

The source of these organisms has never been completely defined. Presumably some colonization occurs from endogenous (eg, gut) flora, as many patients are colonized upon admission to the hospital. This theory is supported by studies that show that newly found gram-negative bacilli in the oropharynx are those predominant among the fecal flora. Furthermore, the predominant species in the fecal flora often change during hospitalization and these organisms are then found in the pharynx. Other patients may be colonized through contamination from the hospital environment (hands of personnel, or ventilatory equipment). The latter is obviously the case when clusters of patients are noted to harbor the same organisms. Waterborne organisms such as *Pseudomonas, Klebsiella, Enterobacter,* and *Acinetobacter* may be particularly important colonizers.

CLINICAL CONSIDERATIONS

Predisposing Factors

As outlined previously, pharyngeal colonization with gram-negative bacilli is an important risk factor for the development of nosocomial pulmonary infections. Certain clinical conditions enhance the probability of colonization and subsequent pneumonia. In addition, some of these states may also impair pulmonary host defenses. Iatrogenic and host factors that have been correlated with risk of nosocomial pulmonary infection due to gram-negative bacilli include: alcoholism, diabetes mellitus, antimicrobial therapy, advanced age, general debility, severe underlying disease, and major surgery. Within these categories, the presence of coma, hypotension, tracheal intubation, acidosis, azotemia, and leukopenia significantly increase the likelihood of colonization and therefore infection.

The correlation of risks for nosocomial infection in general, and for nosocomial respiratory tract infection, specifically, with severity of underlying disease, is particularly striking. The attack rate in one study for respiratory tract infection was 11.6% for patients with fatal underlying diseases, 5.8% for individuals with ultimately fatal diseases, and 1.2% for those with nonfatal disease.

Postoperative patients are also at risk for the development of respiratory tract infection. In this light, nosocomial pneumonia rates among surgical patients have not changed appreciably since the 1940s. It is believed that depressed respiratory clearing mechanisms due to recent endotracheal anesthesia, sedation, diminished cough and gag reflexes, hypoventilation due to pain and discomfort, and patient immobility all add to the likelihood of pulmonary stasis and aspiration. The risk factors for postoperative pneumonia in 520 patients undergoing elective thoracic and upper and lower abdominal surgery has recently been studied by Garibaldi and his colleagues (1981). Lower respiratory tract infection developed in 17.5% of patients studied. The acquisition of pneumonia was highly correlated with preoperative indicators of severity of underlying diseases such as low serum albumin, and high American Society of Anesthesiologists' preanesthesia physical status classification. Smoking, longer preoperative stay, prolonged operative procedures, and thoracic or upper abdominal sites of surgery were important risk factors for postoperative respiratory tract infection. Massive obesity, old age, and male sex were also associated with increased incidence of pneumonia, but statistical significance was lost when these variables were controlled for site and duration of the operative procedure. In general, the risk of postoperative infection would be greatest for an obese male (greater than 250 lb), with significant underlying diseases undergoing a coronary artery bypass procedure. In contrast, the risk for pneumonia should be negligible in a patient who is a nonsmoker undergoing a short lower abdominal procedure. The acquisition of pneumonia by patients such as the latter should alert the physician or the hospital infection surveillance team to the possibility of a potentially preventable nosocomial infection.

The patient bedded in the intensive care unit runs the greatest risk of acquisition of pulmonary infection. In this setting the use of endotracheal tubes, nasotracheal tubes, and tracheostomies is common. These instruments bypass the upper airway defense mechanisms and predispose to tracheal and bronchial trauma because of the frequent mechanical suctioning they necessitate. The clustering of high-risk patients (for colonization and pneumonia) in intensive care units, compounded by problems of physical crowding and understaffing that are common in many hospitals, may lead to breaks in technique and thereby increase the risk of patient-to-patient spread of respiratory pathogens.

Another group of patients that is at risk for acquisition of nosocomial respiratory tract infection is the so-called immunocompromised host. Patients with leukemia, lymphoma, or conditions that require chemotherapy, corticosteroids, or immunosuppressive therapy, fall into this category. These individuals are also prone to developing infections with unusual pathogens (see below). Pulmonary infection in the immunocompromised host is discussed in detail in Chapter 17.

Induction of general anesthesia and bronchoscopy have been implicated in the development of subsequent pulmonary infection. However, such cases are uncommon and anesthesia and bronchoscopy per se must be considered unusual causes of nosocomial respiratory tract infection.

Infecting Organisms

The bacteria that cause nosocomial respiratory tract infections in 1978, according to the National Nosocomial Infection Study Report issued in 1981, are listed in Table 15-1. This table lists the relative frequency of isolation for each particular pathogen. More than one organism may be isolated from one patient. In the preceding discussion of the pathogenesis of hospital-acquired lower respiratory tract infection, colonization of the pharynx with gram-negative bacilli and subsequent development of pulmonary infection was emphasized. However, upon examination of the table, one can readily see that gram-negative bacilli comprise only slightly less than 50% of all the isolates listed. Gram-positive bacteria make up almost 17% of the organisms listed, and *S. aureus* accounts for over 10% of the total organisms recovered. Perhaps the most striking figure is that in almost one fourth of all cases of nosocomial lower respiratory tract infections reported to the CDC, no pathogen was identified.

Another interesting aspect of Table 15-1 is the lack of anaerobic bacteria listed. If one assumes that aspiration of pharyngeal contents is the most important mechanism in the pathogenesis of hospital-acquired lower respiratory tract infection, anaerobic bacteria should be present in at least some of these infections. Obviously, the vast majority of sputum samples sent to the clinical laboratory are coughed specimens or represent tracheal secretions obtained via suctioning maneuvers. The latter, unlike transtracheal aspirates, are not suitable for anaerobic isolation. In studies utililzing the latter technique, it has been shown that enteric gram-negative bacilli and pseudomonas are much more common among patients who acquire infections in the hospital than those who become infected in the community. However, anaerobes are recovered from both groups, and in some hospitalized patients anaerobic bacteria may be the sole pathogens (approximately 10%). Thus, some proportion of those pulmonary infections listed in Table 15-1, in which no pathogen was isolated, may be due to anaerobic bacteria. In fact, colonization is such a common occurrence among hospitalized patients, the isolation of gram-negative bacilli from a coughed sputum specimen does not necessarily mean that the particular organism is present in the role of pathogen and anaerobic bacteria may be the principal organisms present at the alveolar level more often than is appreciated clinically. *Hemophilus influenzae*, which is also not listed in the table, has been incriminated as a major pathogen in some cases of nosocomial pneumonia. The organism has received more attention in this regard in the United Kingdom than it has in the United States.

It should be kept in mind that organisms other than bacteria may also be important in nosocomial respiratory tract infections. Viruses, for instance, have received little attention in the literature. Influenza A has been shown to be a cause of nosocomial pneumonia during concomitant community outbreaks. Respiratory syncytial virus has also caused problems within hospitals on the pediatric service. The so-called immunocompromised host is particularly prone to infections with unusual organisms.

Table 15-1
Relative Frequency of Selected Pathogens Causing Nosocomial Lower Respiratory Tract Infection*

Pathogens	Percent Isolates
Staphylococcus aureus	10.4
Streptococcus pneumoniae	3.8
Streptococcus (Groups A, B, D)	2.4
Escherichia coli	7.3
Klebsiella sp	10.8
Enterobacter sp	6.7
Proteus-Providencia sp	6.1
Pseudomonas aeruginosa	8.8
Serratia sp	3.3
Other	16.9
No culture, no pathogen	24.2

*Modified from Centers for Disease Control: *National Nosocomial Infections Study Report, Annual Summary 1978,* issued March 1981.

Table 15-2
Some Microorganisms Capable of Producing Pulmonary Infection in the Compromised Host

Bacteria	Fungi
Acinetobacter	*Aspergillus*
Corynebacteria	*Candida*
Enterobacteriacae	*Cryptococcus*
Hemophilus influenzae	*Torulopsis*
Legionella	*Zygomycetes*
Mycobacteria	Helminths
Nocardia	*Strongyloides stercoralis*
Pseudomonas	Protozoa
Staphylococci	*Pneumocystis carinii*
Streptococcus pneumoniae	*Toxoplasma gondii*
Chlamydia	Viruses
*Chlamydia trachomatis**	Cytomegalovirus
	Herpes simplex
	Varicella-zoster

*Suspected but not proven.

Some of the organisms that may be acquired by these patients are listed in Table 15-2. The precise incidence of these infections is unknown. Furthermore, it is often difficult to decide whether these infections originate endogenously from the patient's prehospitalization flora or whether the organism is acquired in the hospital. For example, pneumonia due to disseminated herpes zoster is usually a reactivation of the patient's latent infection that was present prior to hospitalization. On the other hand, pulmonary infection due to *Aspergillus* sp is most likely due to the acquisition of this organism in the hospital. Pneumonia due to *Pneumocystis carinii* may be due to reactivation of latent infection within the host, but reports of clusters of hospitalized patients with this infection suggest rather convincingly that this pathogen may be spread person-to-person in the hospital.

DIAGNOSIS

A diagnosis of nosocomial pneumonia should be considered when there is a new pulmonary infiltrate or extension of an old one in association with new fever, elevation of white blood cell count, and the production of purulent sputum.

Much has been written about specific clinical presentations with certain gram-negative pathogens. For example, *Pseudomonas aeruginosa* is said to cause a nodular bronchopneumonia, *Proteus* sp an upper lobe consolidation with tracheal shift, *Klebsiella* a lobar pneumonia, and *Escherichia coli* and *Enterobacter* sp bronchopneumonia. Although these distinctions are of academic interest, practically speaking they are not consistently found, and it is dangerous to select antimicrobial therapy based solely on roentgenographic appearance. In general it can be said that gram-negative pneumonia usually begins as a patchy alveolar infiltrate and evolves to affect the lower lobes most frequently, but any pulmonary segment may be involved. Necrosis of the pulmonary parenchyma may then occur with the development of empyema and sometimes bronchopleural fistula. If air fluid levels on x-ray or foul-smelling empyema or secretions are noted, then anaerobic or mixed aerobic-anaerobic infection is certain to be present.

The bacteriologic diagnosis of hospital-acquired pulmonary infection can be made by culturing and staining pulmonary secretions obtained in several fashions. Specimens may be obtained through 1) expectoration or suctioning of material from endotracheal tubes, 2) transtracheal aspiration, 3) bronchoscopy, and 4) needle aspiration of pulmonary tissue. The diagnosis also can be confirmed by isolating pathogens from blood or pleural fluid.

Expectorated sputum or tracheal secretions obtained through suctioning are utilized most frequently in most clinical settings. However, such specimens obtained from hospitalized patients who frequently are colonized with gram-negative bacilli are contaminated by oropharyngeal contents when passing through the mouth, and thus may contain several species of potentially pathogenic microorganisms. For this reason, examination of the sputum by gram stain often is more valuable clinically than subsequent culture results. The presence of few and preferably no squamous epithelial cells, abundant polymorphonuclear leukocytes and alveolar macrophages indicates that the specimen originated in the lower respiratory tract and is relatively uncontaminated by upper airway organisms. Bacteria in proximity to leukocytes may be especially significant with regard to the indentity of the etiologic agent or agents.

Bronchoscopy frequently is utilized to obtain pulmonary secretions. In order to avoid contamination with upper airway organisms, shielding procedures have been utilized. In general, contamination cannot be avoided and bronchoscopy adds little to the examination of a good expectorated sputum specimen. However, in patients who have difficulty in raising secretions, bronchoscopy may be helpful.

The technique of transtracheal aspiration bypasses the pharynx and, therefore, circumvents the problem of contamination to some degree. Transtracheal aspiration should be considered in severely ill patients with suspected nosocomial pneumonia in whom the diagnosis is in doubt. Although anaerobic cultures obtained from expectorated sputum or from bronchoscopic specimens are worthless, specimens obtained by transtracheal aspiration are suitable for anaerobic culture. However, recent studies have pointed out that material obtained by transtracheal aspiration may also be contaminated and not completely reflect the flora involved in the infectious process.

Microorganisms isolated from pleural fluid are, of course, pathogenic. Positive blood cultures at the time of pneumonia for an organism also present in the sputum are likewise diagnostic. Needle aspiration of the lung parenchyma is not frequently carried out in immunosuppressed patients in whom unusual opportunistic organisms are suspected. These individuals may also require transbronchial or open lung biopsy for precise diagnosis. In general, in our experience, invasive techniques, such as transtracheal aspiration, lung aspiration, and biopsies, are not necessary in the routine case when a good sputum specimen is available for culture and gram stain, and chest x-ray reveals a new pulmonary infiltrate.

Treatment

Antimicrobial regimens for hospital-acquired pneumonia are outlined in Table 15-3. Initial therapy is based on the examination of the gram stain of expectorated sputum, transtracheal aspiration, pleural fluid or lung tissue. Because a wide variety of gram-negative bacilli, alone or in combination, as well as anaerobic bacteria may be responsible for these infections, it is usually necessary to employ combinations of antimicrobial agents (Table 15-3).

Table 15-3
Initial Treatment of Nosocomial Pneumonia

Standard Coverage

1. Aminoglycoside (gentamicin or tobramycin)
   plus
   1st generation cephalosporin (eg, Cefazolin)
   or
2. 3rd generation cephalosporin (eg, moxalactam, cefoperafone, cefotaxime)
   with or without
   aminoglycoside

Additional Considerations

Problem	Adjustment
1. Suspected aminoglycoside resistance	Substitute amikacin for gentamicin or tobramycin
2. Neutropenic patient or other clinical situations with high probability of pseudomonas infection	Substitute ticarcillin plus tobramycin
3. Highly suspect anaerobes	Clindamycin or penicillin with aminoglycoside

PREVENTION AND CONTROL OF NOSOCOMIAL RESPIRATORY TRACT INFECTIONS

All physicians should be familiar with hospital infection control measures. Prevention of nosocomial respiratory tract infection is based on minimizing transmission of respiratory pathogens within the hospital and subsequent colonization of the patient's pharynx with gram-negative rods. This is best accomplished through the proper conduction of nursing techniques, hospital isolation, and surveillance policies, and care and maintenance of respiratory therapy equipment. The essential elements of effective control of respiratory tract infection have been nicely summarized by Pantelick (1978).

General Measures

General supportive measures, such as maintaining an open airway, frequent turning, coughing, deep breathing, and incentive spirometry plus early ambulation for surgical patients, are important in preventing pooling of lower respiratory tract secretions.

Hand Washing

Ironically, in this age of ultrasophisticated medicine, hand washing remains the single most important measure for preventing all types of nosocomial infections. Contaminated hands of medical personnel are responsible for transmission of nosocomial pathogens from one patient to another in most instances. Hands must be washed before and after direct contact with patients or their secretions and before handling sterile equipment or administering respiratory therapy or diagnostic tests.

Suctioning

Suctioning should *not* be performed routinely, as trauma and invasion of the airways occur. Indications for suctioning include the presence of audible secretions or an increase in the pressure/volume ratio of a ventilatory assist device. Aseptic technique must always be utilized while performing endotracheal suctioning. The following steps should be followed:

- Wash hands prior to the procedure.
- A sterile catheter tray with transparent catheter, glove, and bowl should be utilized.
- Repeated withdrawal and reinsertion of the same catheter are not recommended, and the catheter should be discarded after each use.
- Use sterile water for flushing and irrigation. Single-use disposable ampules are available.

- Use sterile suction bottles and tubing.
- Change tubing and bottles every 12 to 24 hours.
- Suction apparatus should be equipped with high efficiency filters to prevent bacterial contamination of ambient air and machinery.

Tracheostomy Care

As previously discussed, patients with tracheostomies are at increased risk for nosocomial pulmonary infections. Aseptic technique must be adhered to when handling the tracheostomy site. The following points deserve emphasis:

- Wash hands.
- Use strict aseptic technique, including sterile gloves and drapes.
- Cleanse adjacent skin with iodine-iodophor applied to a sterile swab every eight to 12 hours.
- Apply antimicrobial ointment or iodine-iodophor locally.
- Once the tract is stabilized, change the tube every two to four days using a sterile replacement.
- With metal tubes, the inner cannula should be changed every two to four hours when secretions are particularly abundant.
- Apply sterile dressings.
- Provide a high humidity environment to prevent drying of the respiratory mucosa and secretions.

Respiratory Therapy Equipment

As pointed out in a prior section, respiratory therapy equipment, solutions, and medications have been implicated as the source in some nosocomial outbreaks of pulmonary infection. The following recommendations should be adhered to:

- Use sterile medications and solutions; unit-dose is preferred over multidose vials.
- Use sterile distilled water. Discard unused portions daily.
- Empty humidifiers and nebulizers entirely before refilling.
- Use sterile breathing circuits and accessories (may be disposable or reusable).
- Use ultra-high efficiency filters on main flow lines and medication nebulizer air-drive systems on equipment designed or adaptable for such a filter.
- Replace the entire breathing circuit, including humidifiers and nebulizers at least every 24–48 hours on machines used for IPPB or aerosol treatments.

- Replace the entire patient breathing circuits on all machines that are being used for more than one patient, between each patient.
- Cover all preassembled equipment used for emergencies. Reservoirs should *not* be filled in advance.
- Oxygen analyzers, vital capacity gauges and the like should be cleaned and decontaminated according to manufacturer's specifications.

Proper handling of contaminated materials is also important in the prevention of spread of pathogens to other patients, personnel, and the inanimate environment. All component parts including mouthpieces, tubing, masks, nebulizers, humidifiers, and exhalation valves should be placed in plastic bags and sealed at the bedside. Several methods of sterilization are available, including steam autoclaving, gas sterilization with ethylene oxide, pasteurization, liquid chemicals, and the use of disposable products. In general, it is important to adhere to the manufacturer's recommendations for disassembling, cleansing, and sterilizing equipment.

Isolation

With the exception of patients with pulmonary infections due to *S. aureus* or *S. pyogenes*, patients with bacterial pneumonia generally do not require isolation. Both *S. aureus* and *S. pyogenes* can be members of the normal respiratory flora. Thus, the identification of these organisms in cultures of respiratory secretions does not necessarily mean that the patient is infected with them. Colonization with these organisms does not require isolation of these patients. Strict isolation or at least geographic separation may be reasonable for patients who have pneumonia due to *S. aureus* or *S. pyogenes* or highly antimicrobial resistant gram-negative bacteria.

Surveillance

Hospital surveillance of all nosocomial infections should be carried out in order to identify problem areas and take appropriate control measures.

Surveillance of nosocomial respiratory tract infections per se consists of defining the entity, collecting the relevant data systematically, tabulating and analyzing these data, and disseminating the information obtained to all who need to know it (eg, infection control committee, nursing staff, medical staff, hospital administration, community, etc).

As discussed previously, the best definition of nosocomial respiratory tract infection for the purpose of surveillance is that of the CDC. In order to identify cases, one must know where to retrieve the appropriate data to fit the definition. The sources of information most helpful in this regard are the following:

- Microbiology laboratory reports of cultures of respiratory tract secretions.
- Ward rounds with special attention to patients with fever, endotracheal tubes, increased respiratory tract secretions or predisposition to nosocomial respiratory tract infection (coma, immunosuppression, etc).
- Admission office for admission diagnosis of pneumonia in patients recently discharged from the hospital.
- Pharmacy for new antibiotic prescriptions.
- X-ray reports of new or increasing pulmonary infiltrates.
- Autopsy reports.

Once the appropriate data are retrieved from these sources, it should be tabulated and analyzed. Incidence rate (number of infections per specific unit of time, eg, one month) and prevalence rate (number of infections at a specific point in time) should be determined. The hospital location of the infected patient, the use of respiratory equipment, or the presence of other factors that might predispose to nosocomial respiratory tract infection should be recorded. In this fashion problem areas and clusters or point outbreaks of infection can be identified so that corrective and preventive measures can be undertaken.

Experimental Procedures

Instillation of either aminoglycosides or polymyxin into the respiratory tree has been carried out in an attempt at prevention of nosocomial pulmonary infection with gram-negative rods. Results of studies have been mixed. However, in some instances, resistant strains have emerged, and in at least one study mortality was increased in the group of patients who received instillation of polymyxin. This type of procedure cannot be recommended for routine use.

SELECTED READINGS

Aber CR, Bennet JV: Surveillance of nosocomial infections, in Bennett JV, Brachman PS (eds): *Hospital Infections*. Boston, Little Brown Co, 1979.

Britt MR, Schleupner CJ, Sego M: Severity of underlying disease as a predictor of nosocomial infection. *JAMA* 1978;239:1047–1051.

Centers for Disease Control: *National Nosocomial Infections Study Report, Annual Summary 1978*, issued March 1981.

Cross AS, Roup B: Role of respiratory assistance devices in endemic noscomial pneumonia. *Am J Med* 1981;70(3):681–685.

Eickhoff TC: Pulmonary infections in surgical patients. *Surg Clin North Am* 1980;60(1):175–183.

Garibaldi RA, Britt MR, Coleman ML, et al: Risk factors for postoperative pneumonia. *Am J Med* 1981;70(3):677–680.

Johanson WG, Pierce AK, Sanford JP: Changing pharyngeal bacterial flora of hospitalized patients: Emergence of gram-negative bacilli. *N Engl J Med* 1969;281:1137.

Johanson WG Jr, Pierce AK, Sanford JP, et al: Nosocomial respiratory infetions with gram-negative bacilli. *Ann Intern Med* 1972;77:701.

LaForce FM: Hospital-acquired gram-negative rod pneumonias: An overview. *Am J Med* 1981;70(3):664–669.

Lerner AM: The gram-negative bacillary pneumonias. *DM* 1980;27(2):1–56.

Lorber B, Swenson RM: Bacteriology of aspiration pneumonia: A prospective study of community- and hospital-acquired cases. *Ann Intern Med* 1974; 81:329.

Pantelick EL: Infection control in respiratory care. *Infect Control Urol Care* 1978;3:4–6.

Stamm EW: Gram-negative pneumonias: Diagnosis and management. *Drug Therapy* May 1979.

Tillotson JR, Finland M: Bacterial colonization and clinical superinfection of the respiratory tract complicating antibiotic treatment of pneumonia. *J Infect Dis* 1969;119:597–624.

16 *Pneumonia in the Aspiration-Prone Patient*

Bennett Lorber

Aspiration is the process during which matter present in the oropharynx is carried through respiration (inhalation) into the lower tracheobronchial tree. There may be no consequence of aspiration, or it may result in damage to the lung parenchyma; to a large degree, the result of aspiration depends on the type and amount of material aspirated as well as the host's lung clearance mechanisms.

ASPIRATION SYNDROMES

Aspiration is more properly thought of as several aspiration syndromes, implying different etiologies and pathophysiologic mechanisms, and requiring different modes of therapy (Table 16-1).

Chemical Pneumonitis

Acute pneumonia may follow aspiration of many toxic agents, the most common of which is gastric acid. The injury to the lung is virtually instantaneous, resulting in marked hypoxemia and a significant mortality of 30% to 60%. Treatment is to correct hypoxemia and may require early use of positive-pressure ventilatory support. Use of corticosteroids in this form of aspiration remains controversial, but efficacy has not been demonstrated in controlled studies and adverse effects may occur. Bacterial pneumonia is a common complication of acid aspiration, but available data indicate that the use of antibiotics in acid aspiration does not decrease the incidence of infections or improve the outcome.

Reflex Airway Closure

Aspiration of inert fluids (water, saline, nasogastric feedings, gastric contents with $pH < 2.5$) may produce reflex airway closure (laryngospasm) and pulmonary edema with resultant hypoxemia. Treatment is intermittent positive-pressure breathing with 100% O_2 and isoproterenol.

Mechanical Obstruction

Aspiration of inert fluid or particulate matter (partially digested food, hot dogs, peanuts) may produce simple mechanical obstruction.

Table 16-1
Aspiration Pneumonia Syndromes

Type	Inoculum	Clinical Presentation	Therapy
Chemical pneumonitis	Toxic fluids (gastric acid)	Acute dyspnea, hypoxemia; lower lobe infiltrates	O_2, Positive-pressure breathing Intravenous fluids Corticosteroids (?)
Reflex airway closure	Inert fluids	Pulmonary edema	Intermittent positive-pressure breathing with O_2 Isoproterenol
Mechanical obstruction	Inert fluids Particulate matter	Acute dyspnea in patients with no cough reflex Ranges from chronic irritating cough to acute dyspnea, depending on level of airway obstruction	Tracheal suction Extraction of foreign body (Bronchoscopy)
Infection	Oropharyngeal bacteria	Productive cough, fever, infiltrate in dependent pulmonary segment; cavitation is a late complication	Antimicrobial drugs

Cough occurs secondary to bronchial irritation. Wheezing and dyspnea may follow and radiographs show atelectasis. Secondary bacterial pneumonia may occur. Therapy is early tracheobronchial suction and removal of large particulate matter by fiberoptic bronchoscopy.

Aspiration Pneumonia

Aspiration pneumonia is a bacterial pulmonary infection which commonly follows aspiration of a suspension in saliva of the oropharyngeal bacterial flora.

Patients present a picture of pulmonary infection with cough, fever, purulent sputum, and radiographic evidence of an infiltrate, usually in a dependent pulmonary segment. Bacterial aspiration pneumonia may also complicate any of the other aspiration syndromes. Therapy is with antimicrobial drugs.

THE ASPIRATION-PRONE PATIENT

Conditions predisposing to aspiration are shown in Table 16-2. Although aspiration is common in normal individuals during sleep, pulmonary complications in otherwise healthy individuals seldom occur. Individuals prone to develop pulmonary complications are those who because of underlying conditions are likely to aspirate frequently due to: 1) reduced level of consciousness with consequent compromise of glottic closure and cough reflex (eg, stroke victims, anesthesia subjects, patients with seizure disorders); 2) dysphagia secondary to esophageal or neurologic disorders (eg, esophageal carcinoma or scleroderma); or 3) mechanical disruption of the esophageal sphincter due to a nasogastric tube. The volume and character of the inoculum are also important; individuals with poor dental hygiene have increased areas of anaerobiosis and consequently may aspirate larger numbers of anaerobic bacteria than those with normal dentition. Gingivodental disease seems important in pathogenesis since the numbers of bacteria in the aspirated oropharyngeal inoculum may be increased by 100- to 1000-fold in the presence of this condition. In addition, patients who develop bacterial pneumonia following aspiration frequently have impairment of the normal lung clearance mechanisms. For example, aspirated particulate matter may interfere with mucociliary transport, and alcohol and hypoxemia may impair alveolar macrophage function.

PATHOPHYSIOLOGY OF ASPIRATION PNEUMONIA

Most bacterial pneumonias occur following initial oropharyngeal colonization and subsequent aspiration; however, the term aspiration pneumonia is generally reserved for those situations in which pneumonia

Table 16-2
Conditions Predisposing to Aspiration

Altered Level of Consciousness
Alcoholism
Seizures
Drugs
Anesthesia
Central nervous system disorders
Trauma
Dysphagia
Esophageal disorders
Neurologic disorders
Mechanical Disruption of Functional Barriers
Nasogastric tube

due to normal oropharyngeal bacteria develops in an indvidual prone to aspiration.

The rare occurrence of pneumonia following aspiration is evidence that the lung possesses remarkably efficient and effective clearance mechanisms. The process of aspiration and clearance can be thought of as a cycle (Figure 16-1). If the aspirated inoculum is large or contains virulent bacteria the clearance mechanisms may be overcome and pneumonia may occur. Similarly, if the mucociliary apparatus and/or alveolar macrophages cannot function normally, aspiration of relatively avirulent organisms, such as normal mouth flora, may produce pneumonia.

BACTERIOLOGY

Aspiration pneumonia is an endogenous infection; that is, the source of the pathogens in the patient's oropharyngeal flora. The infection is typically polymicrobial, but the component microorganisms vary depending upon whether the infection was community-acquired or hospital-acquired (Table 16-3). If community-acquired, the pathogens include numerous normal obligate anaerobic bacteria that typically reside in gingival crevices and are constantly shed into the saliva. The oropharyngeal flora of hospitalized patients differs from that of normals since these individuals commonly become colonized with facultatively anaerobic pathogens, such as enteric gram-negative rods, pseudomonads, and *Staphylococcus aureus*. Consequently, aspiration pneumonia acquired in the hospital frequently involves these facultative anaerobic bacteria, often in combination with the usual obligate mouth anaerobes. Obligate anaerobic bacterial species isolated from community- and hospital-acquired cases are similar; common isolates are *Fusobacterium nucleatum*, *Bacteroides melaninogenicus*, peptostreptococci, and peptococci. *Bacteroides fragilis* is occasionally found in

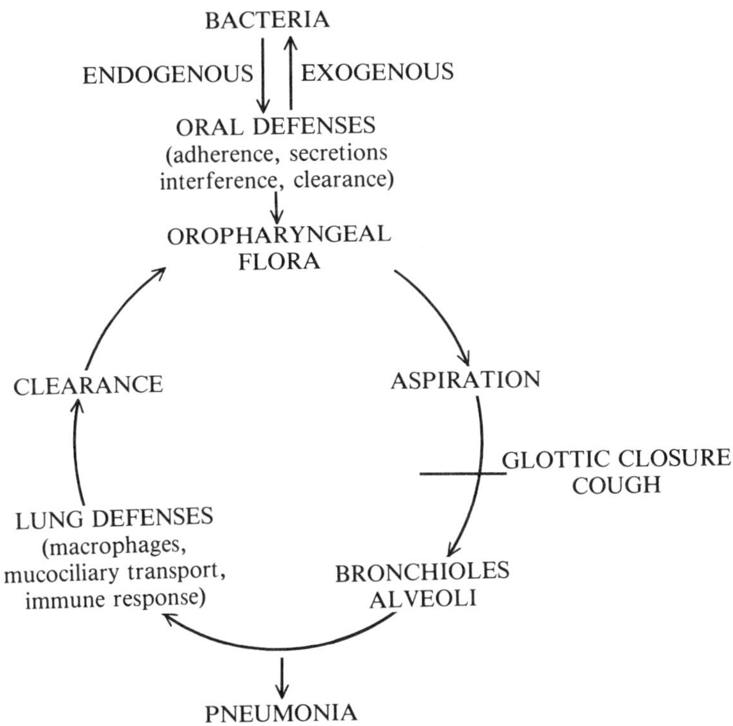

Figure 16-1 Aspiration cycle. The oropharyngeal flora is determined by interaction of endogenous and exogenous bacteria as well as oral defense mechanisms. Aspiration occurs commonly even in healthy individuals. Glottic closure and cough help prevent aspiration of large volumes and particulate matter. Lung defense mechanisms clear aspirated bacteria. If the aspirated inoculum is large or virulent, or if the normal lung defense mechanisms are impaired, pneumonia may result.

Table 16-3
Bacteriology of Aspiration Pneumonia

Types of Bacteria	Community-Acquired (62 patients) *(No.)*	*(%)*	Hospital-Acquired (55 patients) *(No.)*	*(%)*
Obligate anaerobes only	38	61	9	16
Facultative anaerobes only	6	10	21	38
Obligate and facultative anaerobes	18	29	25	46

*Combined data on 117 patients from two prospective studies. (Bartlett 1980; Lorber and Swenson 1974).

these infections (10% to 20%). Facultative anaerobes, usually isolated from community-acquired cases, include nonpathogenic viridans streptococci, but on occasion may include *Streptococcus pneumoniae*, and more rarely *Staphylococcus aureus* and *Klebsiella pneumoniae*. Facultative anaerobes isolated from hospital-acquired cases include *Klebsiella*, *Proteus*, *Pseudomonas* and *Serratia* species, *E. coli* and *S. aureus*.

CLINICAL MANIFESTATIONS

The following case history demonstrates many of the features of bacterial lung infection following aspiration of oropharyngeal flora.

> A 37-year-old man with a history of chronic alcoholism and alcohol withdrawal seizures was admitted to the hospital because of pneumonia. He had been seen in the emergency room four weeks before the present admission following a seizure; a chest radiograph was normal at that time. About two weeks before admission, the patient developed a cough which became productive of purulent sputum. For one week prior to admission he noted fever to 101°F, right-sided pleuritic pain, night sweats and a weight loss of 5 lb. He also noted a foul odor to his sputum over the last few days before admission along with recurrent shaking chills.
>
> On physical examination, the patient appeared ill, older than his stated age, and had a temperature of 102°F, pulse of 100 beats/min, and respiratory rate of 20/min. He had a putrid odor to his breath. The sputum also had a foul odor and was purulent. His oral hygiene was poor with many carious teeth and gingival atrophy. There was evidence of pneumonic consolidation with crackles over the right chest posteriorly. The rest of the examination was unremarkable.
>
> The hemoglobin was 12.4 with normocytic-normochromic indices, and the peripheral leukocyte count was 11,800/mm^3 with a slight left shift. The chest radiograph showed a dense right lower lobe infiltrate with a 4-cm cavity containing an air-fluid level and several smaller cavities.

Lung infection following aspiration may be manifested by bronchopneumonia, lobar pneumonia, necrotizing pneumonia (multiple cavities, $<$ 2 cm each) or lung abscess. Empyema may complicate any of these. Anaerobic bacterial pneumonia may produce an acute illness virtually indistinguishable from pneumococcal pneumonia. Because of the short duration of infection, these patients rarely have cavitation or putrid sputum. Clues to the etiology may be an underlying condition predisposing to aspiration, pneumonia in a dependent lung segment, *recurrent* chills when present (very rare in uncomplicated pneumococcal pneumonia), and growth of normal respiratory flora on routine sputum culture. In many other patients, the onset is insidious. These patients are symptomatic for one to two weeks before seeking medical attention, by which time cavitation, which will occur one to two weeks following aspiration, is commonly present. Sputum becomes fetid once cavitation occurs. Fetid sputum is present in over 50% of anaerobic pulmonary infections following aspiration and is pathognomonic of the presence of anaerobic bacteria. Fever is virtually always present and frequently high; weight loss, night sweats, recurrent rigors and pleuritic pain are all frequent findings.

Laboratory studies are nonspecific. Most patients will have a leukocytosis, and the erythrocyte sedimentation rate may be high (greater than 100 mm/hr). Chest radiographs demonstrate infiltrates that typically are unilateral and occur in dependent pulmonary segments; cavitation and pleural fluid may be seen.

DIAGNOSIS

Anaerobic culture of expectorated sputum is not of value in identifying the bacterial etiology of pneumonia following aspiration because anaerobes, which are always present in the mouth in astronomical numbers, readily contaminate expectorated material. However, the presence of "normal respiratory flora" grown from coughed sputum in a patient prone to aspirate, a clinical picture consistent with aspiration pneumonia, and a sputum gram stain showing many neutrophils and mixed flora suggest the diagnosis. Bacteriologic diagnosis depends on the isolation of the specific microorganisms from uncontaminated specimens, eg, sputum obtained by transtracheal aspiration or pleural fluid, with optimum microbiological techniques to grow anaerobic and aerobic bacteria. Blood cultures very rarely are positive. Because of the hazards of transtracheal aspiration, many patients are treated empirically on the basis of predicted bacteriology.

TREATMENT

Antimicrobial treatment varies depending upon whether the aspiration pneumonia is community- or hospital-acquired since the bacteriology of these infections is different. Penicillin generally has been considered the drug of choice for community-acquired cases and usually is given intravenously in a dose of 5 to 10 million units/day. Larger doses of penicillin (10 to 20 million units/day) have been recommended in those more severely ill. After a good clinical response (defervescence, decreased cough and sputum production, a sense of well-being), penicillin may be given orally at a dose of 750 mg to 1 g every six hours. The oral regimen may be used initially in patients with mild illness. Patients allergic to penicillin or those who appear to be penicillin failures (absence of clinical improvement or progression of pulmonary infiltrate after five days of therapy) should be treated with clindamycin at a dose of 600 mg intravenously every eight hours. After clinical response, clindamycin may be given orally. Patients treated with penicillin should be followed carefully since recent evidence suggests that some organisms commonly involved in these infections, eg, *Bacteroides melaninogenicus*, are becoming increasingly resistent to penicillin, and may be associated with early and late therapy failures. One recent study indicates superiority of clindamycin over penicillin in treatment of anaerobic lung abscess (see Levison et al, 1983).

Hospital-acquired cases should initially be treated with regimens that have activity against aerobic organisms as well as anaerobes. A combination of an aminoglycoside combined with penicillin, clindamycin or a cephalosporin is suggested as initial therapy. Prevalence of specific noscomial pathogens and patterns of antimicrobial resistance at the specific institution should be taken into consideration.

No specific duration of treatment can be recommended. Antimicrobial therapy should be continued until the patient is clinically well, and the chest radiograph is clear or shows a stable residual lesion on two studies two weeks apart. Commonly, this requires three to six weeks of treatment.

Drainage is an important adjunct to antimicrobials, and therapeutic bronchoscopy should be performed in patients who continue to demonstrate fluid in cavities but who cease producing sputum since they may have obstruction due to mucous plugs. Bronchoscopy should also be considered in patients who fail to demonstrate clinical response. Older patients with anaerobic lung infection, particularly smokers and those without a good history of aspiration, may have an underlying bronchogenic carcinoma and appropriate diagnostic studies should be done. Empyema requires chest tube drainage and occasionally thoracotomy with rib resection; repeated thoracenteses generally are not successful in these infections.

Surgery for the pulmonary infection itself, including lung abscess, is virtually never necessary and should be reserved for noncompliant patients with relapse of infection in the same anatomical site. Since these infections are due to endogenous flora, isolation is not necessary.

SELECTED READINGS

Bartlett JG, Finegold SM: Anaerobic infections of the lung and pleural space. *Am Rev Respir Dis* 1974;110:56–77.

Bartlett JG, Gorbach SL, Finegold SM: The bacteriology of aspiration pneumonia. *Am J Med* 1974;56:202–207.

Bartlett JG, Gorbach SL: The triple threat of aspiration pneumonia. *Chest* 1975; 68:560–566.

Bartlett JG: Anaerobic bacterial pneumonitis. *Am Rev Respir Dis* 1979;119:19–23.

Bartlett JG: Aspiration pneumonia. *Clin Notes Respir Dis* 1980;18:3–8.

Green GM: The J. Burns Amberson Lecture: In defense of the lung. *Am Rev Respir Dis* 1970;102:691–703.

Huxley EJ, Viroslav J, Gray WR, et al: Pharyngeal aspiration in normal adults and patients with depressed consciousness. *Am J Med* 1973;64:564–568.

Johanson WG, Pierce AK, Sanford JP: Changing pharyngeal bacterial flora of hospitalized patients. Emergence of gram-negative bacilli. *N Engl J Med* 1969;281:1137–1140.

Levison ME, Mangura CT, Lorber B, et al: Penicillin vs, clindamycin for the treatment of anaerobic lung abscess. *Ann Intern Med* 1983;98:466–471.

Lorber B, Swenson RM: Bacteriology of aspiration pneumonia. A prospective study of community- and hospital-acquired cases. *Ann Intern Med* 1974;81: 329–331.

Lorber B: "Bad breath": Presenting manifestation of anaerobic pulmonary infection. *Am Rev Respir Dis* 1975;112:875–877.

Murray HW: Antimicrobial therapy in pulmonary aspiration. *Am J Med* 1979; 66:188–190.

Wolfe JE, Bone RC, Ruth WE: Effects of corticosteroids in the treatment of patients with gastric aspiration. *Am J Med* 1977;63:719–722.

Wynne JW, Modell JH: Respiratory aspiration of stomach contents. *Ann Intern Med* 1977;87:466–474.

17 *Pulmonary Infections in the Immunocompromised Host*

Jack D. Sobel

The advent of successful organ transplantation and effective chemotherapy for neoplastic and collagen-vascular disease has resulted in a fast-growing population of immunocompromised subjects at risk of acquiring serious infectious complications which may negate any advance in the therapy of these life-threatening diseases. Although alcoholics and diabetics are compromised hosts, in this chapter reference will be made only to immunocompromised patients, ie, patients whose immune mechanisms are defective as a result of either therapy or the basic underlying disease process.

Infection is now the most important cause of morbidity and mortality in the immunocompromised host, especially in acute leukemia in which the risk of death from infection is fourfold greater than that of bleeding. The most common site of infection is the lower respiratory tract. Pneumonia in these patients has proven to be one of the most difficult infections to correctly diagnose and treat. Bodey (1974), in reviewing 50 consecutive autopsies of patients with acute leukemia, noted that 58% of pulmonary infections went unrecognized clinically, and the responsible organisms were isolated in life in only 23% of cases. While several authors have identified the causal organisms in up to 80% of cases, overall successful identification remains low, and all agree that pneumonia is now the leading cause of death in hematological malignancy. Sickles et al (1973) reported the disturbingly high mortality rate of 65% for pneumonia in acute leukemia and several studies indicate that pulmonary infection in the immunocompromised host has a worse prognosis than infection elsewhere.

Pneumonia accounts for as much as 25% to 50% of all infectious deaths among patients with hematological malignancies. Several studies have shown that infection is the leading cause of a new pulmonary infiltrate. Multiple pathogens may be present simultaneously, such as cytomegalovirus and pneumocystis. Several noninfectious processes also may cause pulmonary infiltrates, clinically indistinguishable from infectious processes or infections may be superimposed upon lung previously damaged by neoplasm, radiation therapy or the fibrotic effects of chemotherapy (such as bleomycin and cyclophosphamide) (Table 17-1, Figure 17-1).

Table 17-1
Noninfectious Causes of Pulmonary Infiltrate in Immunocompromised Host

1. Congestive cardiac failure
2. Pulmonary emboli
3. Radiation pneumonitis
4. Pulmonary hemorrhage
5. Underlying malignant process
6. Drug-induced (chemotherapeutic agents)
   - busulfan
   - bleomycin
   - melphalan
   - cyclophosphamide
   - 6-mercaptopurine
   - azathioprine
   - methotrexate
   - nitrofurantoin
   - amphotericin/granulocyte transfusions
7. Leukagglutinin transfusion reaction
8. Nonspecific idiopathic interstitial pneumonitis/fibrosis

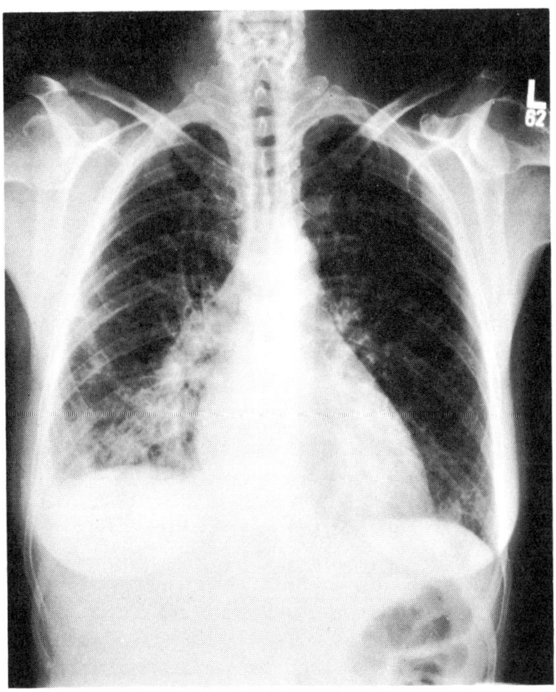

Figure 17-1 A diffuse infiltrate is present in the right lower lobe accompanied by volume loss and blunting of right costo-phrenic angle. This was a 60-year-old woman with bone marrow aplasia and severe pancytopenia. Fever and an infiltrate developed which failed to improve on antibiotic therapy. Open lung biopsy revealed extensive hemorrhage.

Pulmonary infection also is a significant problem in transplant recipients and the lung ranks second only to the operative site and the urinary tract as a source of bacteremia and infection in renal transplant patients (see Chapter 18).

A wide spectrum of infectious agents may cause pulmonary infection in the compromised host including familiar bacterial respiratory pathogens, as well as infrequently encountered, relatively nonvirulent microorganisms that behave as opportunists. These organisms take advantage of the lack of local and systemic resistance and become invasive. The spectrum includes bacteria, mycobacteria, fungi, viruses, protozoa and helminths (Table 17-2).

Table 17-2
Pathogens Causing Pulmonary Infection in Immunocompromised Hosts*

Bacteria	Viruses
Klebsiella pneumoniae	Cytomegalovirus
Escherichia coli	Herpes simplex
Pseudomonas aeruginosa	Varicella-zoster
Serratia sp	Measles
Streptococcus pneumoniae	Adenoviruses
Staphylococcus aureus	
Listeria monocytogenes	Fungi
Mycobacterium tuberculosis	*Aspergillus* sp
Atypical mycobacteria	Zygomycetes
Nocardia sp	*Candida* sp
Legionella sp	*Histoplasma capsulatum*
	Cryptococcus neoformans
Protozoa	*Coccidioides immitis*
Pneumocystis carinii	
Toxoplasma gondii	
Parasites	
Strongyloides stercoralis	

*Incomplete list.

The relative incidence of each infectious agent varies in different parts of the world and within the United States from center to center. Frequently, infections are acquired during hospitalization or may be acquired in the home environment; others still represent not new infection but reactivation of latent foci.

IMMUNOPATHOGENESIS OF PULMONARY INFECTIONS (Table 17-3)

Specific defects in the immune and inflammatory process predispose to specific types of pathogens. Accordingly, pulmonary infections following splenectomy differ considerably from those encountered in neutropenic hosts and, similarly, a different spectrum is found in patients with defective cell-mediated immunity. As shown in Table 17-3, patients with granulocytopenia or defective granulocyte function are mainly prone to pneumonias caused predominantly by gram-negative rods (Enterobacteriaceae and *Pseudomonas* sp) and *Staphylococcus aureus*, as well as opportunist fungi, such as *Aspergillus* sp. and *Zygomycetes*. In contrast, patients with defective cell-mediated immunity are at risk of developing viral pneumonia, especially due to the herpes virus group (cytomegalovirus, herpes simplex) and adenovirus, as well as infections

Table 17-3
Immunodeficient States and Microorganisms Causing Associated Pulmonary Infection

Immunodeficiency State	Microorganism
Neutropenia	
Drug-induced	*Pseudomonas aeruginosa*
Acute myeloblastic leukemia	*Enterobacteriaceae*
Hypersplenism	*Staphylococcus aureus*
Irradiation	*Nocardia* (chronic granulomatous disease)
Defective Neutrophil Function	*Candida* sp
Chronic granulomatous disease	*Aspergillus* sp
Acute leukemia	*Zycomycetes*
Uremia	
Burns	
Diabetic keto-acidosis	
Corticosteroids	
Depressed Cell-mediated Immunity	
Corticosteroids	Cytomegalovirus
Uremia	Herpes simplex
Hodgkin's disease	*Pneumocystis carinii*
Advanced cancer	*Toxoplasma gondii*
Chemotherapy	Fungi
	Mycobacteria
	Nocardia sp
	Listeria monocytogenes
Depressed Humoral Response	
Splenectomy	*Streptococcus pneumoniae*
Multiple myeloma	*Hemophilus influenzae*
Chronic lymphocytic leukemia	*Pneumocystis carinii*
Non-Hodgkin's lymphoma	
Congenital hypogammaglobulinemia	
Irradiation therapy	
Chemotherapy	
Advanced cancer and malnutrition	

caused by *Pneumocystis carinii*, *Toxoplasma*, *Cryptococcus*, *Aspergillus* sp, *Nocardia* sp and mycobacteria. Hypogammaglobulinemia and splenectomy predispose to infections caused by encapsulated microorganisms, including *Streptococcus pneumoniae* and *Hemophilus influenzae*. Furthermore, local pulmonary processes due to underlying disease may favor certain pathogens. For example, in the presence of bronchial obstruction, one should consider infection due to oral anaerobes. The likelihood of opportunistic gram-negative bacillary or fungal infections is enhanced by hospitalization and prolonged use of broad spectrum antimicrobials, corticosteroids and central venous cannulation.

The association between underlying immunodeficiency and the nature of the infectious agent is somewhat simplistic, but it can provide the clinician with valuable information in predicting the nature of invading organisms. When taken together with the clinical and radiological evaluation, these associations can guide the clinician through the difficult maze of decision-making in the management of the febrile immunocompromised patient with a pulmonary infiltrate, and allow the rational selection of relevant diagnostic procedures as well as initial empirical therapy prior to obtaining results of culture and histology. Unfortunately, seriously ill patients often have multiple immunodeficiencies, both as a result of the primary underlying disease, especially in an advanced stage, and intensive chemotherapy. This predisposes to a corresponding wide range of opportunistic organisms.

The most important risk factor is severe neutropenia, especially if prolonged. Numerous studies have correlated the prevalence and severity of pulmonary infection as well as the eventual clinical outcome with the number of circulating granulocytes. Pulmonary infection in the presence of profound granulocytopenia is the most common source of bacteremia in acute leukemia. Fanta and Pennington (1981) have shown in the guinea pig model that granulocytopenia and chemotherapy, which interfere with leukocyte kinetics, profoundly alter the delivery of inflammatory cells to the infected lung as measured by bronchial lavage.

In spite of our increased understanding of pulmonary defense mechanisms, it is still unclear why the lung in particular is the most prevalent site of infection in the compromised host. The answer perhaps lies with the potential exposure of the alveolar surface to inhaled or aspirated environmental microorganisms and enhanced colonization of the upper respiratory tract by respiratory pathogens in these patients. Another major factor in the pathogenesis of lung infection is hospitalization and exposure to hospital flora. These organisms include multiresistant gram-negative bacilli and fungi. Surveillance studies have shown that the compromised host rapidly alters the flora of the oropharynx and upper respiratory tract, acquiring predominantly gram-negative organisms; and, after antibiotic or steroid therapy, *Candida* species are found as well. Colonization results not only from exposure but also from diminished local resistance to colonization which permits the microorganisms to adhere to buccal, pharyngeal and respiratory epithelial cells. Procedures such as suction, intubation and even bronchoscopy in bypassing the natural barriers enhance colonization of the lower respiratory tract. Chemotherapy further contributes by inducing mucosal damage and ulceration, setting the scene for tissue invasion. Bronchogenic pneumonia may result if the number or virulence of the microorganisms can overwhelm the defective defense mechanisms at the alveolar level.

Not infrequently, pulmonary infections in the compromised host are not bronchogenic but metastatic, ie, hematogenous in origin. Twenty-five percent or more of pulmonary infections in hospitalized cancer patients are thought to originate in this manner, resulting in a clinical and radiological picture characterized by a multilobar, miliary and often bilateral interstitial process.

Pneumonia may also result from reactivation of a latent pulmonary focus of infection. Corticosteroids or the primary malignant process impair cell-mediated immunity and permit latent intracellular organisms to proliferate and subsequently to invade adjacent parenchyma. Such infections include tuberculosis, atypical mycobacterial infection, *Pneumocystis carinii* pneumonia and viral infections such as those due to cytomegalovirus and herpes simplex.

The role of splenectomy in predisposing to pulmonary infection in compromised hosts is controversial and is particularly relevant with regard to staging splenectomy in Hodgkin's disease. Several large studies showed no increased risk of pneumonia in splenectomized patients with Hodgkin's disease unless coexistent neutropenia was present. Chilcote et al (1976), however, reported serious infections in 10% of these patients without neutropenia, 50% of which were due to the pneumococcus. Splenectomy becomes a more critical adverse factor in the setting of advanced Hodgkin's disease when the patient receives intensive combined radiotherapy and chemotherapy.

DIAGNOSTIC APPROACH TO THE FEBRILE IMMUNOCOMPROMISED PATIENT WITH A PULMONARY INFILTRATE

Therapy is now available for virtually all the pathogens causing pneumonia in immunosuppressed patients. Since untreated infection may be rapidly fatal, an etiological diagnosis should be made rapidly and accurately to assure administration of appropriate specific therapy and to prevent the hazards of inappropriate therapy. The availability of effective chemotherapeutic agents today should be no justification for the blind empiric use of multiple antimicrobial agents to cover all possible etiologies, although this may be done initially for the rapidly deteriorating, severely hypoxemic patient prior to the availability of results from diagnostic procedures.

Clues to the diagnosis may be based upon the epidemiological setting. Community-acquired pneumonia, especially in the absence of severe granulocytopenia or in cancer patients in remission, is still frequently caused by *S. pneumoniae* or other common respiratory pathogens. Similarly, an accurate history of recent travel and exposure must be taken in order not to miss regional pathogens such as *Histoplasma capsulatum* and *Coccidioides immitis*. Likewise, recent hospitalization or chemotherapy would suggest nosocomial infections due to resistant gram-negative bacteria, fungi, and other opportunistic organisms. Surveillance of nosocomial infections is also essential to document unusual clustering of pulmonary infections in immunocompromised hosts. A careful history may identify possible noninfectious mechanisms such as recent chemotherapy, pulmonary irradiation, pulmonary emboli or congestive failure due to excessive fluid administration or transfusions.

The rate of onset and progression of the pulmonary infection also is useful in the differential diagnosis (Rubin, 1980). Clinical manifestations of pulmonary infection in immunocompromised patients varies from acute onset of respiratory distress and a rapid downhill course to a subacute or chronic disease with minimal fever or respiratory symptoms. Acute onset of severe symptoms would suggest bacterial or *Aspergillus* infection, pulmonary hemorrhage, pulmonary emboli, or a leukagglutinin reaction. A subacute onset over a few days suggests infection due to viruses or *Pneumocystis* and occasionally *Nocardia*. A subacute to chronic course over one to several weeks would suggest infection due to mycobacteria, *Nocardia*, or fungi as well as tumor, radiation pneumonitis or drug-induced disease.

Sputum examination in the immunocompromised host is generally disappointing. Frequently no sputum is produced or, in the neutropenic patients, the sputum lacks polymorphonuclear cells. Representative sputum specimens should be studied for the presence of legionella-like organisms with fluorescent antibody as well as with appropriate stains for acid-fast bacilli and fungi. Sputum culture may be falsely positive or negative and therefore may be less useful than blood cultures in identifying the etiologic agent. However, detection of certain organisms, such as *M. tuberculosis*, *N. asteroides*, *C. neoformans* or *Aspergillus fumigatus*, should be considered to have clinical significance.

Infection is often disseminated at the time of presentation and therefore blood cultures, cerebrospinal fluid examination and a careful search for skin lesions to biopsy may provide the etiological diagnosis. Skin testing for tuberculosis in this clinical setting is generally unhelpful because of the frequent presence of cutaneous anergy, but the absence of tuberculin reactivity may be meaningful if the patient is reactive to an anergy panel. Although one may submit serological tests for antibody to *Toxoplasma*, *Candida*, *Cryptococcus* and other fungi, these tests, together with viral serology for cytomegalovirus, herpes simplex and varicella-zoster virus are rarely contributory in the initial phase of investigation. Cryptococcal antigen usually can be detected in body fluids in disseminated cryptococcosis, but failure to detect this antigen does not rule out isolated pulmonary cryptococcal disease.

Unfortunately, clinical manifestations of pulmonary infection are frequently nonspecific. To complicate matters, in the severely neutropenic patient with pulmonary infection, the signs of pulmonary consolidation may be absent or unimpressive, or grossly underestimate the extent and severity of the pathological process. Except for fever, the clinical findings may be few and subtle in these patients.

Although radiography may be the most sensitive means of defining pulmonary involvement, it is perilous to make an etiological diagnosis and therapeutic decision based upon a radiological pattern alone. Moreover, noninfectious causes of a pulmonary infiltrate in the immunocompromised host are clinically indistinguishable from infectious processes (Table 17-1). A miliary pattern might suggest tuberculosis but also could be caused by disseminated fungal infection or toxoplasmosis. Cavitation similarly has numerous causes, including *M. tuberculosis*, anaerobic bacteria, *Nocardia*, *Pseudomonas*, Enterobacteriaceae or *S. aureus*. Nevertheless, certain patterns on x-ray are more characteristic of some processes than of others. A dense segmental consolidation suggests bacterial infection, pulmonary hemorrhage or pulmonary emboli. In contrast, a diffuse interstitial or peribronchial pattern suggests viral or *Pneumocystis carinii* infection, drug-induced or radiation pneumonitis. It cannot be sufficiently emphasized, however, that diagnosis based upon radiological appearance alone is fraught with danger.

After the preliminary investigation, if an etiological agent is apparent or suggestive (pneumococcal or gram-negative bacillary pneumonia), appropriate antibiotics should be administered. Usually, however, the cause of the pulmonary process is still unknown. Under these circumstances, more invasive diagnostic procedures are required that have risks and may contribute to the patient's deterioration. Available today are a number of invasive procedures that differ in diagnostic yield as well as risk. The sequence and timetable for the diagnostic investigation is determined primarily by the clinical status of the patient, bearing in mind that time is never on the side of infected immunocompromised patients. The diagnostic workup also will depend upon the facilities and expertise available in the specific institution. There is no master plan suited for all patients. In the non-neutropenic patient in which the clinical course of pulmonary infection is not rapidly progressive, it is prudent to elect less invasive procedures initially and resort to more invasive procedures, proceeding from the least to the most hazardous, in a stepwise manner. In the neutropenic or the critically ill patient, procedures must be selected immediately that are most likely to provide useful information without jeopardizing the clinical status of the patient. In this context, delaying open lung biopsy in order to perform procedures with a lower yield may only result in a patient too ill to survive the open lung biopsy when other diagnostic procedures have failed.

Transtracheal aspiration (TTA) is the next logical procedure when sputum examination is unhelpful or when no sputum is obtained. TTA is particularly useful in bacterial infections, but is not recommended for diagnosis of suspected *Pneumocystis carinii* infection. TTA has the advantage of bypassing the contaminated oropharynx and sampling a region that is normally sterile. Consequently, most organisms seen on gram stain or culture generally are pathogens, although tracheobronchial colonization can give false-positive results. TTA should not be done in the presence of a bleeding diathesis, hypoxemia ($PaO_2 < 50$ mmHg), or in uncooperative patients.

Fiberoptic bronchoscopy, including bronchial washings, brushings, and transbronchial biopsy, has enjoyed considerable success in the investigation of the febrile compromised patient with pulmonary infiltrates. Compared to the risks, the probability of obtaining useful information that will alter patient management is high. Overall, diagnostic information, including detection of both infectious and noninfectious etiologies, in different studies was obtained in 55% to 84% of patients. Morbidity of biopsy in experienced hands is low (< 5%). Occasionally, pneumothorax and pulmonary hemorrhage are complications. In general, platelet transfusion is given when prebiopsy platelet counts of less than 50,000/mm^3 are present. In uremic patients because of platelet dysfunction, in spite of increased expertise and platelet transfusion, pulmonary hemorrhage after biopsy is common (45%). Fiberoptic bronchoscopy is of limited value in the diagnosis of bacterial pneumonia because of mouth flora contamination of the lower respiratory tract as a result of passage of the endoscope.

Transbronchial biopsy is useful with both focal and particularly with diffuse infiltrates, and most etiological agents can be identified. This procedure is especially valuable in diagnosing infection due to *Pneumocystis*, mycobacteria, *Nocardia*, and fungi. In 25% to 50% of cases, however, lung specimens obtained by transbronchial biopsy reveal a nonspecific pneumonitis in which no specific causal agent is seen or cultured. The results of the transbronchial biopsy may be falsely negative because of the small amount of tissue obtained. If the transbronchial biopsy is unrevealing, consideration should be given to an open lung biopsy.

Another invasive procedure used to obtain lung tissue is percutaneous transthoracic needle aspiration. Needle lung biopsy may be accomplished by aspiration, cutting needle, suction-excision or trephine drill techniques that have resulted in varying degrees of success and complications. The complications include pneumothorax (the most common), hemoptysis, air embolism, empyema or seeding of the needle tract with neoplasm. Gram-positive and gram-negative bacteria, including *L. pneumophila*, fungi, *Nocardia*, mycobacteria and *Pneumocystis carinii*, have been isolated by these techniques. Bandt et al (1972), using an 18-g thin-walled spinal needle with fluoroscopic guidance, recovered the causative organism in 76% of attempts at aspirating localized lesions in immunocompromised hosts. This procedure was accompanied by a 30% pneumothorax in one of 22 patients with no significant bleeding, ie, very low and acceptable morbidity. Similar results were reported by Zavala (1976) in a review of pulmonary biopsy techniques; needle aspiration achieved a 78% to 87% diagnostic accuracy, but the frequency of pneumothorax was almost 50%. Less than 20% of the latter complications required insertion of a chest tube. The use of a cutting needle has an unacceptably high rate of hemorrhage and pneumothorax that does not justify its use in immunocompromised patients.

In general, percutaneous needle aspiration has a lower yield in diffuse lung disease; however, Chaudhary et al (1977) achieved extremely good results in the diagnosis of *Pneumocystis carinii* infection using this technique in leukemic children. In a series of 202 patients with suspected *Pneumocystis* pneumonia, diagnosis was confirmed in 121 by needle aspiration and only six false-negatives confirmed at autopsy. Pneumothorax occurred in 37% of patients, less than a third of whom required a chest tube. While additional data in the immunocompromised patient is as yet sparse, this method in experienced hands offers an encouraging alternative to open lung biopsy, but more information is needed.

Open lung biopsy is, at present, the procedure most likely to be diagnostic. In major centers, the procedure should take no longer than 30 minutes and offers the maximum control over bleeding and pneumothorax. Open biopsy is often performed early in the seriously ill neutropenic patient with hematological malignancy whose survival is dependent upon avoidance of delay in diagnosis.

Diagnostic procedures have to be evaluated in terms of how often therapy was changed as a result of the procedure so as to contribute to patient survival. Invasive procedures by permitting termination of inappropriate, ineffectual empiric antimicrobial therapy contribute to reduced patient morbidity by decreasing side effects, toxic sequelae and superinfection. It permits the clinician to manage the critically ill patient with greater confidence and fewer logistic problems. The data proving diminished mortality are less convincing. In spite of invasive procedures, a specific diagnosis is often only made at postmortem. Autopsy studies confirm that the diagnosis most often missed is that of invasive fungal infection presenting as either local or diffuse disease. Furthermore, it is extremely uncommon for bacterial infection to result in either a diffuse interstitial infiltrate or remain undiagnosed using more conservative methods of diagnosis.

A management strategy can thus be formulated. In the febrile cancer patient with a localized pulmonary infiltrate or cavitation, if a diagnosis is not immediately available on sputum examination, a transtracheal aspiration should be performed, provided that no contraindication exists. Treatment with broad spectrum antibiotics also should be started at once, pending the results of culture studies. Currently, a combination of a β-lactam antibiotic, such as piperacillin, mezlocillin, or a "third generation" cephalosporin (eg, moxalactam) and an aminoglycoside (gentamicin, tobramycin or amikacin) are recommended. If no answer is forthcoming from the transtracheal aspiration or if the clinical picture fails to improve promptly within a 48- to 72-hour course, an attempt to obtain lung tissue for diagnosis must be made. The choice of procedure depends upon the expertise of pulmonary consultants available, as well as the rate of the clinical deterioration and progression of the infiltrate. Rapid deterioration should mandate an open lung biopsy. If the progression is less dramatic, fiberoptic bronchoscopy, brushings and transbronchial biopsy can be undertaken. Once the diagnosis is established, specific therapy is administered. However, it may be prudent while awaiting a definitive answer to add erythromycin as therapy for legionellosis. It also may be reasonable to add a sulfonamide or trimethoprim-sulfamethoxazole for treatment of possible nocardiosis pending results of the histologic and microbiologic studies. If the condition of a leukemic or granulocytopenic patient does not permit open lung biopsy, then erythromycin and amphotericin B should be promptly started.

Patients with a diffuse infiltrate have a greater chance of being infected with *Pneumocystis carinii*. Transbronchial or open lung biopsy in these patients should be performed immediately. Only patients too ill to tolerate biopsy should receive trimethoprim-sulfamethoxazole empirically. If *P. carinii* is not confirmed by brushings or by histological stains of lung tissue, or if there is further deterioration, amphotericin B is indicated as empiric therapy of possible invasive fungal infection.

Finally, if after initial clinical improvement, fever with or without a new infiltrate appears, it should not be assumed that recurrence of symptoms is due to the original etiological mechanism as a second infectious agent may be responsible. It is essential to reinvestigate the unfortunate patient. This may cause considerable emotional distress to both the patient and the clinician, hence the necessity of a team approach to this difficult management problem.

BACTERIAL PNEUMONIA

The most common cause of a pulmonary infiltrate in the immunocompromised patient is bacterial infection. The most frequently encountered gram-negative bacilli include *E. coli*, *Klebsiella pneumoniae*, *Pseudomonas* sp, as well as *Enterobacter*, *Serratia* and *Proteus* species. Gram-positive cocci are less frequently encountered, although *S. pneumoniae* should still be considered in community-acquired disease and *S. aureus* remains a not infrequent cause of nosocomial pneumonia mainly in children. Mixed infections sometimes occur involving anaerobic organisms, especially in the presence of endobronchial obstruction.

The radiographic pattern of bacterial pneumonia, like the clinical picture, is characterized by its lack of specificity. Cavitation occasionally occurs due to anaerobes, *S. aureus* or *Pseudomonas*, *Serratia* or other gram-negative bacilli. Rarely are diffuse bilateral interstitial changes due to acute bacterial infection.

Management is based upon the overwhelming likelihood of a bacterial etiology among immunocompromised patients, mandating the immediate selection of antibacterial agents, pending the results of preliminary diagnostic studies. Broad spectrum bactericidal agents are administered parenterally in full therapeutic doses. The selection must be based upon knowledge of the antimicrobial sensitivity pattern prevailing in the specific institution. In the absence of a major antimicrobial resistance problem, most authors recommend starting with a broad spectrum β-lactam antibiotic active against *P. aeruginosa* and an antistaphylococcal penicillin combined with an aminoglycoside. The greater in vitro activity and extended spectrum of the newer semisynthetic penicillins (piperacillin, azlocillin, mezlocillin) and the new cephalosporins (cefoperazone, cefotaxime, moxalactam, etc) suggest they may be ideal antimicrobial agents in the immunocompromised host. If gentamicin resistance is a problem in the institution, amikacin should be selected initially.

The most important principle guiding therapy is that single agents are not recommended, and that potentially synergistic combinations should be selected in an attempt to improve the poor results obtained in gram-negative bacillary pneumonia.

Recently, a number of nosocomial outbreaks as well as sporadic cases of *Legionella pneumophila* pneumonia in renal transplant recipients, makes it essential to consider this organism in the differential diagnosis of febrile immunocompromised host with lung infiltrate. Clinical experience has shown that *Legionella* infection is difficult to differentiate from other gram-negative bacillary pneumonias. Clinical characteristics that suggest diagnosis include: prior corticosteroid administration, temperature $> 39.2°$ C, diarrhea, obtundation, lack of symptoms of upper respiratory tract involvement, hematuria, impaired liver function, negative routine bacterial cultures and a failure to respond to therapy with β-lactam antibiotics and an aminoglycoside. The clinical course in the compromised host tends to be more fulminant and cavitation has been described in this setting (Figure 17-2).

Specific diagnosis can be made by culture of *Legionella* from respiratory secretions, lung tissue, pleural fluid or blood using charcoal yeast extract or F-G medium, or a biphasic blood culture medium. Direct immunofluorescence may be used to demonstrate the organism in secretions from the respiratory tract, pleural fluid or lung tissue. Retrospective serologic diagnosis may be made by a fourfold rise in reciprocal titer to $\geq$ 128 or a single titer of $\geq$ 256 by indirect immunofluorescence.

Erythromycin 2 to 4 g/day remains the treatment of choice, and it has been recommended that more prolonged therapy for three weeks be given in the immunocompromised host. Erythromycin, with or without rifampin, should not be used routinely and empirically in the initial antibiotic regimen, but should be reserved for those in whom the possibility of Legionnaires' pneumonia is seriously considered. Although cross-infection and person-to-person spread of legionellosis is unproven, it is prudent to utilize "secretion" precaution for these patients.

Another species of *Legionella* recently described as a pulmonary pathogen in compromised hosts is *Legionella micdadei* (Pittsburgh pneumonia agent). All cases of *L. micdadei* infection reported to date have been in immunosuppressed patients, primarily recipients of renal homografts. Most cases have been nosocomial and usually occur three weeks after use of increasing doses of corticosteroids. The mode of spread is unknown. Clinically, the pneumonia resembles that due to *L. pneumophila*, with progressive pulmonary infiltrates without symptoms of upper respiratory tract involvement, but only in a minority of patients is cough present. Pleuritic chest pain is common. The course has been complicated by acute renal failure, refractory hypoxia and pulmonary abscesses found at autopsy. Effective therapy includes erythromycin, rifampin and trimethoprim-sulfamethoxazole.

MYCOBACTERIAL INFECTION

Earlier studies found a relatively high frequency (up to 20%) of tuberculosis in cancer patients, particularly in lymphoma, chronic lymphatic leukemia and Hodgkin's disease. During the past two decades, tuberculosis has been reported in less than 1% of such patients. Thus, unless a specific suspicion is present, the empiric inclusion of antituberculosis therapy in the initial empiric regimen for therapy of the febrile compromised host is unjustified.

Particularly at risk are the elderly population with healed primary

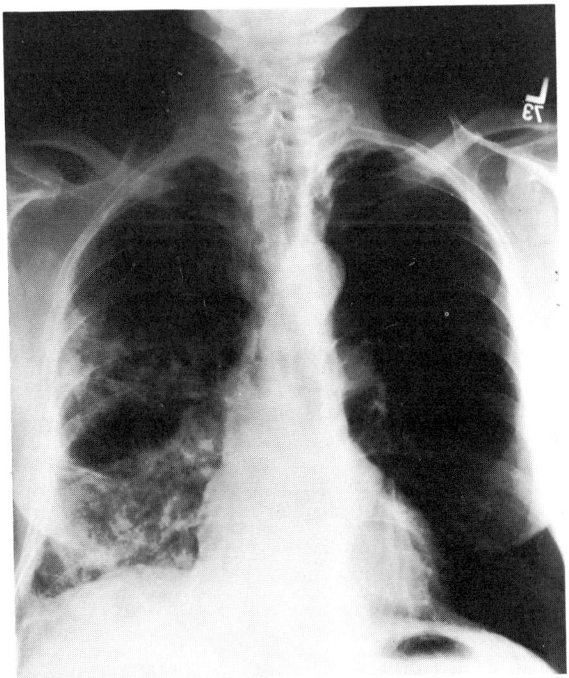

A

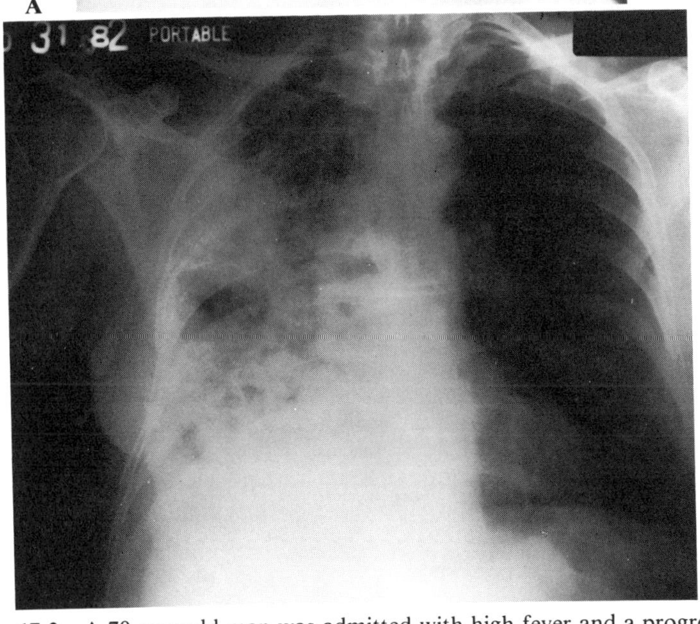

B

Figure 17-2 A 70-year-old man was admitted with high fever and a progressive pneumonia with an initial infiltrate present in his right lower lobe **A**. The pneumonia progressed in spite of therapy of multiple broad spectrum antibiotics **B**. An open lung biopsy was performed and *Legionella bozemanii* was cultured. Erythromycin IV was started, with slow but eventual resolution of the infiltrates.

lesions which might still harbor viable mycobacteria. Patients with lymphoma, especially Hodgkin's disease, remain at high risk as do patients with primary pulmonary neoplasia. Another group susceptible to reactivation are patients on chronic hemodialysis. Therapy used to treat underlying disease, such as antineoplastic chemotherapy, irradiation and corticosteroids increase the risk of reactivation of tuberculosis.

Radiographic manifestations are variable and include upper lobe cavitation, lobar consolidation and miliary pattern. In general, pulmonary tuberculosis in immunocompromised patients tends to be more extensive than in normal hosts. Similarly, extrapulmonary disease is more frequent. Tuberculosis is often missed because it is not considered and not because of difficulties in obtaining diagnostic specimens. Mortality of tuberculosis in cancer patients is high (approximately 17%) and may reach 40% to 50% in those with lymphoma.

Prior to administration of immunosuppressive agents, patients should be tested routinely for tuberculin reactivity and have chest and abdominal radiographs performed. Tuberculin reactors as well as subjects with old, healed, calcified mediastinal or abdominal lymph nodes, should receive 300 mg of isoniazide daily for at least a year and some authors believe for as long as the immunosuppression is given.

In spite of its infrequency, clinicians must remain constantly on guard to exclude tuberculosis in any febrile immunocompromised patient and diagnosis of tuberculosis should be sought in all tissue and respiratory secretions.

Several recent studies have emphasized that with the decline in *Mycobacterium tuberculosis* infection there has been an increasing number of pulmonary infections in immunocompromised patients due to atypical mycobacteria that are frequently resistant to antituberculous agents. Most frequently identified are *M. kansasii* and *M. fortuitum*. Recently, disseminated *M. avium-intracellulare* complex infection has been frequently identified in patients with acquired immunodeficiency syndrome (AIDS).

NOCARDIA

Nocardia infections continue to be a significant problem in immunocompromised patients, especially those with lymphoma or hematologic malignancy and following organ transplantation. Neutropenia does not appear to be a major predisposing factor and is present in less than 25% of patients with nocardiosis. In contrast, corticosteroid therapy is a major risk factor.

In most cases, the portal of entry is the respiratory tract (70%), less commonly infection originates in the skin (27%) and rarely in the gastrointestinal tract (3%). In a recent outbreak of *Nocardia* infection in a renal transplant unit, six recipients acquired infection, air and dust samples were positive, and patient-to-patient transmission was considered responsible for spread. Only after closure of the unit and fumigation with formaldehyde was the outbreak controlled. Dissemination from the lung to the brain, skin, subcutaneous tissue, spleen, kidney, heart, liver, bone and lymph nodes occurs in slightly less than one third of patients.

Although several species of *Nocardia* have been incriminated, *N. asteroides* is by far the most frequent pulmonary pathogen. *N. asteroides* is a gram-positive, weakly acid-fast bacillus that grows aerobically but often at a slow rate, resulting in the diagnosis being missed when negative cultures are discarded after only a few days of incubation. This factor contributes to the difficulties in diagnosis. Often, multiple sputum specimens must be processed before a positive culture is obtained. Higher yields have been obtained by direct-needle aspiration or biopsy of the pulmonary lesions. Occasionally, pleural fluid and blood cultures may be positive.

The clinical picture varies from an acute and fulminant course to a chronic one. Fever and cough are present; the latter may be dry or productive. The more chronic course is often accompanied by night sweats. Pulmonary involvement varies from single to multiple areas of consolidation which may undergo cavitation resulting in multiple subpleural abscesses. Other manifestations include lobar consolidation, diffuse bronchopneumonia, miliary lesions and thin-walled cavitary lesions.

Sulfonamides, 10 g/day, in divided doses remain the mainstay of therapy. Prior to their introduction, mortality of 70% was described and since their use, mortality has declined to 45% but remains high when disease is disseminated, especially to the brain. Treatment should be prolonged for at least three to six months and in the severely immunosuppressed host, for as long as 12 months, to prevent relapse. A number of other antimicrobial agents have been used in combination with sulfonamides, including erythromycin, ampicillin, tetracycline, cycloserine and aminoglycosides. There is no convincing evidence that these agents, even when used in combination, are superior to sulfonamides alone, although good results have been obtained with the combination of trimethoprim-sulfamethoxazole in a dose of 5 to 10 mg of trimethoprim/kg per day and five times as much sulfamethoxazole to yield a peak serum level of sulfamethoxazole of 75 to 150 μg/mL.

FUNGAL PNEUMONIA

Although pulmonary infections due to fungi are less frequent than those due to bacteria, fungal pneumonia is nevertheless common in immunocompromised patients and is associated with a much worse prognosis. Thus, in patients with a hematological malignancy, particularly acute nonlymphocytic leukemia, fungi cause about 30% of fatal infections and 15% to 20% of fatal pneumonias. Similarly, renal transplant recipients are prone to fungal lung infections, the incidence of which is related to the frequency of rejection episodes and the intensity of immunosuppressive therapy.

Of the various risk factors, granulocytopenia, especially when prolonged, is the most important predisposing factor, followed by corticosteroid administration, prolonged administration of broad spectrum antibiotics, central intravenous lines, and finally suppression of cell-mediated immunity by either the primary disease process or chemotherapy.

By far, the most prevalent fungus in this setting is *Aspergillus*. Less frequently encountered are *Candida*, *Mucorales* and *Torulopsis*. A moderate increased frequency of pneumonia due to *Cryptococcus neoformans* and *Histoplasma capsulatum* is described, but pulmonary blastomycosis, coccidioidomycosis, and *Sporothrix* infection remains infrequent in the immunocompromised host.

Aspergillus

A. fumigatus, *A. niger* and *A. flavus* are well known for their predilection to infect lung tissue. *A. fumigatus* is the most common offender.

Aspergillus sp are ubiquitous in nature, especially in soil and in the hospital atmosphere. This makes human exposure inevitable. *Aspergillus* readily colonizes the human respiratory tract either as a saprophyte, allergen or as an invasive pathogen. The clinical spectrum that results depends primarily upon the status of the host: atopic, nonatopic, or immunosuppressed.

Aspergillus hypersensitivity in lung disease includes: extrinsic asthma, extrinsic allergic alveolitis and allergic bronchopulmonary aspergillosis. *Aspergillus* lung disease also includes a noninvasive chronic form characterized by fungus ball formation in a preexisting pulmonary cavity. Invasive pulmonary aspergillosis is a progressive life-threatening necrotizing pneumonia characterized by hyphal proliferation in lung parenchyma and invasion of blood vessels resulting in hemorrhagic infarcts. This fulminant process occurs almost exclusively in immunosuppressed hosts. Rarely, invasive disease occurs in the absence of immune deficiency, but even then, underlying obstructive lung disease usually is present.

The most important risk factor for invasive aspergillosis is severe granulocytopenia, usually associated with acute nonlymphocytic leukemia. The risk of invasive aspergillosis is approximately 20 times greater in acute leukemia than in lymphoma or organ transplantation. Other predisposing factors include high-dose corticosteroid and azathioprine therapy.

The onset of invasive disease is sudden and dramatic, simulating acute bacterial pneumonia. Fever, toxicity, and dyspnea are present, accompanied by a mild, usually nonproductive cough. A fulminant downhill course usually results in fatal respiratory failure in one to two weeks. Pleuritic pain and a pleural rub may be present which suggests a diagnosis of pulmonary infarction. In 10% to 25% of patients, signs of extrapulmonary dissemination to brain, heart, gastrointestinal tract, liver, or spleen occur.

On chest x-ray, the earliest lesions are often single or multiple nodules (Figure 17-3). Infiltrates may be wedge shaped and peripherally placed, resembling multiple infarcts. Occasionally, more extensive consolidation and cavitation may occur. The cavitating pneumonia should not be confused with a fungus ball due to *Aspergillus* colonization of a preexisting cavity.

In the febrile immunocompromised patient with a pulmonary infiltrate not responding to antibacterial therapy, invasive aspergillosis must be immediately considered, because successful treatment requires early diagnosis.

Sputum cultures are rarely helpful in diagnosis and, in one large study, only 9% of subjects with positive sputum cultures had *Aspergillus* pneumonia, whereas less than 10% of subjects with invasive pulmonary aspergillosis had positive sputum cultures. For this reason, many experienced clinicians feel reluctant to institute amphotericin B therapy for presumptive invasive pulmonary aspergillosis based on positive sputum culture alone and require histologic evidence or tissue culture confirmation. In contrast to this approach, Aisner et al at the Baltimore Cancer Institute have adopted the view that isolation of *Aspergillus* in sputum in an immunocompromised host, in the absence of an alternative diagnosis, is in itself justification for the immediate administration of amphotericin B. These investigators have demonstrated that in neutropenic leukemic patients, surveillance nasal cultures positive for *Aspergillus* sp predict the subsequent development of invasive pulmonary or disseminated *Aspergillus* infection. Blood cultures are rarely positive for *Aspergillus* even when hematogenous dissemination is present. Serology generally has not been helpful. If the patient can tolerate it, some procedure to obtain lung tissue for culture and histology should be undertaken. Lung tissue obtained at biopsy should be stained with periodic acid—Schiff and silver methenamine stains—to demonstrate the acutely branching septate hyphae of *Aspergillus*. If a biopsy cannot be performed, empirical treatment with amphotericin B in high doses (0.5 to 0.6 mg/kg/day) should be started. Such a trial can be considered unsuccessful if no clinical response occurs after seven days of full-dose therapy. A full therapeutic dose should be given shortly after a 1-mg test dose. One cannot gradually increase the daily dose of amphotericin B to therapeutic levels in leukemic patients with invasive fungal disease. The optimal dosage and

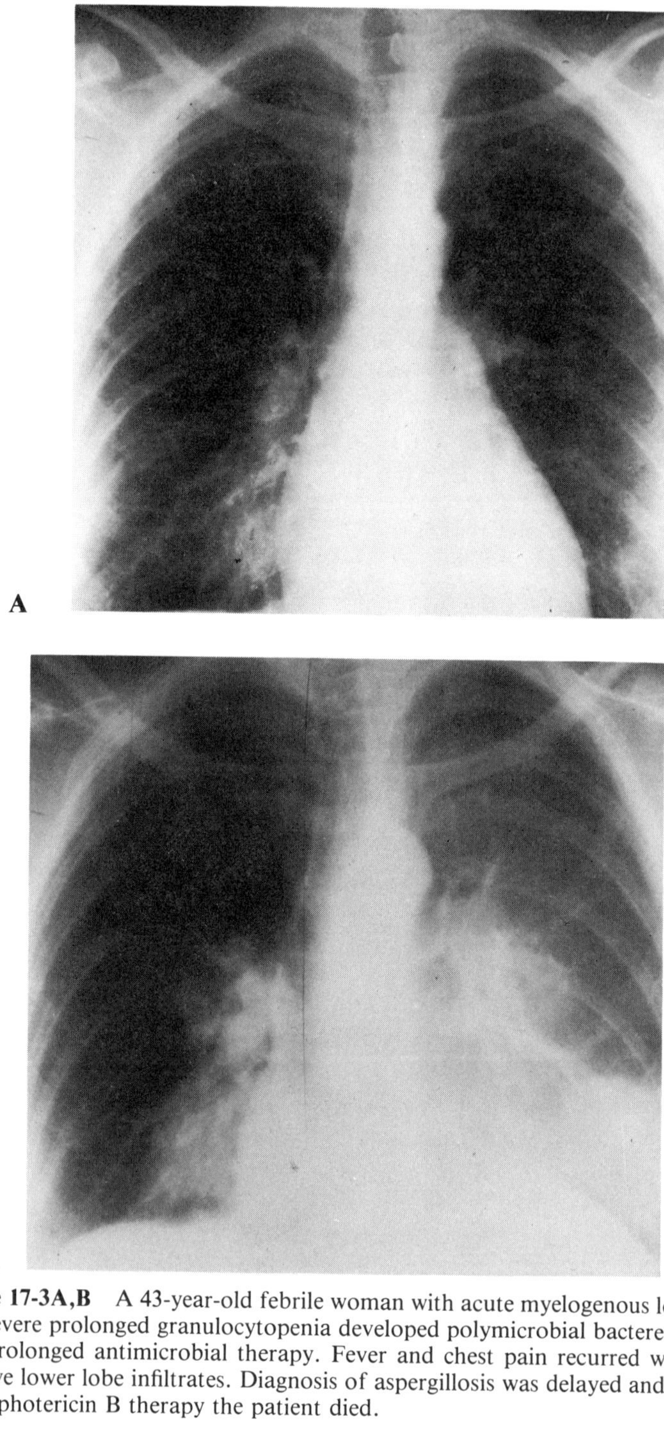

Figure 17-3A,B A 43-year-old febrile woman with acute myelogenous leukemia and severe prolonged granulocytopenia developed polymicrobial bacteremia and had prolonged antimicrobial therapy. Fever and chest pain recurred with progressive lower lobe infiltrates. Diagnosis of aspergillosis was delayed and in spite of amphotericin B therapy the patient died.

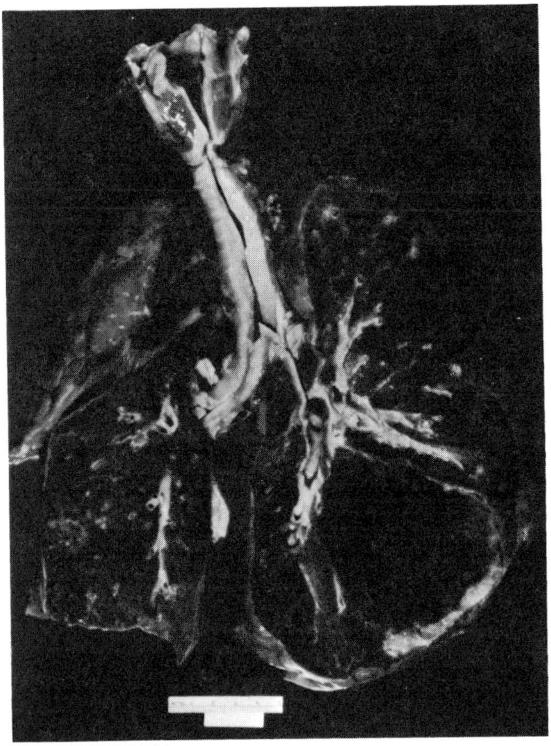

Figure 17-3C Gross pathology specimen of lungs, showing characteristic pulmonary infarcts and extensive hemorrhage.

duration of therapy with amphotericin are unknown. At present, clinical parameters remain the best guide regarding duration of therapy.

Aspergillus appears relatively insensitive to 5-fluorocytosine. Miconazole and ketoconazole are also relatively inactive against *Aspergillus*. One in vitro study showed synergy with amphotericin B and rifampin.

Granulocyte transfusion in grancytopenic patients may be helpful but are not essential for success. Recovery from marrow suppression associated with a rise in granulocyte count constitute the most important favorable prognostic sign. The overall mortality in spite of therapy exceeds 80% in leukemic subjects. Survival figures are better in transplant recipients in which the risk factors, such as immunosuppressive medication, can be withdrawn.

Surgical resection has been traditionally advised for the compromised host with an asymptomatic mycetoma or fungus ball because of the risk of invasion. Recent studies, however, have shown that observation alone may be adequate.

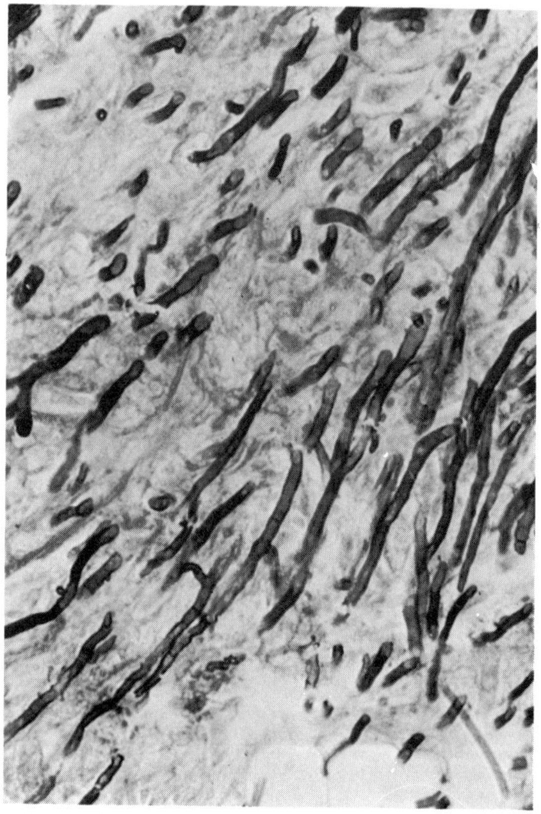

Figure 17-3D The typical acute branching septate hyphae of *Aspergillus* can be seen in the histological preparation.

Candida

Candida pneumonia may be acquired by two routes: 1) bronchogenic spread may follow aspiration of upper respiratory secretions, or 2) hematogenous dissemination to the lung may occur as part of multiple organ involvement, including kidneys, skin, and fundi. The primary source for hematogenous dissemination usually is ulceration of the gastrointestinal tract, often asymptomatic, or central intravenous lines used for parenteral nutrition. It is striking, however, that although *Candida* often are cultured from sputum and respiratory secretions, *Candida* pneumonia is infrequent. The lungs appear relatively resistant to direct parenchymal invasion by *Candida*. *Candida albicans* is the most common species isolated, followed by *C. tropicalis* and *C. parapsilosis*, the latter commonly associated with hyperalimentation.

The type of patient who develops *Candida* pneumonia almost invariably is the immunosuppressed hospitalized patient with hematological malignancy and granulocytopenia, who has received broad spectrum, parenteral antibiotics. The patient develops fever, is extremely ill and a new pulmonary infiltrate is observed which fails to respond to antibacterial agents. There may be concomitant evidence of *Candida* stomatitis or esophagitis. Chest x-ray findings are somewhat variable and include nonspecific infiltrates, nodules, bronchopneumonia, and abscess formation. Hematogenous disease results in multilobar nodule formation and there may be evidence of infiltrates in the optic fundi and skin.

Confirmation of the diagnosis of *Candida* pneumonitis is extremely difficult for the following reasons: isolation of *Candida* from sputum, transtracheal and bronchoscopic specimens are common and usually reflect upper or lower airway colonization or contamination. Positive blood cultures are present in no more than 25% to 33% of patients with disseminated disease and are rarely positive in primary bronchogenic *Candida* pneumonia. Furthermore, when blood cultures are positive, they may represent transient candidemia related to indwelling intravenous devices, which may resolve rapidly after removal of the catheter. In spite of these difficulties, positive blood cultures in the immunocompromised host, especially when multiple and in the absence of a catheter should suggest dissemination.

Use of serology for the diagnosis of *Candida* infection has been disappointing. Even newer, more sensitive techniques, such as the passive hemagglutination test, demonstrates a fourfold increase in titer only inconsistently. When a rise in titer does occur, it is suggestive in retrospect, but a negative response does not rule out invasive *Candida* infection.

Newer diagnostic methods include detection of antigenemia and the specific use of mycelial-phase antigens to differentiate invasion from colonization. Preliminary results are encouraging; however, antigenemia, when present, does not distinguish between disseminated candidiasis and transient candidemia associated with intravenous catheters. Accordingly, initiation of therapy must rely heavily upon clinical judgment based on data obtained from clinical and autopsy studies, which shows that about 50% of autopsied patients with hematological malignancy had unsuspected disseminated *Candida* infection.

Intravenous amphotericin B remains the mainstay of therapy, although the optimal dose and duration of therapy is still uncertain. Whereas, low-dose and short-term therapy with amphotericin may be appropriate for *Candida* esophagitis, *Candida* pneumonia in a severely granulocytopenic host requires immediate high-dose therapy (0.4 to 0.6 mg/kg/day) after a 1-mg test dose if the critically ill patient is to have any chance of survival. 5-Fluorocytosine is active in vitro against *Candida* and is less toxic than amphotericin. It is tempting to use this orally administered agent whenever the question of *Candida* infection is raised. Unfortunately, numerous failures due to emergence of resistance have been described when this agent is used alone. The use of miconazole and ketoconazole alone or in combination with amphotericin is currently being assessed.

The prognosis for invasive candidiasis remains extremely poor in patients with malignancy; only 58% of subjects with solid tumors and 29% with acute leukemia survive this infection.

Although prophylactic oral nonabsorbable nystatin is prescribed in granulocytopenic hosts, its efficacy remains unproven and recent reports suggest that nystatin resistance is now more frequent and may be related to its widespread use.

Torulopsis glabrata

Although related to *Candida albicans*, these yeasts do not produce pseudohyphae. They are also found as commensuals in the normal respiratory and gastrointestinal tracts and are part of vaginal flora. Infection can only be documented by isolation of these yeasts from a normally sterile site or by histological identification in human tissue. *T. glabrata* mainly has caused fungemia as a complication of intravenous hyperalimentation, although rare reports of pneumonia due to this organism exist. There is no typical radiological picture of *Torulopsis* pneumonia, and infection is often mixed with other fungi and bacteria. Amphotericin B and 5-fluorocytosine are active in vitro against this yeast.

Zygomycosis

Zygomycosis refers to infection with any of several genera of the order *Mucorales*, namely *Absidia*, *Mucor* and *Rhizopus*, all of which result in similar clinical manifestations, and is virtually found only in diabetics and in severely immunocompromised hosts. Infection is rare and present in less than 3% of leukemic patients at autopsy. Pneumonia usually occurs in granulocytopenic leukemic patients, and is less frequently associated with lymphoma and organ transplantation. Pathologic specimens demonstrate the marked tendency of these fungi to grow across tissue planes, including organ boundaries in a manner similar to *Aspergillus*, and also to invade blood vessels resulting in organ infarction and hemorrhage. Clinically, an acutely ill patient shows progressive bronchopneumonia and cavitation unresponsive to antibacterial therapy. Unfortunately, there are only isolated survivors after antifungal therapy. The small hope of recovery depends upon early diagnosis and administration of amphotericin B, possibly combined with resection of infarcted lung. Diagnosis usually requires lung biopsy. There are no specific in vitro tests to facilitate the diagnosis.

Cryptococcus neoformans

In contrast to *Aspergillus* and *Candida*, the prevalence of cryptococcal disease is only slightly increased in the immunocompromised host. One half of all patients with a disseminated form of cryptococcal disease, namely cryptococcal meningitis, have no apparent underlying disease. When infection does occur in immunocompromised patients, dissemination is more common and infection is more difficult to eradicate. Severe, resistant infection is most commonly seen in patients with defects in cell-mediated immunity. Neutropenia is not a significant risk factor with regard to *Cryptococcus*.

The clinical spectrum of pulmonary cryptococcosis is highly variable, and most cases in the immunocompromised host are thought to represent reactivation of latent foci of infection. Because of its tendency for dissemination to extrapulmonary sites, pulmonary symptoms alone are uncommon in this patient population. In contrast to normal hosts, about one third of whom are asymptomatic, a higher proportion of immunocompromised patients with pulmonary cryptococcosis have symptoms which include fever, night sweats, weight loss, cough and pleuritic chest pain. Chest x-ray may reveal either a single mass lesion that occasionally cavitates, lobar or segmental consolidation or multiple poorly localized infiltrates (Figure 17-4).

Since the recovery of *Cryptococcus* from sputum in patients with chronic obstructive airways disease may represent bronchial colonization only, a definitive diagnosis of pulmonary cryptococcosis requires demonstration of the organism in pulmonary tissue. Nevertheless, recovery of cryptococci from sputum of immunocompromised patients should be interpreted as indicating active infection. Identification of cryptococci in needle aspirates of a pulmonary mass, a skin lesion or pleural fluid is an indication for therapy in the compromised host.

Cryptococcal antigen detection in the serum or cerebrospinal fluid is usually diagnostic of cryptococcal disease. False-positive reaction may occur, but the test is helpful in the early diagnosis of cryptococcal meningitis before other laboratory tests (India ink or culture) are positive. However, the test may be negative in an infection restricted to the lung. The presence of cryptococcal antibody is only suggestive evidence of active cryptococcal infection. In contrast to normal hosts, immunocompromised patients with pulmonary cryptococcosis, even if asymptomatic, should be treated with amphotericin B, both to prevent and eradicate silent metastatic foci. 5-Fluorocytosine should be combined with amphotericin B in an attempt to achieve synergistic activity.

PARASITIC PNEUMONIA

Toxoplasma gondii

Toxoplasma gondii is an obligate intracellular parasite which causes a variety of relatively mild self-limited clinical syndromes in the normal

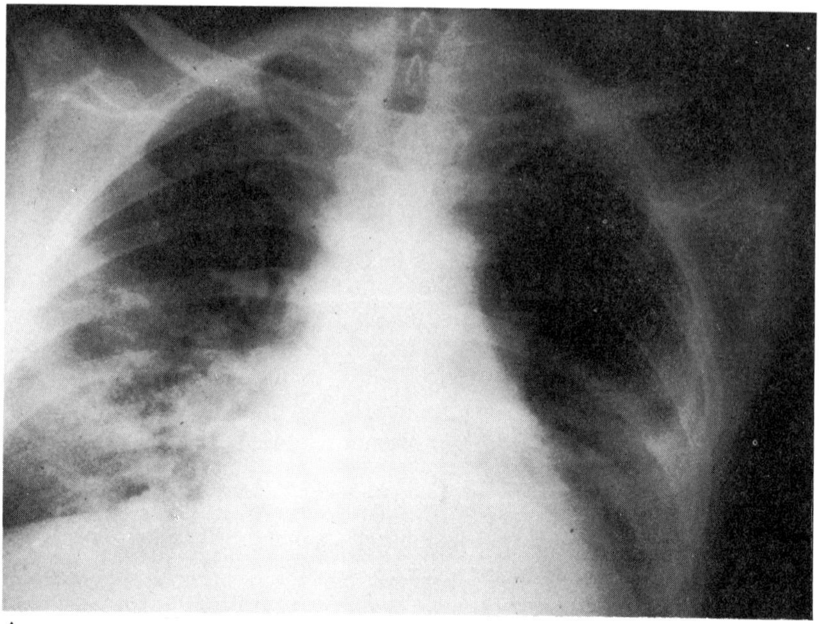

A

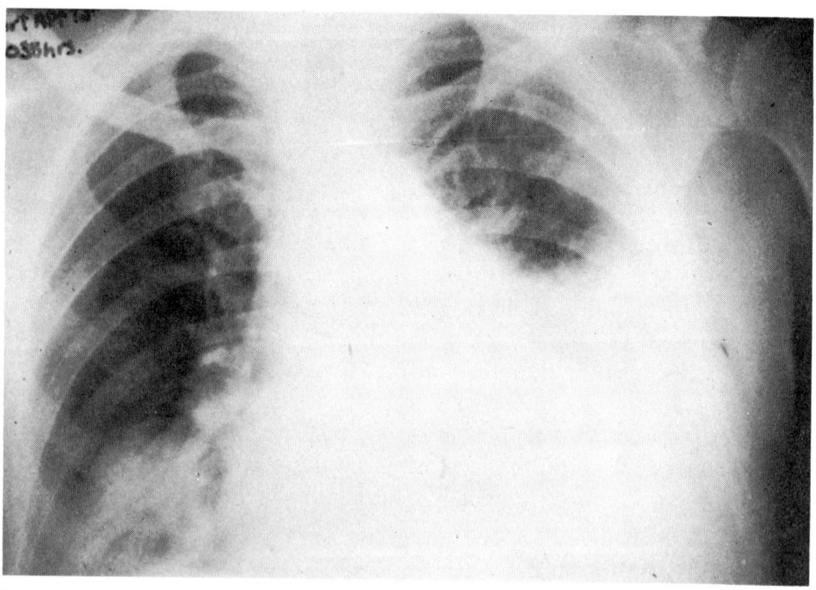

B

Figure 17-4A,B Diffuse, poorly localized infiltrates and pleural effusions in two renal transplant patients due to severe bilateral cryptococcal pneumonia.

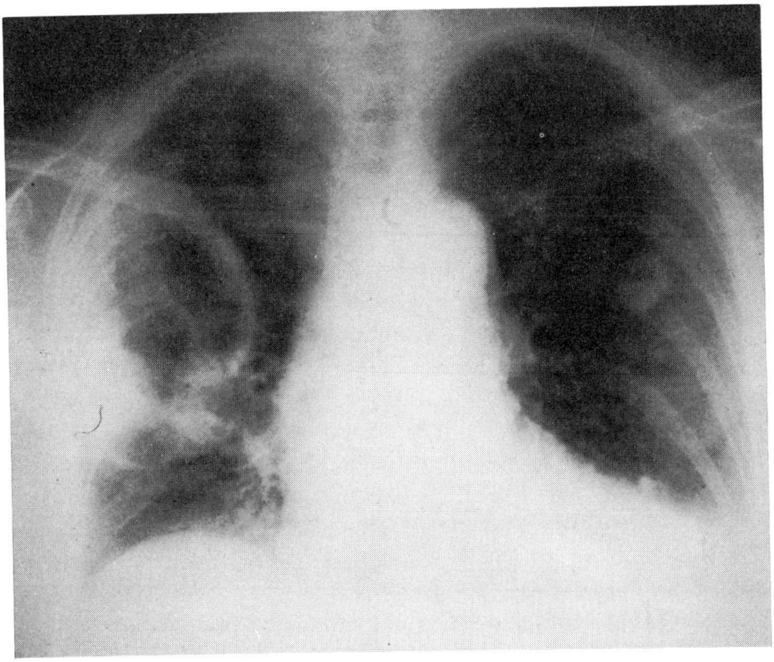

Figure 17-4C A chest radiograph in a 65-year-old woman receiving prednisone for temporal arteritis revealed nodular and cavitating pulmonary lesions due to cryptococcal infection.

host, but has the ability to cause devastating infection, including pneumonia, in the immunocompromised host. The organism exists in three forms, trophozoite, tissue cyst and oocyst. The trophozoites are the rapidly proliferating form seen in tissues during acute infection. They enter all types of tissue cells, except erythrocytes, by the process of endocytosis. Trophozoites do not grow on artificial media. After endocytosis, trophozoites multiply and, after the host cell ruptures, are released to invade additional cells. The intracellular location protects the *Toxoplasma* from antibodies and complement. Cell-mediated immunity is apparently crucial in controlling infection.

Tissue cysts represent the latent form of infection and are found mainly in the brain and skeletal or heart muscle where they evoke a minimal inflammatory response. Oocysts are produced in epithelial cells of the digestive tract in cats and are excreted in cat feces.

Infection after birth is most likely to occur by ingestion of cysts in undercooked meat, usually pork or lamb, or food contaminated with oocysts from cat feces. Occasionally, infection is acquired by blood transfusion and very rarely by heart transplantation.

The prevalence of infection varies geographically. In the United States, serological tests have shown antibody present in 17% to 35% of

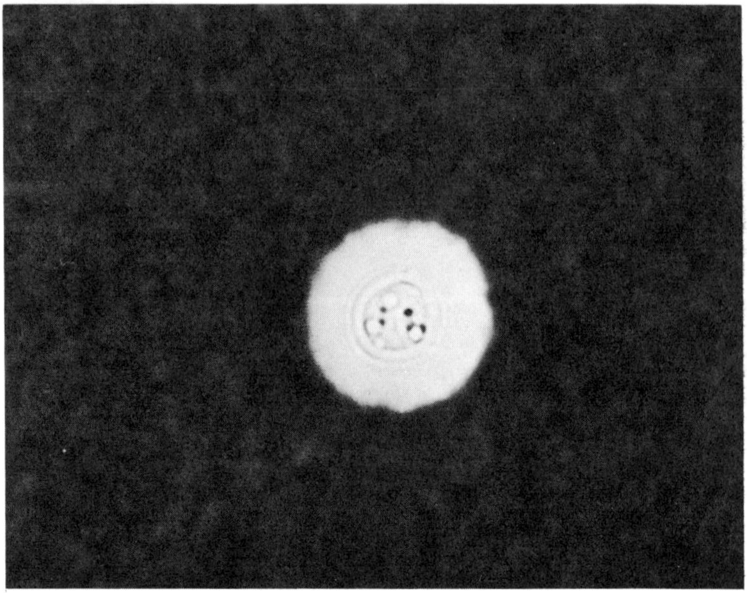

Figure 17-4D India ink preparation of *Cryptococcus neoformans* with large clear capsule found in sputum.

the population. Infection in the normal host usually is asymptomatic. Clinical manifestations usually are mild and resolve spontaneously in most cases within one to three months. Most commonly, asymptomatic lymphadenopathy occurs in the cervical region. At times, toxoplasmosis may be indistinguishable from infectious mononucleosis caused by the Epstein-Barr virus with generalized lymphadenopathy, fever, malaise, pharyngitis and splenomegaly.

In the immunocompromised host, *Toxoplasma* are capable of producing a rapidly fatal disseminated infection. Infection in this setting may result from reactivation of latent infection or recent acquisition of organisms. Most frequently, the immunocompromised patients have a lymphoreticular malignancy, particularly Hodgkin's disease or, less frequently, leukemia, solid tumors, collagen-vascular disease or have had an organ transplantation. The central nervous system is most commonly involved with a diffuse meningoencephalitis or, less commonly, a localized lesion, mimicking brain abscess. Pneumonia occurs in about one third of patients, but rarely are the lungs alone involved. The pneumonia usually is an antibiotic-unresponsive interstitial process and tends to be severe. Histology often reveals intense inflammation, interstitial hemorrhage and an alveolar exudate.

Serological tests for the detection of *Toxoplasma* antibody constitute the primary means of diagnosis of acute and chronic infection. IgM antibodies detected by indirect immunofluorescence or the ELISA technique are extremely useful in diagnosis of recent infection, even in the immunocompromised host. A fourfold increase rise in IgM antibody titer establishes the diagnosis of acute infection. In most cases, maximum titers usually exceed 1:1000. IgG antibodies may be detected by indirect immunofluorescence or the Sabin-Feldman test.

A definitive diagnosis of acute toxoplasmosis also can be made by demonstration of trophozoites in tissues or body fluids. Recognition of trophozoites in histologic sections is difficult but can be facilitated by Giemsa, Wright or immunofluorescent staining. The presence of cysts in tissue usually represents subacute or chronic infection, but does not exclude the possibility of acute infection. In specialized centers, organisms may be isolated by injection into mouse peritoneal cavity.

Pyrimethamine combined with sulfadiazine is the standard treatment. Both drugs are used because the combination is synergistic against *Toxoplasma gondii*. In the immunocompromised host as opposed to normal subjects, therapy is always indicated, as most immunocompromised patients will die if untreated. Early therapy results in about an 80% response rate. Folinic acid supplementation should be considered to prevent the development of bone marrow suppression or megaloblastic anemia.

Pneumocystis carinii

P. carinii was first recognized as a pulmonary pathogen in neonates and infants during the Second World War. Its role as a major cause of respiratory morbidity and mortality in the immunocompromised host has been established over the last two decades. It is responsible for 45% of cases of interstitial pneumonia among immunocompromised patients. Only rarely does dissemination to extrapulmonary sites occur.

Two forms of the organism can be distinguished, the trophozoite and the cyst, which contains four to eight trophozoites. Fully developed cysts rupture and release trophozoites into surrounding tissue.

It is not as yet clear whether human disease is due to reactivation of a latent infection or due to primary infection. Considerable controversy exists as to whether person-to-person spread occurs, although animal studies have documented aerosol transmission. Recent data using an immunofluorescent antibody assay suggests that infection is widespread and occurs early in life, with the prevalence of antibodies to *P. carinii* being 75% to 80% by the age of 4. Nevertheless, the prevalence of clinical disease varies considerably on a geographical basis. The reason for this discrepancy is still unknown.

The most important predisposing factor to *P. carinii* infection is immunodeficiency. Most frequently, infection occurs in the presence of defective cell-mediated immunity, but humoral factors also appear to be important. Treatment with corticosteroids has been the usual predisposing factor in most series of *P. carinii* pneumonitis. Paradoxically, pneumonia which may appear after steroid therapy is being reduced. Other risk factors include acute lymphocytic leukemia, often in remission, lymphoid malignancy, and congenital immunodeficiency. Recently, apparently healthy homosexuals have been described as developing recurrent *P. carinii* pneumonia as part of the acquired immunodeficiency syndrome.

The typical clinical picture is that of acute, rapidly progressive dyspnea, cyanosis, nonproductive cough and bilateral pulmonary infiltrates. Some patients have a more indolent course. *P. carinii* is uncommonly found in sputum and tracheal aspirates. Auscultation of the lungs reveals few physical signs, and the leukocyte count generally is not helpful.

Pulmonary infiltrates tend to be symmetric and to have a predominantly perihilar interstitial pattern early and a diffuse alveolar pattern late (Figure 17-5). In severe infection, extensive consolidation with air bronchograms may be seen. Atypical radiologic presentation is not uncommon, with a unilateral predominance, lobar distribution, nodular densities, abscess formation and initially even a normal chest x-ray may be reported. If untreated, death due to rapidly progressive respiratory failure is the usual outcome. In treated patients, multiple episodes of pneumocystosis have been described, which probably represent relapse rather than reinfection.

Histology demonstrates the presence of cysts and trophozoites within the cytoplasm of cells attached to the alveolar walls. Subsequently, alveoli become filled with intense foamy exudate and mononuclear cell infiltration. Clusters of cysts are identified within the alveoli by their outer double-layered wall containing two to eight internal bodies. Specific stains are, however, required. Recommended is Gomori's methenamine silver nitrate impregnation and Gram-Weigert stains for demonstration of the cyst wall (Figure 17-5B). With the Giemsa and methylene blue stains, sporozoites within the cysts and trophozoites can be identified. Care must be taken with improper staining, otherwise red cells or yeast can be mistaken for *P. carinii*.

The diagnosis of *P. carinii* pneumonia rests upon morphologic identification of organisms in tissues and secretions. Whereas percutaneous lung aspiration is useful in children, the most widely used and successful methods are fiberoptic bronchoscopy, together with bronchial washings, brushings and transbronchial biopsy, as well as open lung biopsy. Brushings and transbronchial biopsy appear to be about 80% to 90% as sensitive as open lung biopsy, although even the latter method is not infallible. At present, no reliable serological test is available for diagnosis of acute *P. carinii* infection in immunocompromised patients.

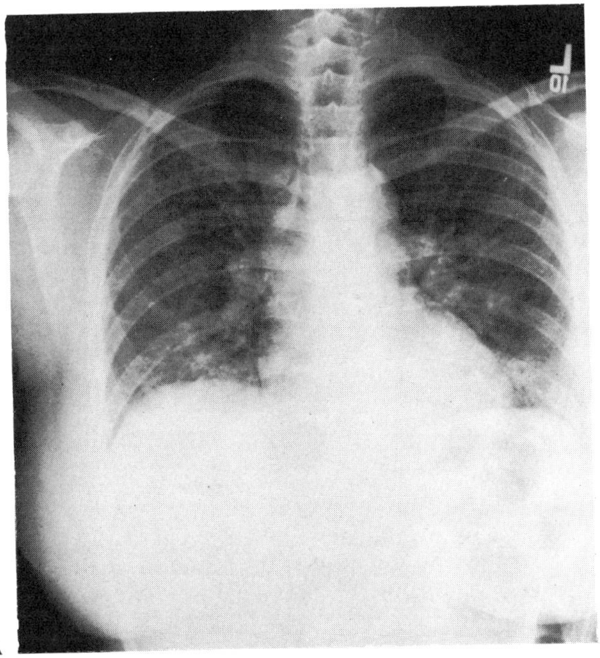

A

B

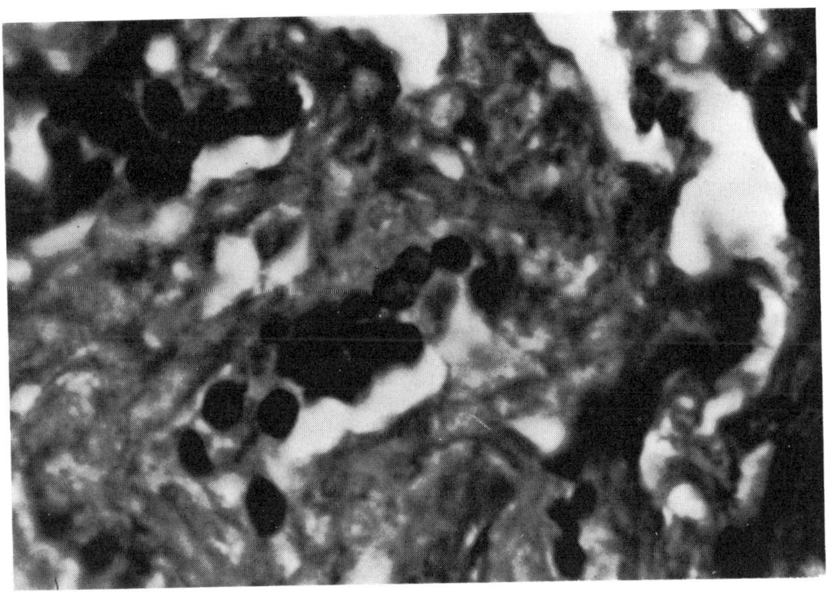

Figure 17-5 A 43-year-old woman with acquired immunodeficiency syndrome presented with recurrent bouts of *Pneumocystitis carinii* infection. Chest radiograph revealed a diffuse symmetrical interstitial pattern **A**. Lung biopsy revealed multiple cyst forms with silver methenamine stain **B**.

Pentamidine isethionate was the first useful therapeutic agent for *P. carinii* infections with an overall response rate of approximately 40%. If the patient survived one week, recovery rates increased to 60% to 70%. Complications include azotemia, hypoglycemia, hypocalcemia, abnormal liver function tests, skin reactions, hypotension and pain at the site of infusion. Unfortunately, the incidence of adverse reaction was so high (50%) that pentamidine has now been replaced by trimethoprim-sulfamethoxazole (TMP-SMZ). Controlled studies in humans have shown that TMP-SMZ is as effective as pentamidine, if not more so, with significantly less toxicity. Dosage recommended is 20 mg of TMP and 100 mg of SMZ per kilogram of body weight per day in four equal doses given by mouth or intravenously.

In view of the efficacy, ready availability and relative lack of toxicity of TMP-SMZ, this therapy is frequently given to patients with *P. carinii* pneumonia without obtaining a tissue diagnosis. This approach is fraught with potential hazard. First, empiric treatment can obscure the histologic diagnosis and complicate management in the event of subsequent lung biopsy. Second, because of the broad spectrum of its activity, empiric TMP-SMZ might obscure the diagnosis of *Nocardia* and other bacterial infection.

VIRAL INFECTIONS

The major viral respiratory pathogens in the immunocompromised are cytomegalovirus, varicella-zoster, herpes simplex, adenovirus and measles. In general, viral pneumonia is much less frequent than bacterial or fungal pneumonia except after organ transplantation, in which an interstitial pneumonia due to cytomegalovirus develops in 30% to 50% of patients within four months after receiving the graft.

Cytomegalovirus

By far, the most important virus associated with pulmonary infection in the immunocompromised host is cytomegalovirus. Although usually isolated together with other respiratory pathogens, predominantly *P. carinii*, there is good evidence that cytomegalovirus alone can produce serious pneumonia.

Disease due to cytomegalovirus may result from primary viral infection or reactivation of latent infection during immunosuppression. Primary infection may occur following transplantation of a cytomegalovirus-infected kidney in nonimmune recipients. It has been established that most immunosuppressed patients with a primary infection and perhaps 25% to 30% of those with evidence of reactivation are symptomatic, ie, fever, leukopenia, atypical lymphocytes, pneumonia or hepatitis. Reactivation also can occur as asymptomatic viral shedding.

In immunocompromised patients, cytomegalovirus pneumonia varies in severity. Fever, a nonproductive cough, dyspnea and hypoxemia occur. The mortality rate approximates 50% to 60%. The radiological picture typically shows an interstitial infiltrate, predominantly in the lung periphery; however, other patterns have been described. Because virus can be recovered from patients in the absence of demonstrable disease, the presence of cytomegalovirus-positive cultures in symptomatic patients is difficult to evaluate. Serological evidence of infection occurs in 25% to 33% of asymptomatic adults with neoplasia and, unfortunately, disease may also occur without serologic confirmation.

Optimally, the diagnosis of cytomegalovirus pneumonia requires both histological demonstration of typical intranuclear inclusions of cytomegalovirus-infected cells and a positive culture of lung tissue for this virus. Therapy, including the use of adenine arabinoside and interferon, to date remains disappointing. Preliminary studies using interferon prophylactically in bone marrow transplantation recipients have been encouraging.

Varicella-Zoster (V-Z)

Primary V-Z infection rarely causes pneumonia in children, but occurs in 16% to 33% of adults with primary V-Z infection. Usually, varicella pneumonia is mild, but occasionally may be life-threatening in normal patients. In contrast, a severe form of progressive varicella may be seen with extremely prominent skin lesions, pneumonia, hepatitis and meningoencephalitis in immunocompromised hosts.

Limited cutaneous reactivation of latent V-Z infection (ie, zoster or shingles) occurs in patients with Hodgkin's disease (15% to 40%) and less frequently in patients with non-Hodgkin's lymphoma, renal transplantation, acute leukemia and solid tumors, and may become disseminated in these patients. Dissemination usually is limited to the skin, but occasionally life-threatening V-Z pneumonia may accompany the cutaneous dissemination.

V-Z pneumonia is characterized by high fever, nonproductive cough, progressive dyspnea, chest pain and hemoptysis. Physical examination reveals few findings in contrast to the symptoms and x-ray picture. A widespread small nodular infiltrate in a peribronchial distribution occurs (see Figure 1 in Chapter 45). The diagnosis usually is not difficult because of the skin lesions, but secondary bacterial infection may complicate the picture. Death in varicella pneumonia usually is secondary to respiratory insufficiency.

Adenine-arabinoside is thought to favorably alter the course of V-Z infection in immunocompromised patients and may have a role in the treatment of V-Z pneumonia. Similarly, interferon and acyclovir may also improve the outcome of V-Z pneumonia.

In immunosuppressed patients, zoster-immune globulin if given within 72 hours of exposure may prevent or reduce the severity of varicella pneumonia in both nonimmune children and adults.

Herpes Simplex

Herpes simplex rarely causes pneumonia, although tracheitis is not uncommon in immunosuppressed hosts. Pneumonia, when it occurs, usually accompanies herpes simplex infection in the upper respiratory tract, suggesting contiguous spread or aspiration. Interstitial or bronchopneumonia develops with a fulminant course, the diagnosis rarely being made antemortem. Lung biopsy reveals intranuclear inclusions and the virus may be isolated from tissue culture of the biopsy. Therapy of herpes simplex pneumonia with adenine-arabinoside may be successful in view of the encouraging therapeutic results of adenine-arabinoside in herpes simplex encephalitis.

Adenovirus

A recent study described 15 immunocompromised patients with adenovirus pneumonia. Clinical features included high fever, myalgia, malaise, cough, tachypnea and gastrointestinal symptoms. Radiological confirmation of pneumonia was present in 80%. Most commonly, a bilateral alveolar or interstitial pattern was observed and in 20% a pleural effusion was present. The virus was isolated from throat, urine, lung tissue and occasionally blood. Nine of the 15 patients died, confirming the severity of adenovirus infection in immunocompromised hosts.

Influenza Virus

It is uncertain whether immunocompromised hosts are more susceptible to influenza than normal individuals. Nevertheless, it is still advisable to recommend influenza vaccination on an annual basis in immunocompromised patients.

ACQUIRED IMMUNODEFICIENCY SYNDROME (AIDS)

By December 1982, over 800 cases of AIDS had been reported to the Communicable Disease Center, USPHS. Although the vast majority of cases have occurred in previously healthy homosexually active men, particularly in New York City and San Francisco, other groups involved include intravenous drug abusers, hemophiliacs and heterosexual Haitian immigrants. About 5% of cases belong to no known risk group. Several infants have been described with AIDS developing within the first six months of life. One of the infants received blood products at birth from a man who was subsequently found to have AIDS; the other infants were born to mothers who had AIDS, were Haitian or were intravenous drug abusers. Also, clusters of sexually related cases have occurred among homosexual men in Southern California. Although the etiology of AIDS is unknown, this distribution of cases suggests that AIDS is caused by an infectious agent transmitted sexually or by exposure to blood or blood products. Transmission of the agent from mother to infant in utero or shortly after birth could account for the early onset of AIDS in some infants.

The earliest clinical manifestations include fever, generalized lymphadenopathy, malaise, lethargy and weight loss. After a variable period, often lasting several months, severe, fulminant infections caused by opportunistic microorganisms occur. These infections, previously seen only in severely immunodeficient hosts, include: *Pneumocystis carinii* pneumonia, which often relapses after appropriate chemotherapy; oral, esophageal and disseminated candidiasis; herpes simplex infection (Figure 17-6); disseminated *Mycobacterium avium-intracellulare* infection; cerebral toxoplasmosis; multifocal leukoencephalopathy thought to be due to a papovavirus; cryptococcal meningitis; and severe, protracted diarrhea due to an intestinal protozoan parasite, *Cryptosporidium*. Males with AIDS have developed cutaneous and visceral Kaposi's sarcoma.

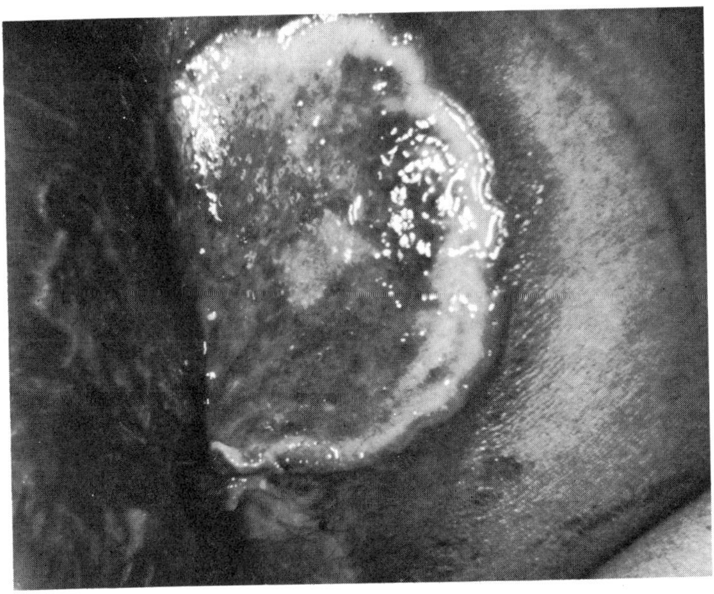

Figure 17-6 A 29-year-old homosexual with acquired immunodeficiency syndrome and recurrent opportunistic infections developed a chronic progressive ulcer in perianal area. Both *Mycobacterium avium-intracellulare* complex and herpes simplex were cultured from the lesion.

The immune defects in patients with AIDS include profound lymphocytopenia, T-lymphocyte depletion and dysfunction, reversal of the normal helper/suppressor T-lymphocyte ratio.

Although the pulmonary manifestations caused by these opportunistic pathogens have been described in this and other chapters, a number of differences should be stressed. Prior to the recognition of AIDS, *Pneumocystis* pneumonia in adults almost always had been observed in patients who were immunosuppressed by the nature of their recognized underlying disease, eg, those receiving corticosteroids or having lymphoreticular malignancies. Physicians should be aware now of the possibility of these infections developing in previously healthy individuals with undiagnosed AIDS.

The natural history and response to appropriate chemotherapy in AIDS has been extremely poor. Many patients with *P. carinii* infection have not responded to trimethoprim-sulfamethoxazole, pentamidine, or both. Perhaps patients with AIDS would benefit from prophylactic use of trimethoprim-sulfamethoxazole, as is done in leukemic children. In addition, no suitable agent is as yet available to treat cryptosporidiosis or disseminated infection due to *M. avium-intracellulare*.

SELECTED READINGS

Aisner J, Murillo J, Schimpff SC, et al: Invasive aspergillosis in acute leukemia: Correlation with nose cultures and antibiotic use. *Ann Intern Med* 1979; 90:4–9.

Bodey FR, Pare JAP, Fraser RG: Pulmonary disease in the compromised host. *Medicine* 1974;53:255–293.

Bandt PD, Blank N, Castellino RA: Needle diagnosis of pneumonitis: Value in high risk patients. *JAMA* 1972;220:1578.

Chaudhary S, Hughes WT, Feldman S, et al: Percutaneous transthoracic needle aspiration of the lung. Diagnosing *Pneumocystitis carinii* pneumonitis. *Am J Dis Child* 1977;131:902–907.

Chilcote RR, et al: Septicemia and meningitis in children splenectomized for Hodgkin's disease. *N Engl J Med* 1976;295:798–800.

Fanta CH, Pennington JE: Fever and new lung infiltrates in the immunocompromised host. *Clin Chest Med* 1981;2:19–39.

Greenman RL, Goodall PT, King D: Lung biopsy in immunocompromised hosts. *Am J Med* 1975;59:488–496.

Matthay RA, Greene WH: Pulmonary infections in the immunocompromised patient. *Med Clin North Am* May 1980;64:529–552.

Ramsey PG, Rubin RH, Tolkoff-Rubin NE, et al: The renal transplant patient with fever and pulmonary infiltrates—Etiology, clinical manifestations and management. *Medicine* 1980;59:206–222.

Rubin RH: The cancer patient with fever and pulmonary infiltrates: Etiology and diagnostic approach, in Remington JS, Swartz MN (eds): *Current Clinical Topics in Infectious Diseases, vol 1*. New York, McGraw-Hill, 1980.

Sickles EA, Young VM, Greene WH, et al: Pneumonia in acute leukemia. *Ann Intern Med* 1973;79:528–534.

Singer C, Armstrong D, Rosen PB, et al: Diffuse pulmonary infiltrates in immunosuppressed patients—A prospective study of 80 cases. *Am J Med* 1979;66: 110–120.

Williams DM, Krick JA, Remington JS: State of the art. Pulmonary infection in the compromised host. *Am Rev Respir Dis* 1976;114:359–394,593–617.

Zavala DC: Pulmonary biopsy. *Ann Intern Med* 1976;21:21–45.

18 *Pneumonia in the Transplant Patient*

George H. Talbot

Organ transplantation has opened new frontiers in medicine's quest for improvement in the human condition. However, transplant procedures have also opened a Pandora's box of undesirable side effects and outcomes, with infections among the most prominent of these. This chapter reviews the etiology, epidemiology, chronology, and management of pulmonary infections complicating transplantation. Renal allograft recipients will be discussed in greatest detail since they are the most commonly encountered group. Shorter sections will be devoted to bone marrow and cardiac transplant recipients.

THE RENAL TRANSPLANT RECIPIENT

Lower respiratory tract infection is a major cause of morbidity and mortality in this patient population. Reported attack rates have varied, but range from less than 5% to 35% of patients at risk. Mortality has been as high as 50% overall. Certain subgroups emerge as being at particularly high risk of developing pulmonary infection and of succumbing to it.

Host Defense Deficiencies

The renal transplant recipient often suffers from severe deficiencies in a wide range of host defense mechanisms. These defects arise not only as a consequence of the transplantation procedure and its attendant immunosuppressive therapy, but also as a result of the patient's underlying illness and chronic maintenance hemodialysis.

Host defense deficiencies characteristic of individuals with chronic renal insufficiency who are undergoing maintenance hemodialysis have been reviewed in detail by Goldblum and Reed (reference cited). Particularly relevant features are outlined in Table 18-1. Most important are structural and functional abnormalities in the respiratory tract itself. In addition, defects in the urinary tract, gastrointestinal tract, and skin may provide portals of entry which allow spread of potential pathogens to the lungs by indirect routes. Furthermore, once these physical barriers have been transgressed, abnormal granulocyte number and function, subnormal immunoglobulin levels, and impaired T-cell function predispose the host to severe, even life-threatening infection.

Although some of these deficiencies may be reversed by an adequately functioning allograft, quite often the process of transplantation substitutes new problems for old. During the immediate perioperative

Table 18-1
Host Defense Abnormalities of Renal Transplant Recipients

Pre-Transplantation

Physical Barriers
- Respiratory tract (decreased pulmonary clearance, altered nasopharyngeal flora, pulmonary edema)
- Mucocutaneous (repeated vascular access site cannulation, increased carriage of *S. aureus*)
- Gastrointestinal tract (alterations in secretion of gastric acid, in mucosal integrity, and in gastrointestinal flora)
- Urinary tract (repeated instrumentation)

Granulocytes
- Abnormalities in function (depressed adherence and chemotaxis)

Lymphocytes
- Depression in cell-mediated immunity
- Depression in immunoglobulin production

Weeks 1 through 4 Post-Transplantation

Physical Barriers
- Further compromise by invasive procedures (endotracheal intubation, assisted ventilation, intravenous therapy, intra-arterial monitoring, urinary tract instrumentation)
- Alteration in normal flora (replacement by hospital organisms)

Granulocytes
- Impaired adherence and chemotaxis

Lymphocytes
- Continued mild impairment

Months 2 through 6

Physical Barriers
- Continued, but less significant, compromise

Granulocytes
- Transient or persistent granulocytopenia

Lymphocytes
- Lymphopenia with severe depression of cell-mediated immunity
- Subnormal immunoglobulin production

After 6 Months

Physical Barriers
- Relatively intact

Granulocytes
- Relatively normal in number and function

Lymphocytes
- Mild defects in T- and B-cell function

period, the patient usually experiences violation of the respiratory tract (endotracheal intubation and assisted ventilation), the urinary tract (instrumentation), and the integument (intravascular catheters). Prolonged postoperative antimicrobial prophylaxis encourages colonization of multiple body sites by drug-resistant nosocomial microorganisms. The patient's nutritional status may be compromised by the surgery and its complications.

Most importantly, those medications essential for continued allograft survival have broad and potentially profound immunosuppressive effects. Corticosteroids impair both granulocyte function and T-cell mediated immunity. The basic regimen of prednisone 2 mg/kg/day, with tapering over several months, is often augmented by pulses of high-dose intravenous methylprednisolone. Azathioprine, administered at 1.5 to 3.0 mg/kg/day as another mainstay of many post-transplantation regimens, may occasionally accentuate bone marrow depression despite careful prospective monitoring of peripheral granulocyte and platelet counts. In some centers, antithymocyte, or antilymphocyte, globulin is given to selected allograft recipients in the immediate post-transplant period; such therapy potentiates depression of lymphocyte-mediated immunity.

At least one infectious sequela of the above-mentioned host defense abnormalities may itself contribute to immunosuppression. Cytomegalovirus (CMV) infection, both primary and secondary (reactivation), can produce profound impairment of cell-mediated immunity, thereby further increasing host susceptibility to those infections dependent on normal T-cell function for prevention or control. For some patients, this CMV-induced immunosuppression may be the most important factor determining outcome.

The foregoing discussion suggests that the post-transplantation period is not characterized by uniform immunosuppression, and indeed this is true. Immediately postoperatively, the patient is placed at risk simply by the invasive nature of the surgery and its ancillary procedures. The same risk factors for nosocomial lower respiratory tract infections that apply to any hospitalized patient also apply to this population. Although high-dose prednisone therapy may depress granulocyte function early postoperatively, it is not until approximately three to four weeks into the life of the allograft that the combination of corticosteroids and azathioprine takes its full toll on cell-mediated immunity, thereby creating the proper predisposing factors for those lower respiratory tract infections characteristic of this population. In part, because of this exogenous immunosuppression, CMV disease reaches its peak frequency during the second through the fourth months following transplantation, at which time it exerts its own immunosuppressive effect. This coincidence of peaks of exogenous and endogenous immunosuppression makes this period particularly hazardous for the transplant recipient. Beyond four to six months, the intensity of corticosteroid and azathioprine therapy is almost invariably reduced, save for intermittent pulses of methylprednisolone for acute rejection episodes. Therefore, the patient with a properly functioning allograft who has survived to the six-month mark will have improved, though not necessarily entirely normal, cell-mediated immunity. Subtle defects in humoral immunity may also persist, but granulocyte number and function generally are normal.

Chronology of Post-Transplantation Pneumonia

The chronology of post-transplantation lower respiratory tract infection correlates well with the nature and intensity of immunosuppression. This sequence has been reviewed by Ramsey et al (1980) and Rubin et al (1981). The reader wishing an elegant and exhaustive review of this topic is referred to these sources.

The allograft recipient is susceptible to bacterial lower respiratory tract infections throughout the postoperative period, but their peak incidence occurs in months two through four (see Table 18-2). Proportionately, however, primary bacterial pneumonias are more frequent than nonbacterial pneumonias early (within the first four weeks following transplantation), when they are nosocomial in origin, and late (after six months), at which time they are often community-acquired. In contrast, CMV pneumonia, an unusual event during the first postoperative month, is the most common lower respiratory tract process in months two through four, after which it diminishes in frequency. *Candida, Cryptococcus, Aspergillus*, and *Nocardia* are likewise rare in the immediate postoperative period, but begin to appear after the fourth week, sometimes following on the heels of CMV pneumonia. The incidence of these "opportunistic" pathogens decreases after four to six months, but cases may occur sporadically for the life of the transplant.

In absolute terms, then, the renal allograft recipient is at highest risk for bacterial and nonbacterial lower respiratory tract infection during postoperative months two through four.

At this juncture, it is important to note that not all chest roentgenographic abnormalities represent infection. During the immediate postoperative period, a variety of noninfectious processes, such as pulmonary edema, pulmonary embolism with or without infarction, and aspiration of gastric contents, may mimic lower respiratory tract infection. In one series, 28% of pulmonary disease episode were noninfectious in origin. These will not be discussed further, but the clinician would do well to include them in the differential diagnosis.

In summary, lower respiratory tract infections presenting in the first month or after the sixth month are likely to be bacterial in origin, whereas those appearing in the interim often are either of viral or fungal

Table 18-2
Pneumonia in Renal Transplant Recipients

Time	Major Host Defense Abnormalities	Pathogens	Onset	Chest X-ray	Clinical
0–30 Days	Impaired physical barriers, allowing direct or indirect access to the lungs	Nosocomial bacteria, including gram-negative rods	Acute	Lobar pneumonia or bronchopneumonia	Bacteremia; hypoxemia; exclude pulmonary embolism and pulmonary edema
30–120 Days	1. Depressed cell-mediated immunity	Nosocomial bacteria	As above	As above	As above
		CMV	Subacute	Diffuse interstitial or intra-alveolar infiltrates	Multisystem disease with leukopenia and thrombocytopenia; hypoxemia
	2. Impaired antibody production	*Nocardia* *Aspergillus*	Subacute	Nodular infiltrates, sometimes cavitary	Pleuritic chest pain; hemoptysis; minimal hypoxemia
	3. Transient, occasionally severe, leukopenia				
	4. Variable impairment of physical barriers	*Candida*	Subacute	Nodules or bronchopneumonia	Fungemia; colonization at multiple sites
After 120 Days	Minimal deficiencies in cell-mediated immunity and antibody production	Community-acquired bacteria: *S. pneumoniae*, *H. influenzae*, *S. aureus*	Acute	Lobar pneumonia or bronchopneumonia	Bacteremia or hypoxemia

etiology. Additional clinical clues suggesting the correct diagnosis are discussed further below.

Clinical and Epidemiological Clues to Etiology

Bacteria Bacterial pneumonia occurring within 30 days of transplantation is most commonly due to hospital-acquired organisms, often gram-negative rods. The pattern of nosocomial lower respiratory tract infection previously observed within a particular transplant unit may allow a reasonably accurate prediction of etiology in any single patient. For instance, the group at the Massachusetts General Hospital observed temporal and spatial clustering of *Pseudomonas aeruginosa* pneumonia that resolved when burn patients were physically segregated from the transplant recipients. In other institutions, *Klebsiella, E. coli, Enterobacter,* and *Serratia* are more frequent pathogens. *Legionella* has proved especially troublesome for some centers. Although gram-positive cocci, such as *Staphylococcus aureus* and *Streptococcus pneumoniae*, are occasionally encountered within the first post-transplant month, these organisms are more commonly community-acquired, and, as such, tend to appear late. *Hemophilus influenzae* pneumonias have also been noted more than six months postoperatively.

In general, the clinical presentation of these pneumonias in transplant patients is similar to that observed in other patient populations. The onset is acute to subacute, rarely insidious. The patient may be mildly ill, or die rapidly with fulminant disease. Feverishness, rigors, breathlessness, cough, and on occasion chest pain are prominent symptoms. Examination reveals an anxious, tachypneic individual with evidence of pulmonary consolidation, although rales alone may be the first finding. The cough is often productive unless the patient is neutropenic, is infected with an organism less frequently associated with purulent sputum, or is physically incapable of coughing. Corticosteroid therapy seems at times to attenuate the severity of the symptoms and signs. Arterial hypoxemia, sometimes accompanied by overt cyanosis, occurs in a majority of patients. Chest roentgenographic abnormalities include lobar infiltrates or patchy bronchopneumonia. Diffuse bilateral infiltrates occasionally are observed.

Although the clinical presentation and the epidemiologic context may suggest the identity of the etiologic agent, laboratory confirmation is required to ensure optimal management. Gram stain and culture of expectorated sputum may reveal the diagnosis. If not, transtracheal aspiration or bronchoscopy may be necessary. Blood cultures are helpful when positive. Despite extensive diagnostic procedures, empiric therapy may be necessary. This and other aspects of antibiotic therapy are discussed elsewhere.

Fungi The fungi most commonly implicated in pneumonias in this population include *Aspergillus* and *Nocardia* (not truly a fungus, but often included in this category). *Candida* and *Cryptococcus neoformans* are also observed. Once again, the epidemiologic context in a particular transplant unit may prove helpful. Clusters of invasive pulmonary aspergillosis, often attributed to hospital construction or renovation, have been reported. *Aspergillus fumigatus* has been the most frequent isolate. Similarly, "epidemic" nocardiosis has been described in at least one center.

In contrast to bacterial pathogens, the fungi tend to cause pneumonia of more insidious onset. In other respects, however, the clinical presentation may be similar to bacterial lower respiratory tract infection, with fever, shortness of breath, cough, and hemoptysis. Pleuritic chest pain is observed in *Nocardia* and *Aspergillus* pneumonias. Clues to a fungal versus bacterial etiology include the absence of significant hypoxemia until late in the course of disease and, in invasive pulmonary aspergillosis and nocardiosis, the finding of multiple rounded infiltrates which may progress to cavitation.

Blood cultures may be positive in patients with pulmonary candidiasis, nocardiosis, or cryptococcosis, but are rarely revealing in cases of invasive aspergillosis. Gram stain and culture of expectorated sputum is variably helpful. *Candida* may be seen and may grow, but more often than not this is the result of contamination by oral thrush. Gram staining may also show *Nocardia* organisms; however, these can be overlooked and the culture will be falsely negative unless it is held in the laboratory long enough to grow. *Cryptococcus neoformans* and *Aspergillus* are rarely seen on gram stain. A culture positive for the former is good evidence for the presence of disease. Although *Aspergillus* may appear as laboratory contaminant, even a single positive culture should not be disregarded if the clinical context is suggestive.

Serologic methods for diagnosis of these infections are discussed in the chapters dealing with these pathogens. At present, the only widely available potentially helpful method is the determination of cryptococcal antigen. When performed on a serum sample, a positive result is helpful, but a negative result does not exclude the disease.

Although these indirect methods may at times provide a diagnosis early enough in the course of illness to direct therapy, more often they do not. In this instance, lung biopsy is indicated. Bronchoscopy with transbronchial biopsy usually is successful, but open lung biopsy may be necessary if the closed procedure is unrewarding. Specifics of management are discussed in other chapters.

Viruses Although viral pneumonia in the transplant patient occasionally is due to adenovirus, influenza, or herpes simplex, the most common offender by far is cytomegalovirus. In fact, CMV is the leading cause of primary infectious pneumonias in this group. Conversely, 40% of all patients with CMV disease develop pneumonia. Furthermore, the effects of CMV infection are not limited to end-organ dysfunction alone, but include potentially life-threatening potentiation of corticosteroid and azathioprine-induced depression of cell-mediated immunity. This immunosuppression no doubt contributes to the 50% mortality of CMV pneumonia. The major risk factors for development of CMV disease are 1) the immunosuppressive therapy necessary for allograft survival, 2) the presence or absence of latent CMV in the recipient, and 3) the presence or absence of CMV in the transplanted kidney. Factors 2) and 3) can be assessed by performing CMV titers.

Given the invariable presence of immunosuppressive therapy, the patient's risk is determined in a relatively predictable fashion by his CMV status and that of the donor. If both are seronegative, CMV disease is unlikely (0% to 30%). However, if the recipient is seronegative, and the donor is seropositive, infection occurs in as many as 80% of individuals. When both are seropositive, the rate is intermediate, and presumably due to reactivation of recipient CMV rather than to a primary infection.

The spectrum of CMV infection in these individuals is broad. It may range from subclinical illness to a catastrophic, ultimately fatal multisystem disease. Pneumonia is a virtually invariable finding in this latter group of patients. Other clinical manifestations of CMV disease include prolonged fever, worsening renal function, pancreatitis, gastrointestinal bleeding, hepatitis, leukopenia, and thrombocytopenia. Peterson et al (1980) found that fever of more than seven days' duration and gastrointestinal bleeding were specific for CMV-induced illness in the transplant population. In this and other studies, leukopenia was associated with a high frequency of superinfection (pulmonary and nonpulmonary) as well as with ultimate mortality.

CMV pneumonia commonly develops in an insidious fashion, often following several days of fever with no obvious source. Nonspecific presenting complaints include fatigue, rigors, headache, arthralgias, and myalgias. Pulmonary signs and symptoms, usually absent at the onset of illness, appear relatively late in the course of fever—two weeks in Peterson et al's series. Dry cough and tachypnea are frequently the only objective abnormalities referable to the respiratory tract at this time.

Chest x-ray classically reveals diffuse interstitial or intra-alveolar infiltrates, but virtually any pattern can be seen, including multiple or solitary nodules, wedge-shaped lesions suggestive of embolism, and atelectasis. Pleural effusions, when present, are minimal, and not necessarily due to CMV. Not infrequently, the roentgenographic abnormalities are in part due to bacterial or fungal superinfection.

Hypoxemia is present in a majority of patients at some time during their illness. Individuals with severe disease invariably demonstrate a reduced partial pressure of oxygen. Hypocapnia is universal, barring underlying chronic lung disease or other reasons for CO_2 retention.

CMV infection is an important determinant of patient outcome. Peterson et al (1980) noted that 25% of patients who developed overt CMV disease died, as opposed to only 6% of those who did not. Pneumonia usually is a manifestation of severe illness, and consequently mortality is even higher in the subgroup developing CMV lower respiratory tract infection. A significant percentage of this mortality is due to complicating bacterial and fungal infection (vide infra).

CMV should be included in the differential diagnosis for virtually every febrile renal transplant patient with a pulmonary infiltrate. In the context of a clinical syndrome compatible with CMV, a firm diagnosis of CMV disease can be established if 1) cultures of urine, buffy coat, respiratory secretions, or tissue specimens grow CMV or 2) a fourfold rise in titer to CMV is detected by complement fixation or indirect fluorescent antibody tests. Histopathologic demonstration of intranuclear inclusions is consistent with, but not diagnostic of, CMV disease, since other herpes viruses may produce similar patterns.

In most instances, laboratory confirmation of clinical suspicion of CMV pneumonia is delayed. Cultures may take as long as two to four weeks to turn positive. Serologic and histopathologic techniques also have inherent delays. This situation may prove frustrating, and is compounded by the unfortunate fact that no effective antiviral agent is yet available for treatment of this illness. Aside from appropriate supportive management of complications such as respiratory failure and bacterial superinfection, the essential and only step in the therapy of CMV pneumonia is prompt and dramatic reduction in the dose of immunosuppressive drugs. This maneuver, if performed early in the course of disease, may be life-saving. Several series document improved patient survival when this approach is routinely employed. Loss of the transplanted kidney is of course viewed with concern, but this outcome is obviously preferred to that of the patient's demise. In fact, reduction of immunosuppression may at times result in salvage of the kidney since CMV itself can cause significant renal dysfunction. In the future, prophylaxis with interferon or other agents may allow prevention of CMV disease.

Other Infections

Early series emphasized that *Pneumocystis carinii* was commonly encountered in this population. Recent reports suggest that this organism is less frequent, perhaps as a result of the use of trimethoprim-sulfamethoxazole as prophylaxis for urinary tract infection. When *P. carinii* does cause illness, it is often in association with antecedent CMV infection. The presentation, course, laboratory and chest x-ray findings, and management of renal transplant recipients with *P. carinii* pneumonia parallel those of patients with other underlying illnesses and will not be discussed further here.

Toxoplasmosis or reactivation tuberculosis is the cause of pulmonary infiltrates in some transplant patients. These illnesses should be considered if other diagnoses cannot be established.

Pulmonary Superinfection

The clinician treating a normal host usually assumes that any pulmonary process has but a single etiology; most of the time he will be correct. However, this assumption clearly does not hold when one deals with renal transplant recipients. In this group, pulmonary infiltrates may have multiple causes, both infectious and noninfectious. This concept especially applies throughout the evolution of a primary pulmonary process, during which time bacterial or fungal superinfection occurs in upwards of 50% of patients. For instance, Ramsey et al (1980) reported this complication in 42% of their patients. It was particularly common among patients with CMV pneumonia (50%) and pulmonary embolism (89%). Peterson et al (1980) noted superinfection in 24% of their transplant recipients with CMV pneumonia. CMV-induced leukopenia probably plays a role in this phenomenon.

The organisms responsible for this lethal complication include nosocomial gram-negative bacilli, *Candida* and *Aspergillus* species, and *Pneumocystis carinii*. Superinfection may or may not be accompanied by a clear-cut, abrupt change in clinical status. Similarly, roentgenographic findings may not allow distinction between progression of the underlying process and the appearance of an intercurrent illness. Only a high index of suspicion and judicious repetition of appropriate tests will allow antemortem diagnosis. Often the clinician must rely on his judgment and on empiric antimicrobial therapy, but at best the salvage rate is poor. Ramsey et al (1980) reported only one survivor in a group of 23 patients with pulmonary superinfection.

Diagnosis and Management

Pneumonia should be a diagnostic consideration in all febrile renal allograft recipients. At the onset of fever, a careful history and physical examination should be performed with special attention to symptoms and signs of lower respiratory tract infection. A chest x-ray should be obtained on the vast majority of febrile patients, especially if they have been transplanted within the preceding four months.

When the chest x-ray confirms the presence of a pulmonary process, the clinician may construct a hypothesis as to its etiology by utilizing the clues described above and outlined in Figure 18-1. The direction of the workup will depend on the nature of the postulated process and the

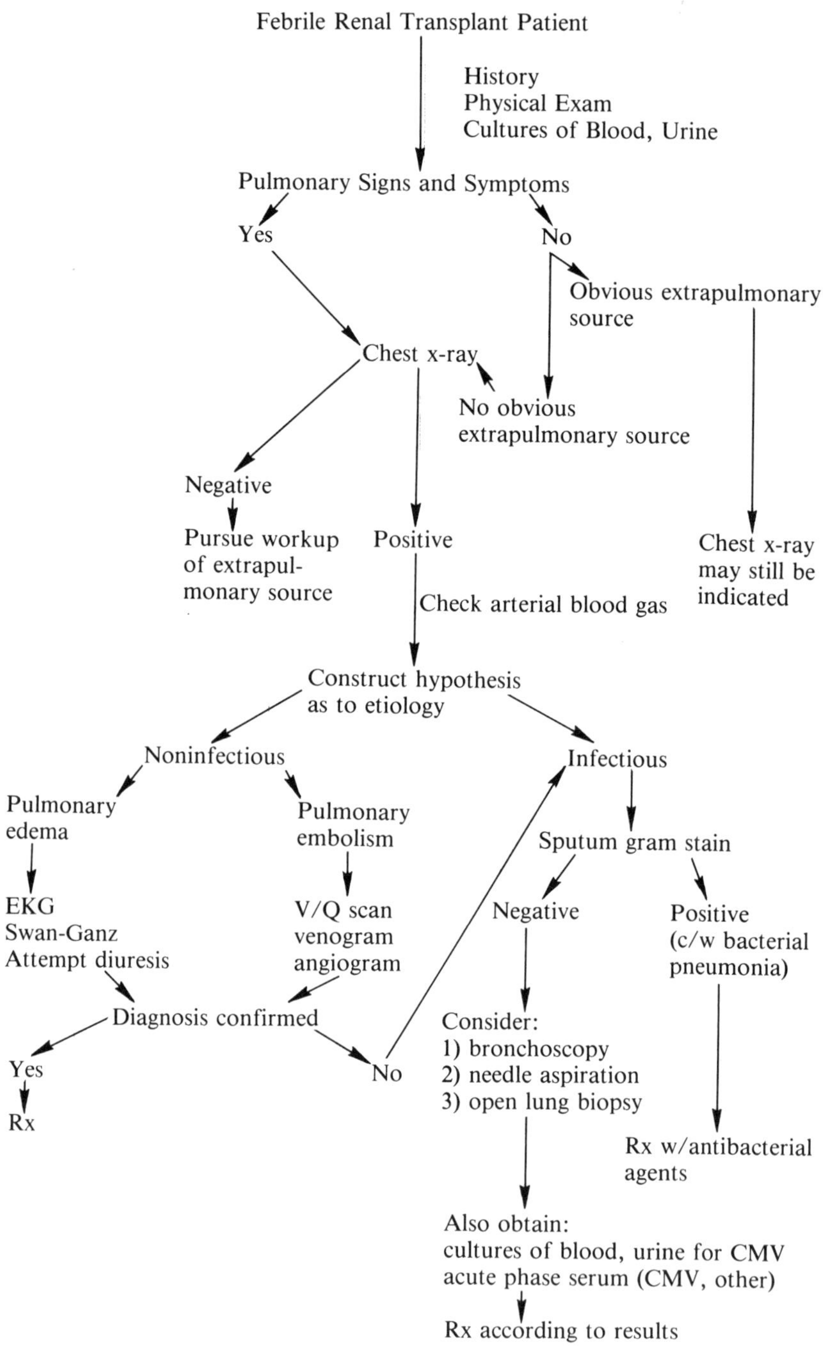

Figure 18-1 Management of pneumonia in the febrile renal transplant patient.

severity of the patient's illness. In all circumstances, the evaluation should be prompt, since inappropriate delay may prove fatal.

The initial differential diagnosis should include noninfectious as well as infectious etiologies. As noted, pulmonary embolism and pulmonary edema are to be considered, the former particularly in the first eight weeks postoperatively. Of these two conditions, embolic disease may be particularly difficult to diagnose since it may mimic other conditions and the underlying thrombosis may be silent. Ventilation-perfusion scanning, venography, or pulmonary angiography may be helpful in establishing the diagnosis.

More often than not the first clinical evaluation suggests that infection is at fault. In that instance, cultures of blood, urine, sputum, and other sites as clinically indicated should be obtained. Gram stain of expectorated sputum may be diagnostic in as many as 75% of patients with bacterial pneumonia. Care must be taken to obtain an adequate specimen that reveals a predominance of polymorphonuclear neutrophils and a relative absence of squamous epithelial cells on staining.

If this first simple maneuver reveals a likely diagnosis, the evaluation may be stopped at that point and appropriate antimicrobial therapy instituted. The choice of agents will depend upon the type of organisms seen and the epidemiologic context (nosocomial versus community acquisition).

When the sputum gram stain is nondiagnostic or unobtainable, more invasive procedures are necessary. Transtracheal aspiration is still favored in some institutions, but in many others bronchoscopy with washings, brushings and transbronchial biopsy is the method of choice. If the lesion is located peripherally, transthoracic needle aspiration may be preferred. Specimens should be obtained for the following tests:

- Gram stain and routine culture
- Acid-fast bacillus stain and culture
- Fungal culture (including *Nocardia*)
- Viral culture
- Cytology (for herpes virus inclusions)
- Fungal and *Pneumocystis* stains
- Direct immunofluorescence for herpes simplex and/or *Legionella pneumophila*
- *Legionella* culture; modified gram stain

In addition to these invasive tests, the following also may be indicated:

- CMV culture of blood and urine
- Acute and convalescent titers for CMV, other viruses as clinically indicated, *Legionella, Mycoplasma*

- Cryptococcal antigen
- Toxoplasmosis titer

Therapy is selected depending upon the results of these tests and upon the clinical context. Specifics of therapy are discussed elsewhere. If the initial attempt at diagnosis fails, the clinician has three choices: 1) repeating the bronchoscopy, 2) proceeding directly to open lung biopsy, or 3) empiric treatment with antimicrobial agents. Generally one prefers to establish a diagnosis, but the approach to each patient must be made on an individual basis.

Once a diagnosis has been established and therapy initiated, the clinician must remain vigilant, not only for the predictable and unpredictable side effects and toxicities of the treatment regimen, but also for the appearance of superinfection. A clear-cut change in the clinical course, or even apparent progression of the original problem, may call for judicious repetition of diagnostic maneuvers and alteration of the initial antimicrobial regimen.

THE BONE MARROW TRANSPLANT RECIPIENT

During the last decade, allogenic bone marrow transplantation has been performed on increasing numbers of individuals with aplastic anemia and acute leukemia. Autologous grafting occasionally is employed for treatment of far-advanced nonhematologic malignancies. The price exacted by the intense pretransplantation immunosuppression necessary for successful engraftment is serious infection, including pneumonia. The incidence of lower respiratory tract infection in this population reaches 50%. Considerably more than one half of affected patients die. Mortality rates vary depending on the etiologic organism(s), but may be as high as 80% for individuals with fungal and bacterial processes.

Host Defense Deficiencies

The bone marrow transplant recipient is afflicted by significantly greater host defense impairment than his counterpart who has received a renal allograft. As a consequence of underlying disease (which may be particularly debilitating for the patient with acute leukemia) and its therapy with a broad range of chemotherapeutic agents, these patients may enter the transplantation protocol with severe dysfunction of their cell-mediated, humoral, and polymorphonuclear responses to infection. Preparation for transplant induces still further host defense compromise.

Several different regimens may be employed to prepare the patient for marrow engraftment. One such conditioning program involves administration of cyclophosphamide and total body irradiation. Common to these protocols is the intent to ablate all leukemic cells. The invariable result is profound lymphopenia, causing pronounced impairment of humoral and cellular immunity, as well as intense granulocytopenia. Alveolar macrophage dysfunction also occurs. Invasive procedures further compromise host defenses by disrupting the skin and mucous membranes, while prolonged, broad-spectrum antibiotic therapy reduces normal flora, allowing colonization by fungi or resistant bacteria.

Reconstitution of normal host defenses depends on two major factors: 1) successful engraftment of the transplanted marrow, and 2) the absence of significant graft-versus-host disease (GVHD). Failure of engraftment essentially dooms the patient to death from infection or bleeding. Conversely, when all goes well, granulocyte levels reach 1000/mm^3 in an average of three weeks. Despite this apparent manifestation of restored host defenses, humoral and cell-mediated immunity often remain markedly impaired for another three months. These abnormalities may persist even longer in patients developing GVHD. They are probably due in part to the agents used to prevent or treat GVHD: methotrexate, corticosteroids, and antithymocyte globulin.

One especially important defect demonstrated in long-term survivors (> seven months post-transplant) is impaired opsonic activity for *Streptococcus pneumoniae*. This can be due to either low serum antibody levels or low complement levels. The etiology of this particular abnormality is not clear. The common practice of administering antimicrobial prophylaxis (often trimethoprim-sulfamethoxazole) for the first five months post-transplant may account for the late appearance of *S. pneumoniae* infections.

Chronology of Post-Transplantation Pneumonia

The chronology of lower respiratory tract infection in bone marrow transplant recipients differs from that in renal allograft recipients. The extensive review by Winston et al (1979) suggests that a major difference is the earlier appearance of fungal pneumonia in the former group. In that series, the median time of onset for fungal pneumonia was day 8 after transplantation, for bacterial pneumonia day 44, and for viral pneumonia day 74. *Pneumocystis carinii* pneumonias clustered at the end of the third month. Idiopathic interstitial pneumonias, an important cause of morbidity and mortality in this population, had a median onset at day 85. As noted above, there is in addition an apparent tendency for pneumococcal pneumonias to occur late, ie > seven months post-transplant.

Characteristics of Pneumonia in the Marrow Transplant Recipient

The pathogens implicated are essentially identical to those causing problems for renal allograft recipients. Nosocomial gram negative rods,

Aspergillus and *Candida* species, CMV, and *Pneumocystis carinii* are most common. Furthermore, each of these infections tends to produce similar clinical and radiographic manifestations regardless of whether it is a bone marrow or renal allograft recipient that is afflicted.

One process particularly frequent in the marrow transplant group is interstitial pneumonia. Although this illness often is due to CMV or *P. carinii* infection, the diagnosis commonly remains obscure, even after lung biopsy or postmortem examination. Allogenic grafting and GVHD appear to be predisposing factors for interstitial pneumonia in general. Prophylactic white blood cell transfusions have been demonstrated to increase the risk of CMV-induced disease for patients who are CMV-seronegative. CMV immune plasma appears to decrease the incidence of symptomatic CMV infection in marrow transplants, especially when leukocyte transfusions are not used. The reader wishing a more detailed discussion of these issues is referred to the references cited.

Diagnosis and Management

The principles of diagnosis and management outlined above for renal transplant recipients generally apply to the marrow transplant patient. Prompt diagnosis, by invasive methods if necessary, is absolutely essential. In fact, bronchoscopy, needle aspiration, or open lung biopsy usually are indicated since the marrow graft recipient, unlike the renal transplant patient, will rarely produce a diagnostic expectorated sputum. This difficulty may result from the patient's inability to produce sputum in the absence of polymorphonuclear leukocytes, or, if sputum is produced, from its contamination by oropharyngeal flora. Noninvasive methods (eg, serology) may prove helpful in certain patients, but often the information arrives after a delay long enough to diminish its usefulness.

When a diagnosis is established, therapy can be chosen on a rational basis. Antimicrobial regimens of choice for specific pathogens are discussed elsewhere in this book. Often, however, therapy must be initiated empirically. Virtually all patients receive broad-spectrum antibacterial agents effective against the local nosocomial flora. Lack of response and/or evolution of a characteristic radiographic abnormality may dictate addition of other drugs such as amphotericin B or high-dose trimethoprim-sulfamethoxazole. More precise guidelines for managing the severely immunocompromised patient with lower respiratory tract infection are outlined in Chapter 17.

THE CARDIAC TRANSPLANT RECIPIENT

Cardiac transplantation is rarely performed in the United States; only a limited number of centers have the resources necessary to undertake this difficult procedure. Although much of the reported data comes from but a single institution, it is clear that pulmonary infection is a major cause of morbidity and mortality in this patient population.

Host Defense Deficiencies

Cardiac transplant patients receive an immunosuppressive regimen similar to that employed to prevent renal allograft rejection. Azathioprine, corticosteroids, and antithymocyte globulin have been the mainstays of treatment, although cyclosporin A now offers an alternative. Therapy is initiated in high doses, with gradual reduction over the first few postoperative months. Acute rejection episodes can be treated with either increased oral prednisone or a combination of intravenous methylprednisolone and antithymocyte globulin. This latter regimen seems particularly immunosuppressive, and has been shown to increase the overall infection rate in patients receiving it.

In addition to drug-induced deficiencies of humoral and cell-mediated immunity, the cardiac transplant patient is further compromised by abnormalities in local pulmonary defenses. Antecedent congestive heart failure, cardiopulmonary bypass, the thoracic incision, intubation, and respiratory support may all contribute to the genesis of infection.

Finally, these patients are predisposed to CMV infection, which may exert additional immunosuppressive effects, as described above. Rand et al (1978) have demonstrated an increased incidence of pulmonary superinfections in cardiac recipients who have primary CMV infection.

Chronology and Etiology of Postcardiac Transplant Pneumonia

Most lower respiratory tract infections in this group of patients occur more than a month after surgery. This similarity to the chronology of postrenal transplantation pneumonias is obvious. The clinician can expect a peak frequency of infection during the first few postoperative months, followed by a declining incidence that parallels the tapering of immunosuppressive therapy. However, patients remain at relatively high risk for the life of the transplant, and particularly so when increased medication is needed to combat threatened rejection.

The etiologic organisms are the same as those described for other transplant recipients. *Aspergillus* and *Nocardia* seem to have been particularly troublesome at Stanford.

Diagnosis and Management

Pertinent aspects have been discussed above.

SUMMARY

1. The chronology of post-transplantation pneumonia can be predicted from a knowledge of the chronology of post-

transplantation immunosuppression.

2. Renal allograft recipients are at particularly high risk during months two through four following transplantation. Bone marrow transplant patients are highly susceptible throughout the initial four post-transplant months, including the first 30 days. Cardiac transplant recipients more closely resemble the former patient group.
3. Infectious agents likely to be encountered include those commonly considered as "opportunistic" invaders: nosocomial gram-negative rods, *S. aureus*, CMV, *Aspergillus, Candida, Nocardia*, and *Pneumocystis carinii.*
4. Attack rates are high, as is morbidity and mortality.
5. Proper management includes rapid diagnosis, prompt initiation of appropriate antimicrobial agents and, when possible, reduction in the intensity of immunosuppressive therapy.

SELECTED READINGS

Renal Transplants

Goldblum SE, Reed WP: Host defenses and immunologic alterations associated with chronic hemodialysis. *Ann Intern Med* 1980;93:597–613.

Ho M, Dowling JN: Cytomegalovirus infection in transplant and cancer patients in Remington JS, Swartz MN (eds): *Current Clinical Topics in Infectious Diseases*, vol 1. New York, McGraw-Hill Book Company, 1980.

Hirsch MS, Schooley RT, Cosimi AB, et al: Effects of interferon-alpha on cytomegalovirus reactivation syndromes in renal-transplant recipients. *N Engl J Med* 1983;308:1489–1531.

Lichtenstein IH, MacGregor RR: Mycobacterial infections in renal transplant recipients: Report of five cases and review of the literature. *Rev Infect Dis* 1983;5:216–226.

Moore FD, Kohler TR, Strom TB, et al: The declining mortality from pneumonia in renal transplant patients. *Infect Surg* January 1983: 13–19.

Peterson PK, Balfour HH, Marker SC, et al: Cytomegalovirus disease in renal allograft recipients: A prospective study of the clinical features, risk factors, and impact on renal transplantation. *Medicine* 1980;59:283–300.

Ramsey PG, Rubin RH, Tolkoff-Rubin NE, et al: The renal transplant patient with fever and pulmonary infiltrates. *Medicine* 1980;59:206–222.

Rubin RH, Wolfson JS, Cosimi AB, et al: Infection in the renal transplant patient. *Am J Med* 1981;70:405–411.

Vincenti F, Amend W, Feduski NJ, et al: Improved outcome following renal transplantation with reduction in the immunosuppression therapy for rejection episodes. *Am J Med* 1980;69:107–115.

Bone Marrow Transplants

Atkinson K, Storb R, Prentice RL, et al: Analysis of late infections in 89 long-term survivors of bone marrow transplantation. *Blood* 1979;53:720–731.

Cline MJ (moderator): Bone marrow transplantation in man. *Ann Intern Med* 1975;83:691–708.

Hersman J, Meyers JD, Thomas ED, et al: The effect of granulocyte transfusions on the incidence of cytomegalovirus infection after allogeneic marrow transplantation. *Ann Intern Med* 1982;96:149–152.

Meyers JD, Spencer HC Jr, Watts JC, et al: Cytomegalovirus pneumonia after human marrow transplantation. *Ann Intern Med* 1975;82:181–188.

Meyers JD, Flournoy N, Thomas ED: Nonbacterial pneumonia after allogeneic marrow transplantation: A review of ten years' experience. *Rev Infect Dis* 1982;4:1119–1132.

Winston DJ, Schiffman G, Wang D, et al: Pneumococcal infections after human bone marrow transplantation. *Ann Intern Med* 1979;91:835–841.

Winston DJ, Gale RP, Meyer DV, et al: Infectious complications of human bone marrow transplantation. *Medicine* 1979;58:1–31.

Winston DJ, Ho WG, Young LS, et al: Prophylactic granulocyte transfusions during human bone marrow transplantation. *Am J Med* 1980;68:893–897.

Winston DJ, Pillard RB, Ho WG, et al: Cytomegalovirus immune plasma in bone marrow transplant recipients. *Ann Intern Med* 1982;97:11–18.

Winston DJ, Territo MC, Ho WG, et al: Alveolar macrophage dysfunction in human bone marrow transplant recipients. *Am J Med* 1982;73:859–866.

Cardiac Transplants

Gurwith MJ, Stinson EB, Remington JS: *Aspergillus* infection complicating cardiac transplantation. *Arch Intern Med* 1971;128:541–545.

Krick JA, Stinson EB, Remington JS: *Nocardia* infection in heart transplant patients. *Ann Intern Med* 1975;82:18–26.

Mason JW, Stinson EB, Hunt SA, et al: Infections after cardiac transplantation: Relation to rejection therapy. *Ann Intern Med* 1976;85:69–72.

Rand UH, Pollard RB, Merigan TC: Increased pulmonary superinfections in cardiac-transplant patients undergoing primary cytomegalovirus infection. *N Engl J Med* 1978;298:951–953.

Stinson EB, Beiber CP, Griepp RB, et al: Infectious complications after cardiac transplantation in man. *Ann Intern Med* 1971;74:22–36.

19 *Streptococcus pneumoniae*

Arnold Lentnek
Jack L. LeFrock
Abdolghader Molavi

Pneumococcal pneumonia is the most common bacterial pulmonary infection in adults. For the medical profession as well as the lay public, it is the paradigm of what is usually, simply called pneumonia. Growth in our understanding of the pneumococcus and its interactions with body defense mechanisms mirrors the growth in our understanding of many other bacterial-host relations.

Accurate descriptions of acute, presumably pneumococcal, pulmonary infection are found in classical Greek texts and in the writings of Maimonides. The specific association of this infection with *Streptococcus pneumoniae* was originally noted by Friedlander in 1883, only two years after the organism was described by Pasteur. During the early 20th century, the discovery of distinct pneumococcal serotypes and of the protective role of type-specific antibody led to the use of type-specific antisera for treatment of pneumocoçcal pneumonia and the development of multivalent polysaccharide vaccines. When mass production of penicillin was developed in 1943, further investigation of the pathogenesis and immunology of pneumococcal infection seemed unnecessary. More recently, however, the appearance of pneumococci resistant to penicillin, as well as the recognition of continuing high mortality among certain high-risk groups despite "adequate" penicillin therapy, has led to a renewal of interest in both the immunobiology of pneumococcal disease and the use of immunoprophylaxis.

Microbial Characteristics

For many years the lancet-shaped gram-positive pneumococcus was afforded a unique genus and referred to as *Diplococcus pneumoniae*. On the basis of DNA-RNA homology studies, as well as capsular and cell-wall antigenic structure, it has been reclassified with the genus *Streptococcus* and appears structurally most similar to group A streptococci. In direct smears of pathologic material the organism is frequently found in pairs, aligned on the long axis. Short-chain formation is more likely to occur in broth culture or in the presence of type-specific antibody. Because it produces autolytic enzymes, the organism may stain gram-negative after prolonged incubation.

Pneumococci, lacking cytochromes, utilize oxygen through a flavoprotein enzyme system in which the end product is hydrogen peroxide. Since pneumococci also lack catalase and peroxidase to dispose of this bactericidal compound a source of catalase must be incorporated into the culture medium. This requirement usually is satisfied by adding sheep red blood cells, a rich source of catalase, to the agar. Pneumococcal growth is also pH-sensitive, and lactic acid is the dominant end product of its fermentation. Occasional (5% to 10%) isolates require CO_2 for growth on agar. Accordingly, the organism is best grown in an enriched CO_2 atmosphere at pH 7.8. Within these limitations, pneumococci grow rapidly on a variety of bacteriologic media. On blood agar, virulent (encapsulated) pneumococci form circular, glistening, dome-shaped colonies, the centers of which may collapse after 48 hours of incubation due to autolysis. The basis for such autolysis is the production of an enzyme (N-acetylmuramyl-l-alanine amidase) that splits the bond between muramic acid and alanine in the peptidoglycan portion of the cell wall. This enzyme may normally play a roll in cell division and separation. When pneumococci are grown aerobically, hyaluronidase production causes α-hemolysis ("greening") on the blood agar; when they are grown anaerobically, production of oxygen-labile pneumolysin will cause β-hemolysis. The umbilicated morphology of pneumococcal colonies are sufficiently characteristic to be used as an indicator for further testing in cultures of specimens eg, sputum that frequently contain other α-hemolytic streptococci as contaminants.

Pneumococci usually are differentiated from other streptococci by their sensitivity to ethyl hydrocupreine hydrochloride (Optichin), a sensitivity not shared by other streptococcal species. Accordingly, an Optichin-impregnated paper disk is placed on a agar plate inoculated with the organism and the plate is then incubated overnight. A clear zone of inhibited growth occurs around colonies of pneumococci. This procedure is employed in most clinical laboratories to identify this organism. Pneumococci also can be identified by the bile solubility test. Since the autolytic amidase in pneumococci is activated by various surface-active agents, including bile and bile salts, addition of bile (10% deoxycholic acid) to a saline suspension of pneumococci will cause lysis of the organisms.

The Quellung reaction is frequently employed for rapid indentification of pneumococci in clinical specimens. This reaction depends upon the fact that the polysaccharide capsule of pathogenic pneumococci will undergo swelling and changes in light refraction when mixed with type-specific antisera. "Omni-serum" (obtainable only from Statens Seruministut, Copenhagen, Denmark) contains a mixture of all 84 known pneumococcal serotypes. Loopfuls of bacteria in suspension, Omni-serum, and methylene blue (to better define the capsule) are mixed on the surface of a glass slide and compared to a bacterial suspension mixed with saline under oil immersion. Capsular swelling indicates a positive reaction.

One of the more sensitive methods to detect pneumococci in clinical specimens, now rarely employed, utilizes the extraordinary virulence of the pneumococcus for mice. A small inoculum of sputum or other material containing pneumococci, when injected intraperitoneally in mice, causes death within 48 hours, and a pure culture of pneumococci can be obtained from heart blood. Since few other bacteria are so virulent for mice, this animal can thus serve as a highly sensitive, differential "culture medium" for isolation of pneumococci.

Thus far, 84 distinct serotypes of pneumococci have been identified, based on the specific antigenic composition of the pneumococcal capsule. This high-molecular-weight polysaccharide capsule is intimately involved with the organism's invasive potential. Nonencapsulated pneumococci (R, or rough, strains) are rarely virulent. Unfortunately, two systems of serotyping of nomenclature, Danish and American, have been developed. Not all serotypes are equally represented in infectious processes. Only 14 serotypes account for nearly 85% of pneumococcal infections, a fact utilized in the development of polysaccharide vaccines. These differences in pathogenicity have yet to be fully explained.

Epidemiology

The human nasopharynx is the natural habitat of the pneumococcus; there is no recognized environmental source or animal reservoir. Both asymptomatic nasopharyngeal carriage and clinically overt pneumococcal pneumonia display considerable seasonal variation, with peak rates in the winter and early spring. During this period, nasopharyngeal carriage may be as high as 60% in some closed populations. A similar seasonal variation occurs with other organisms that often inhabit the pharynx, such as *Hemophilus influenzae* and *Neisseria meningitidis*. Such variability may reflect closer person-to-person contact during these periods, as well as the high frequency of concomitant viral infections during the winter months.

The annual rate of pneumococcal infections has been estimated as only 2.1 cases/1000 population, but very high rates, ranging from 40 to 200 cases/1000 population, have been noted in certain closed populations, such as military recruits and South African gold miners, as well as in such occupational groups as painters and welders. The annual incidence in persons over age 40 is three to four times greater than in persons under age 20.

Although pneumococcal pneumonia is clearly transmissible and outbreaks occasionally have been seen in closed populations, there is considerable evidence that asymptomatic carriers are more important in disseminating the organism than are patients with acute illness. Carriage rates are high among urban families, children (and adults in families containing children), school classes, orphanages, and military populations. In most instances, however, community-acquired pneumococcal disease occurs sporadically in asymptomatic carriers whose systemic or local pulmonary defense mechanism has become impaired. Only rarely can a single serotype be implicated in an outbreak of infection.

Pathogenicity

The clinical syndromes produced by pneumococcal infection are a consequence of direct invasion of susceptible tissue. Pneumococci elaborate a variety of extracellular toxins, including pneumolysin, neuraminidase, and purpura-producing factor, but the pathologic importance of these materials is unclear. The ability of the host to prevent or ameliorate direct bacterial invasion determines whether or not infection will occur, as well as the severity and outcome of the process.

The primary determinant of pneumococcal pathogenicity is probably the polysaccharide capsule. Unencapsulated (R, rough) strains are avirulent for both man and experimental animals, while certain encapsulated (S, smooth) strains, such as Types 1, 3, 4, 14, and 78, are very frequently associated with invasive disease. Moreover, mortality from pneumococcal disease can be correlated with the capsular serotype, eg, approximately 20% (51% with bacteremia) for Type 3 but less than 2% (10% with bacteremia) for Type 2.

The molecular basis for the differences in type virulence is poorly understood, but is at least partially related to the amount of capsular polysaccharide produced and the capsule's ability to impair macrophage and granulocyte phagocytosis. During the early stages of infection, in the absence of capsule-specific antibody, phagocytosis proceeds slowly and inefficiently, dependent upon opsonization of bacteria via direct stimulation of the alternative (properidin) complement pathway. A C-polysaccharide on the bacterial surface is responsible for this type of complement activation. As this form of opsonization is inefficient, most of the organisms remain extracellular; thus inflammation progresses, and the patient remains clinically ill. After five to seven days of illness, type-specific anticapsular antibody appears, opsonization is enhanced and the rate of phagocytosis markedly increases. This phenomenon is closely correlated with the clinical "crisis," characterized by an abrupt fall in temperature and an improvement in the patient's sense of well-being. In addition to determining the course of clinical infection, an absence of anticapsular antibody also is closely correlated with asymptomatic nasopharyngeal carriage and may explain the higher rate of pneumococcal carriage among children. Some strains of pneumococci, however, have been recovered from the nasopharynx despite the presence of type-specific antibody. Such strains produce large amounts of IgA protease, which inactivates the secretory immunoglobulin IgA1. IgA protease may therefore be responsible for the continued nasopharyngeal carriage of these organisms despite the anticapsular antibody.

Local defense mechanisms—including the epiglottal reflex, the viscous mucus lining the bronchial tree, the cilia of the respiratory epithelium, and the cough reflex—all play major roles in determining whether organisms in the nasopharynx will reach the alveoli and initiate tissue invasion. Conditions that impair these local defenses or result in increased fluid accumulation in the lung (such as decreased consciousness, exposure to noxious gases or anesthetics, congestive heart failure, or preexisting pulmonary viral infection) all increase the patient's susceptibility to pneumococcal pneumonia.

Since containment of the infection is primarily dependent upon elaboration of anticapsular antibody, activation of complement, and subsequent engulfment and disposal of the organism by phagocytic cells, conditions which impair one or more of these mechanisms have been associated with increased severity of pneumococcal infection but not necessarily with increased frequency of infection. Patients with lymphoma, hypogammaglobulinemia, hemoglobinopathies, hyposplenism, chronic renal failure, alcoholic cirrhosis, or diabetes mellitis with acidosis all experience more severe, if not more frequent, episodes of pneumococcal infection. Both the frequency and severity of infection is increased in the elderly.

Clinical Diseases

Sir William Osler's classic description of pneumococcal pneumonia—written in 1892, only 11 years after the initial description of the pneumococcus—is relevant and lucid today:

> Abruptly, or preceded by a day or two of indisposition, the patient has a severe chill, lasting from 10 to 30 minutes. In no acute disease is an initial chill so constant or so severe. The fever rises quickly. There is pain in the side, often of an agonizing character. A short, dry painful cough soon develops and the respirations are increased in frequency. When seen on the second or third day the patient presents an appearance which may be quite pathognomonic. He lies flat in bed, often on the affected side; the face is flushed, particularly the cheeks; the breath is hurried; the alae nasi dilate with every inspiration, the eyes are bright, the expression is anxious, and there is a frequent short cough which makes the patient wince and hold his side. The expectoration is blood-tinged and extremely tenacious. The temperature rises rapidly to 104°F or 105°F. The pulse is full and bounding and the pulse-respiration ratio much disturbed. Examination of the lung shows the physical signs of consolidation—blowing breathing, and fine rales. After persisting for from seven to ten days, the crisis occurs, and with a fall in the temperature the patient passes from a condition of extreme distress and anxiety to one of comparative comfort.

Although this remains the classic description of pneumococcal pneumonia, not all patients experience this syndrome. In elderly or debilitated patients chills and rigors may be absent and fever only moderately elevated, while confusion or stupor may be the principal finding. In patients with underlying chronic pulmonary disease the presenting finding may be rapidly progressive pulmonary failure, with only minimally increased sputum production and temperature. Prior use of antipyretics may also modify the initial signs, with some patients experiencing low grade, recurrent chills and fever. At the other extreme, patients anatomically or functionally asplenic may present with shock, hypotension, and a hemorrhagic exanthem reflecting disseminated intravascular coagulation. A well-described phenomenon is the occasional misdiagnosis of pneumococcal right lower-lobe pneumonia as acute cholecystitis, owing to the fever, right upper-quadrant pain, and jaundice which may be seen in both conditions. Herpes labialis may appear in up to 30% of patients with pneumococcal pneumonia.

The white blood count usually reveals leukocytosis, with an increase of granulocytes and immature forms. Some patients—especially the elderly, the immunocompromised, and those with depressed bone marrow function—may present with leukopenia due to margination and extravascular migration of granulocytes. Anemia and indirect hyperbilirubinemia occasionally are noted, probably secondary to production of pneumolysin.

The most common local complication of pneumococcal pneumonia is pleural effusion, which occurs in up to one third of patients. In the preantibiotic era frank empyema was relatively common, occurring in nearly one patient in 10. Empyema is now rare, and although the pleural effusion often has the chemical characteristics of an exudate, gram stain and culture of the material usually fails to reveal an organism, and no specific therapy usually is required. Nonetheless, diagnostic aspiration of pneumococcal pleural effusion routinely is indicated to identify the approximately 1% of patients in whom frank empyema will develop.

Pneumococcal pericarditis was a relatively common and often fatal complication of pneumococcal pneumonia in the preantibiotic era, but it too is now rarely seen. Its presenting syndrome resembles other forms of purulent pericarditis, with fever, tachycardia, chest pain, and often a pericardial friction rub. Two thirds of such patients have a concomitant empyema. Pericardiocentesis establishes the diagnosis. Therapy with appropriate antibiotics should be supplemented with drainage, either through a pericardial window or by pericardiectomy, to reduce the risk of late constrictive pericarditis.

Other extrapulmonary foci of infection may include the meninges, joints, or endocardium. These areas do not respond as promptly to antibiotic therapy as does pulmonary infection, perhaps due to inefficient phagocytosis of bacteria and poor penetration of antibiotic. Because bacterial multiplication is slowed at these sites, β-lactam antibiotics such as penicillin may not be as effectively bactericidal as they are in the lung. Many of these extrapulmonary suppurative foci respond only when antibiotic therapy is combined with some form of drainage that removes the bulk of the necrotic exudate and large numbers of bacteria.

One of the most remarkable features of pneumococcal pneumonia is the completeness of histologic resolution, even when several lobes are completely consolidated. On rare occasions, however, especially with infections caused by Type 3 pneumococci or in situations involving bronchial obstruction, abscesses may form. Clinically, one sees persistent fever, tachycardia, and leukocytosis, while the chest x-ray demonstrates a cavity in the involved segment.

In the absence of these complications, patients usually defervesce after one or two days of antibiotic therapy, although resolution of fever is occasionally delayed, especially in the elderly or in those with an underlying immunocompromised state. Fever persisting beyond one week after initiation of antibiotic therapy requires a careful search for a pathologic complication or for the possibility of drug fever.

Diagnostic Tests

The diagnosis of pneumococcal pneumonia is based on the clinical syndrome, along with the demonstration of *S. pneumoniae* in pulmonary secretions by gram stain and culture. The adequacy of expectorated sputum for diagnosis is the subject of considerable controversy. Although the finding of gram-positive, lancet-shaped diplococci intermixed between sheets of polymorphonuclear leukocytes has a good correlation, with growth of *S. pneumoniae* in secretions obtained by fiber-optic bronchoscopy, such "clean" specimens are often difficult to obtain in the elderly, debilitated, disoriented and/or dehydrated patient who is most likely to present with severe pneumococcal pneumonia. Expectorated sputum from such patients is likely to be contaminated with oropharyngeal secretions and contain many squamous epithelial cells intermixed among the bacteria. If the gram stain demonstrates organisms compatible with pneumococci, a Quellung reaction test with Omni-sera should be performed to differentiate pneumococci from other streptococcal species. When an adequate sputum specimen cannot be obtained, some authorities have advocated obtaining a nasopharyngeal culture. There is a high positive correlation between specific pneumococcal types isolated from cultures of the nasopharynx and of sputum from patients with pneumococcal pneumonia. However, for the critically ill, in which accurate, rapid information is crucial to the patients' care, sputum obtained via transtracheal aspiration or direct transthoracic lung puncture is the specimen of choice.

In all but the most mild forms of the disease, the patient's blood should be cultured. A blood culture positive for pneumococci is helpful both to establish the diagnosis and to provide prognostic information. Approximately 25% of patients with pneumococcal pneumonia have bacteremia, although the incidence varies with the serotype. Within each serotype, bacteremia is associated with an approximate doubling of mortality. Bacteremia is especially likely to occur in patients with functional or anatomic asplenism, hypogammaglobulinemia, or hepatic cirrhosis.

Counterimmunoelectrophoresis (CIE) to detect pneumococcal capsular polysaccharide antigen can be helpful in establishing a definitive diagnosis. This procedure, when performed either directly on sputum, pleural fluid, blood or urine, has the advantage of being rapid and highly specific; it may give positive results for several days after initiation of antibiotic therapy. However, antigen has been detected in blood in only about two thirds of bacteremic cases, and much less frequently in nonbacteremic cases. Detection of antigen in pleural fluid or sputum in patients with pneumonia is helpful, but sputum can also be positive for pneumococcal antigen in individuals whose bronchi are colonized by pneumococci. Polysaccharide antigens of pneumococcal Types 7 and 14 are not reliably detected by CIE.

The chest x-ray, although not specific, may be highly suggestive of pneumococcal pneumonia. Pneumococcal infection usually begins in the right middle lobe or one of the lower lobes. In most patients the process remains confined to a single lobe or even a single pulmonary segment, but in approximately 30% two or more lobes may be involved. Radiologic resolution is considerably slower than is clinical improvement and often takes two to three weeks. In patients with underlying chronic pulmonary disease the resolution of the infiltrate may be even slower.

Therapy

For nearly 40 years, penicillin has been the mainstay of therapy for pneumococcal infection. The vast majority of strains are exquisitely sensitive to this agent, with a minimum inhibitory concentration (MIC) of 0.02 μg/mL or less. For most patients, intramuscular procaine penicillin in doses of 300,000 to 600,000 units at 12-hour intervals is recommended. It usually is inadvisable to rely on oral therapy for acutely ill patients. However, patients with minimal infection who are otherwise healthy and able to retain oral medications can be safely treated with an initial intramuscular dose of procaine penicillin G followed by oral penicillin V (250 mg every six hours) for 10 days. At the other extreme, for patients experiencing overwhelming disease with potential cardiovascular collapse, penicillin G should be administered only intravenously, in doses of 5 to 10 million units/day, at least until the possibility of extrapulmonic spread of infection can be confidently ruled out.

More recently, this clear-cut situation has been clouded by two developments. Since 1967, rare isolates of pneumococci have been recovered in Australia, New Guinea, England, Canada, and the United States which have displayed relative resistance to penicillin G. Patients receiving long-term penicillin prophylaxis (often for rheumatic fever) have also been found to harbor these strains. The MICs of these organisms have ranged from 0.1 to 2.0 μg/mL. Although this remains well below clinically achievable serum concentrations of penicillin, several instances of delayed response or failure of penicillin therapy in pneumococcal meningitis caused by these strains of "intermediate sensitivity" have been reported. In pneumococcal infection, especially at sites where penicillin may penetrate poorly, delay in response to therapy occasionally may be due to such strains.

In May 1977 an outbreak of pneumococcal infection involving highly penicillin-resistant strains of Types 6A and 19A (American Type 57) was reported in South Africa. Unlike the earlier reported strains, these were resistant not only to penicillin but also to tetracycline, erythromycin, chloramphenicol, and clindamycin. Moreover, they became resistant to rifampin when this drug was used prophylactically to prevent further spread of the infection. These strains were reliably sensitive only to vancomycin. Similar sensitivity patterns, involving different serotypes, have since been reported from several areas in the United States as well. The pathogenic potential of these highly resistant strains has been well demonstrated. However, thus far they have been reported only in a few well-defined outbreaks, and the degree to which they will become established in the general community has yet to be determined. For now, at least, pneumococcal isolates should be assumed to be penicillin-sensitive.

Penicillin-resistant strains can be detected by use of a disk-diffusion test. These strains produce zones of inhibited growth of ≤ 12 mm in diameter around a 1 μg oxacillin disk on sheep blood agar plates after incubation in air for 18 to 24 hours at 35°C.

Penicillin-sensitive pneumococci are also sensitive to virtually all other clinically available penicillin congeners, including ampicillin, nafcillin, methicillin, and carbenicillin, to name only a few. However, none is more active against the pneumococcus than is penicillin, and some, such as methicillin, are considerably less active. Since all these agents display extensive cross-reactivity with penicillin in the penicillin-allergic patient, the only indication for their use may be during the early stages of infection, before a definitive diagnosis is established.

Cephalothin and other cephalosporin cogeners are effective alternatives to penicillin for the penicillin-allergic patient, although 8% to 15% of such patients will demonstrate cross-sensitivity to cephalosporins. Since these agents penetrate the meninges unreliably, physicians should be alert to signs or symptoms of meningitis in patients with pneumococcal disease treated with them. Cephalothin should be administered in doses of 1 g every four hours. Cefazolin, owing to its longer half-life, may be administered every eight hours. Both erythromycin (250 mg every six hours) and vancomycin (500 mg every 12 hours) are useful alternatives to penicillin therapy. In the absence of specific sensitivity data, tetracycline and its cogeners should not be used to treat pneumococcal infection, since up to 10% of organisms may prove resistant. Pneumococci usually are quite resistant to aminoglycosides (kanamycin, gentamicin, amikacin, and tobramycin).

Although often relegated to the role of supportive therapy, administration of intravenous fluids and electrolytes to the frequently dehydrated, septic patient with overwhelming pneumococcal pneumonia is of crucial importance. Similarly, tracheal suctioning to clear inspissated secretions and administration of oxygen to correct hypoxia frequently are life-saving maneuvers which will "buy time" until the antimicrobial agent exerts its effect. With appropriate therapy, the response is often dramatic. A crisis, characterized by rapid defervescence and amelioration of symptoms, occurs within 48 hours in approximately one half of the patients. For the rest, fever and symptoms resolve more gradually (lysis) over a five- to seven-day period. Occasionally, a secondary rise in temperature will follow the crisis, only to subside spontaneously within one or two days.

If the expected resolution of signs and symptoms fails to occur promptly, several possibilities must be considered. The initial infection may have been nonpneumococcal and caused by an organism resistant to penicillin, eg, *Staphylococcus, Klebsiella,* or *Hemophilus influenzae*. Alternatively, the patient may have developed an extrapulmonic complication of pneumococcal pneumonia (meningitis, empyema, endocarditis), which may require modification of the antibiotic dose or drainage of the involved area. Especially in instances in which the pulmonic infiltrate fails to resolve, the possibility of infection behind a bronchial obstruction (either an endobronchial tumor or a foreign body) must be considered. Finally, if most signs and symptoms of infection have resolved but the patient remains persistently febrile, the possibility of drug-induced fever should be considered.

SELECTED READINGS

Austrian R, Douglas RM, Schiffman G: Prevention of pneumococcal pneumonia by vaccination. *Trans Assoc Am Phys* 1976;89:184.

Austrian R, Gold J: Pneumococcal bacteremia with especial reference to bacteremic pneumococcal pneumonia. *Ann Intern Med* 1964;60:759.

Bisno AL: Hyposplenism and overwhelming pneumococcal infection: A reappraisal. *Am J Med Sci* 1971;262:101.

Coonrod JD, Rytel MW: Detection of type-specific pneumococcal antigens by counterimmunoelectrophoresis. II. Etiologic diagnosis of pneumonia. *J Lab Clin Med* 1973;81:778.

Hodges RG, MacLeod CM: Epidemic pneumococcal pneumonia. III. Pneumococcal carrier studies. *Am J Hyg* 1946;44:207.

Jacobs MR, Koornhof HJ, Robins-Browne RM, et al: Emergence of multiply resistant pneumococci. *N Engl J Med* 1978;249:735.

Jay SJ, Johanson WG Jr, Pierce AK: The radiographic resolution of *Streptococcus pneumoniae. N Engl J Med* 1975;293:798.

Roberts RB: Streptococcus Pneumonia, in Mandell GL, Douglas RG, Bennett MD (eds): *Principles and Practice of Infectious Diseases.* New York, John Wiley and Sons, 1970, pp 1589–1604.

20 *Pneumococcal Pneumonia Prevention*

Richard V. McCloskey

Antimicrobial therapy has decreased the mortality of pneumococcal pneumonia, but fatal outcome may still attend bacteremic pneumococcal pneumonia.

Since the pathophysiology of fatal pneumococcal infections is obscure and treatment not always successful, prophylaxis of pneumococcal infection offers the best way to reduce the risk of fatality among patients most likely to die if infected.

Prophylaxis against pneumococcal infections by active immunization dates to the early studies of Wright and co-workers (1914) using heat and carbolic acid-treated pneumococcal cultures. These early attempts preceded the identification of pneumococcal polysaccharide types. Subsequent studies by MacLeod and colleagues (1945) documented the antigenicity of a polysaccharide vaccine of Types 1, 2, 5, and 7. This vaccine was effective in preventing pneumonia and reducing the carrier rate for the types included in the vaccine.

Since these early studies, purified pneumococcal capsular polysaccharide vaccines have been proved to induce antibody production, and are effective in preventing pneumococcal disease. A vaccine containing six types reduced pneumococcal infection by 76% and a dodecavalent vaccine reduced such infection by 92%.

The contemporary pneumococcal polysaccharide vaccine containing 14 types was licensed in United States in 1977, and has recently been expanded to include nine additional types. Local erythema and induration at the injection site usually are mild and occur in about one half of the people who receive the vaccine. Anaphylactoid reactions are rare. Protection against infection develops within two weeks after vaccination. Immunity will last at least five years after vaccination in those having an adequate initial antibody response after vaccination.

Antibody Response

Methods that have been used to measure the pneumococcal antibody produced by this vaccine include radioimmunoassay (RIA), indirect hemagglutination (IHA), and the enzyme-linked immunosorbent assay (ELISA) techniques. The latter method has not been widely used in clinical studies. Currently, the only reliable quantitative technique is the

RIA. Most of the studies of vaccine-induced pneumococcal antibody responses have used the RIA to study the antibody response. Most authors define antibody response as postvaccination antibody levels that are 50% to 100% greater than prevaccination levels. The antibody level that is protective is not well defined, although an antibody content of 250 ng to 300 ng of antibody nitrogen per mL is thought to be protective. Antibodies from one vaccine serotype do not cross-react or cross-protect with another vaccine serotype regardless of the level of antibody nitrogen achieved after vaccination. Influenza virus vaccine can be administered simultaneously with pneumococcal vaccine without significant reduction in antibody response to either vaccine and without an increase in side reactions. Each dose of 14-valent pneumococcal vaccine is 0.5 mL and contains 50 μg each of the following capsular polysaccharides (Danish pneumococcal serotypes) 1, 2, 3, 4, 6a, 7f, 8, 9n, 12f, 14, 18c, 19f, 23f, and 25.

Initial trials that clearly demonstrated the effectiveness of the current vaccine were originally performed with populations of healthy, young persons. Clinicians are more concerned with the protective effect of such a vaccine in populations of patients who may be at a high risk for disease or for increased severity of pneumococcal infection. Some of these conditions are indicated in Table 20-1. To the types of disorders mentioned in that table, we should probably also add patients with cardiac insufficiency, leukopenic patients, and the institutionalized elderly.

Table 20-1
High-Risk Patient Populations: *Streptococcus pneumoniae* Infection

	Pneumococcal Infection Increased in:		
Condition	*Incidence*	*Severity*	*Adequate Antibody Response*
Traumatic asplenia	Yes	Yes	Yes
Sickle cell disease	Yes	Yes	Variable
Splenectomized, Hodgkin's disease	Yes	Yes	Variable
Multiple myeloma	Yes	Yes	No
Splenectomized, marrow transplant	Yes	Yes	?
Splenectomized, renal transplant	Yes	Yes	Variable
Nephrotic syndrome	Yes	Yes	Variable
Elderly, congestive heart failure	Yes	Yes	Yes
Systemic lupus erythematosus	No	No	Yes
Chronic renal failure	No	No	Variable
Diabetes mellitus, insulin dependent	No	No	Yes

Modified from Landesman and Schiffman, 1981.

Data in patients at high risk of morbidity and mortality due to pneumococcal infection suggest that the antibody response to vaccination in certain of these groups may be low (children under 2 years of age, the elderly, and immunocompromised patients). Some individuals may produce protective levels of antibody to only some of the polysaccharide types in the vaccine.

Vaccine Failure

In addition to a poor antibody response to vaccination, host defenses other than antibody may be ineffective because of the immunosuppressive effect of an underlying illness or its therapy. Vaccine failure may also occur because infection caused by types of *Streptococcus pneumoniae* not contained in the vaccine are not prevented by immunization because of the lack of cross-reactivity between the types of specific polysaccharides. Capsular polysaccharide types were selected for inclusion in the vaccine because these types account for approximately 75% of the isolates of *Streptococcus pneumoniae* from patients who have bacteremic pneumococcal infections in general hospital populations. However, serotypes included in the vaccine may represent a smaller percentage (45% to 65%) of the serotypes responsible for pneumococcal pneumonia. This is especially important if a significant proportion of pneumococcal disease in a semi-closed population (eg, those in nursing homes) is caused by serotypes that are not represented in the vaccine. In this case, the effectiveness of the vaccine in reducing pneumococcal pneumonia in the immunized population will be correspondingly decreased. These considerations have led to somewhat tentative recommendations for use of the vaccine in the United States (see Public Health Service Advisory Committee on Immunization Practices, 1978). It is apparent, however, that the pneumococcal vaccine offers to high-risk patients a degree of partial protection with little accompanying toxicity and, therefore, should be viewed as part of a prophylaxis program to prevent high mortality pneumococcal disease in these groups (see Centers for Disease Control, 1981).

Recommendations for Vaccination in High-Risk Populations

Recommendations concerning high-risk patient populations and pneumococcal vaccine are as follows:

1. For healthy patients who have undergone splenectomy, the risk of pneumococcal sepsis is small, but the mortality is high. Since antibody response to vaccination in these patients is essentially the same as in normals, these patients should be vaccinated.

2. For young patients with homozygous sickle cell disease, the risk of pneumococcal infection is greatest in those under 2 years of age when antibody response to vaccination is poor. Vaccination of those over 2 years of age has resulted in satisfactory antibody response and a decreased incidence of pneumococcal infection. Therefore, to prevent pneumococcal disease in these patients, continuous penicillin prophylaxis and pneumococcal vaccine is recommended for those under 2 years of age and vaccination for those over 2 years of age. A combination of both methods will probably be found to give optimal prevention from pneumococcal infection for children with sickle cell disease because of suboptimal antibody response to vaccination found in very young children.
3. Patients with Hodgkin's disease, who have had splenectomy and immunosuppression chemotherapy and/or radiation therapy, do have increased risk for severe infection caused by encapsulated organisms, particularly *Streptococcus pneumoniae.* Administration of pneumococcal vaccine is an obvious means of prophylaxis for these patients. It is clear that pneumococcal vaccine is reduced in effectiveness if it is administered after chemotherapy or radiation therapy. Therefore, if possible, pneumococcal vaccine should be administered at least two weeks prior to initiation of chemotherapy or irradiation. Antibody duration in patients with Hodgkin's disease is not clearly known, but it is probably shorter than that reported for normals. For this reason, most authorities do not recommend pneumococcal vaccine prophylaxis as the sole method of controlling pneumococcal infection in splenectomized patients with Hodgkin's disease.
4. Patients with multiple myeloma are at increased risk for developing pneumococcal infection. Unfortunately, the presence of multiple myeloma itself impairs antibody synthesis. Therefore, pneumococcal vaccine is unlikely to generate protective antibody levels in patients with myeloma. Although the vaccine frequently is given because of its low toxicity, benefit for the patient with myeloma may be small. Penicillin prophylaxis would seem to be more efficacious in these patients.
5. Pneumococcal disease occurs frequently and severely in patients who have had bone marrow transplantation. The antibody response and efficacy of pneumococcal vaccine in patients with bone marrow transplants is not known, but vaccination is reasonable under these circumstances.

6. Patients with chronic renal failure who have been splenectomized and those with renal transplants are a high-risk group for both the occurrence and severity of pneumococcal disease. Antibody response is abnormally low during the first six months following transplantation. Although antibody response may be suboptimal, patients with chronic renal failure who have been splenectomized, or who are expected to receive a transplant within six months, should be vaccinated. Otherwise, renal transplant recipients should be vaccinated six months after transplantation.
7. Insulin-dependent diabetics are not a high risk group for the development of pneumococcal pneumonia and pneumococcal disease. When pneumococcal infection develops, there is no evidence that it is of greater severity than in normal persons if ketoacidosis is not simultaneously present. Insulin-dependent diabetics do develop antibody response to pneumococcal vaccine equal to that of normals. Since there is little to indicate that these patients are at increased risk for pneumococcal disease, vaccination of well-controlled diabetics without any other underlying medical problem is unlikely to be useful.
8. Children with nephrotic syndrome are clearly at risk for pneumococcal infection—particularly and peculiarly for pneumococcal peritonitis. The response to pneumococcal vaccine is suboptimal and may not reach protective levels for some of the serotypes in the vaccine. As with other high-risk groups, pneumococcal vaccine alone is probably not sufficient to produce optimal protection from pneumococcal disease.
9. The elderly respond to the vaccine with antibodies thought to be in the protective range, but the duration of protection is unknown. The package insert for pneumococcal vaccine does recommend it for the elderly and for those with chronic cardiopulmonary disease. The minimal toxicity combined with the morbidity and mortality of pneumococcal disease in the elderly population makes vaccination a reasonable preventive maneuver. Because of the occurrence of outbreaks of pneumococcal disease in the institutionalized elderly, vaccination of the entire closed population is recommended.
10. Since the safety of the vaccine has not been evaluated in pregnancy, vaccination should be withheld until delivery.

The high-risk patients discussed above may experience more rapid antibody decline than normal patients. This, in combination with the possible suboptimal initial antibody response, makes the duration of protective antibody levels less than that of normal controls. Revaccination has been suggested to obtain a booster response. Initially, the recommendation was to revaccinate at intervals of five years. However, severe local and systemic reactions have been common among adults given a second dose when presumably levels of circulating antibody were high. Since antibody levels usually are not available, revaccination has become problematic. In fact, the United States Public Health Service currently recommends pneumococcal vaccination be given only once to adults. Data on revaccination of children are not yet sufficient to provide a basis for comment.

SELECTED READINGS

Amman AJ, Addiego J, Wara DW, et al: Polyvalent pneumococcal-polysaccharide immunization of patients with sickle cell anemia and patients with splenectomy. *N Engl J Med* 1977;297:897–900.

Austrian R: Pneumococcal infection and the pneumococcal vaccine. *N Engl J Med* 1977;297:938–939.

Centers for Disease Control: Pneumococcal polysaccharide vaccine. *Morbid Mortal Weekly Rep* 1981;30:410–419.

Kass EH (ed): Assessment of the pneumococcal polysaccharide vaccine. *Rev Infect Dis* 1981;3(suppl).

Landesman SH, Schiffman G: Assessment of the antibody response to pneumococcal vaccine in high-risk populations. *Rev Infect Dis* 1981;3:S184–S196.

MacLeod CM, Hodges RG, Heidelberger M, et al: Prevention of pneumococcal pneumonia by immunization with specific capsular polysaccharides. *J Exp Med* 1945;82:445–465.

Public Health Service Advisory Committee on Immunization Practices: Pneumococcal polysaccharide vaccine. *Morbid Mortal Weekly Rep* 1978;27:25–26.

Smit P, Oberholzer D, Hayden-Smith S, et al: Protective efficacy of pneumococcal polysaccharide vaccines. *JAMA* 1977;238:2613–2616.

Weibel RE, Vella PO, McLean AA, et al: Studies in human subjects of polyvalent pneumococcal vaccines. *Proc Soc Exp Biol Med* 1977;156:144–150.

Wright AE, Morgan WP, Cantab MB, et al: Prophylactic inoculation against pneumococcal infection. *Lancet* 1914;1:1–10,89–95.

21 *Streptococcus pyogenes (Group A Streptococci)*

Jack L. LeFrock
Abdolghader Molavi
Arnold Lentnek

Before the antimicrobial era, pneumonia due to group A β-hemolytic streptococci (*Streptococcus pyogenes*) was not uncommon in children after measles, varicella or pertussis, or in adults after influenza. It was also occasionally observed in healthy persons. Overall, it accounted for 3% to 25% of all bacterial pneumonias in children and 5% in adults. During the influenza pandemic of 1918–1919, severe streptococcal pneumonia, often culminating in death, assumed epidemic proportions in many areas of the world. The incidence of streptococcal pneumonia decreased markedly as penicillin came into use.

Group A streptococci cause a great variety of other infections, most of which are suppurative (pus-producing). These include pharyngitis, otitis media, meningitis, brain abscess, pyoderma, peritonitis, and rare puerperal sepsis. Nonsuppurative complications of group A streptococcal infections are rheumatic fever and acute glomerulonephritis.

Microbial Characteristics

Group A streptococci are gram-positive cocci which may be found in pairs but more commonly as chains in clinical specimens. The cells within the chain are attached by intercellular bridges, at which point cell-wall synthesis occurs. They are facultative anerobes with an optimum growth temperature of 37°C. Unlike *Staphylococcus aureus* they are catalase-negative. Of the streptococci, *S. pyogenes* is the most important human pathogen. It produces pinpoint, convex, β-hemolytic colonies on the surface of blood agar; it is sensitive to bacitracin (1% to 4% resistant) and contains group A carbohydrate in its cell wall. This group antigen provokes an antibody response in infected individuals, but has not been demonstrated to play a direct role in pathogenicity. In addition to the group antigen, the outermost layer of the cell wall is composed of several antigenic proteins, the most important of which is M protein, the major virulence factor. This protein forms a layer of slender projections (fimbriae) extending out radially from the cell wall. The M protein may be one of 63 antigenic types which form the basis for serotyping group A streptococci. However, some strains are M protein deficient and thus nontypable. (Strains lacking M protein are avirulent.) Both the M protein and the nonantigenic hyaluronic acid capsule have an antiphagocytic property.

S. pyogenes produces enzymes (streptokinase, hyaluronidase, proteases, nucleases, and diphosphopyridine nucleotidase) which enhance its pathogenicity and help it to meet its nutritional requirements in the human host. It also produces hemolysins and toxins.

Epidemiology

Streptococcal pneumonia usually is endemic, but may become epidemic, as it did during World War I. Its incidence appears to increase from age 5 or 6 to young adulthood. Like pneumococcal and staphylococcal pneumonia, it occurs most frequently during the winter. Streptococcal respiratory infection is spread by large droplets expelled from the nose and throat of infected persons living in crowded conditions.

Pathogenicity

S. pyogenes enters the lungs by inhalation and/or aspiration and, under the influence of gravity, passes to the most dependent portions. Thus, it is almost invariably localized to the lower lobes. Streptococcal pneumonia frequently follows a viral infection of the respiratory tract.

Two forms of streptococcal pneumonia have been described. Interstitial bronchopneumonia, the more common form, accounts for about 75% of cases in children. The pathologic picture is one of thickening bronchiolar walls, necrosis of the mucosal lining, purulent engorgement of the lymphatics, and microabscesses with rupture through the pleura. The other form is lobar pneumonia, similar to that of pneumococcal pneumonia.

Among the lesions associated with streptococcal pneumonia is an intense reddening of the entire respiratory tract. In some patients the larynx and adjacent structures may be involved with ulceration. The major pulmonary complications include bronchopleural fistula, empyema, pneumothorax, pneumatoceles, bronchiectasis, "trapped" lung and persistent atelectasis. These complications have been found in 18% of children and in 1% to 10% of young adults surveyed.

Extrapulmonary complications include anemia, which probably results from serosanguinous drainage and intravascular hemolysis. Thrombocytopenia, either separately or as part of purpura fulminans, may be a complication of streptococcal bacteremia. Biopsy-proven acute glomerulonephritis has been reported but not acute rheumatic fever. Purulent pericarditis is seen in less than 10% of cases.

Empyema is found in most (66% to 86%) adult cases and in all pediatric cases. The effusion is initially serous, then serosanguinous, which rapidly becomes fibrinopurulent. This thick effusion makes chest drainage difficult. Empyema develops as the infecting organisms extend in a retrograde manner by way of occluded lymphatics to the pleural surface, where they initiate an inflammatory, exudative response in the pleural space. Early in the course of the infection, peribronchial or lobular lesions are seen in the lung, but the pleura remains smooth and glistening. Subsequently, however, the pleura nearly always becomes thickened and its surface is covered by a fibrin layer.

An apparent predominance of left-sided empyemas can be explained by the poorer bronchial drainage from the lower lobe of the left lung, resulting in a more protracted infection in that area. Bronchial involvement is part of the pathologic picture of this type of pneumonia, and exudation into the bronchial lumen is a usual finding. Drainage of the involved bronchi seems to be essential for proper resolution. Bronchiectasis has been known to favor this site, possibly for the same reason.

Clinical Diseases

Although streptococcal pneumonia frequently is secondary to some other acute illness, especially measles or influenza, it may apparently begin suddenly in individuals without recent illness. A history of a previous upper respiratory infection frequently is obtained.

Onset usually is sudden. Fever, shaking chills, restlessness, cough, dyspnea, cherry-red cyanosis, and blood-streaked sputum are the outstanding manifestations. Respiratory symptoms are severe because of the diffuse interstitial location of the disease. The physical and x-ray findings indicate an extensive bronchopneumonia. Pleuritic pain is a frequent premonitory of empyema formation. Empyema is a common and early feature, occurring within 48 to 72 hours after onset.

Signs or symptoms of pharyngitis are present in about two thirds of patients. Surprisingly, in only 19% of these patients can streptococci be recovered by culture of throat specimens. Fever, which usually is higher than 38.5°C. (102°F) at the onset, remains for a week or more despite appropriate antimicrobial therapy. Persistence of fever should therefore be regarded as another characteristic of streptococcal pneumonia.

Leukocyte counts vary considerably but are between 10,000 and 20,000 mm^3 in about one half of the patients; the higher the count, the more likely the patient is to have empyema. Nearly one third of patients are anemic. Bacteremia is unusual; when it occurs, the prognosis is poor.

Radiographic examination of the infection usually reveals lower lobe bronchopneumonia. When empyema is present, underlying parenchymal lesions are often obscured.

Diagnostic Tests

The striking characteristic of streptococcal pneumonia, which distinguishes it from all other kinds of infectious pneumonia, is the remarkable tendency for early involvement of the pleura with the formation of clinically significant empyema.

The diagnosis is confirmed when group A β-hemolytic *Streptococcus* is cultured from the sputum or pleural fluid. If satisfactory specimens are obtained before antimicrobial drugs are given, the yield is high. Positive blood cultures are found in 2% to 12% of cases but may be positive in 55% to 100% of severely ill patients. Gram stains of sputum and pleural fluid specimens may give an early clue to the presence of *S. pyogenes*, but it may easily be overlooked because streptococcal chains often fragment and appear as gram-positive diplococci or cocci.

Sensitivity to a 0.02-unit bacitracin-impregnated disc on the surface of blood agar is used for routine identification but is by no means specific, since other streptococci may be bacitracin-sensitive. Final identification can be made with group A specific antisera. Antistreptolysin O titers of 250 Todd units or greater are found on admission or develop shortly thereafter in virtually all patients with streptococcal pneumonias.

Therapy and Prevention

The antimicrobial treatment of choice for streptococcal pneumonia is penicillin G, 1 to 2 million units every four hours intravenously. For patients with known penicillin sensitivity, either clindamycin or cephalothin administered intravenously is a good alternative. Empyemas should be drained by intubation of the chest as early as possible. They should not be managed by frequent thoracentesis because the fluid may be difficult to aspirate and because loculations form quickly.

SELECTED READINGS

Basiliere JL, Bistrang HW, Spencer WF: Streptococcal pneumonia: Recent outbreaks in military recruit populations. *Am J Med* 1968;44:580–589.

Burmeister RW, Overholt EL: Pneumonia caused by hemolytic streptococcus. *Arch Intern Med* 1963;111:367–375.

Keefer CS, Rantz LA, Rammelkamp CH: Hemolytic streptococcal pneumonia and empyema. A study of 55 cases with special reference to treatment. *Ann Intern Med* 1941;14:1533–1550.

Kevy SV, Lowe BA: Streptococcal pneumonia and empyema in childhood. *N Engl J Med* 1961;264:738–743.

Molten RA: Group A beta-hemolytic streptococcal pneumonia. *Am J Dis Child* 1977;131:1366–1371.

Welch CC: Beta-hemolytic streptococcal pneumonia—Report of an outbreak in a military population. *Am J Med Sci* 1961;242:157–165.

22 *Group B Streptococci*

Alan R. Spitzer
Stephen Baumgart
Richard A. Polin

Streptococcus agalactiae, group B *Streptococcus* (GBS), was first isolated in 1887 by Nocard and Mollereau from a case of bovine mastitis. Five serologically detectable types of human group B streptococci (1a, 1b, 1c, 2 and 3) with unique polysaccharide and protein antigens have since been identified, all of which can be either normal inhabitants of the genitourinary, gastrointestinal and respiratory tract of man or pathogens responsible for serious infections in infants and adults. GBS is either the leading cause of serious bacterial infection in the newborn or is second only to *Escherichia coli.*

Two clinical presentations of neonatal group B streptococcal infections have been described. Early onset disease (1 to 3/1000 live births) begins in the first few days of life (usually the first 24 hours) and presents as fulminant sepsis with respiratory distress and shock. Group B streptococci responsible for early onset disease are acquired from the maternal genital tract prior to, or during labor and delivery. Blanc has designated the sequence of events responsible for early onset infections as the "ascending amniotic infection syndrome." Infection begins with colonization of the maternal genital tract. Pathogenic bacteria spread upward through the cervix into the amniotic cavity resulting in chorioamnionitis. Susceptible infants either inhale or swallow infected amniotic fluid and develop generalized sepsis. Late onset group B streptococcal disease generally presents as meningitis which occurs between the tenth day and fourth month of life. The origin of group B streptococci responsible for late onset disease is unknown, but sources may include nursery personnel, other colonized infants, parents and siblings.

Epidemiology

The reported incidence of group B streptococcal carriage has varied between series due perhaps in part to variation in the body site sampled (nasopharynx, vagina, rectum), and in the laboratory methodology used to isolate and identify the microorganisms. Lancefield and Hare in 1935 reported a vaginal carrier rate of only 2.3% in the puerperium. Recent studies, however, that used selective media have demonstrated colonization rates varying from 20% to 30% both in pregnant and nonpregnant women. Factors known to enhance colonization of the genital tract with GBS include: age less than 20 years, three or fewer pregnancies, first half of the menstrual cycle, the presence of an intrauterine device, and sexual activity. For unknown reasons, Mexican American women have a lower carriage rate than other ethnic groups. Three kinds of group B streptococcal vaginal carriers may be identified during pregnancy: transient carriers, intermittent carriers, and chronic carriers. Therefore, a single positive culture during pregnancy will not reliably predict who will be culture positive at delivery. Rectal colonization among obstetrical patients may exceed the vaginal carrier rate (16.8% to 29.1%). Badri et al (1977) has suggested that vaginal colonization may represent contamination from a gastrointestinal source. Nasopharyngeal carriage is the least common site for maternal colonization. Infants born to culture-positive women acquire the organism approximately 70% of the time. The estimated attack rate for GBS disease in culture-positive infants is 1% to 2%, but is higher in association with prematurity, prolonged rupture of membranes or signs of maternal sepsis. Infants can also acquire the organism postnatally from other infants and nursery personnel, and up to 65% of infants may be colonized in the nasopharynx prior to discharge from the nursery. The duration of rupture of membranes has no effect on the incidence of neonatal colonization, and infants born by cesarean section frequently are culture-positive.

Immunology

Host immunity to group B *Streptococcus* has been studied with respect to immunologic factors related to prevention of invasive disease rather than colonization. The presence of type-specific antibody against major polysaccharide or protein determinants, an intact classical and alternate complement pathway, and functionally normal polymorphonuclear leukocytes all appear to be important for preventing infection.

Prior to the time of birth, the fetus makes very little of its own antibody and IgG is actively transported from the maternal circulation. Transplacental transfer of antibody from the mother accounts for the rarity of neonatal infection with group B *Streptococcus*. In order to identify infants prone to develop Type 3 group B streptococcal disease, Baker and Kasper (1976) compared antibody titers in mothers and infants who were asymptomatically colonized with GBS to a group of women who delivered septic infants. Seventy-six percent of the mothers who delivered asymptomatic infants had serum antibodies directed against GBS, whereas, the seven infected neonates and their mothers had not demonstrable titer.

In a subsequent investigation, Baker et al (1977) evaluated a larger group of mothers and once again demonstrated 100% concordance between maternal and neonatal antistreptococcal antibody titers. An additional finding in this study was that mothers with invasive streptococcal disease developed antibody titers to the capsular polysaccharide of GBS during convalescence; however, antibody was absent from 10 infants who had recovered from bacteremia, septicemia or meningitis. This is in agreement with data obtained from children under age 1 year who have little or no antibody response to *Hemophilus influenzae* capsular antigen.

Clinical Presentation

Respiratory distress is the most common manifestation of early onset group B streptococcal infection and generally indicates that the infant has a pneumonic process. Clinical signs of respiratory distress usually are present at birth or within 12 to 15 hours of birth. Pulmonary involvement occurs in approximately 40% of infants with early onset GBS infection. The radiographic appearance and histopathology of group B streptococcal pneumonia in term infants is similar to that noted in older children and adults. In contrast, the chest radiographs of preterm infants with streptococcal pneumonia frequently mimic the radiographic appearance of the respiratory distress syndrome (RDS) (Figure 22-1). Small lung volumes are apparent with a reticulogranular appearance to the lung fields bilaterally. Air bronchograms may also be seen. Histopathologically, these infants have findings consistent with both diseases: infiltrative inflammation characteristic of bronchopneumonia plus the presence of hyaline membranes in alveolar ducts and respiratory bronchioles.

During the neonatal period, the signs of pneumonia are variable and include apneic episodes, grunting, cyanosis, tachypnea, and retractions. The tachypnea and retractions signify that lung compliance has been reduced. Grunting is caused by forceful expiration of air through a partially closed glottis, and is noted in infants with a number of respiratory diseases. This partial valsalva maneuver is thought to maintain positive end expiratory pressure and stabilize the functional residual capacity of the lung. Cyanosis uniformly is present in neonates with group B streptococcal pneumonia and may not be relieved by an increase in the inspired oxygen concentration. Cyanosis results from mismatching of ventilation and perfusion in the pulmonary parenchyma, plus right-to-left shunting through the foramen ovale (persistent fetal circulation). In addition to the signs of respiratory distress, there are many other signs associated with streptococcal sepsis, which unfortunately are neither specific for group B streptococcal infection nor indeed for an infectious process.

Diagnosis

Some of the mortality and morbidity of early onset group B streptococcal pneumonia results from difficulty in distinguishing it from the

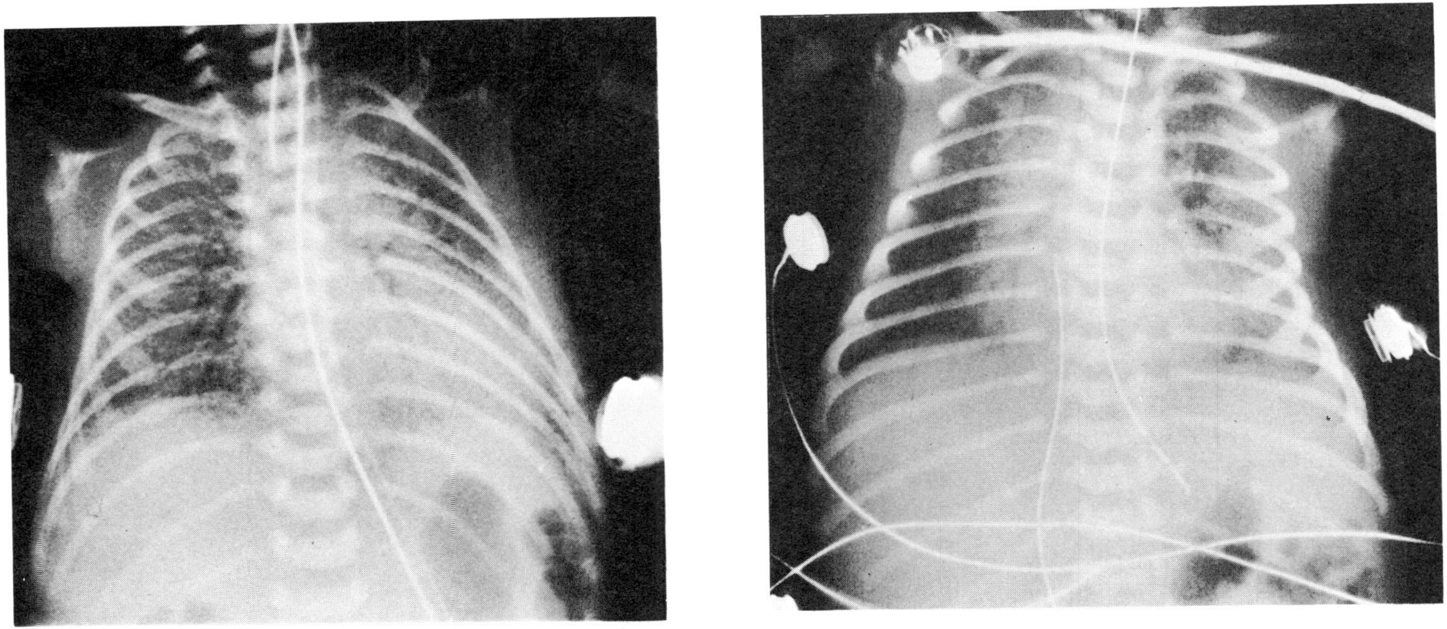

Figure 22-1 Typical radiographic appearance of respiratory distress syndrome (left) is compared with group B streptococcal pneumonia (right). Note similar loss of lung volumes, diffuse and hazy reticulogranular appearance to lung fields and air bronchograms in the perihilar region. The only difference noted by radiographer was the presence of a small pleural reaction in the bases of the radiograph depicting pneumonia. (Courtesy of Henrietta Rosenberg, MD, Children's Hospital of Philadelphia, Department of Radiology.)

respiratory distress syndrome or aspiration pneumonias. Perinatal factors known to increase the likelihood of an infectious process include rupture of membranes more than 24 hours before delivery, maternal fever, uterine tenderness, foul smelling or cloudy amniotic fluid, and genital colonization with group B *Streptococcus*. However, early onset sepsis is known to occur in infants with no maternal predisposing factors, and in infants delivered by cesarean section. The clinician must rely on laboratory tests and culture specimens to distinguish respiratory distress syndrome or aspiration pneumonia from an acute bacterial infection. Positive blood cultures are present in the majority of infants with GBS infection. The cerebrospinal fluid and urine are always cultured in addition to the blood because of a 30% incidence of meningitis and 10% incidence of pyelonephritis in early onset bacterial infections. Surface cultures of the ear, axilla, groin, or umbilicus are not helpful diagnostically because they represent colonization with group B *Streptococcus* and are not indicative of invasive disease. When a specimen can be obtained directly from the trachea, there is good correlation between the identification of gram-positive cocci in the aspirate and documented bacteremia. A gram stain of the gastric contents is not as informative as a tracheal aspirate because bacteria in a gastric aspirate represent organisms that were colonizing or infecting the amniotic cavity, not necessarily those infecting the fetus. However, the presence of gram-positive cocci in a gastric aspirate does increase the suspicion of a group B streptococcal infection. Three components of the white blood count are helpful in distinguishing sepsis from hyaline membrane disease: 1) a low total neutrophil count, 2) an increase in the ratio between immature neutrophils and total neutrophils, or 3) an increase in the absolute band count (Table 22-1). Leukocytosis is not a reliable indicator of infection.

Table 22-1
Neutrophil Values Predictive of Bacterial Infection in the Neonate

	Diagnostic Values	Postnatal Age
1. Neutropenia	< 1800 cells/mm^3	Birth
	< 7200 cells/mm^3	12 hours
	< 3600 cells/mm^3	48 hours
	< 1800 cells/mm^3	By 60 hours
2. Increase in the number of immature neutrophils	> 1100 cells/mm^3	Birth
	> 1400 cells/mm^3	12 hours
	> 800 cells/mm^3	By 60 hours
3. Increase in the ratio between immature forms and mature neutrophils	$> .20$	

Adapted from Manroe et al, 1979.

Table 22-2
Recommended Drugs and Dosages for Treating Infections with Group B Streptococcus

Infection	Drug	Dose	Duration
Bacteremia (without meningitis)	Ampicillin Penicillin G	150–200 mg/kg/day 200,000 units/kg/day	14 days*
Meningitis	Ampicillin Penicillin G	300–400 mg/kg/day 400,000 units/kg/day	14 days*

*After achieving negative blood or cerebrospinal fluid cultures *on* therapy.

In addition to a positive blood, urine or cerebrospinal fluid culture, definitive identification of group B *Streptococcus* can be made by identifying bacterial antigen in these body fluid specimens. Three assays have been developed, all of which have proven reliable for antigen detection: latex particle agglutination, staphylococcal coagglutination, and counterimmunoelectrophoresis. If meningitis is present, group B streptococcal antigen can be detected in almost 100% of the infected infants. Serum has been GBS antigen positive in 43% of early onset infections and concentrated urine is antigen positive in 85.7%.

Therapy

Every infant with suspected group B streptococcal sepsis or pneumonia should initially receive broad spectrum antimicrobial coverage consisting of ampicillin plus an aminoglycoside antibiotic (kanamycin or gentamicin). Once positive identification of a specific group B *Streptococcus* organism is made, the drug of choice is penicillin. The minimal inhibitory concentration for group B *Streptococcus* is higher than group A *Streptococcus* and ranges from 0.02 to 0.4 μg/mL. Dosage recommendations for penicillin are shown in Table 22-2. The duration of therapy should be 10 to 14 days for uncomplicated bacteremia or pneumonia, 14 days after the cerebrospinal fluid has been sterilized for meningitis, 14 days for septic arthritis, and four weeks or longer for osteomyelitis. Despite therapy, about 50% of newborns with early onset infection die, and mortality is greater in preterm infants.

SELECTED READINGS

Ablow RC, Driscoll SG, Effmann EL, et al: A comparison of early-onset group B streptococcal neonatal infection and the respiratory distress syndrome of the newborn. *N Engl J Med* 1976;294:65.

Anthony BF: Carriage of group B streptococci during pregnancy: A puzzler. *J Infect Dis* 1982;145:789.

Anthony BF, Eisenstadt R, Carter J, et al: Genital and intestinal carriage of group B streptococci during pregnancy. *J Infect Dis* 1981;143:761.

Anthony BF, Okada DM: The emergence of group B streptococci in infections of the newborn infant. *Annu Rev Med* 1977;28:355.

Anthony BF, Okada DM, Hobel CJ: Epidemiology of group B streptococcus: Longitudinal observations during pregnancy. *J Infect Dis* 1978;137:524.

Anthony BF, Okada DM, Hobel CJ: Epidemiology of the group B streptococcus: Maternal and nosocomial sources for infant acquisitions. *J Pediatr* 1979;95: 431.

Badri MS, Zawaneh S, Cruz AC, et al: Rectal colonization with group B streptococcus: Relation to vaginal colonization in pregnant women. *J Infect Dis* 1977;135:308.

Baker CJ: Group B streptococcal infections in neonates. *Pediatrics Rev* 1979;1:3.

Baker CJ: Summary of the workshop in perinatal infections due to group B streptococcus. *J Infect Dis* 1977;136:137.

Baker CJ, Barrett FF, Gordon RC, et al: Suppurative meningitis due to streptococci of Lancefield group B. *J Pediatr* 1973;82:724.

Baker CJ, Edwards MS, Kasper DL: Role of antibody to native type III polysaccharide of group B streptococcus in infant infection. *Pediatrics* 1981;68: 544.

Baker CJ, Kasper DL: Correlation of maternal antibody deficiency with susceptibility to neonatal group B streptococcal infections. *N Engl J Med* 1976; 294:752.

Baker CJ, Kasper D, Tager IB, et al: Quantitative determination of antibody to capsular polysaccharide in infection with type III strains of group B streptococcus. *J Clin Invest* 1977;59:810.

Baker CJ, Webb BJ, Kasper DL, et al: The natural history of group B streptococcal colonization in the pregnant woman and her offspring. II. Determination of serum antibody to capsular polysaccharide from type III, group B streptococcus. *Am J Obstet Gynecol* 1980;137:39.

Dillon HC Jr, Gray E, Pass MA, Gray BM: Anorectal and vaginal carriage of group B streptococci in pregnant women. *J Infect Dis* 1982;145:794.

Edwards MS, Baker CJ: Prospective diagnosis of early onset group B streptococcal infection by countercurrent immunoelectrophoresis. *J Pediatr* 1979;94: 286.

Edwards MS, Kasper DL, Baker CJ: Rapid diagnosis of type III group B streptococcal meningitis by latex particle agglutination. *J Pediatr* 1979;95:202.

Franciosi RA, Knostman JD, Zimmerman RA: Group B streptococcal neonatal and infant infections. *J Pediatr* 1973;82:707.

Hemming VG, Hall RT, Rhodes PG, et al: Assessment of group B streptococcal opsonins in human and rabbit serum by neutrophil chemiluminescence. *J Clin Invest* 1976;58:1379.

Hoogkamp-Korstanje JAA, Gerards LJ, Cats BP: Maternal carriage and neonatal acquisition of group B streptococci. *J Infect Dis* 1982;145:800.

Howard JB, McCracken GH Jr: The spectrum of group B streptococcal infections in infancy. *Am J Dis Child* 1974;128:815.

Katzenstein A, David C, Braude A: Pulmonary changes in neonatal sepsis due to group B beta-hemolytic streptococcus: Relation to hyaline membrane disease. *J Infect Dis* 1976;133:430.

Lillien LD, Harris VJ, Pildes RS: Significance of radiographic findings in early-onset group B streptococcal infection. *Pediatrics* 1977;60:360.

Pass MA, Gray BM, Khare S, et al: Prospective studies of group B streptococcal infection in infants. *J Pediatr* 1979;95:437.

Shigeoka AO, Hall RT, Hemming VG, et al: Role of antibody and complement in opsonization of group B streptococci. *Infect Immun* 1978;21:34.

Shigeoka AO, Hall RT, Hill HR: Strain specificity of opsonins for group B streptococcal types II and III. *Infect Immun* 1979;23:438.

Siegel JD, McCracken GH Jr: Detection of group B streptococcal antigens in body fluids of neonates. *J Pediatr* 1978;93:491.

Stechenberg BW, Schreiner RL, Grass SM, et al: Countercurrent immunoelectrophoresis in group B streptococcal disease. *Pediatrics* 1979;64:632.

Vollman JH, Smith WL, Ballard ET, et al: Early onset group B streptococcal disease: Clinical, roentgenographic, and pathologic features. *J Pediatr* 1976; 89:199.

Yow MD, Leeds LJ, Thompson PK, et al: The natural history of group B streptococcal colonization in the pregnant woman and her offspring. I. Colonization studies. *Am J Obstet Gynecol* 1980;137:34.

23 *Staphylococcus aureus*

Arnold Lentnek
Jack L. LeFrock
Abdolghader Molavi

Although *Staphylococcus aureus* accounts for less than 5% of all bacterial pneumonias in adults, its importance as a respiratory pathogen greatly exceeds the relative infrequency of its occurrence. Unlike pneumococcal pulmonary infection, mortality in staphylococcal pneumonia is high (up to 50% in some series) despite good antibiotic therapy; and since extensive tissue destruction and healing with fibrosis is the rule in survivors, there is considerable long-term morbidity. The role of *S. aureus* as predominantly a secondary pathogen in patients already compromised by viral infection or by a preexisting staphylococcal bacteremia further compounds the difficulty of treatment and has spurred the search for alternative modes of antibiotic therapy.

Predominantly a pathogen of skin and adjacent tissues, *S. aureus* was first isolated in 1880 by Alexander Ogston, a surgeon studying the pathogenesis of subcutaneous abscesses. Shortly thereafter, invasive *S. aureus* was differentiated from the more ubiquitous but less pathogenic *S. albus* (renamed *S. epidermitis*) by the coagulase test. Unlike pneumococci, staphylococci lack highly antigenic, serotypically distinctive capsules to aid in their differentiation, and it was not until 1942 that Fisk discovered a method of subclassifying staphylococci through differences in their susceptibility to various lytic bacteriophages.

The introduction of penicillin in the mid-1940s had a biphasic effect on staphylococcal infections. Initially, many dramatic responses were recorded. However, the proliferation and dissemination of naturally occurring penicillinase-producing strains, first within hospitals and later in the general population, led to a pandemic of staphylococcal infection during the 1950s which diminished only with the introduction of methicillin, cephalosporins, and other penicillinase-resistant penicillins in the late 1950s and early 1960s.

Microbial Characteristics

The gram-positive staphylococcus is a nonsporulating, nonmotile organism of approximately 1 μm in diameter, slightly larger and rounder than a *Streptococcus*. *S. aureus* belongs to the family Micrococcaceae, within which it is distinguished from the less pathogenic *S. epidermitis* and *S. saphrophyticus* by its production of coagulase. It grows well either aerobically or anaerobically on simple laboratory media as well as in blood agar to form small, slightly raised, golden yellow colonies, usually surrounded by a zone of β-hemolysis due to release of β-hemolysis. Because cell division occurs in three planes, organisms are typically found in grapelike clusters when grown in liquid media. (Selective media incorporating either 7.5% sodium chloride or tellurite glycine agar can be used to screen out other bacteria.) In smears of pathologic material these clusters, as well as tetrads, pairs, and occasionally short chains, are commonly seen. Since staphylococci may remain viable within leukocytes for some time after ingestion, whereas streptococci generally are rapidly killed and digested, it is not uncommon to observe intraleukocyte gram-positive cocci in specimens taken from staphylococcal infections.

Staphylococci are extremely hardy organisms that resist long periods of drying, wide temperature extremes (replication may occur at 10°C to 45°C), and high salt concentrations. Although growth is most rapid in the presence of oxygen, the organisms are facultative anaerobes and will grow slowly in strictly anaerobic environments. They produce catalase, unlike streptococci, and thus break down hydrogen peroxide, an ability which may be of pathologic importance in patients with impaired granulocyte hydrogen peroxide production, such as those with chronic granulomatous disease of childhood.

Unlike the *Pneumococcus*, there is no satisfactory serologic classification system for staphylococci. For epidemiologic purposes *S. aureus* are subclassified on the basis of their susceptibility patterns to various strains of lytic bacteriophage. Four such phage groups (1 through 4) have been identified, with numerous phage types within each group. In a geographically localized outbreak most of the involved organisms will be of the same phage type. Certain phage types, such as 80/81, frequently have been associated with hospital epidemics and are said to be epidemiologically virulent strains, but the basis for their enhanced virulence remains undefined.

Epidemiology

Although *S. aureus* is widely distributed in nature, no significant focus in wild or domestic animals exists, and the organisms infect man primarily. In view of their hardiness it is not surprising that staphylococci can be recovered from a large variety of inanimate surfaces. Nonetheless, it is doubtful that fomites are significant in the acquisition and spread of staphylococcal infections. Rather, asymptomatic carriers appear to play a pivotal role.

Pathogenic staphylococci are normally acquired by a high percentage of healthy infants within several days or occasionally weeks of birth.

The unbilical stump, the stool, and the perineum are the areas of most frequent colonization. Such infants may be responsible for occasional epidemics in nurseries. In adults, carriage in the anterior nares is more common, although the nasopharynx, rectum, and perineum may occasionally be colonized as well. Contrary to popular belief, persistent colonization of otherwise normal skin is rare; *S. aureus* cultured from the skin probably represent a transient population which is continually repopulated from the nose. Approximately 30% of adults are persistent nasal carriers of *S. aureus*; another 50% may harbor the organism intermittently; in some 20% staphylococcal nasal carriage is virtually never found. At any one time 20% to 40% of adults are nasal carriers. Rates are higher among diabetics and narcotics addicts and are increased by prolonged hospitalization, especially in the setting of antibiotic administration. However, in most instances the conditions facilitating or halting nasal carriage remain poorly understood. Some strains of staphylococci, especially those associated with methicillin resistance, seem to be poorly adapted to nasal colonization.

The staphylococcal carrier spreads infection in one of two ways: by direct autoinoculation, or by transmission to others in the immediate environment. Staphylococcal carriers incur staphylococcal postoperative wound infections at a rate severalfold higher than noncarriers. They also have a higher incidence of spontaneous skin infections. Epidemiologic studies have demonstrated a high correlation between the phage type carried in the anterior nares and the phage type subsequently recovered from wound or cutaneous infections. Similar autoinoculation has been demonstrated in heroin addicts with staphylococcal endocarditis, as well as in patients with staphylococcal phlebitis secondary to intravenous catheters.

The carrier may also spread staphylococci to his skin, clothing and bedding. Susceptible individuals coming in contact with such carriers or their fomites, are at high risk of acquiring and becoming infected with the same phage type. Accordingly, medical personnel, especially those with direct, frequent patient contact, have a considerably higher rate of staphylococcal carriage than does the general population. In addition to becoming actively colonized, medical personnel also may occasionally serve as passive intermediaries, transferring organisms from an asymptomatic carrier to another susceptible individual without themselves acquiring the disease or becoming persistently colonized. Airborne spread has also been demonstrated, as in the case of "cloud babies," infants who widely disseminate staphylococci because of a concomitant viral upper respiratory infection superimposed upon an asymptomatic staphylococcal carrier state. Epidemiologic patterns similar to those in hospitals may exist within any closed population group, such as families, day care centers, and other domiciliary institutions.

Staphylococcal carriage is not seasonal. However, since much of staphylococcal pneumonia in infants and adults occurs after viral respiratory infection (see below), the incidence of staphylococcal pneumonia reflects that of the initiating viral infection and generally is greatest during the winter and early spring.

Pathogenicity

Unlike the *Pneumococcus*, which produces its characteristic clinical syndromes predominantly through direct invasion of tissue, staphylococcal infection results in extensive tissue necrosis by elaborating a variety of exotoxins and enzymes. Pathologically, the characteristic features of staphylococcal infection are suppuration and abscess formation. After invasion, small vessels thrombose, fibrin is deposited in the area, and the site becomes avascular, necrotic, and surrounded by fibroblasts. The involved tissues become hypertonic, edematous, tense, and painful; the center liquifies, forming the thick yellow pus characteristic of staphylococcal infection.

Mediators of this sequence of events include enzymes such as coagulase, hyaluronidase, staphylokinase (plasminogen inactivator), catalase, and lipolytic enzymes. The pathogenic role of these enzymes has been only partially defined. Lipolytic enzymes, for example, may permit the *Staphylococcus* to overcome the bactericidal lipids of the skin. Coagulase and staphylokinase, acting in tandem, probably mediate local blood vessel thrombosis, while hyaluronidase appears to be important in producing the central liquification necrosis characteristic of staphylococcal lesions. Most staphylococci also possess a surface component, designated protein A, which nonspecifically binds IgG antibody at the Fc fragment end, rather than at the usual Fab fragment end. This reverse attachment appears to render the immunoglobulin functionally ineffective and may partially account for the observation that humoral antibody offers little protection against either staphylococcal colonization or infection.

Pathogenic staphylococci also produce a variety of exotoxins, only some of which have been characterized. Of the four hemolysins, alpha toxin (or hemolysis) has been the most intensively studied. It has a hemolytic effect on rabbit erythrocytes, is cytotoxic and cytolytic to a wide variety of cell types, and is dermonecrotic. Beta toxin causes damage to the plasma membrane of erythrocytes, leukocytes, and macrophages. Gamma and delta toxins seem to cause similar effects but have distinct cell-type specificities and different electrophoretic and chemical properties. Exfoliative toxin, whose production appears to be mediated by a bacteriophage, is responsible for the syndrome of toxic epidermal necrolysis (scalded skin syndrome) seen predominantly in children. Phage group 2 staphylococci appear to be exclusively responsible.

Staphylococci also produce a variety of enterotoxins which cause nausea and vomiting when ingested in small amounts. Their production also is often mediated by a temperate phage, which can be passed from one toxigenic strain to another. Six staphylococcal enterotoxins have been identified.

Protection against staphylococcal infection appears to be primarily related to the presence of intact integumen, serosal, or mucosal surfaces. The inoculum of staphylococci needed to produce a localized skin infection, for example, can be reduced nearly 1000-fold if there is a break in the skin and if a foreign body, such as a loosely tied suture, is present. Most adults possess high serum antibody titers to a variety of staphylococcal antigens, but such high titers have not correlated well with either protection from infection or diminution of the carriage state. Accordingly, immunization as a means of enhancing staphylococcal resistance has met with little success.

Although seemingly normal adults can be infected with virulent staphylococci, most patients with overwhelming staphylococcal infection have an identifiable preexisting depression of host defenses. Staphylococcal pneumonias often follow a pulmonary viral infection (often influenza, measles, or varicella), mucoviscidosis, or breach of a normal host barrier, as by tracheostomy, parenteral drug abuse, or surgery. Common denominators of all these conditions include impairment of the cough reflex, depression of mucociliary clearance of bronchial secretions, alterations in the viscosity and antibacterial properties of bronchial mucus, and depression of alveolar macrophage function.

Clinical Disease

Staphylococcal pneumonia may present as any one of several distinct syndromes, depending upon the patient's age (infant versus adult) and the route of spread (hematogenous versus orotracheal aspiration). In children, staphylococcal pneumonia is seen predominantly during the first two years of age, especially in the neonatal period. Most cases present during the winter and early spring when viral respiratory illness is prevalent. Staphylococcal pneumonia usually appears shortly after a presumably minor upper or lower respiratory infection or during recovery from measles infection. Many of the young patients or members of their families have a history of minor staphylococcal skin infection. Rather than the gradual improvement expected after a viral respiratory illness, the child deteriorates. Nonspecific findings such as failure to feed, irritability, vomiting, diarrhea, and low-grade fever mark the initiation of staphylococcal infection. Staphylococcal skin lesions often are found peripherally. The deterioration progresses to tachypnea, grunting respirations, and cyanosis, usually over a two- to four-day period, but occasionally much more rapidly. The cough is initially dry and nonproductive, but later may become markedly purulent, with production of large amounts of thick yellow sputum. Pleural effusion with dullness to percussion and decreased breath sounds on physical exam develops in most children, and as many as 40% may develop pneumothorax, a complication that may be increased by glucocorticoid therapy. The pneumonia usually begins as a unilateral process (right more commonly than left), but progression to bilateral infection occurs in one quarter of the patients. In older children, leukocytosis is common, with white blood cell counts of 15,000 to 20,000, but counts below 5000 are common in neonates and indicate a poor prognosis. Blood cultures demonstrate staphylococci in approximately 20% of children. Chest x-rays initially show patchy infiltrates, which characteristically progress to form small pneumatoceles. Pleural effusion, empyema, and pneumothorax are also common. In young children this clinical picture may be mimicked by a variety of other bacterial pathogens, including pneumococci, *Klebsiella*, and *Hemophilus influenzae*. Primary tuberculosis occasionally produces a similar syndrome.

Staphylococcal pneumonia in adults, as in children, commonly appears as a complication of viral (usually influenza) infection. Postinfluenza bacterial pneumonias are most commonly due to pneumococci, with *S. aureus* and *H. influenzae* accounting for most of the remainder. The illness presents in a characteristic biphasic manner. The patient usually has experienced a "flulike" illness with malaise, myalgias, fever, and a dry, irritating, nonproductive cough. After five to seven days of illness, the fever resolves and the patient begins to feel better, only to suddenly deteriorate with acute staphylococcal suprainfection. In fulminating cases this deterioration can be dramatic, with a sudden onset of multiple, shaking chills leading to high fever, disorientation, and coma. Peripheral vascular collapse, hypoxia, and cyanosis rapidly appear. However, specific signs and symptoms of pulmonary infection may not be prominent; cough, increased sputum production, dyspnea, and chest pain may be minimal during the early stages, leading the clinician away from the correct diagnosis. Patients with underlying chronic pulmonary disease, congestive heart failure or especially mitral regurgitation are especially prone to staphylococcal suprainfections. As in children, concomitant pneumonia and peripheral staphylococcal skin lesions may be a helpful diagnostic clue. In debilitated or elderly adults, primary staphylococcal pneumonia may develop without an antecedent viral respiratory illness. The onset may be either sudden and dramatic or insidious; many such patients present simply with mental confusion and no signs or symptoms of pulmonary infection. Sputum production is often scanty, and the diagnosis may be difficult to establish.

Chest x-rays in adults with staphylococcal pneumonia often demonstrate patchy, widely scattered infiltrates, frequently with an intense pleural reaction. Frank consolidation is uncommon and pneumatoceles are rare, but empyema is found in approximately 10% of adult patients. Abscess formation, often in multiple areas, occurs in approximately 25%.

Bacteremic staphylococcal pneumonia occurs under very specific circumstances. Usually, there is a clearly identifiable source of continuous staphylococcal bacteremia. Transient bacteremia does not usually result in attachment of the organism to respiratory tissue, although a syndrome compatible with bacteremic staphylococcal pneumonia has been documented in heroin addicts with no evidence of underlying endocarditis or phlebitis. Such cases may result from injection of virulent *S. aureus*, as well as injury to pulmonary tissue from impurities in the heroin.

The common sources of persistent staphylococcal bacteremia include infected intravenous lines or hemodialysis access sites and bacterial endocarditis, especially on the right side of the heart, as seen in drug addicts, and in patients with prosthetic cardiac valves. Symptoms of the underlying bacteremia predominate, and the patient presents with chills, fever, malaise, weakness, and impaired consciousness. Attention usually is drawn to the pulmonary process only by the appearance of localized pleuritic chest pain, minimal and nonproductive cough, dyspnea, or by the findings on a incidental chest x-ray. The x-ray is characterized by multiple peripheral infiltrates that resemble embolic lesions and frequently progress to necrosis and abscess formation. Empyema is common, and pleural effusions are seen in approximately one third of patients. Pneumatoceles are rare in adults.

Diagnostic Tests

Diagnosis of staphylococcal pneumonia is based on recovery of *S. aureus* from pulmonary secretions in a patient with a compatible clinical syndrome. Unfortunately, beneath this straightforward statement are many diagnostic pitfalls. Productive cough and increased sputum production are often not present in patients with acute staphylococcal pneumonia, especially in infants and in adults with bacteremic infection. Even in adults whose pneumonia results from aspiration of oropharyngeal staphylococci, purulent sputum may appear only several days after the onset of infection—a diagnostic delay which usually cannot be accepted in a patient desperately ill with staphylococcal pneumonia. Moreover, interpretation of expectorated sputum in staphylococcal pneumonia is subject to many misinterpretations: gram-positive cocci normally found in the oropharynx may mimic the staphylococci, while even isolation of staphylococci from expectorated sputum may represent merely oropharyngeal colonization. There is no readily available equivalent of the pneumococcal Quellung reaction to differentiate *S. aureus* from the other gram-positive cocci normally a part of mouth flora.

Despite these drawbacks, examination and culture of expectorated sputum remains the most common diagnostic maneuver when staphylococcal pneumonia is suspected. If an uncontaminated sample of expectorated sputum cannot be obtained, transtracheal aspiration or fiberoptic bronchoscopy are acceptable alternatives. Gram stain of the sample should demonstrate sheets of polymorphonuclear leukocytes and many large gram-positive cocci, often in clusters, tetrads, or short chains. In contrast to oblong or lancet-shaped pneumococci and streptococci, the staphylococci will appear slightly larger and perfectly round. The finding of many intracellular gram-positive cocci further helps distinguish staphylococci from other oropharyngeal flora. As staphylococci frequently colonize the respiratory tract in patients hospitalized for other conditions or in those receiving antibiotics, recovery of rare or moderate numbers of staphylococci in sputum culture is not diagnostic of staphylococcal pneumonia.

In view of the frequency of pleural effusions, thoracentesis often is helpful for diagnosis as well as therapy. In contrast to pneumoccal infection, in which pleural effusions often represent a sterile sympathetic reaction to an adjacent focus of inflammation, such effusions in staphylococcal pneumonia usually represent true empyema. The organism usually can be seen on gram stains and recovered in culture from such samples. Blood cultures also are frequently helpful in establishing a diagnosis. Overall, approximately 25% of affected patients have positive blood cultures; the percentage is considerably higher in patients with bacteremic pneumonia and in children.

When bacteremic staphylococcal pneumonia is suspected, counterimmunoelectrophoresis to demonstrate serum antibody to a staphylococcal cell-wall component, teichoic acid, is a rapid and specific test. Eighty percent of patients with underlying staphylococcal endocarditis have detectable antibodies at the time of hospitalization. Unfortunately, this sensitivity is observed only in staphylococcal endocarditis. One half of patients with transient staphylococcal bacteremia have positive tests, and in nonbacteremic staphylococcal pneumonia the rate falls to 15%.

The chest x-ray, while not diagnostic, may be highly suggestive of staphylococcal infection. Characteristic patchy infiltrates appear bilaterally in approximately 30% of patients, progress rapidly, and are associated with early formation of small abscesses. Pneumatoceles are frequently seen in children while, in adults, rapidly progressing pleural effusions are common. These effusions are often loculated in intralobar tissues and are therefore occasionally difficult to detect and aspirate.

Therapy

Although antimicrobial agents play a pivotal role in the treatment, response to antibiotics is not as dramatic as is seen in other forms of bacterial pneumonia. This slow response of staphylococcal infection has been attributed to several characteristics: 1) because staphylococcal abscesses are avascular, antibiotics may penetrate poorly into them; 2) the depressed growth rate of bacteria within an abscess may render the organisms less susceptible to antibiotic-mediated cytolysis; 3) the low pH of an abscess cavity may decrease the activity of many antibiotics; and 4) enzymes released from degenerating granulocytes within the abscess may partially inactivate the antibiotic. Detection and drainage of loculated effusions and abscesses are therefore extremely important and may be life-saving.

β-Lactam antibiotics are considered the drugs of choice in treating staphylococcal infections. Since the vast majority of community and hospital-acquired strains of *S. aureus* produce penicillinase, the choice should, initially at least, be limited to β-lactam antibiotics that are not inactivated by staphylococcal β-lactamase. Methicillin, nafcillin, oxacillin, cloxacillin and dicloxacillin all meet this criterion and are approximately equally effective. The risk of nephritis is higher with methicillin than with other drugs. Either nafcillin or oxacillin, 2 g intravenously every four hours, is the regimen of choice. Nafcillin is metabolized predominantly in the liver and therefore may be especially useful for patients with renal impairment.

In addition to production of penicillinase, two other forms of staphylococcal resistance to penicillin have been found. Methicillin-resistant strains (a generic term indicating resistance to all β-lactamase-resistant penicillins such as oxacillin, cloxacillin, dicloxacillin and nafcillin) share a chromosomally linked trait which usually affects a small percentage of organisms in a culture and may become apparent only when the organism is grown under special conditions (at 30°C in high concentrations of sodium chloride). These strains also are always resistant to penicillin G and cephalosporins in vitro, and are frequently resistant to other antibiotics. Infection due to such strains are best treated with vancomycin. Although methicillin resistance is less widespread in the United States than in Europe and the organisms are believed to be less virulent than methicillin-sensitive *S. aureus*, several large outbreaks have been reported in this country.

Penicillin tolerance is a newly described phenomenon wherein the serum minimal inhibitory concentration (MIC) is in the sensitive range, but the minimum bactericidal concentration (MBC) indicates resistance; thus the drug is bacteriostatic not bactericidal. Such staphylococci have decreased activity of an enzyme that appears necessary for penicillin-mediated bacteriolysis. Tolerant strains can be killed by aminoglycosides, cycloserine, or rifampin. Some evidence indicates that tolerant strains may be clinically important in patients with staphylococcal endocarditis who respond slowly to therapy, but their role in staphylococcal pneumonia remains undefined.

For patients allergic to penicillin, a first-generation cephalosporin is considered the drug of choice. The second- and third-generation cephalosporins are less active against *S. aureus*. Cross-reactions to cephalosporins occur in 8% to 15% of patients with documented penicillin allergy, but a cephalosporin generally can be safely administered to such patients as long as a syringe containing epinephrine is at hand. However, if the patient has experienced a recent immediate-type penicillin reaction, cephalosporins should be avoided.

For patients in whom β-lactam antibiotics are contraindicated, vancomycin is a useful alternative. This drug also is effective against methicillin-resistant strains. The combination of a penicillinase-resistant penicillin and either gentamicin or tobramycin displays synergistic activity against many strains of *S. aureus* in vitro. Such combinations have been suggested for treatment of overwhelming staphylococcal infections, predominantly staphylococcal endocarditis, but their efficacy for staphylococcal pneumonia has yet to be demonstrated.

Prevention

Considerable attention has been devoted to prevention of staphylococcal spread and to amelioration of the staphylococcal carrier state. In fact, many environmental procedures now considered routine in hospital care are a result of concepts introduced during the 1950s to contain the epidemic of hospital-acquired staphylococcal infection then so common. The need for frequent hand washing to decrease transmission of the organism from one patient to another, as well as from nasal carriers to patients, cannot be overemphasized. In special situations, such as staphylococcal outbreaks in newborn nurseries, washing with germicidal soaps or disinfectants, such as chlorhexidine (Hibiclens) or povidone iodine (Betadine), can be justified; but, in general, handwashing with ordinary bar soap is sufficient to markedly reduce the rate of staphylococcal transmission.

Although most staphylococci are transmitted by direct contact, droplet spread from patients with staphylococcal pneumonia has been well documented. It seems prudent to recommend that patients with staphylococcal pneumonia not be placed in the same room with patients at high risk of developing other staphylococcal infections.

Other than hand washing, efforts to control the spread of staphylococci from carriers have not proven very effective. Systemic antibiotics do not eliminate the carrier state, and attempts to produce an antistaphylococcal vaccine have been unsuccessful. Topical antibacterial ointment, usually bacitracin, may transiently reduce nasal shedding but does not appear to effect any long-term alteration in the frequency of nasal carriage or the titer of organisms shed. Bacterial interference, using a relatively nonvirulent strain of staphylococci (502A) to replace a more virulent one, has met with varying success; but infections, usually minor, have been reported even with this supposedly avirulent organism. In general, these techniques have little applicability to sporadic cases of staphylococcal pneumonia. They generally are used to curtail a well-defined, single phage-type outbreak of staphylococcal infection within a confined group or within a specified environment. In view of the high risk of development of staphylococcal suprainfection, patients with viral pneumonia probably should not be hospitalized at all unless the seriousness of their condition demands admission. For those requiring hospitalization, compulsive hand washing remains the single most effective procedure to reduce the rate of staphylococcal spread.

SELECTED READINGS

Cohen JO (ed): *The Staphylococci.* New York, Wiley Interscience, 1972.

Fekety RR: The epidemiology and prevention of staphylococcal infection. *Medicine* 1964;43:593.

Hendren WH III, Haggerty RJ: Staphylococcic pneumonia in infancy and childhood. *JAMA* 1968;168:6.

Klimek JJ, Marsik FJ, Bartlett RC, et al: Clinical, epidemiologic and bacteriologic observations of a methicillin-resistant *Staphylococcus aureus* at a large community hospital. *Am J Med* 1976;61:340.

Lindsay MI Jr, Herrmann EC Jr, Morrow GW Jr, et al: Hong Kong influenza: Clinical, microbiologic and pathologic features in 127 cases. *JAMA* 1970; 214:1825.

Musher DM, McKenzie SO: Infections due to *Staphylococcus aureus. Medicine* 1977;56:383.

Rebhan AW, Edwards, HE: Staphylococcal pneumonia: A review of 329 cases. *Can Med Assoc J* 1960;82:513.

Sabath LD, Wheeler N, Laverdiere M, et al: A new type of penicillin resistance. *Lancet* 1977;1:443.

Smith IM: *Staphylococcus aureus*, in Mandell GL, Douglas RG, Bennett MD (eds): *Principles and Practices of Infectious Diseases.* New York, John Wiley and Sons, 1979, pp 1530–1552.

Tuazon CV, Sheagren JN: Teichoic acid antibodies in the diagnosis of serious infections with *Staphylococcus aureus. Ann Intern Med* 1976;84:543.

24 *Bacillus anthracis and Other Bacillus Species*

Jack L. LeFrock
Abdolghader Molavi
Arnold Lentnek

Anthrax has been known since antiquity and was described in the *Iliad* and in the collection of Hippocratic texts by Pliny and Galen. The epidemiology is hinted at in the Bible: ". . . and it shall become fine dust over the land of Egypt and become boils breaking out in sores in man and beast throughout the land of Egypt" (*Exodus* 9:9).

The study of anthrax led to the development of modern bacteriology, serology and immunology. Starting in 1863 with Davaine who first saw the microorganism, many great men such as Koch, Pasteur and Vallery-Radot worked with this microorganism. Anthrax is a zoonotic disease which occurs in three forms in humans: cutaneous, accounting for 95% of cases seen in the United States; inhalation, accounting for 5%; and gastrointestinal, which has never been reported in the United States.

Microbial Characteristics

Bacillus anthracis is a gram-positive, encapsulated, sporulating rod (3 to 5 μm long) with square ends. It is the largest bacterium that infects man. Lack of motility, slow fermentation of gelatin, and pathogenicity for animals distinguish it from many other organisms that have a similar appearance (*B. subtilis* group) but do not usually produce human disease. Sporulation does not occur in vivo, but the spores may live in soil for 15 to 20 years. The spores, which are the infective form, are quite resistant to disinfectants and low heat but can be destroyed by boiling for 10 minutes or by exposure to dry heat (140° C) for three hours. *B. anthracis* colonies are raised, opaque, and grayish-white when cultured on blood agar. The anthrax bacillus has at least 23 demonstable antigens, including those associated with the cell wall, cytoplasm, spore, capsule, and toxin.

Only the capsule and toxin are associated with pathogenicity. The toxin is a thermolabile protein or lipoprotein made up of at least three components, which individually have little toxicity. When combined, they are immunogenic, edema-producing, dermonecrotizing, and lethal.

Epidemiology

Eighty percent of cases in the United States are industrial in origin, secondary to contact with goat hair, wool, hides, skins, and bones originating in Asia, the Middle East, or Africa. Agricultural cases result from contact with diseased animals or from self-inoculation with veterinarian anthrax vaccine. Inhalation of *B. anthracis* spores occurs when aerosols are created during the processing of infected materials. There have been no reports of human-to-human transmission.

Pathogenicity

Inhalation anthrax is not primarily a pneumonic disease. *B. anthracis* spores are ingested as inert particles by macrophages in the alveoli. After phagocytosis, the spores are carried to the regional lymph nodes where they germinate. The vegetative forms then multiply and produce toxin. This process is accompanied by hemorrhage and edema of the lymph nodes and the surrounding mediastinal connective tissue. Dissemination occurs through the bloodstream to the lungs, causing a hemorrhagic pneumonitis. The pleural effusion that occurs is perhaps caused by lymphatic obstruction. Seeding may also occur to the meninges (resulting in hemorrhagic meningitis), spleen, and gastrointestinal tract.

Clinical Disease

The course of inhalation anthrax is characterized by two stages. The initial stage is marked by the insidious onset of a mild fever, malaise, fatigue, myalgia, and nonproductive cough. Except for fever, few objective findings are noted except that rhonchi may be heard. This initial stage typically lasts for a few days.

The second stage is manifested by the acute onset of dyspnea, respiratory failure, and subsequent cyanosis. The patient usually appears toxic, with high fever and diaphoresis. Stridor may result from extrinsic obstruction of the trachea by enlarged mediastinal nodes. Subcutaneous edema of the chest and neck also may be present. On examination, moist, crepitant rales and signs of pleural effusion are observed. The chest x-ray shows mediastinal widening, resulting from node enlargement, as well as patchy, nonsegmental opacities probably related to hemorrhagic edema. The white blood count usually is normal.

Even with therapy inhalation anthrax has a very poor prognosis.

Diagnostic Tests

Diagnosis of inhalation anthrax is very difficult. The first stage is often mistaken for influenza or bronchitis; the second stage resembles cardiac failure or a cerebrovascular accident. One needs a high index of suspicion to make the diagnosis. If a person has had contact with infected material, especially imported from the Middle or Far East, and if he presents with severe dyspnea after a few days of a mild febrile illness, associated with acute widening of the mediastinum, one should suspect anthrax.

Isolation of *B. anthracis* from sputum, pleural fluid, cerebrospinal fluid, or blood is definitive. Cultures must be taken before treatment because specific therapy inhibits the recovery of *B. anthracis*. Demonstration of mediastinal widening by roentgenography is highly suggestive of inhalation anthrax when there is a history of exposure.

Therapy

Penicillin in high doses (20 million units/day) is the treatment of choice. For penicillin-allergic patients, erythromycin, chloramphenicol, or tetracycline is an alternative. However, despite seemingly appropriate antimicrobial therapy, treatment usually is unsuccessful.

Prevention

Individual awareness of the danger of potentially contaminated materials is the key to prevention of anthrax. Control programs should include education of employees; decontamination of potentially contaminated raw materials, if possible, and effective regular cleaning of equipment and work areas. Vaccination may be effective in preventing infection in those occupationally exposed.

OTHER BACILLUS SPECIES

Although *Bacillus cereus* has many morphologic and biochemical similarities to the more virulent anthrax bacillus, it has rarely been incriminated in infections in humans. Like other nonpathogenic members of this genus it generally is considered a saprophyte or contaminant when identified in cultures of clinical material. However, it has caused necrotizing pneumonia in the compromised host, and has produced both primary pneumonia and endocarditis in drug abusers.

B. cereus and *B. subtilis* have been recovered from blood cultures of drug abusers with right-sided endocarditis. As part of this syndrome, pneumonitis resulting from septic emboli to the lungs may occur.

The pathogenicity of *B. cereus* has been attributed to its production of an extracellular toxin that produces massive thrombi in pulmonary vessels. *B. cereus* usually is sensitive to aminoglycosides, chloramphenicol, erythromycin, and clindamycin.

SELECTED READINGS

Amidi S, Dutz W, Kohout, E, et al: Anthrax in Iran. *Z Tropenmed Parasitol* 1977;24:250.

Bell JH: On woolsorter's disease. *Lancet* 1980;1:871.
Brachman PS, Plotkin SA, Bumford FH, et al: An epidemic of inhalation anthrax. The first in the twentieth century. *Am J Hyg* 1960;72:6–23.
Butz W, Kohaut E: Anthrax. *Pathol Annu* 1971;6:209.
Coronrod JD, Leadley PJ, Eickhoff TC: *Bacillus cereus* pneumonia and bacteremia. *Am Rev Respir Dis* 1971;103:711–714.
Plotkin SA, Brachman PS, Utell M, et al: An epidemic of inhalation anthrax, the first in the twentieth century. I. Clinical features. *Am J Med* 1960;29:992–1001.
Ross JM: The pathogenesis of anthrax following the administration of spores by the respiratory route. *J Pathol Bact* 1957;73:485–494.
Tuazon CU, Murray HW, Levy C, et al: Serious infections from Bacillus species. *JAMA* 1979;241:1132–1140.
Vessal K, et al: Radiological changes in inhalation anthrax. *Clin Radiol* 1975; 26:471.
Weller PF, Nicholson A, Braslow N: The spectrum of Bacillus bacteremias in heroin addicts. *Arch Intern Med* 1979;139:293.

25 *Nocardia Species*

Jack L. LeFrock
Abdolghader Molavi
Arnold Lentnek

Three *Nocardia* species can cause infections in man: *N. asteroides, N. brasiliensis* and *N. caviae.* Systemic involvement is due almost entirely to *N. asteroides*, a pulmonary opportunist with a predilection to cause brain abscesses. As *Nocardia* are not normal inhabitants of the oropharynx or intestinal tract, their isolation from sputum, exudate, or any other specimen should be considered as indicating an infection.

Microbial Characteristics

Nocardia are branching, filamentous, irregularly staining, beaded gram-positive, nonspore-forming bacteria. Morphologically, they resemble *Actinomyces* which are, however, anaerobic; whereas, *Nocardia* are obligately aerobic. *Nocardia* usually are weakly acid fast and, due to ease of complete decolorization, may be missed by the routine Kinyoun-modified Ziehl-Neelson method for demonstrating acid-fast bacteria. Use of a weaker decolorizer (1% H_2SO_4) or reducing the decolorizing time with acid ethanol to one to two minutes, instead of the usual five minutes, can overcome this problem. *Nocardia* grow aerobically on many routine media (eg, blood agar) and Sabouraud's agar but require at least four days of incubation to form visible colonies. These become irregularly folded and yellow to deep orange or chalky white in color and are composed of filaments that break up into bacillary and coccoid forms.

Nocardia produce acid from carbohydrates oxidatively and use a wide variety of compounds, including hydrocarbons, as a source of carbon. The cell wall contains diaminopimelic acid, arabinose, galactose, and nocardomycolic acid. Variable hydrolysis of casein, tyrosine, and xanthine is used to differentiate species. *N. asteroides* does not hydrolyze any of these substrates.

Epidemiology

Nocardia inhabit the soil and are not normally found in the oral or nasal cavities or the intestinal tract. Men and other animals become infected most often by inhaling nocardial organisms. There is no proof of man-to-man, animal-to-man, or animal-to-animal transmission. The incidence of nocardosis is highest in males, and between the ages of 20 and 50 years.

Pathogenicity

Nocardia do not produce toxins. The cellular products are not antiphagocytic, although the filamentous growth makes phagocytosis difficult. They can produce hypersensitivity, which could prompt an inflammatory response. However, their ability to survive and metabolize in tissue is probably the principal mechanism causing inflammation and necrosis.

One half of the reported cases have been in normal hosts. The other half occur in people with diminished host defenses, particularly patients with neoplasia of the lymphoreticular system, hematologic or malignant diseases, pulmonary alveolar proteinosis, or sarcoidosis. Transplant patients are at risk. About 20% of *Nocardia* infections occur in patients receiving corticosteroids. Neutropenia is not an important predisposing factor; approximately 25% of patients are neutropenic.

The portal of entry and site of initial lesions usually is the lung. The pneumonitis advances to tissue necrosis. The resultant abscesses may extend and coalesce with neighboring abscesses. The sputum tends to be thick and purulent. In tissues, true granulomas are quite uncommon and sulfur granules are rare.

Direct extension from the lungs into the pleural cavity may go on to penetrate the chest wall, yielding draining sinuses. Lymphohematogenous spread or bacteremia arising from the erosion of blood vessels gives rise to metastatic infection in 30% of the patients. Metastatic spread to brain, joint, bone, skin, kidney, liver, or eye can occur from relatively small or inconspicuous pulmonary lesions. Brain and subcutaneous tissues are the most frequent sites of dissemination.

Clinical Disease

Infection may be subclinical to severe and be either chronic or fulminant. The onset usually is subacute but progressive. The usual clinical symptoms are fever, night sweats, and productive cough. The sputum occasionally is blood-tinged, thick, purulent or mucopurulent, but not foul-smelling. Chest pain commonly results from extension of the process to the pleural surface. Leukocytosis may or may not be present. Anemia of chronic infection develops as the disease persists.

Because nocardiosis often develops in patients with other diseases, the clinical features of the infection are superimposed on, and sometimes confused with, those of the underlying disorder. The clinical course of nocardiosis often is more fulminant in immunosuppressed patients than in those without associated diseases.

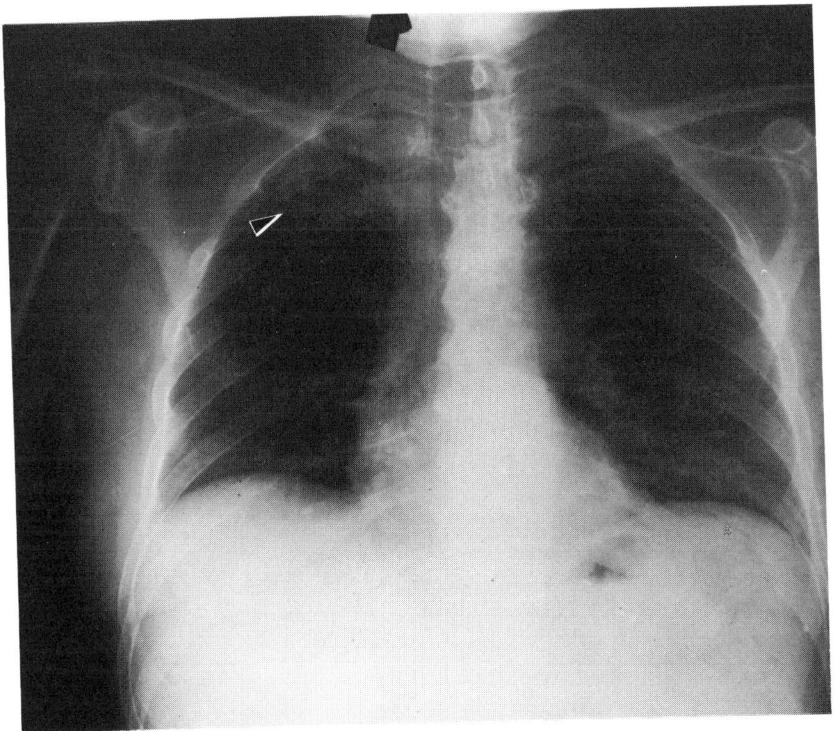

Figure 25-1 Chest radiograph, which shows right upper lobe cavities (arrow) in a patient with pulmonary nocardiosis.

The radiologic findings (Figure 25-1) in pulmonary nocardiosis may show the following patterns: 1) infiltrates or lobar consolidation, with or without necrosis and scarring; 2) a thick-walled cavity; 3) single or multiple large nodules; or 4) a miliary micronodular pattern associated with one of the foregoing.

In the presulfonamide era, 75% of patients with nocardiosis succumbed; now, with appropriate treatment, 60% to 75% recover. Several factors that adversely affect the prognosis have been defined: less than three weeks' duration of symptoms, treatment with corticosteroids or cytotoxic drugs, and the presence of disseminated nocardiosis, especially central nervous system involvement.

Diagnostic Tests

Definitive diagnosis of nocardiosis depends on isolation and cultural identification of the microorganisms. Although many attempts have been made to develop serologic studies and skin tests, none is of clinical value.

Prompt diagnosis and treatment are essential, especially in the compromised host. The diagnostic workup for these patients, including the selection of noninvasive and invasive procedures, is discussed in detail in Chapter 17.

Even though *Nocardia* grows well on a variety of common laboratory media, it is sometimes difficult to isolate from patients with nocardiosis. Many problems can preclude recovery: 1) the specimen may be contaminated with other bacteria that grow more rapidly on the culture medium used; 2) growth on blood agar is slow, and the plates may be discarded before colonies appear; 3) although *Nocardia* will grow on most media used for identification of mycobacteria, the concentration procedures ordinarily used to isolate tubercle bacilli often kill *Nocardia.* To increase chances of recovery, multiple specimens should be taken for culture and the laboratory notified that *Nocardia* is suspected so that appropriate media and incubation time are chosen.

The presence of *Nocardia* can be inferred by finding characteristic gram-positive, weakly acid fast, branching filaments in sputum or aspirated pus. *Actinomyces* have similar morphologic characteristics but are nonacid-fast.

The differential diagnosis of pulmonary nocardiosis includes the pyogenic, necrotizing pneumonias, actinomycosis, aspiration lung abscess, pulmonary tuberculosis, and the deep mycoses.

Therapy

The drug of choice is any of the sulfonamides. It makes little difference which preparation is used—sulfadiazine or sulfisoxazole—as long as peak serum concentrations of 10 to 20 mg/100 mL are achieved. Dosages recommended are: po 6 to 12 g of sulfadiazine or an equivalent amount of sulfamethoxazole or sulfisoxazole daily for an adult. Trimethoprim-sulfamethoxazole has been shown to be synergistic against *Nocardia* and has been used successfully in a dose of 5 to 10 mg of trimethoprim/kg/day in divided doses. To prevent relapse, especially in the compromised host, prolonged therapy (eg, up to 12 months) is required. Surgical drainage of abscesses and empyema should be performed.

SELECTED READINGS

Goodman JS, Koenig MG: Nocardia infections in a general hospital. *Ann NY Acad Sci* 1970;175:552.

Krick JA, Stinson EB, Remington JS: Nocardia infection in heart transplant patients. *Ann Intern Med* 1975;82:18.

Palmer L, Harvey RL, Wheeler JK: Diagnostic and therapeutic considerations in *Nocardia asteroides* infection. *Medicine* 1974;53:391.

Wallace RJ, Septimus EJ, Williams TW Jr, et al: Use of a trimethoprim-sulfamethoxazole for treatment of infections due to Nocardia. *Rev Infect Dis* 1982;4:315–325.

Yang LS, Armstrong D, Blevins A, Lieberman P: *Nocardia asteroides* infection complicating neoplastic disease. *Am J Med* 1971;50:356.

26 *Enterobacteriaceae, Pseudomonas aeruginosa and Acinetobacter*

Abdolghader Molavi
Jack L. LeFrock

Pneumonias caused by a few species belonging to the family Enterobacteriaceae and by *Pseudomonas aeruginosa* and *Acinetobacter calcoaceticus* are considered together in this chapter because of the common circumstances in which they occur and the similarities in their clinical and radiologic features. Pulmonary pathogens among the Enterobacteriaceae include *Klebsiella pneumoniae*, *Escherichia coli*, *Enterobacter* sp, *Proteus* sp, and *Serratia marcescens.* Together with *P. aeruginosa* and *A. calcoaceticus* var *anitratus* they will be referred to here as aerobic gram-negative bacilli (AGNB).

AGNB account for only a small percentage of community-acquired pneumonias, most often in patients with chronic obstructive lung disease, alcoholism, or diabetes mellitus. However, they frequently are the cause of pulmonary infection in patients who acquire pneumonia in the hospital (nosocomial pneumonia) and in those who are immunocompromised. Serious underlying disease usually is present, and despite antimicrobial therapy the overall mortality approaches 30%. In a study of adult patients with malignancies, pneumonia due to AGNB was the most common proximate cause of death among patients with solid tumors, and it was second only to septicemia among patients with acute leukemia and malignant lymphoma. Two of every three deaths from pneumonia are due to these organisms.

Epidemiology

Community-acquired pneumonia caused by AGNB is relatively infrequent, accounting for 0.5% to 5% of cases of bacterial pneumonia. The incidence increases with the age of the population surveyed and with the presence of underlying chronic diseases. Among persons 65 years of age or older living at home or requiring domiciliary care in nursing homes, AGNB account for a significant proportion of bacterial pneumonias.

Lower respiratory tract infections are the leading cause of mortality among hospital-acquired infections, although they rank third in incidence behind urinary tract and wound infections. Nosocomial pneumonias occur in only 0.5% to 0.8% of hospitalized patients, but 40% to 50% of these infections are caused by AGNB. In university-affiliated teaching hospitals the incidence is significantly higher than in community hospitals, partly because university hospitals tend to be tertiary care centers to which patients with more complicated illnesses are referred. Within a given hospital, nosocomial pneumonias occur with equal frequency in medical and surgical services. Among patients admitted to intensive care units, the incidence is much higher, approximately 10% to 22%.

Among adults and children with cancer, including hematologic malignancies, the lungs are the single most commonly documented site of infection. Up to 90% of all bacterial pneumonias in such patients are caused by AGNB. Similarly, in renal transplant patients more than 70% of bacterial pneumonias are due to these organisms.

Microbial Characteristics

Organisms of the family Enterobacteriaceae are small, aerobic or facultatively anaerobic, gram-negative, nonspore-forming bacilli which inhabit the intestinal tract of man and animals, soil, water, and decaying matter. They are commonly motile, by means of peritrichous flagella, although two genera (*Klebsiella* and *Shigella*) are characteristically nonmotile. Most species possess fimbriae (pili) which play a role in attachment to the host cells, and in bacterial conjugation and transfer of genetic material. Some species have a well-defined capsule or a loose coating referred to as the slime layer; others lack either structure.

Enterobacteriaceae grow readily on unsupplemented nutrient media over a wide range of temperatures. On nondifferential media, such as blood agar, the genera cannot be distinguished. Most species appear as moist, smooth, gray colonies; hemolysis, if it occurs, is usually of the beta type. A variety of differential and selective media are utilized for isolation and preliminary identification of various groups.

Enterobacteriaceae are biochemically diverse and complex. By definition, they all ferment glucose with production of acid or of acid and gas and, except for some strains of *Erwinia,* reduce nitrates to nitrites. They are broadly divided into two groups: lactose fermenters (which include *Escherichia*, *Klebsiella*, and *Enterobacter*) and slow or nonlactose fermenters. The genera and species are differentiated by their biochemical properties, such as fermentation of carbohydrates, presence or absence of enzymes, and ability to utilize substrates and products formed during growth.

The major antigenic components of the bacterial cell—the O or somatic antigen, the H or flagellar antigen, and the K or capsular antigen—are useful for serologic typing and further subdivisions. O antigens are the polysaccharide side chains of the lipopolysaccharide component of the outer membrane. H antigens are the flagellar protein antigens found in the motile members of the family. K antigens are surface polysaccharides that usually contain acidic groups, although some are protein in nature. When well developed, they form microscopically distinct capsules. K antigens promote pathogenicity by interfering with phagocytosis. K antigens also promote adherence to host epithelial cells and thus give the organism an advantage on initial contact with the host. Serotyping is used to establish the precise identification of strains isolated during outbreaks and epidemics.

Enteric bacilli are relatively sensitive to drying but can survive for extended periods with adequate moisture. They can tolerate cold for prolonged periods. These organisms produce no spores and are thus easily destroyed by heat or by low concentrations of common germicides or disinfectants.

The microbiologic characteristics of individual genera of the family Enterobacteriaceae and *P. aeruginosa* and *A. calcoaceticus* will be described below in separate sections on pneumonia caused by these organisms.

PATHOGENESIS

There are three routes by which AGNB can reach and infect the lower respiratory tract (Figure 26-1). The most common and most significant is direct extension of pharyngeal flora, usually by aspiration. Occasionally, the organisms reach the lung by hematogenous spread from an

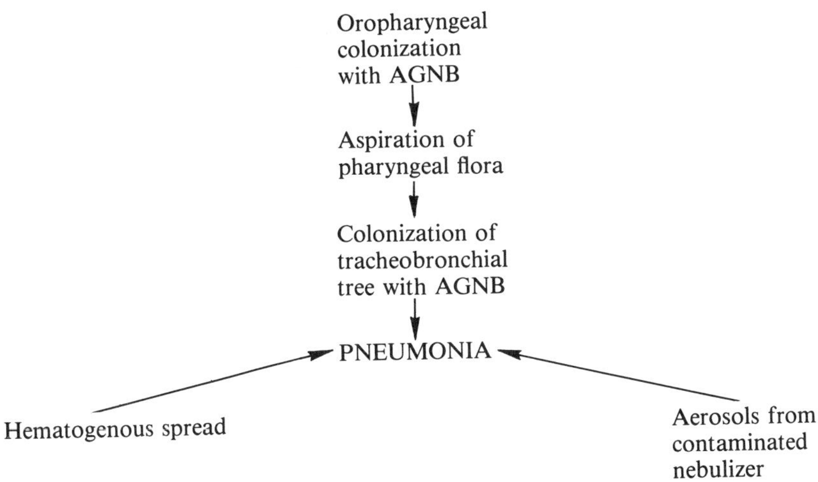

Figure 26-1 Routes of infection leading to AGNB pneumonia.

extrapulmonary focus. Least commonly, the lower respiratory tract is inoculated directly by inhalation of aerosols from a contaminated nebulizer. Airborne spread does not play a significant role.

Aspiration Aspiration of oropharyngeal flora is the most common route. The following sequence of events appears to be involved: 1) colonization of the oropharynx with AGNB; 2) aspiration of oropharyngeal secretions and subsequent colonization of the lower respiratory tract by these organisms; and 3) impaired clearance of the pathogens, resulting in infection of the pulmonary parenchyma.

The oropharynx of healthy individuals is not a suitable environment for growth of AGNB. The ability of bacteria to adhere to buccal epithelial cells, as well as the host's ability to block attachment by coating organisms with specific IgA or nonspecific glycoproteins, is important in determining whether colonization of the oropharynx is successful. Ordinarily, a small proportion of healthy persons harbor AGNB in significant numbers in their oropharynx at any given time. The colonization is transient, but its duration has not been defined. Using selective broth media, low numbers of AGNB were detected in the pharynx of 18% of healthy men who had not been hospitalized for at least three months prior to examination and who had not received antimicrobial agents in the preceding four weeks.

Chronic alcoholism and diabetes mellitus are two of the most common underlying diseases associated with community-acquired AGNB pneumonias. The prevalence of AGNB in the pharyngeal flora of ambulatory alcoholics (35% to 50%) and diabetics (36%) is significantly higher than in the healthy population. This is probably the major reason for their susceptibility to pulmonary infections caused by AGNB. Epileptics and narcotic addicts, while prone to episodes of unconsciousness and the associated risk of aspiration, do not have high rates of pharyngeal colonization by AGNB or of pneumonia caused by these organisms. The mechanism responsible for increased pharyngeal colonization among alcoholics and diabetics is not clear.

In chronically or severely ill patients, colonization of the oropharynx by AGNB is more prevalent (60% to 75% of patients). The reason for this increase is not known. Colonization is accompanied by significantly greater adherence of AGNB to the epithelial cells of upper respiratory tract, possibly due to alterations in the cells or to factors in the pharyngeal secretions of ill patients.

In hospitalized patients who are not severely ill the prevalence of AGNB in the pharyngeal flora approximates 30% to 40%. Most patients who become colonized do so within the first five days of hospitalization, suggesting the existence of a susceptible population, but the likelihood of colonization increases with increasing hospital stay. Factors predisposing to colonization include treatment with antimicrobial agents, exposure to inhalation therapy equipment, endotracheal intubation, presence of a nasogastric tube, and impaired mentation.

AGNB that colonize the oropharynx of hospitalized patients usually are derived from their indigenous enteric flora. However, clustering of patients colonized with the same species suggests that some bacteria are transmitted from patient to patient or from reservoir to patient. AGNB may be carried on the hands of hospital personnel and transferred to patients during daily care procedures unless scrupulous aseptic practices are observed. Opportunities for such transmission range from nonsterile suctioning of the oropharynx or tracheobronchial tree to contamination of bedside articles, water (ice), and food.

Within a given hospital there is often a periodic variation in the predominant AGNB causing oropharyngeal colonization and nosocomial pneumonia. The explanation for these fluctuations remains unclear. Certain organisms, particularly *P. aeruginosa*, appear to have a propensity for causing pneumonia later in the hospital stay.

Microaspiration of pharyngeal secretions occurs normally in a significant proportion of healthy individuals, especially during sleep. The frequency and quantity of microaspiration increases in hospitalized patients with tracheostomies, endotracheal intubations, or altered states of consciousness (due to cerebrovascular accident, drug overdose, alcoholic stupor, seizure, shock, hepatic coma, encephalitis, or anesthesia). Tracheostomy, endotracheal intubation, and bronchoscopy also allow direct inoculation of bacteria into the lower respiratory tract.

Despite repeated microaspiration, pulmonary clearance mechanisms normally ensure sterility of the tracheobronchial tree beyond the first bronchial division. Removal of small particles impinging on the walls of the trachea and bronchi is facilitated by the mucociliary lining. Bacteria reaching normal alveoli are phagocytized by alveolar macrophages; their growth is also inhibited by the relative dryness of the alveoli.

Any anatomic or physiologic derangement of these coordinated defenses increases the lungs' susceptibility to infection. Factors that impair mucociliary clearance (chronic obstructive lung disease, hypercarbia, smoking, alcoholism, or acute respiratory tract infections) or depress alveolar macrophage defense (immunosuppressive agents, acidosis, prior viral infections, or normal aging) predispose to development of AGNB pneumonia once colonization of the lower respiratory tract has occurred.

Immunocompromised patients present a complex array of disordered host defenses. The cytotoxic and immunosuppressed agents administered to these patients produce subtle metabolic effects which impair the phagocytic and bactericidal capacity of alveolar macrophages. The functional impairment of these cells and the granulocytopenia that is common in these patients account for their predisposition to AGNB pneumonia.

Hospitalization itself does not predispose patients to pneumonia. Rather, the hospitalized patient is an altered host and thus more susceptible to pulmonary infection. Patients in whom nosocomial pneumonias most commonly occur are 1) obtunded patients whose gag reflex and cough are ineffective; 2) patients with underlying pulmonary disease or heart failure whose pulmonary clearance mechanisms are impaired; 3) patients receiving mechanical ventilatory support or inhalation therapy via tracheostomy or endotracheal tubes; 4) patients with chronic debilitating illness requiring prolonged hospitalization; and 5) patients with impaired host defenses, particularly those with granulocytopenia. The high frequency of nosocomial AGNB pneumonia reflects both the frequency with which AGNB colonize the oropharynx of hospitalized patients, and the associated frequency of aspiration among these individuals.

The bacteriology of aspiration pneumonia differs strikingly according to whether aspiration occurred outside or within the hospital. AGNB are relatively common in those who acquire infection in the hospital while they are rare in community-acquired aspiration pneumonia.

Most AGNB pneumonias are monomicrobial, but occasionally two (or more) species may simultaneously affect the same region of the lung. Usually such cases follow aspiration and are nosocomial.

Hematogenous spread AGNB pneumonia may occur via bacteremic spread from an extrapulmonary focus of infection. The usual sources of seeding are the urinary, gastrointestinal, and female genital tracts, and burn wounds. Except for infections resulting from intravenous drug abuse, in which large numbers of organisms might be injected along with particulate material, bacteremia is an infrequent source of AGNB pulmonary infection. *E. coli* and *P. aeruginosa*, more commonly than other AGNB, cause pneumonia by the hematogenous route.

Inhalation of contaminated aerosols Since nearly all the gases utilized in respiratory therapy are 100% dry, they must be humidified before being delivered to patients. To accomplish this, either humidifiers or nebulizers are employed. Humidifiers saturate the gas with water vapor, usually by bubbling it through water. Aerosols are not generated. Nebulizers of all designs (jet, centrifugal, ultrasonic) produce aerosols and, in addition, saturate the gas with water vapor.

The water in the nebulizer reservoir may become contaminated with AGNB, which can then multiply and contaminate the aerosols generated by the nebulizer. The size of the aerosol particles is the major factor in determining the depth to which they will penetrate the respiratory tract. Particles below 2 μm in size can penetrate terminal bronchioles and alveoli. In the terminal lung units the main defense is the clearing capacity of alveolar macrophages, which are less effective against AGNB than against pneumococci. Furthermore, patients who receive inhalation therapy often are elderly and suffer from transient or chronic metabolic disorders, which may inhibit diapedesis and/or the phagocytic efficiency of the alveolar macrophages.

Nebulizer reservoirs may become contaminated from many sources. These include the oxygen or compressed air itself; the room air, which usually is added through the diluter ports to decrease the concentration of inspired oxygen; the inside of the reservoir container, which may become contaminated during cleaning or replenishing of the fluid; the water used to fill the reservoir; or an inadequately sterilized nebulizer jet, which may serve as a nidus for reinoculation of the reservoir. The condensate in the plastic delivery tubing that connects the nebulizer to the face mask may become contaminated with organisms from the patients' nose and mouth and retroflux into the reservoir. Finally, a contaminated medication may be added directly to the nebulizer.

The varying ability of species to proliferate in the nebulizer reservoir is important in determining the organisms that predominate. Outbreaks of pneumonia due to *K. pneumoniae*, *P. aeruginosa*, *S. marcescens*, *P. cepacia*, *Enterobacter agglomerans*, and *A. calcoaceticus* var *anitratus* have occurred due to contaminated nebulizers and mist tents. In recent years, improvements in the general care and handling of inhalation therapy equipment have decreased the incidence of pneumonia by this route.

Clinical Features

The clinical manifestations of AGNB pneumonia resemble those produced by other bacterial pathogens. Fever, chills, or chilly sensation, and malaise are commonly present. Fever may be sustained, remittent, intermittent, or at times hectic; the pattern does not correlate with a specific etiology. Respiratory symptoms, including cough, sputum production, dyspnea, and pleuritic chest pain, also are frequently present.

Early in the disease process, definite signs of pulmonary involvement may be lacking or may manifest only as fine, crackling rales. When consolidation develops, the typical findings of dullness to percussion, increased vocal fremitus, and bronchial or tubular breath sounds are easily elicited. A pleural friction rub may be audible over the involved area. Dullness to percussion associated with decreased vocal fremitus and diminished breath sounds suggest pleural effusion or empyema.

The radiologic features of AGNB pneumonia vary considerably depending upon the underlying conditions, the etiologic organism, the pathogenetic mechanism, and the stage of infection. X-rays cannot establish an etiologic diagnosis, although patterns correlated with particular organisms have been described. *Klebsiella* infections, for example, frequently demonstrate lobar consolidation with preference for the upper lobes, whereas *P. aeruginosa* infections show bronchopneumonia or widespread hematogenous dissemination.

Pulmonary infiltrates that appear as a result of hematogenous spread often produce a distinctive x-ray pattern. The infiltrates are patchy, occasionally with small areas of radiolucency, and are distributed widely in the peripheral lung fields.

In hospitalized patients the appearance on x-ray of a new infiltrate associated with fever, leukocytosis, and purulent sputum suggests nosocomial pneumonia, which is often caused by AGNB. Not infrequently, the patient's underlying disease process dominates the clinical picture, obscuring the development of a newly acquired pneumonia. Radiologically, nosocomial pneumonias usually begin as patchy, nonlobar, alveolar infiltrates, most commonly in the lower lobes. Pleural effusion usually is absent, and widespread multilobar involvement is rare. Microabscesses and empyema may subsequently develop.

In patients with granulocytopenia the clinical picture of AGNB pneumonia is characterized by a lack of the symptoms and signs usually found in patients with otherwise normal host-defense mechanisms. Sputum, if present, may not be purulent, and chest pain is uncommon. Because an impaired inflammatory response usually is found in association with granulocytopenia, physical findings are initially minimal, and the chest x-ray may be normal. Only after a few days do the physical findings of pneumonitis become apparent. At this point infiltrates develop, usually bilaterally and predominantly at the bases. Lobar pneumonia and abscess formation are infrequent, and empyema is uncommon.

Diagnosis

An AGNB etiology should be suspected in all patients who develop pneumonia in the hospital, particularly elderly or debilitated patients, or those receiving mechanical ventilation, or immunosuppressive or cytotoxic therapy. In community-acquired pneumonias AGNB should be particularly suspected if the patient is diabetic or alcoholic, or has chronic obstructive lung disease.

The clinical and radiologic features of AGNB pneumonias are not pathognomonic. A presumptive diagnosis can be made if the expectorated sputum contains many polymorphonuclear leukocytes amid a monotonous array of gram-negative rods of the same length, width, and staining characteristics. The presumptive diagnosis can guide therapy until culture results are available.

Frankly purulent sputum specimens should be selected for microscopic examination and culture. Specimens containing large numbers of neutrophils with very few (less than 10) epithelial cells per low-power ($\times 100$) field are accurate samples of lower respiratory tract secretions with minimal contamination by oropharyngeal flora. Large numbers of epithelial cells reflect significant contamination of the sputum with oropharyngeal flora. Since AGNB may be part of the normal pharyngeal flora, particularly in hospitalized patients and in "healthy" alcoholics and diabetics, isolation of AGNB from a sputum specimen is not pathognomonic.

When one has only an expectorated sputum specimen, examination of a gram-stained smear yields more information than culture results. Bacteria within or adjacent to leukocytes provide a clue to the etiologic agent. Most gram-negative bacilli can be easily recognized on gram-stained smears, but speciation can never be established by the appearance alone. Some AGNB can easily be misinterpreted. For instance, *Acinetobacter* may appear as a small, gram-negative coccus or diplococcus and be misinterpreted as a *Neisseria* or *Hemophilus* species.

Transtracheal aspiration, if performed properly, is a safe technique for sampling lower respiratory tract secretions. The procedure does carry some risk and should be reserved for patients with complicated pneumonias from whom sputum cannot be obtained or whose sputum specimens are uniformative or uninterpretable.

Transtracheal aspiration should be performed only by experienced or well-supervised physicians and only on cooperative patients in whom the cricothyroid membrane is easily identified. The procedure should not be done if the patient has hemorrhagic diathesis, severe cough, or significant hypoxemia or hypercarbia. Platelet count, prothrombin time, and partial thromboplastin time must be normal before the procedure is attempted. For several minutes after the procedure, pressure should be maintained over the cricothyroid puncture to minimize subcutaneous emphysema and soft-tissue bleeding. Thereafter, the patient should be kept at bed rest for six hours to minimize sucking air through the tracheal lesion into subcutaneous tissue or the mediastinum.

Despite these precautions, complications may appear. Mild hemoptysis may occur during and after the procedure. Subcutaneous emphysema, usually localized, develops in 5% to 10% of patients and is related to the amount of coughing during and after the procedure. Extensive subcutaneous emphysema of the neck, face, and chest wall and pneumomediastinum have been described. In rare infections of the paratracheal puncture site, the etiologic agent is usually, but not always, the organism recovered from the transtracheal aspirate. Bradycardia and cardiorespiratory arrest have very rarely been observed, usually in the presence of hypoxemia and hypercarbia.

Material obtained by transtracheal aspiration should be gram stained and cultured aerobically and anaerobically. A negative transtracheal aspirate in the presence of bacterial pneumonia usually is due to prior antimicrobial therapy. False-positive results usually are due to tracheobronchial colonization, especially in patients with chronic bronchitis.

Percutaneous needle aspiration of the lung is a relatively safe, simple procedure which can provide uncontaminated material from lung parenchyma for microbiologic and cytologic examination. Its highest yield is from localized or cavitary peripheral lung infiltrates. This procedure is used more commonly with infants and children, for whom transtracheal aspiration is considered dangerous. With adults, it usually is employed in immunocompromised patients when other diagnostic procedures have failed to reveal the etiology of pulmonary infiltrates.

Fiberoptic bronchoscopy and bronchial brushing are performed for diagnostic purposes in immunosuppressed patients with pulmonary infiltrates when the sputum specimen is uninterpretable or inadequate, particularly if there is a high risk of bleeding. Since passage of a bronchoscope through the oropharynx can contaminate any sample that may be obtained, the gram-stained smears and culture results should be interpreted with caution. Application of the new plugged, telescoping, brush-in-catheter system to obtain uncontaminated lower respiratory secretions is under investigation.

Bacteremia occurs in up to one third of patients with AGNB pneumonia, and blood cultures should always be obtained. Pleural effusion, if present, should be aspirated and examined for cells, sugar, protein, lactate dehydrogenase activity, and pH. A gram-stained smear should be examined microscopically and the specimen cultured aerobically and anaerobically.

Definitive diagnosis of AGNB pneumonia can be made by one of the following criteria: 1) isolation of the same predominant organism from two consecutive specimens of sputum or bronchial washings obtained by bronchoscopy, with gram-stained smears supporting the diagnosis; 2) isolation of the same organism from blood and sputum in close temporal proximity; 3) isolation of the organism from pleural fluid in a patient with pulmonary infiltrate; 4) isolation of the organism from a lung biopsy or needle aspiration of the lung; and 5) isolation of the organism from a transtracheal aspirate.

Pulmonary infiltrates, especially in hospitalized patients and immunocompromised hosts, may be of noninfectious etiology. In the former group atelectasis, pulmonary infarction, or pulmonary edema may be associated with fever and leukocytosis and should be distinguished from pnemonia. In immunocompromised hosts the possibility of malignant disease, intrapulmonary hemorrhage, drug-induced pulmonary disease, or radiation pneumonitis also should be considered.

Treatment

Despite the availability of antibiotics effective against AGNB, the overall mortality rate of pneumonia caused by these organisms has been high. These poor results largely reflect the underlying host conditions;

however, poor penetration of aminoglycosides into respiratory secretions may also be a contributory factor.

Once a presumptive diagnosis of AGNB pneumonia is made, antibiotic therapy must be started. Controversy exists as to the "best"empiric therapy in such cases. The combination of an aminoglycoside and an antipseudomonal penicillin (carbenicillin, ticarcillin, mezlocillin, azlocillin, piperacillin) would not be the regimen of choice to treat infection with *K. pneumoniae.* A cephalosporin plus an aminoglycoside would not be the regimen of choice for *P. aeruginosa* or *Acinetobacter* infections.

The third generation cephalosporins are highly active against most enteric bacilli, and the minimal inhibitory and bactericidal concentrations are in most cases remarkably low. In patients who are not neutropenic or who are not likely to be infected with *P. aeruginosa* a third-generation cephalosporin (cefotaxime, cefoperazone, moxalactam, etc) administered in full dosage (8 to 12 g/day in four to six divided doses for cefotaxime or 6 g/day in three divided doses for cefoperazone and moxalactam) either alone or preferably in combination with an aminoglycoside, would provide adequate coverage until cultures reveal the etiologic organism. However, these regimens would not be optimal for *Acinetobacter.* In neutropenic patients and those in whom *P. aeruginosa* is a likely pathogen the combination of an antipseudomonal penicillin and an aminoglycoside should be used. When the causative agent has been identified and its susceptibility determined, the antibiotic regimen should be modified when indicated. Combined use of two antibiotics is justified if the combination has a known synergistic effect against the causative organism.

In hospital-acquired aspiration pneumonia a mixture of anaerobes and aerobes (most commonly AGNB) is found in nearly half of the cases, and, in one-third, aerobes (usually AGNB) are the exclusive pathogens. Treatment should therefore include clindamycin in addition to an aminoglycoside. Alternatively, cefoxitin alone or preferably combined with an aminoglycoside may be used.

Aminoglycosides are administered intramuscularly or intravenously at a loading dose of 2 mg/kg gentamicin, tobramycin, or netilmicin, or 7.5 mg/kg amikacin, irrespective of the state of renal function. To patients with normal renal function, subsequent doses of 1.5 to 1.7 mg/kg gentamicin, tobramycin or netilmicin, or 5 mg/kg amikacin are administered every eight hours. For patients with renal impairment, the dosage should be adjusted.

Aminoglycosides are only sparingly distributed into the adipose tissue. In obese patients the dosage should be calculated on the basis of the ideal weight plus 50% of the adipose weight (actual body weight − ideal body weight).

Since the toxic and therapeutic doses of aminoglycosides differ only slightly and there is considerable interpatient variation in the serum concentrations produced by a given dose, it is important to monitor serum concentrations in all patients, especially those with impaired renal function. This is doubly important for patients with unstable renal function whose serum creatinine is changing from day to day. For gentamicin, tobramycin and netilmicin, peak serum levels should be 6 to 10 μg/mL, and trough levels of greater than 2 μg/mL should be avoided. For amikacin, peak levels of 18 to 30 μg/mL are considered therapeutic and trough levels greater than 10 μg/mL are excessive and toxic.

With severely ill patients, it may be worthwhile to determine minimal inhibitory and bactericidal concentrations and to investigate the synergistic activity of the combinations employed (if any), and to measure the serum bactericidal titers, which should be 1:8 or higher at peak serum concentrations.

Uncomplicated AGNB pneumonias should be treated for two to three weeks, guided by clinical and radiologic responses. If there are complications such as abscess or empyema, treatment should be continued for longer periods.

For empyema, adequate drainage of the pleural fluid is essential. Repeated needle aspiration may be adequate if the fluid is thin, free-flowing, and of small quantity, but such cases are rare. In most cases continuous, closed-tube drainage is necessary. This should be instituted immediately if the empyema fluid 1) is thick and purulent, 2) shows organisms on gram-stained smears, 3) has a pH below 7, 4) reaccumulates rapidly, or 5) has a sugar concentration less than 40 mg/100 mL. More than one chest tube may be needed if the empyema is loculated and not free flowing. In addition to parenteral administration of aminoglycosides, daily instillation into the pleural space is recommended by some clinicians. Immediately after instillation, the chest tube is clamped for three to four hours. Clinical improvement is accompanied by a gradual decrease in the volume of fluid drained daily and disappearance of organisms from the fluid.

Prevention

Efforts to prevent respiratory tract infection by AGNB should be directed toward 1) preventing oropharyngeal colonization by these organisms and 2) eliminating contamination of respiratory support equipment, particularly nebulizer reservoirs.

In the hospital, rigorous hand washing and other procedures designed to prevent transmission of AGNB are of major importance for minimizing the colonization of susceptible patients, particularly those in intensive care units. The value of prophylactic antibiotics (polymyxin B, aminoglycosides) administered intratracheally via aerosols to prevent colonization of the tracheobronchial tree is uncertain at best. Furthermore, there is a distinct hazard of the emergence of resistant organisms when aerosolized antibiotics are used for prolonged periods.

Every effort should be made to reduce microbial contamination of inhalation therapy equipment, ventilators, humidifiers, and nebulizers. Proper and regular disinfection and sterilization of these devices is important to prevent pulmonary infection with nosocomial pathogens. An active surveillance program should be maintained to detect outbreaks associated with such equipment.

On both medical and surgical services a conscientious effort to minimize the use of techniques, instruments, tubes, or drugs that compromise host pulmonary defense mechanisms or predispose patients to colonization with AGNB can decrease the incidence of nosocomial pneumonia.

Proper positioning of obtunded and comatose patients to prevent aspiration—and frequent sterile suctioning of secretions, particularly for patients with endotracheal intubation or tracheostomy—are important prophylactic measures for nosocomial pneumonia. Regular monitoring of respirtory flora, particularly in intubated patients, will facilitate a prompt, appropriate choice of therapy for pulmonary infections should they occur.

KLEBSIELLA PNEUMONIAE

K. pneumoniae is the most frequent cause of community-acquired pneumonia (ie, primary pneumonia) due to AGNB. It also accounts for a significant proportion of pneumonias acquired in the hospital.

Microbial Characteristics

The genus *Klebsiella* includes four species: *K. pneumoniae*, *K. oxytoca* (previously designated *K. pneumoniae*, indole positive), *K. rhinoscleromatis*, and *K. ozenae*. The most commonly isolated species is *K. pneumoniae* (Friedländer's bacillus), so-named because it can cause pneumonia. Similar infections are caused by *K. oxytoca*. The remaining species are not pulmonary pathogens.

All *Klebsiella* are characteristically encapsulated and, in contrast to the closely related *Enterobacter*, are nonmotile. They ferment a wide range of sugars, producing acid and gas. These organisms tend to be somewhat shorter and thicker than other enterobacteria. On gram-stained smears they are seen in pairs, end-to-end, or arranged singly. On solid media they form large mucoid colonies. This appearance is due to the prominent polysaccharide capsule, which can often be seen on gram-stained smears of clinical material and is believed to enhance the virulence of the organism.

Klebsiella possess K (capsular) and O (somatic) antigens, of which the polysaccharide K antigen is the most useful for serologic typing. Approximately 80 K antigens and 11 O antigens have been described. No single serotype of *K. pneumoniae* is more virulent than others, nor is one more frequently associated with infections. Nevertheless, serologic typing provides a useful marker for investigating apparent epidemics caused by this organism.

Epidemiology

K. pneumoniae is found in the oropharynx of 1% to 6% of healthy persons. Its prevalence in the pharyngeal flora increases in hospitalized patients, alcoholics, and diabetics. The organism is part of the fecal flora of man and animals and is found in soil and water.

Primary *Klebsiella* pneumonia accounts for approximately 1% of community-acquired bacterial pneumonias. It is seven to nine times more frequent in men than women and occurs most commonly in the middle-aged and elderly. A common coexisting condition is alcoholism (66% of cases). In nonalcoholic patients a predisposing condition—chronic obstructive pulmonary disease or, less frequently, diabetes mellitus—usually is present. The disease is endemic throughout the year, and there is no occupational predilection.

K. pneumoniae is responsible for a significant proportion of pneumonias that develop in nursing home residents. It is one of the most common gram-negative bacilli causing pulmonary infection in immunocompromised hosts, particularly those with granulocytopenia. Nearly one third of AGNB pneumonias in patients with cancer are caused by this organism.

Pathogenesis and Pathology

Pulmonary infections due to *K. pneumoniae* usually arise from aspiration of oropharyngeal secretions. Rarely, the infection is acquired from a contaminated nebulizer.

Primary *Klebsiella* pneumonia usually produces a lobar consolidation, but infection may be lobular or occasionally bronchopneumonic. The right upper lobe is most commonly involved. At autopsy, the involved lung is reddish gray, granular, and fibrotic. The pleura is thickened by an adherent fibrinous exudate, and empyema may be present. Hilar lymph nodes are enlarged and matted to adjacent structures.

Microscopically, the alveoli are filled with an inflammatory exudate composed primarily of polymorphonuclear leukocytes. The dominant histologic lesion is necrosis of alveolar septae, producing multiple small or large abscesses.

Clinical Features

The onset of primary *Klebsiella* pneumonia usually is abrupt (90%

of cases), with rigors (60%), fever, productive cough (90%), pleuritic chest pain (80%), and dyspnea. Early prostration is a usual feature. Occasionally, the acute onset is preceded by a nondescript upper respiratory infection. Rarely, epigastric pain and vomiting may be the initial symptoms. The characteristic sputum is tenacious and brick-red, consisting of a thick homogenous mixture of blood and pus. It is seen in up to 50% of patients. In some patients the sputum is thin, resembling currant jelly. Frank hemoptysis may occur.

On examination the patient appears acutely ill, febrile, dyspneic, and often cyanotic. Scleral icterus may be present. Herpes labialis is uncommon (12%). Clinical examination reveals signs of lobar consolidation. There may be loss of lung volume, as manifested by ipsilateral tracheal shift, narrow retracted intercostal spaces, and elevation of the hemidiaphragm secondary to bronchial obstruction with tenacious secretions. Involvement of more than one lobe is not uncommon.

The characteristic radiologic feature of primary *Klebsiella* pneumonia is lobar consolidation, most commonly in the right upper lobe, with bulging interlobar fissure. Occasionally, lobular involvement or bronchopneumonic infiltrates are seen. In nearly one half of the patients more than one lobe is involved. Abscess formation with either multiple small or large abscess cavities is found in 16% to 50% of patients. Empyema is relatively common (up to 66%), but pyopneumothorax is unusual.

Leukocytosis is common, but a normal or even decreased white cell count with a shift to the left is found in some patients. Blood cultures are positive in approximately 25% of cases.

Gram-stained smears of sputum show many polymorphonuclear leukocytes with numerous gram-negative encapsulated rods, which usually are thick, short, and arranged singly, in pairs (diplobacillus), or in short chains.

Therapy

K. pneumoniae is sensitive to cephalosporins, aminoglycosides, and chloramphenicol. Strains resistant to first- and second-generation cephalosporins, chloramphenicol, and even gentamicin and tobramycin are being reported with increasing frequency. However, all strains remain sensitive to amikacin and third-generation cephalosporins. The antimicrobial regimen of choice depends upon the local prevalence of resistant strains.

For a suspected *Klebsiella* pneumonia, treatment should begin with a third-generation cephalosporin alone or combined with an aminoglycoside. The antibiotic regimen may be modified when sensitivity data become available. Treatment should be continued for at least two to three weeks, depending on the clinical and radiologic responses. Prolonged therapy is required when multiple abscesses are present.

Prognosis

Untreated *Klebsiella* pneumonia is fatal in over 50% of cases. Antimicrobial therapy reduces mortality significantly. The risk factors associated with high mortality are serious underlying disease, advanced age, bacteremia, and leukopenia. Inadequate removal of tenacious pulmonary secretions is a significant factor contributing to mortality.

Chronic Klebsiella Pneumonia

Although primary *Klebsiella* pneumonia usually presents acutely, rarely does it occur as a subacute or chronic infection. The exact incidence of these chronic forms is difficult to establish, but they are much less frequent than the acute pneumonia.

The disease is characterized by a protracted, relatively benign course. Low grade fever, cough with copious purulent sputum, and weight loss are the usual symptoms. The disease may go on for several weeks or months. Chest x-rays show thin-walled cavities, with or without fluid, usually involving one or both upper lobes. Fibrosis and retraction of the involved lobes may later develop. Clinically and radiologically the disease resembles tuberculosis.

PSEUDOMONAS AERUGINOSA

P. aeruginosa is common cause of nosocomial pneumonia and pneumonia in patients with granulocytopenia. Community-acquired *Pseudomonas* pneumonia is relatively rare.

Microbial Characteristics

P. aeruginosa is a gram-negative, nonspore-forming bacillus which appears as straight or slightly curved rods on gram-stained smears. The organism is motile by means of polar flagella. Strains isolated from clinical specimens frequently possess pili, which may promote attachment to host cells and play a role in resistance to phagocytosis.

P. aeruginosa has simple nutritional requirements. It requires no growth factors and can use atmospheric carbon dioxide as its sole carbon source and ammonium as its sole nitrogen source. It is a nonfermentative, obligate aerobe that derives its energy from oxidative reactions. Clinical isolates grown on blood agar frequently are β-hemolytic. Most but not all cultures have a characteristic fruity odor.

Two pigments, pyocyanin (bluish-green) and fluorescein (greenish-yellow), are produced both in vitro and in vivo. These are responsible for the blue-green diffusible color associated with cultures of *P. aeruginosa* and with pus produced during infection.

P. aeruginosa elaborates a number of bacterial products that are potentially significant in infection. Two hemolysins (a phospholipase C and a glycolipid) are produced. In pneumonia the phosholipase may contribute to invasiveness by destroying the pulmonary surfactant and attacking the pulmonary tissue, producing atelectasis and necrosis. A number of proteolytic enzymes, including protease, elastase, and collagenase, are also produced. Elastase digests elastin, which is found in arterial walls, and may be important in the pathogenesis of necrotizing vasculitis. Pyocins, the bacteriocins of *P. aeruginosa*, are strain-specific proteins that are lethal to other strains. A polysaccharide slime layer covers the cell wall. Unlike the pneumococcal capsule, this slime is not firmly bound to the cell surface.

The O (somatic) antigens of *P. aeruginosa* are used to serotype the organism for epidemiologic purposes. Phage typing and pyocin typing, however, may also be necessary for complete characterization of isolates during an epidemic. Neither the pathogenicity nor the virulence of the organism is related to its serotype.

Epidemiology

P. aeruginosa is ubiquitous in the environment but is found primarily in water, vegetation, and moist soil. A variety of vegetables, including the tomato, radish, celery, carrot, cabbage and lettuce, may harbor the organism. Man is not a major habitat, but it is isolated in low numbers from the oropharynx of up to 5% of healthy adults, is frequently carried on the skin (axillary and anogenital areas) of normal people, and may be transiently part of the colonic flora in 5% to 24% of individuals.

Almost any alteration of health status, particularly hospitalization and antimicrobial or immunosuppressive therapy, is associated with an increased carriage rate of *P. aeruginosa*. The organism usually is part of the bacterial flora of hospitals, particularly in intensive care units. It thrives in moist environments, such as sinks, disinfectants (notably the quaternary ammonium compounds), ventilators, and nebulizers. Spread among patients occurs primarily from the hands of hospital personnel, who carry the organism from patient to patient or from reservoir to patient. Sinks for hand washing are a frequent repository for *P. aeruginosa*. It is difficult to determine whether the contaminated sink is an end stage of environmental contamination or a reservoir for colonization and infection. Airborne spread by splatter from contaminated sinks appears to be restricted to a radius of about 6 feet. This suggests that droplets carrying the organism are relatively large and settle rapidly.

Patients with cystic fibrosis frequently have persistent colonization of their respiratory tracts with *P. aeruginosa*. In those who are newly or intermittently colonized the organism is almost always nonmucoid, but as colonization becomes chronic, the strain becomes mucoid. The slime of mucoid isolates differs both physically and biochemically from the slime of nonmucoid strains, but the serotype does not change. Mucoid strains are better able to resist phagocytosis by neutrophils and are rarely isolated from patients without cystic fibrosis.

P. aeruginosa is unique among human pathogens in that it infects, not only other vertebrates, both warm- and cold-blooded, but also lower animals, terrestrial and aquatic, including insects. Despite its many potential virulence factors it rarely produces infection in normal persons. However, it commonly infects patients with compromised host defense mechanisms and/or structural lung disease, and it is one of the most frequent causes of nosocomial pneumonia.

Community-acquired *Pseudomonas* pneumonia usually occurs in patients with chronic lung or heart disease or cystic fibrosis. Conditions predisposing hospitalized patients to *Pseudomonas* pneumonia include inhalation therapy, breach of airway by tracheostomy or endotracheal tube, exposure to antimicrobial agents, and compromised host defenses, particularly neutropenia, due to hematologic malignancies or cytotoxic therapy.

Pathogenesis and Pathology

Pneumonia due to *P. aeruginosa* usually begins with aspiration of oropharyngeal secretions containing the organism. This may occur in a hospitalized patient whose pharynx is colonized by *P. aeruginosa*. Outside the hospital it may develop in elderly, debilitated patients with underlying cardiopulmonary disease.

Pseudomonas pneumonia can also be acquired via bacteremia from an extrapulmonary focus. Bacteremic *Pseudomonas* pneumonia is characteristically hospital-acquired and affects patients with serious underlying disorders that impair host defenses, particularly hematologic malignancies. Granulocytopenia, immunosuppressive therapy, assisted ventilation via tracheostomy or endotracheal tube, and prior antibiotic therapy are common conditions for these patients. Rarely, the disease may be community-acquired by healthy persons, and occasionally it occurs secondary to *Pseudomonas* endocarditis in illicit intravenous drug users.

Outbreaks of *Pseudomonas* pneumonia secondary to inhalation therapy with contaminated nebulizers have been reported. *P. aeruginosa* can multiply in distilled water, which is used in nebulizers.

Patients with cystic fibrosis have impaired mucociliary clearance and eventually develop chronic pulmonary infection. In recent years *P. aeruginosa* has become the predominant pathogen in these patients. An unusual feature is the tendency of such infections to remain limited almost exclusively to the lungs.

The dominant histologic lesion in *Pseudomonas* pneumonia is necrosis of the alveolar walls, producing multiple small or large abscesses scattered throughout the affected lung. In other areas focal hemorrhages may be present. The alveolar inflammatory exudate contains both polymorphonuclear and mononuclear cells. Invasion of the arterial walls, with thrombosis of vessels and nodular bland infarcts, may be seen in bacteremic pneumonia. In the nonbacteremic type, pulmonary vessels are patent with no evidence of necrotizing vasculitis.

Clinical Features

Nonbacteremic *Pseudomonas* pneumonia usually manifests by chills, fever, dyspnea, and cough productive of yellow-green sputum. Apprehension, toxicity, confusion, and cyanosis are common. Relative bradycardia and reversal of diurnal variation in body temperature may be present. The chest x-ray shows diffuse bronchopneumonia, which is often bilateral. Infiltrates are nodular, usually with multiple small areas of radiolucency (microabscesses). Nodules may enlarge and coalesce. A pleural effusion or empyema commonly is present.

Patients with bacteremic *Pseudomonas* pneumonia generally are quite ill, with fever, dyspnea, and marked toxicity. Ecthyma gangrenosum may be evident. The chest x-ray may initially show pulmonary vascular congestion or a pattern consistent with early pulmonary edema. However, septal lines are absent, and there is no evidence of left heart failure. The radiologic picture progresses rapidly to a necrotizing bronchopneumonia, often with a small pleural effusion and abscess formation.

Therapy

P. aeruginosa is resistant to most antimicrobial agents, including ampicillin, first- and second-generation cephalosporins, chloramphenicol, and tetracyclines. Some strains susceptible in vitro to third-generation cephalosporins (cefotaxime, cefoperazone, moxalactam, etc) may develop resistance during therapy. The organism is uniformly sensitive to polymyxins, but these agents are not effective against infections outside the urinary tract, and their toxicity is forbidding.

P. aeruginosa is susceptible to aminoglycosides and antipseudomonal penicillins (carbenicillin, ticarcillin, mezlocillin, azlocillin, and piperacillin). Resistance to gentamicin varies with geographic location, but in most areas of the United States it is low. Tobramycin is more active than gentamicin and may be effective against some gentamicin-resistant strains. Amikacin is effective against many strains resistant to gentamicin and tobramycin. Azlocillin and piperacillin are the most active penicillins against *P. aeruginosa*; mezlocillin and ticarcillin are two- to fourfold less active. Carbenicillin is the least active of these compounds against *P. aeruginosa*.

For treatment of *Pseudomonas* pneumonia, the combination of an aminoglycoside and an antipseudomonal penicillin is recommended. Both in vitro and clinical evidence supports the use of a two-drug versus a one-drug regimen, particularly for neutropenic patients.

Prognosis

Untreated *Pseudomonas* pneumonia has a very high mortality rate. Development of antibiotics with better activity against this organism has decreased the rate, but the overall figure is still about 35%. The prognosis varies with the patient's underlying condition. Bacteremic *Pseudomonas* pneumonia in neutropenic patients is almost uniformly fatal.

The unsatisfactory prognosis of patients with *Pseudomonas* pneumonia, even with currently available antibiotics, has led to consideration of immunoprophylaxis for patients at high risk of respiratory infection by this organism. Vaccines incorporating *P. aeruginosa* lipopolysaccharide antigens appear to produce a local protective response in the respiratory tissue of guinea pigs. Evaluation of these vaccines in humans awaits further investigation. Since protection against *P. aeruginosa* infection is type-specific and since all serotypes are potentially pathogenic, an effective vaccine would have to incorporate multiple serotypes.

ESCHERICHIA COLI

Escherichia coli is a gram-negative motile bacillus of the family Enterobacteriaceae. Most strains ferment lactose. The O (somatic), H (flagellar), and K (envelop) antigens are used to serotype an isolate for epidemiologic purposes. Some of these antigens cross-react with those of other enterics. One hundred and sixty-four O, 75 H, and 103 K antigens have been identified.

E. coli is part of the normal flora of the intestinal tract of man and animals. It is the predominant facultatively anaerobic rod in the colon; approximately 10^8 organisms are found per gram of feces.

Although *E. coli* pneumonia is sometimes community-acquired, most cases are nosocomial. The disease may arise by aspiration of oropharyngeal secretions containing the organism or via hematogenous spread from an extrapulmonary focus of infection, usually in the genitourinary or gastrointestinal tract.

The presenting manifestations of *E. coli* pneumonia include fever, chills, pleuritic chest pain, productive cough, and dyspnea. Most or all of these symptoms usually are present. In the bacteremic form symptoms referable to the primary site of infection also are evident.

Chest x-rays usually reveal lower-lobe bronchopneumonia, which may be unilateral or bilateral. Abscess formation is rare, but empyema is not uncommon. Pathologically, the alveoli are filled with an inflammatory exudate composed predominantly of mononuclear cells.

E. coli usually is sensitive to ampicillin, antipseudomonal penicillins, cephalosporins, aminoglycosides, or chloramphenicol. Up to 30%

of strains may be resistant to ampicillin and first- or second-generation cephalosporins. A third-generation cephalosporin (cefotaxime, cefoperazone, moxalactam, etc), alone or combined with aminoglycoside, is the regimen of choice for initial therapy. When the sensitivity pattern becomes available, the antibiotic regimen may be changed if indicated. The length of therapy is judged by clinical and radiologic responses; it should be at least two weeks.

PROTEUS

The genus *Proteus* includes two clinically important species: *P. mirabilis*, which is indole-negative, and *P. vulgaris*, which is indole-positive. Two other indole-positive species previously included in this genus, *P. morganii* and *P. rettgeri*, are now classified as *Morganella morganii* and *Providencia rettgeri*, respectively. These two species have traditionally been lumped with *P. vulgaris* as "indole-positive *Proteus*" in clinical reports and so are included in the following discussion.

P. mirabilis and *P. vulgaris* are characteristically motile and produce a unique pattern of growth on agar, called swarming. Isolated colonies are surrounded by concentric circles of a thin, translucent film caused by cyclic appearance of highly motile organisms bearing hundreds of flagella. Both species, as well as *M. morganii* and *P. rettgeri*, are lactose-nonfermenters and produce a powerful urease that hydrolyzes urea to ammonia and carbon dioxide.

Organisms of the *Proteus* group are widely distributed in nature and constitute and important part of the flora of decomposing organic matter of animal origin. They frequently are present in the intestinal tract of man and animals and are common in garden soil and on certain vegetables.

The most common site of *Proteus* infection is the urinary tract. Pneumonia is uncommon and usually develops by aspiration of oropharyngeal secretions containing the organisms. Rarely, it may be acquired via bacteremia arising from an extrapulmonary focus. The infection may be community-acquired or nosocomial.

Community-acquired *Proteus* pneumonia usually occurs in persons with underlying conditions, particularly chronic obstructive lung disease or diabetes mellitus. The patients are moderately ill, with chills, fever, pleuritic chest pain, dyspnea, and cough productive of tenacious yellow sputum. Chest x-rays show dense lobar infiltrations, usually with multiple abscesses. The right upper lobe is more commonly involved, and the associated volume loss produces ipsilateral tracheal shift. The radiologic appearance resembles that of primary *Klebsiella* pneumonia.

P. mirabilis usually is sensitive to ampicillin, antipseudomonal penicillins, cephalosporins, and aminoglycosides. The treatment of choice is a penicillin or a cephalosporin. *P. vulgaris*, *P. rettgeri*, and *M. morganii* are resistant to ampicillin and first-generation cephalosporins, but usually sensitive to antipseudomonal penicillins, second- and third-generation cephalosporins (cefamandole, cefoxitin, cefotaxime, moxalactam, etc), and aminoglycosides. Among the aminoglycosides, amikacin usually is effective against strains resistant to gentamicin and tobramycin. For initial therapy of pneumonia caused by indole-positive species, a third-generation cephalosporin, alone or combined with an aminoglycoside, is recommended. The antibiotic regimen may be modified depending upon the sensitivity pattern of the isolate. Treatment is continued for two weeks or longer, guided by the clinical and radiologic responses.

ENTEROBACTER

The genus *Enterobacter* includes five species: *E. cloacae*, *E. aerogenes*, *E. agglomerans*, *E. gergoviae*, and *E. sakazakii*. All have been isolated from clinical specimens, but most isolates are *E. cloacae*.

In contrast to *Klebsiella*, all *Enterobacter* species are motile. They are also less often and less heavily encapsulated. All strains have O (somatic) and H (flagellar) antigens; some also have K (capsular) antigens.

Enterobacter species are found in the intestinal tract of man and animals and in soil, water, and vegetation. They survive on the hands of hospital personnel and are easily transferred from one patient to another.

Enterobacter pneumonia may be community-acquired or nosocomial. It commonly arises by aspiration of oropharyngeal flora; occasionally is may develop via bacteremia from an extrapulmonary focus of infection. Symptoms include fever, dyspnea, cough, and occasionally chest pain. The sputum is yellow and purulent. Chest x-rays show bronchopneumonia, usually involving more than one lobe.

Enterobacter usually is sensitive to antipseudomonal penicillins, cefamandole, third-generation cephalosporins, and aminoglycosides. It is resistant to ampicillin, first-generation cephalosporins, and cefoxitin. For initial therapy of *Enterobacter* pneumonia, a third-generation cephalosporin (cefotaxime, cefoperazone, moxalactam, etc) combined with an aminoglycoside is recommended. The antibiotic regimen may be modified, depending upon the sensitivity pattern of the isolate. Treatment should be continued for at least two weeks.

SERRATIA MARCESCENS

S. marcescens is a small, gram-negative bacillus of the family Enterobacteriaceae. Most strains are motile and slow lactose fermenters; capsules are not ordinarily formed. Production of an extracellular deoxyribonuclease helps to differentiate the species from other enterobacteria. Approximately 5% of clinical isolates produce a nondiffusible red pigment, prodigiosin. An isolate can be typed serologically with O and H antisera and by determining bacteriocin (marcescens) production and susceptibility.

S. marscescens is widely distributed in nature. It has been isolated from water and soil and has a predilection for growth on foodstuffs, especially of the starchy variety, where the pigmented colonies are easily mistaken for drops of blood. The organism occasionally is found in human feces. It is an opportunistic pathogen, capable of producing a variety of infections in hospitalized patients. The organism thrives in moist environments and can contaminate medical equipment, such as ventilators, intermittent positive-pressure breathing machines, and nebulizers. It can be easily transmitted from patient to patient on the hands of personnel. Spread via an inadequately sterilized fiberbronchoscope has been reported.

S. marscescens pneumonia frequently is nosocomial and usually related to inhalation therapy with a contaminated nebulizer. Chronic cardiopulmonary disease is a major predisposing factor.

The clinical features of *S. marcescens* pneumonia include fever, chills, and productive cough. Pseudohemoptysis related to prodigiosin occasionally has been reported. The predominant radiologic finding is focal or diffuse, patchy bronchopneumonia. Small radiolucent areas corresponding to small abscesses at necropsy occasionally are seen. Large abscesses rarely occur. Small effusions may be present, but empyema is uncommon.

S. marcescens is sensitive to aminoglycosides, third-generation cephalosporins (cefotaxime, moxalactam, etc), chloramphenicol, and trimethoprim-sulfamethoxazole. Among the aminoglycosides, amikacin is the most active; resistance to gentamicin and tobramycin is not uncommon. Twenty percent of strains are sensitive to carbenicillin or ticarcillin, and the combination of an effective aminoglycoside with one of these penicillins has a synergistic effect against those strains. Most strains are sensitive to cefotaxime and moxalactam, and the minimal inhibitory concentrations are relatively low. Trimethoprim-sulfamethoxazole is quite active in vitro and may act synergistically with other antibiotics against the organism, but the clinical efficacy of such combinations is not known.

The initial choice of antibiotic for treatment of *S. marcescens* pneumonia depends upon the susceptibility pattern of the isolate in a particular hospital. In the absence of susceptibility data the initial regimen should be a third-generation cephalosporin, alone or combined with an aminoglycoside. The antibiotic regimen can be modified later if indicated. If the isolate is susceptible to carbenicillin or ticarcillin and an aminoglycoside, combined therapy can be used. Treatment is continued for two weeks or longer, guided by the clinical and radiologic responses.

ACINETOBACTER

A. calcoaceticus is a nonfermentative, gram-negative, nonmotile bacterium which is typically coccoid to coccobacillary. The oval coccobacilli may show bipolar staining, giving the organism a diplococcal appearance resembling *Neisseria*. Some strains exhibit moderate pleomorphism, including bacillary and filamentous forms. *A. calcoaceticus* is oxidase-negative (in contrast to *Neisseria*, which is oxidase-positive) and frequently encapsulated. It is a strict aerobe, growing well on ordinary media. It can grow in salt solutions, with ammonia as the nitrogen source and acetate as the only carbon source. It will not use carbohydrates as a carbon source.

A. calcoaceticus includes two biochemically distinct varieties, *anitratus* and *lwoffi*. The *anitratus* variety forms acid from glucose; the *lwoffi* variety does not. All reported *Acinetobacter* pulmonary infections have been due to the *anitratus* variety.

A. calcoaceticus var *anitratus* is widely distributed in nature. It is commonly found in soil and fresh water. It can be isolated from the skin of up to 25% and the throat of up to 7% of normal persons, but pulmonary infections are infrequent. The infection usually is acquired by aspiration of oropharyngeal secretions and much less commonly by inhalation of aerosols from contaminated nebulizers.

Acinetobacter pneumonia usually is nosocomial, principally in intensive care units. It occurs most frequently in patients who have been supported with prolonged ventilatory assistance via endotracheal tubes or tracheostomy, particularly patients who have received antimicrobial therapy. Chronic obstructive pulmonary disease and recent major surgery are significant predisposing factors. The pneumonia may involve one or multiple lobes. Bronchopneumonia (often bilateral) is the most common pattern on chest x-rays, but occasionally a lobar consolidation is seen. Abscess formation is uncommon; pleural effusions and rarely empyema may occur. Bacteremia occurs in some patients and may be associated with septic shock and circulatory collapse. The mortality rate is high (36%); death usually is attributable to inappropriate antimicrobial therapy.

Community-acquired bacteremic pneumonia caused by *A. calcoaceticus* is relatively uncommon. It is a fulminant disease with a high mortality and occurs in older persons with chronic disease, especially alcoholism. The onset is abrupt, with chills, fever, pleuritic chest pain, productive cough, and rapid prostration. The patients usually present acutely ill with respiratory distress and severe hypoxemia. The radiologic findings are not distinctive. The infiltrates, which may be lobar or bronchopneumonic, usually progress rapidly to bilateral involvement, even with adequate antibiotic therapy. Pleural effusions occur in about one half of the patients and may be empyemas. Shock occurs in up to half of the cases. The mortality rate is high (up to 43%); death generally occurs within the first three days. Factors that predict a fatal outcome are neutropenia, empyema, and inappropriate antimicrobial therapy.

A. calcoaceticus var *anitratus* usually is resistant to chloramphenicol, ampicillin, and cephalosporins. Sensitivity to tetracyclines is variable. The most effective antimicrobial agents are the aminoglycosides, among which amikacin is the most active. The organism is also sensitive to antipseudomonal penicillins and trimethoprim-sulfamethoxazole. Synergism occurs in vitro with the combination of an aminoglycoside and an antipseudomonal penicillin. If the diagnosis of *Acinetobacter* pneumonia is established, combined use of an aminoglycoside, preferably amikacin, and an antipseudomonal penicillin is recommended.

SELECTED READINGS

Balikian JP, Herman PG, Godleski JJ: *Serratia* pneumonia. *Radiology* 1980;137:309–311.

Feely TW, DuMoulin GC, Hedley-Whyte J, et al: Aerosol polymyxin and pneumonia in seriously ill patients. *N Engl J Med* 1975;293:471–475.

Garb JL, Brown RB, Garb JR, et al: Differences in etiology of pneumonias in nursing home and community patients. *JAMA* 1978;24:2169–2172.

Glew RH, Moellering RC, Kunz LJ Jr: Infections with *Acinetobacter calcoaceticus* (Herellea vaginicola). Clinical and laboratory studies. *Medicine* 1977;56:79–97.

Graybill JR, Marshall LW, Charache P, et al: Nosocomial pneumonia. A continuing major problem. *Am Rev Respir Dis* 1973;108:1130–1140.

Hahn HH, Beaty HN: Transtracheal aspiration in the evaluation of patients with pneumonia. *Ann Intern Med* 1970;72:183–187.

Iannini PB, Claffey T, Quintiliani R: Bacteremic *Pseudomonas* pneumonia. *JAMA* 1974;230:558–561.

Johanson WG, Pierce AK, Sanford JP, et al: Nosocomial respiratory infections with gram-negative bacilli. *Ann Intern Med* 1972;77:701–706.

Johanson WG Jr, Woods DE, Chaudhuri T: Association of respiratory tract colonization with adherence of gram-negative bacilli to epithelial cells. *J Infect Dis* 1979;139:667–673.

Lerner AM: The gram-negative bacillary pneumonias. *DM* 1980.

Mackowiak PA, Martin RM, Jones SR, et al: Pharyngeal colonization by gram-negative bacilli in aspiration-prone persons. *Arch Intern Med* 1978;138:1224–1227.

Manfredi F, Daly WJ, Behnke RH: Clinical observations of acute Friedlander pneumonia. *Ann Intern Med* 1963;58:642–653.

Meltz DJ, Grieco MH: Characteristics of *Serratia marcescens* pneumonia. *Arch Intern Med* 1973;132:359–364.

Pennington JE, Reynolds HY, Carbone PP: Pseudomonas pneumonia, a retrospective study of 36 cases. *Am J Med* 1973;55:155–160.

Pierce AK, Sanford JP: Bacterial contamination of aerosols. *Arch Intern Med* 1973;131:156–159.

Reyes MP: The aerobic gram-negative bacillary pneumonias. *Med Clin North Am* 1980;64:363–383.

Rudin ML, Michael JR, Huxley EJ: Community-acquired *Acinetobacter* pneumonia. *Am J Med* 1979;67:39–43.

Sanford JP, Pierce AK: Lower respiratory tract infections, in Bennett JV, Brachman PS (eds): *Hospital Infections*. Boston, Little, Brown and Co, 1979, pp 255–286.

Sickles EA, Young VM, Green WH, et al: Pneumonia in acute leukemia. *Ann Intern Med* 1974;79:528–534.

Spencer CD, Beaty HN: Complications of transtracheal aspiration. *N Engl J Med* 1972;286:304–306.

Stamm WE: Nosocomial pneumonia, in Fishman AP (ed): *Pulmonary Diseases and Disorders*. New York, McGraw-Hill, Inc, 1980, pp 1041–1051.

Tillotson JR, Lerner AM: Characteristics of pneumonia caused by *Escherichia coli*. *N Engl J Med* 1967;277:115–122.

Tillotson JR, Lerner AM: Characteristics of nonbacteremic Pseudomonas pneumonia. *Ann Intern Med* 1968;68:295–307.

Valdivieso M, Gil-Extremera B, Nornoza J et al: Gram-negative bacillary pneumonia in the compromised host. *Medicine* 1977;56:241–254.

27 *Pseudomonas pseudomallei*

Jack L. LeFrock
Arnold Lentnek
Abdolghader Molavi

Melioidosis is an infection of man and animals with a protean clinical spectrum. First described by Whitmore and Krishnaswami in 1912, melioidosis bears a striking resemblance to glanders, both clinically and pathologically, but it is epidemiologically dissimilar.

Microbial Characteristics

Pulmonary melioidosis is caused by *Pseudomonas pseudomallei*, a bipolar-staining, gram-negative rod that is motile and grows well on most laboratory culture media. A nonsporulating, oxidase-positive, obligatory aerobe, it does not produce pigment, which distinguishes it from *Pseudomonas aeruginosa*. However, after incubation for three to four days, the colonies frequently assume a rough, wrinkled appearance, which is a clue for presumptive identification of *P. pseudomallei*. Identification is confirmed by agglutination or fluorescent antibody reactions.

Epidemiology

This disease is endemic in humid tropical climates and may be more prevalent than is currently suspected. Some endemic areas exist in Malaysia, Madagascar, Guam and Australia. Sporadic cases have been reported from Korea, the Philippines, Central and South America, the West Indies and Turkey. Europeans and Americans acquire the infection only after traveling in endemic areas. Asymptomatic infection can persist for many years before clinical disease appears. American soldiers exposed in Vietnam have developed this disease months or even years after their return to the United States.

P. pseudomallei is a natural saprophyte that can be isolated from soil, stagnant streams, ponds, rice paddies, and market produce in endemic areas. Although rodents and domestic animals are susceptible to melioidosis, they apparently are not a reservoir for human disease. Man-to-man transmission has not been described. Humans mainly acquire the disease from infectious soil or water through contamination of skin, abrasions, ingestion, or inhalation. Inapparent infection, as determined by serologic evidence, also occurs.

Clinical Disease

The respiratory infection can vary from a mild bronchitis to an overwhelming, necrotizing pneumonia. The typical patient with pulmonary melioidosis presents with either an abrupt or subacute illness consisting of fever, productive cough, weight loss, and a history of visiting an endemic area sometime in the past. Dull or pleuritic chest pain is common, and tachypnea may be out of proportion to the fever and to the findings on physical or x-ray examination. Chest x-ray discloses upper lobe infiltrates and/or cavitations suggesting granulomatous disease. The cavities usually are single but occasionally multiple and varying in size; they rarely contain air-fluid levels.

Narcotic addicts can present with the septicemic form of the disease. The onset may be abrupt, and the dominant symptoms depend upon the site of major involvement. Chest x-rays most commonly show irregular nodular densities throughout the lungs. These enlarge, coalesce, and often undergo cavitation as the disease progresses.

Diagnostic Tests

The signs and symptoms of pulmonary melioidosis differ little from those of other lower respiratory infections. Fever, productive cough, chest pain, and hemoptysis predominate. These symptoms plus substantial weight loss in a person who has been in an endemic area should alert the physician to the possibility of melioidosis. Physicians examining returnees from Southeast Asia must be especially aware of the possibility of melioidosis in any unexplained pulmonary disease or febrile illness. A condition that appears to be tuberculosis but fails to yield a positive sputum culture might prove to be melioidosis if the patient has been in Southeast Asia.

The specific diagnosis depends on isolation of *P. pseudomallei* from the sputum or blood and on serologic evidence. Sputum cultures have been positive in 74% of patients studied with this disease. Serologic titers have been valuable in establishing a presumptive diagnosis. The indirect hemagglutination and complement fixation tests demonstrate significant antibody titers in most patients. A fourfold or greater rise in titers in paired sera is required for diagnosis of acute infection. Of the two tests, the indirect hemagglutination test appears to be a little more specific. A titer of 1:8 by the complement fixation test or 1:40 by the indirect hemagglutination test during the acute illness are significant, but may indicate old or new disease. Both tests may cross-react with *Pseudomonas mallei*.

Therapy and Prevention

Individuals with low titer, positive serologic results but with no clinical evidence of infection do not require treatment. In active infection, the choice of antibiotics should be based upon sensitivity studies. The following can be used: chloramphenicol, tetracyclines, sulfonamides, kanamycin, and a trimethoprim-sulfamethoxazole combination. However, no single antimicrobial agent has been effective against all strains of *P. pseudomallei*. The most efficacious drugs currently used to treat melioidosis are bacteriostatic and not always successful in eradicating the organisms.

For the patient who is extremely toxic, two agents have been recommended for the first 30 days. Therapy should be continued for at least 30 days and, in patients with extrapulmonary suppurative lesions, for six months to one year.

There is no active immunization or other preventive measures except those based on good hygienic practices.

SELECTED READINGS

Everett ED, Nelson RA: Pulmonary melioidosis: Observations in thirty-nine cases. *Am Rev Respir Dis* 1975;112:331.

Flemma RJ, DiVincent FC, Dotin LN, et al: Pulmonary Melioidosis. *Am Thorac Surg* 1969;7:491.

Hall WH, Manion RE: Antibiotic susceptibility of *Pseudomonas pseudomallei*. *Antimicrob Agents Chemother* 1973;4:193.

James AE, Dixon GD, Johnson HF: Melioidosis: A correlation of the radiologic and pathologic findings. *Radiology* 1967;89:230.

Sanford JP, Moore WL: Recrudescent melioidosis: A Southeast Asian legacy. *Am Rev Respir Dis* 1971;104:452.

Zimmerman JE: Acute septicemic melioidosis. *JAMA* 1970;213:2266.

28 *Pseudomonas mallei*

Matthew E. Levison

Pseudomonas mallei causes glanders, which is primarily an equine infection rarely transmitted to man.

Microbial Characteristics

P. mallei is an aerobic, nonmotile gram-negative bacillus. An antigen (mallein) that is released upon lysis is used for a diagnostic skin test of delayed hypersensitivity. The organism produces a fatal infection in guinea pigs and hamsters in laboratory testing.

Epidemiology

Glanders, once a common disease in horses, mules and donkeys, has been eradicated from the United States as a result of strict control measures. This disease is now mainly seen in the Middle East, Africa, and Asia. The disease is transmitted to persons handling infected animals or laboratory workers through skin abrasions, implantation on the conjunctiva, by ingestion or inhalation. Person-to-person spread also may occur.

Clinical Manifestation

After an incubation period of several days, glanders may begin either abruptly with chills, fever and prostration, or in a more indolent fashion. At point of entry a nodule forms which subsequently ulcerates and is associated with regional lymphadenitis and suppurative subcutaneous nodules along the lymphatics which may ulcerate to form cutaneous fistulae. Ulcerating abscesses may occur in the nose and mouth at portals of entry or as a result of hematogenous dissemination. Metastatic lesions also may occur in the lungs and other viscera. Other metastatic manifestations include intramuscular and subcutaneous abscesses, meningitis, osteomyelitis and septic arthritis. The acute disease is rapidly fatal in two to three weeks if untreated. A chronic recurrent form of glanders occurs with an insidious onset of low grade fever and draining abscesses. The chronic form may become fulminant with bacteremia and death. Pulmonary involvement occurs as pneumonia and abscesses. Pleural effusions and empyema may occur, as may hilar adenopathy.

Diagnosis

P. mallei can be recovered from cultures of exudate, sputum and blood in ordinary nutrient media. A fourfold rise in agglutinating antibodies (to 1:64 or higher) or complement-fixing antibodies (to 1:20 or higher) occurs during the two to four weeks of illness. Cross-reactions occur with *P. pseudomallei*.

Treatment

Sulfadiazine, 100 mg/kg daily, is given in divided doses by mouth for at least three weeks.

Prevention

Destruction of infected horses identified by mallein reactivity or by serology can eliminate glanders.

SELECTED READING

Howe C, Miller WR: The pseudomallei: A review. *J Infect Dis* 1971;124: 598–606.

29 *Yersinia pestis*

Jack L. LeFrock
Abdolghader Molavi
Arnold Lentnek

Yersinia pestis, the cause of bubonic plague, has produced rare cases of pneumonic plague. Plague is primarily a disease of rodents; man is only incidentally involved, usually when bitten by a flea that had ingested blood of a bacteremic rodent.

Microbial Characteristics

Y. pestis is a plump (0.5 to 0.8 μm by 1.5 to 2.0 μm), gram-negative, nonmotile, nonsporulating, nonlactose-fermenting, pleomorphic bacillus. A bipolar or safety-pin appearance is seen with Giemsa or Wayson's (carbolfuchsin-methylene blue) stain. Like the enteric bacteria, it is a facultative anaerobe and grows on simple media. However, growth is slow, requiring 48 hours to form visible colonies. *Y. pestis* is antigenically complex and has a protein capsule that resists phagocytosis. It produces both an endotoxin and a protein toxin which is released on cell death. The role of the protein toxin in human infection is not known.

Epidemiology and Pathogenicity

Y. pestis normally causes a disease of wild rodents called sylvatic plague. In the United States sylvatic plague occurs in Texas, New Mexico, Utah, California and Arizona.

A flea-rodent cycle is required to perpetuate the disease. The permanent reservoirs of infection are rodents; these include prairie dogs, ground squirrels, wood rats, field mice, gerbils and wild rabbits. Most human disease in the United States occurs along the Pacific coast and the Southwest. Plague can be transmitted to man in several ways: through a flea bite, via aerosols generated by patients with pneumonic plague or by direct contact with tissues of infected animals.

Pulmonary involvement may occur in two distinct syndromes: 1) secondary pneumonia due to the hematogenous dissemination in bubonic (ie, acute lymphadenitic) plague, and 2) primary pneumonia due to inhalation of bacilli from aerosols generated by pneumonic patients. In epidemics of plagues, initial cases appear as bubonic plague, of whom as many as 5% develop secondary lesions in the lungs. The plague bacillus then may spread to other individuals by inhalation. Primary pneumonic plague rarely has been documented in the United States. One case occurred at Lake Tahoe, California, in 1980, and resulted from exposure to a kitten with plague pneumonia.

Clinical Disease

Bubonic plague has an incubation period of one to 12 days followed by an abrupt onset of chills, fever, headache, vomiting, marked prostration and delirium. Rarely is the flea bite noticeable. Regional lymphadenitis appears with the onset of the fever. Secondary plague pneumonia may occur several days after onset of fever and lymphadenitis.

The incubation period for primary pneumonic plague is shorter, ie, two or three days. Rigors, malaise, and headache is followed within 24 hours by cough productive of mucoid or bloody sputum, dyspnea and cyanosis. The sputum contains numerous bacilli. Signs of consolidation are minimal, and chest x-ray reveals rapidly progressing pneumonia. If not treated, death results in three or four days. However, with early diagnosis and appropriate antibiotics, recovery is the rule.

A third clinical form of plague occurs, ie, primary septicemic plague with marked constitutional symptoms, but without detectable lymphadenopathy. Death supervenes due to endotoxic shock before localization becomes clinically apparent, unless effective antibiotics are administered.

Diagnostic Tests

Pneumonic plague must be distinguished from the pneumococcal and other bacterial pneumonias (eg, tularemic) as well as from anthrax, psittacosis, mycoplasma, and other causes of atypical pneumonia. Epidemiologic factors and bacteriologic studies will aid in the differentiation.

Sputum, blood (about 5% have positive cultures) or pus aspirated from the buboes should be cultured on blood, MacConkey or deoxycholate agar, nutrient agar, and meat infusion broth. Confirmation is based on agglutination with specific *Y. pestis* antiserum and staining by fluorescent antiserum. All specimens should be handled with extreme care.

Serologic diagnosis is of aid only for retrospective confirmation. Specific antibodies appear in the serum of convalescent patients and can be detected in the second week by complement fixation, agglutination, or passive hemagglutination tests.

Therapy

Treatment must begin within 24 hours after onset to be effective. Streptomycin, 30 mg/kg body weight per day, should be given in three equal doses, or tetracycline, 30 to 50 mg/kg/day, given as four equal doses for 10 days. Chloramphenicol is an alternative potent antiplague agent and should be given intravenously in initial doses of 6 to 8 g daily; the dose should be reduced to 3 to 4 g when the patient improves.

Patients commonly develop laboratory evidence of disseminated intravascular coagulation for which heparin is not indicated.

Prevention

A few streptomycin-resistant strains were isolated in Vietnam, but no therapeutic failures have been attributable to drug resistance. Drug resistance may pose a threat in the future, however, because transfer of drug resistance factors (R factors) from *Escherichia coli* to *Y. pestis* has been demonstrated.

All contacts of patients with pulmonary involvement, whether primary or secondary, should be quarantined and given either tetracycline (15 to 20 mg/kg/day in four equal portions) or a sulfonamide (40 mg/kg/day in four equal portions) for seven days. Chemoprophylaxis is also recommended for household contacts of fleaborne plague because about 5% of such contacts would otherwise develop plague. Close observation of all contacts is essential. If febrile or plaguelike illness develops, immediate hospitalization and streptomycin therapy is indicated. Strict isolation is recommended for all patients with plague. This may be discontinued after 48 to 72 hours of specific antimicrobial therapy, except for patients with open draining lesions or pneumonia.

In plague-endemic areas, handling wild mammals should be avoided. Vaccination is advisable for laboratory personnel working with *Y. pestis* and for those working in high-risk occupations in plague-endemic areas.

SELECTED READINGS

Finegold MJ: Pathogenesis of plague: A review of plague deaths in the United States during the last decade. *Am J Med* 1968;45:549.

Palmer DL, Kisch AL, Williams RC Jr, et al: Clinical features of plague in the United States: The 1969–1970 epidemic. *J Infect Dis* 1971;124:367.

Reed WP, Palmer DL, Williams RC Jr, et al: Bubonic plague in the Southwestern United States. *Medicine* 1970;49:465.

30 *Francisella tularensis*

Jack L. LeFrock
Abdolghader Molavi
Arnold Lentnek

Tularemia is a generalized infection due to *Francisella tularensis.* About one third of all cases show evidence of pneumonia. The disease received its name from the place where it was discovered: Tulare County, California.

Microbiologic Characteristics

F. tularensis (*Pasteurella tularensis*) is a small (0.2 to 0.3 μm by 0.3 μm by 0.7 μm), pleomorphic, gram-negative, nonmotile, obligate aerobe that appears as short rods or coccobacilli. Capsules are not produced, and faint bipolar staining can be observed. This organism grows slowly and is fastidious, requiring cysteine for growth. Only one serotype of *F. tularensis* is recognized.

A polysaccharide antigen produces immediate-type hypersensitivity (wheal and flare) in an immune individual; a protein antigen produces delayed hypersensitivity. Another protein antigen shared with *Brucella* accounts for immunologic cross-reactions. The cell wall contains endotoxin.

Epidemiology

F. tularensis is widely distributed throughout the United States, especially the Southeastern region, and has been reported in Canada, Central Europe, Scandinavia, Japan, and Russia. The infection is common among mammals (rabbits, ground squirrels, opossums, beavers, skunks, coyotes, sheep, dogs, and cats) and birds (pheasants, grouse, and quail). The organism has been isolated from wood ticks, rabbit ticks, fleas, lice, deer flies, mosquitoes, and horseflies—all of which presumably act as arthropod vectors. The organisms are transmitted transovarially in ticks, which thus serve as a continual reservoir of infection.

Humans of all races and ages and both sexes are uniformly susceptible, but person-to-person transmission is extremely unusual. In the United States the disease most commonly occurs in the winter months in hunters who skin infected game animals, especially rabbits, and in persons who have been bitten by infected ticks, horseflies, or deer flies in the spring and summer months. The disease has also been reported after ingestion of partially cooked, infected meat. It can be contracted by inhaling droplets containing viable bacilli or by drinking water contaminated with bacilli.

Pneumonic tularemia occurs among bacteriologists and clinical laboratory workers and researchers who, in working with the organism, produce and inhale infectious aerosols.

Pathogenicity

The portal of entry may be the skin, eye, nasopharynx, intestinal tract or lung. After entry, *F. tularensis* reaches the blood via the regional lymphatics. Pneumonia can be initiated either by an alveolar localization of relatively few minute infectious particles that have been inhaled or by hematogenous dissemination. Inflammation occurs around the site of deposition of bacteria in the lung, giving rise to granulomas and necrosis of the alveolar walls. Thus, many small areas of bronchopneumonia may be evident as patchy infiltrates throughout the lung fields.

Clinical Diseases

The incubation period is three to seven days; clinical disease may take one of several forms. An ulcer may be evident at the portal of entry in the skin (ulceroglandular) or the eye (oculoglandular) accompanied by regional lymphadenitis. Lymphadenitis may also occur without an evident portal of entry (glandular type). An intestinal portal of entry is associated with pronounced diarrhea, abdominal pain, nausea, vomiting, melena and hematemesis. Tularemia may occur without an evident portal of entry or lymphadenitis (typhoidal type). Pneumonia can occur with any of the various clinical types, subsequent to bacteremia, or as primary tularemic pneumonia.

In addition to symptoms of systemic invasion characterized by headache, fever, myalgias, and prostration, patients with tularemic pneumonia have an initial persistent nonproductive cough. Later, mucoid or bloody sputum is produced, and in severe cases is accompanied by pleuritic pain, dyspnea or cyanosis. Despite extensive pulmonary involvement, the physical findings may be minimal.

Roentgenographic findings are similar to those for other bronchopneumonias. Usually there are multiple areas of consolidation and rarely signs of typical lobar pneumonia. Pleural effusion may occur.

Diagnostic Tests

A thorough history is needed to aid in the diagnosis of tularemia. Contact with rabbits, ticks, or other known vectors should alert one to the possibility of tularemia in a patient with an acute febrile illness. Fluorescent antibody staining can rapidly and specifically identify *F.*

tularensis in exudates and tissues. Examination of gram-stained smears usually is unrewarding. Specimens for culture include material from the initial skin lesion and aspirates of enlarged regional lymph nodes. Blood cultures rarely are positive.

Cultures of sputum, gastric aspirate, pleural fiuid, and bronchial secretions may be obtained from patients with pneumonic tularemia. Gastric washings collected early in the morning are an excellent source for recovery of *F. tularensis.* The organism may take two to four days to grow in culture media. If *F. tularensis* is present, intraperitoneal inoculation of guinea pigs with clinical specimens will cause death in five to ten days. Granulomatous lesions will be found in the spleen and liver, and the organisms can be isolated from the heart blood, spleen and liver of the infected guinea pig. The identity of isolates from patients and guinea pigs can be confirmed by agglutination with specific antiserum. However, unless the laboratory has appropriate facilities, attempts at isolation of *F. tularensis* or inoculation of laboratory animals is not recommended because of the hazard of infecting laboratory personnel. Therefore, the diagnosis usually is confirmed serologically. Agglutinins are first detectable in patients 10 to 14 days after onset of the disease. The titer rises abruptly to 640 or greater within the next week, reaching a maximum (generally in excess of 1280) around the fourth to eighth week of illness. Because of cross-reactivity, parallel agglutination tests should be done with *Brucella. Brucella* titers are generally one fourth to one sixth of the tularemia titer.

The pneumonitis of tularemia can be mistaken for any of the atypical pneumonias, including Q fever, *Mycoplasma* pneumonia or psittacosis. With paired serum samples, a retrospective serologic diagnosis can be made.

Therapy

Treatment is often dramatically effective when streptomycin, which is rapidly bactericidal, is given intramuscularly (15 mg/kg/day in divided doses for seven to 10 days). Tetracycline or chloramphenicol can control the acute phase of tularemia, but these bacteriostatic agents do not eradicate the organisms and relapses occur. Mortality can occur in up to 30% of untreated patients, but is rare in those treated with specific antimicrobial therapy.

Prevention

Tularemia can be prevented by adequately cooking infected animals and by wearing rubber gloves and glasses when skinning and dressing animals. In those who work outdoors in endemic areas, clothing should be secured around the ankles and wrists to prevent attachment of ticks. Immunization with a live attenuated vaccine reduces severity of infection and may possibly prevent the disease among laboratory personnel working with this organism or among those in other high-risk occupations.

SELECTED READINGS

Kozak AJ, Hall WH, Gerding DN: Cavitary pneumonia associated with tularemic chest. 1978;73:426.

Miller RP, Bates JH: Pleuropulmonary tularemia: A review of 29 patients. *Am Rev Respir Dis* 1969;99:31.

Morgan HJ: Pleuropulmonary tularemia. *Ann Intern Med* 1947;27:519.

Stuart BM, Pullen RL: Tularemic pneumonia: Review of American literature and report of 15 additional cases. *Am J Med Sci* 1945;210:223.

Waverly FW, Barnett TB: Pulmonary tularemia. *Am Rev Respir Dis* 1967;95:584.

31 *Hemophilus influenzae*

Jack L. LeFrock
Abdolghader Molavi
Arnold Lentnek

Hemophilus influenzae is still generally considered an unusual cause of pneumonia, yet it has become increasingly recognized as a cause of bacterial pneumonias in adults. The apparent increase is probably due to improvement in bacteriologic techniques, and perhaps to a true increased incidence.

Microbial Characteristics

H. influenzae are small (0.2 to 0.3 μm by 0.5 to 2.0 μm), gram-negative, pleomorphic rods that vary in appearance from coccobacilli to long filamentous rods. They are nonmotile, grow optimally at 37° C, are facultatively anaerobic, and require both hemin (X factor) and nicotinamide adenine dinucleotide (V factor) for growth.

Strains of *H. influenzae* causing serious systemic illness are almost always encapsulated. Encapsulated *H. influenzae* are divided into six serologic types (a-f), based on the antigenicity of the capsular polysaccharide. The capsular polysaccharide is antiphagocytic and is a major virulence factor. Of the encapsulated strains, Type b is the most frequent cause of meningitis, acute epiglottitis, bacteremia and pneumonia. The capsule from Type b, a polyribosyl-ribitol phosphate, is immunologically related to some of the pneumococcal capsular polysaccharides. Nontypable strains lack a capsule.

H. influenzae produces endotoxin and a lymphocyte blastogenic factor. Early in the growth cycle it also produces a heat-stable ciliostatic factor which causes a loss of cilia, resulting in damage and sloughing of epithelial cells. This process may be important in pathogenicity of pulmonary infection.

H. influenzae Type b produces a thermostable protein (bacteriocin) that is toxic for other *H. influenzae* serotypes, nontypable *H. influenzae*, other *Hemophilus* species, and enteric bacteria. This bacteriocin may be important in helping the organism establish itself in the host's upper respiratory tract.

Epidemiology

H. influenzae frequently is recovered from the upper respiratory tract of healthy adults and children. Most of these isolates are nonencapsulated and nontypable. These strains are also present in the mucoid sputum of 50% to 60% of patients with chronic bronchitis, and some investigators have reported that these strains can cause exacerbations of purulent bronchitis in patients with chronic obstructive lung disease. These strains are frequent causes of otitis media and sinusitis. The role of nonencapsulated strains in pneumonia is unclear, but recently these strains have been reported to cause both nonbacteremic and bacteremic pneumonia in elderly adults.

Encapsulated strains are found less commonly (0.4% to 6%) in the upper respiratory tracts of healthy individuals. Carriage of these strains is more frequent (20% to 60%) among household or other close contacts of a patient with *H. influenzae* meningitis. *H. influenzae* Type b is an important pathogen in those patients who are especially susceptible as a result of age (3 months to about 5 years old), impaired opsonic activity due to splenectomy or sickle cell disease or hypogammaglobulinemia.

Pathogenicity

H. influenzae infections are acquired by aspiration of organisms that colonize the respiratory tract (endogenous) or by inhalation of respiratory secretions from other carriers (exogenous).

Two factors are important in determining the host-parasite relationship: the capsule and serum antibody. *H. influenzae* Type b infections occur primarily in young children (3 months to 5 years of age). Susceptibility to *H. influenzae* Type b was found to correlate with the absence of bactericidal antibody in whole blood in a study by Fothergill and Wright in 1933. Children up to 6 weeks of age are generally thought to be immune to infection because of placental transfer of maternal antibody. Susceptibility to infection increases as maternal antibody is lost and continues for the first 2 to 5 years of life, until immunity is naturally acquired. Immunity, presumably as a result of subclinical infection or by immunization with cross-reacting antigens from other organisms, remains throughout adulthood but decreases in older persons.

Serotype b pulmonary infection in adults is associated with impairment of normal host defense mechanisms, as occurs in the lungs after viral pneumonia or in patients with chronic debilitation of the lower respiratory tract, eg, chronic bronchitis or bronchiectasis. Immunodeficiency diseases, alcoholism, and diabetes also predispose to infection.

However, the simple inverse relationship between bactericidal antibodies and susceptibility to *H. influenzae* Type b infections postulated by Fothergill a half-century ago is now open to doubt. Several surveys of the prevalence of the serum bactericidal antibodies in healthy populations have given conflicting results. In addition, although more sensitive assays for anticapsular *H. influenzae* Type b antibodies have been developed

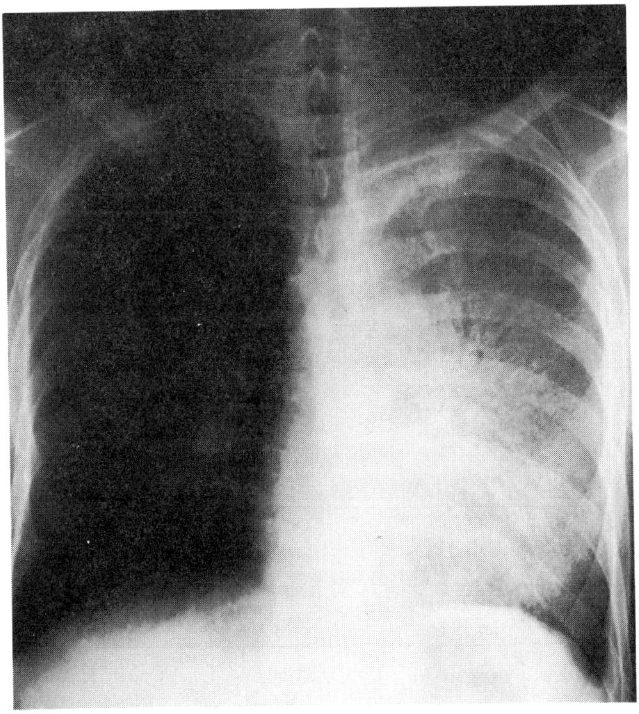

Figure 31-1 Chest radiography of a bacteremic *H. influenzae*, left upper lobar Type b pneumonia.

and have shown that these antibodies apparently vary with age as does serum bactericidal activity, there are still no hard data as to what level of these antibodies is protective.

Clinical Diseases

The clinical symptoms of patients with *H. influenzae* pneumonia, as in other bacterial pneumonias, include fever, chills, cough, purulent sputum production, sore throat, shortness of breath, and at times hemoptysis and pleuritic chest pain. Leukocytosis with a neutrophilic response is seen. A history of recent respiratory tract infection is obtained in 30% to 50% of cases.

Two forms of pneumonia due to *H. influenzae* are recognized, bacteremic and nonbacteremic. The strains causing the bacteremic form are generally encapsulated and are predominantly Type b followed in frequency by Type f. The pneumonia tends to be lobar (Figure 31-1) or segmental and may be complicated by the development of sterile or infected pleural effusions. These patients may also present with a diffuse bronchopneumonia, especially if they have chronic lung disease (as many do) or are alcoholic. Mortality in this group may be high, due to the patients' advanced age and their chronic underlying illnesses.

In the nonbacteremic form the isolates are commonly nontypable. Patients generally present with bronchopneumonic infiltrates in the lower lobes of either lung or of both lungs. Complications are less frequent, multilobar involvement is rare and mortality is low in this form.

H. influenzae (generally nonencapsulated strains) are isolated significantly more frequently from individuals with chronic bronchitis producing purulent sputum than from similar patients with mucoid sputum. The pus disappears from the sputum when *H. influenzae* is eliminated by antibiotic therapy; subsequent relapse is associated with the reappearance in the sputum of *H. influenzae* but not of other pathogens.

Diagnostic Test

Diagnosis of *H. influenzae* pneumonia can be made from gram stains and cultures of sputum, transtracheal aspirates, pleural fluid, and blood cultures. Gram stain of sputum may reveal many granulocytes and small gram-negative coccobacilli which must be distinguished from *Acinetobacter* or meningococci. Specimens must be grown in 5% CO_2, on a primary medium that can support the growth of *H. influenzae*, and then subcultured to chocolate agar. Suspicious organisms should be identified and typed with appropriate antiserum. Serotyping is done by the Quellung test and by agglutination.

If no sputum can be obtained or if the specimen is inadequate for proper examination, a transtracheal aspiration should be performed. A definitive diagnosis can be made only with positive cultures of blood or pleural fluid or by detection of Type b capsular antigen in sputum or pleural fluid by counterimmunoelectrophoresis.

Therapy

Since 1974 the frequency of isolation of ampicillin-resistant *H. influenzae* Type b has steadily increased. The only mechanism of ampicillin-resistance is the production of β-lactamase (Type III a), and is plasmid-mediated. Because of this, all *H. influenzae* type b isolates should be tested for production of β-lactamase. Tests for β-lactamase production exist which are more rapid and easier to perform than the standard antibiotic susceptibility tests. Minimum inhibitory concentrations (MIC) can also be determined.

Ampicillin is the drug of choice for susceptible strains and is given intravenously at a dose of 1 to 2 g every four hours for two to three weeks, depending on the clinical response. If the patient is allergic to penicillin, cefamandole, which shows a consistently low MIC (0.12 to 2.0 μg/mL) for both ampicillin-sensitive and ampicillin-resistant strains, can be used. Other effective agents include chloramphenicol, trimethoprim-sulfamethoxazole, and the tetracyclines, although strains resistant to these drugs have been reported. The third generation cephalosporins (moxalactam, cefoperazone and cefotaxime) are very active against *H. influenzae*, with MIC of < 0.1 $\mu g/mL$. They are about 20 times more active than ampicillin against non-β-lactamase producing strains and are only slightly less active against β-lactamase producing strains. In addition, these agents diffuse into the cerebrospinal fluid. For these reasons, the third generation cephalosporins may become the preferred antibiotics for serious infections due to this organism.

SELECTED READINGS

Berk SL, Holtsclaw SA, Wiener SL, et al: Nontypable *Haemophilus influenzae* in the elderly. *Arch Intern Med* 1982;142:537–539.

Everett A, Rahn A, Adaniya R, et al: *Haemophilus influenzae* in adults. *JAMA* 1977;238:319.

Francis JB, Francis PB: Bulging (sagging) fissure sign in *Hemophilus influenzae* lobar pneumonia. *South Med J* 1978;71:1452.

Fothergill LD, Wright J: Influenzal meningitid. The relation of age incidence to the bactericidal power of blood against the causal organism. *J Immunol* 1933;24:273–284.

Johnson WA, Kaye A, Hook EW: *Hemophilus influenzae pneumonia* in adults: Report of five cases and review of the literature. *Amer Rev Respir Dis* 1968; 97:1117.

Keefer CS, Rammel Kamp CH: *Hemophilus influenzae* bacteremia: Report of two cases recovering following sulfathiazole and sulfapyridine. *Ann Intern Med* 1942;16:1221.

Levin DC, Schwarz MI, Malthay RA, et al: Bacteremic *Hemophilus influenzae* pneumonia in adults. A report of 24 cases and a review of the literature. *Am J Med* 1977;62:219–223.

Musher DM, Wallace RJ Jr: Nontypable *Haemophilus influenzae:* Definitely pathogenic for adults. *Arch Intern Med* 1982;142:448–449.

Quitiliani R, Hymans PJ: The association of bacteremic *Haemophilus influenzae* pneumonia in adults with typable strains. *Am J Med* 1971;50:781.

Tillotson JR, Lerner AM: *Hemophilus influenzae*, bronchopneumonia in adults. *Arch Intern Med* 1968;21:428.

Turck M, May J: *Haemophilus influenzae.* London, English Universities Press, 1967.

Wallace AJ Jr, Musher DM, Martin RR: *Hemophilus influenzae* pneumonia in adults. *Am J Med* 1978;64:87.

32 *Bordetella pertussis*

Jack L. LeFrock
Abdolghader Molavi
Arnold Lentnek

Whooping cough due to *Bordetella pertussis* is characterized by an inflammation of the entire respiratory tract, which produces paroxysmal coughing and the typical inspiratory stridor or "whoop."

Microbial Characteristics

B. pertussis is a gram-negative, small (0.2 μm by 0.5 to 1.0 μm) coccobacillus which is found singly or in pairs. *B. pertussis* frequently shows bipolar staining, is nonmotile, nonsporulating, and obligately aerobic, and has a capsule that does not elicit a Quellung reaction. It is fastidious, and requires potato-glycerol agar with 30% fresh rabbit blood (Bordet-Gengou agar) for primary isolation and growth. No growth occurs on ordinary blood agar. Of the two other *Bordetella* species, *B. parapertussis* can cause an infection similar to *B. pertussis*, and *B. bronchiseptica* occasionally is found in respiratory infections. Both *B. parapertussis* and *B. bronchiseptica* grow on blood agar within 24 to 48 hours.

Epidemiology

Pertussis is spread by droplets from the respiratory tract. It is found worldwide. Seasonal variation is not marked. Within a closed community of susceptibles, the attack rate may be extremely high, approaching 90%. Neonates are often susceptible due to lack of maternal antibodies. Immunity following vaccination or natural infection is not life-long, and attack rates may approach those seen in unimmunized groups when the interval after vaccination is greater than 12 years.

Pathogenicity

The organism has a predilection for ciliated epithelial cells of the respiratory tract. Patchy areas of transient atelectasis and localized emphysema probably are present in most cases. Unless superinfection with other organisms occurs, these appear to be of little consequence to the outcome of the disease process. Most pulmonary superinfections are due to encapsulated organisms, such as *Streptococcus pneumoniae*, *He-*

mophilus influenzae, β-hemolytic streptococci and *Staphylococcus aureus*.

Clinical Disease

A variable period (one to two weeks) of coryza is followed by a phase characterized by violent paroxysms of nonproductive coughing. Each paroxysm of coughing ends with a "whoop," ie, a forced inspiration over a partially closed glottis. Epistaxis, subconjunctival hemorrhages, facial edema and cyanosis can occur secondary to increased venous pressure that accompanies the paroxysms of coughing. Fever is absent unless complicated by superinfection. This phase of paroxysmal coughing is accompanied by a lymphocytosis. The most frequently encountered complication in children under 2 years of age is convulsions, due to anoxia resulting from prolonged paroxysms of coughing. Fever, signs of pneumonia, polymorphonuclear leukocytosis and an elevated erythrocyte sedimentation rate suggest superinfection which probably accounts for most of the mortality associated with pertussis. Death from pertussis and its complications most often occurs in children under 1 year of age.

Diagnostic Tests

In the paroxysmal phase, the characteristic whoop and lymphocytosis usually are diagnostic, but other organisms (*B. parapertussis*, *B. bronchoseptica* and adenoviruses) on occasion can cause a pertussis-like illness. Isolation of *B. pertussis* from the respiratory tract with nasopharyngeal swabs plated onto Bordet-Gengou medium establishes the diagnosis. As disease progresses, however, the chances for obtaining a positive culture decreases. A fluorescent antibody-staining procedure applied directly to clinical specimens or the isolates is now available for rapid identification of *B. pertussis*.

Therapy

Although many antimicrobial drugs have been tried in the treatment of pertussis, there is no evidence that they are clinically beneficial when administered during the paroxysmal stage. Chlortetracycline, chloramphenicol, and erythromycin regularly eliminate *B. pertussis* within a few days from patients with pertussis and from carriers. Of these drugs, erythromycin is least toxic and most effective. In addition to rendering patients noninfectious for public health purposes, erythromycin (35 to 50 mg/kg daily in four divided doses for 14 days) may prevent pertussis in exposed susceptible persons and may abort or attenuate pertussis when given during early phases of the illness. Corticosteroids can significantly lower the severity and duration of pertussis, but may possibly enhance susceptibility to complicating infections.

Prevention

Active immunization effectively prevents pertussis in most individuals and should be started after 6 weeks of age. Both antibody production and protection against *B. pertussis* result. A booster injection should be administered at 1 year of age and again just before the child starts school.

SELECTED READINGS

Oetgen WJ: Pertussoid eosinophilic pneumonia. *Chest* 1977;71:492.
Olson LC: Pertussis. *Medicine* 1975;54:427.

33 *Neisseria meningitidis*

Jack L. LeFrock
Abdolghader Molavi
Arnold Lentnek

The genus *Neisseria* includes two species that are pathogenic in humans: the meningococcus, *Neisseria meningitidis* and the gonococcus, *Neisseria gonorrhoeae.* Meningococcal disease occurs in both epidemic and endemic patterns. Meningococci can play a role as a respiratory pathogen either by 1) hematogenous dissemination to the lung in patients who have meningococcal meningitis or a clinical syndrome consistent with meningococcemia (fever, shock, petechial or purpuric rash and disseminated intravascular coagulation) or 2) in the absence of meningococcemia or meningitis presumably by bronchogenic spread from the upper respiratory tract.

Microbial Characteristics

N. meningitidis is a fastidious, obligately aerobic, gram-negative diplococcus which can be best cultured on blood or chocolate agar at 35°C to 37°C in an atmosphere enriched with 5% to 10% carbon dioxide. Isolation of *N. meningitidis* from a specimen that also contains other organisms (eg, throat swab or sputum) requires use of a selective medium that contains antibiotics, such as Thayer-Martin agar. *N. meningitidis* is distinguished from other *Neisseria* species by its ability to produce acid from glucose and maltose but not sucrose and lactose. (*N. gonorrhoeae* produces acid only from glucose.) Agglutination with antibody to various capsular antigens separates meningococci into nine major groups: A, B, C, D, X, Y, Z, 135, and 29E. Although all serogroups cause clinical infection, meningococcal disease is primarily associated with groups A, B, C, and Y. Serogrouping is primarily of epidemiologic importance.

Epidemiology

The natural reservoir of *N. meningitidis* is the human posterior nasopharynx. The organism is spread via large droplets of contaminated upper respiratory tract secretions. The spread is most efficient when there is close physical contact or crowding in closed populations, such as occurs among groups of military recruits. *N. meningitidis* can be cultured from the nasopharynx of 2% to 15% of healthy individuals during nonepidemic periods. Carriage may rise to 20% to 40% among close contacts of persons with meningococcal disease and to 75% or more in closed populations. Meningococcal disease may occur when a virulent strain is acquired by a susceptible individual (ie, one who lacks bactericidal antibody or perhaps has antimeningococcal antibody of the IgA class capable of blocking the action of protective antibody).

Metastatic meningococcal pneumonia, usually due to groups B and C, may be present in up to 15% of patients with meningococcemia or meningococcal meningitis. Meningococcal pneumonia also has been reported to complicate viral respiratory infection. During the 1910-1919 influenza pandemic, meningococcal lobar pneumonia and bronchopneumonia in the absence of meningococcemia or meningitis was documented at autopsy in numerous reports. Recent reports also have associated meningococcal pneumonia with preceding influenza or adenoviral infections. Primary meningococcal pneumonia, in particular due to group Y, is now recognized as the most common form of meningococcal disease in certain military recruit populations. Since 1970, group Y has emerged as a predominant pathogen in military recruit camps, coincident with the introduction of meningococcal group C vaccine routinely in these training camps. Group Y can cause meningococcemia and meningitis, but primary pneumonia may be the major clinical form of group Y disease. Koppes et al (1977) reported 68 cases of primary meningococcal pneumonia due to group Y in the military recruit population. Though only the third most common serogroup causing disease in the United States civilian population, serogroup Y is the most common isolate in the 15- to 29-year age group of patients with meningococcal disease.

Clinical Diseases

In patients with primary meningococcal pneumonia, there is a gradual onset of symptoms and a history of an antecedent upper respiratory infection. Patients present with cough, sore throat, chest pain, chills, fever, and rales. Pleuritic chest pain and small pleural effusions occur in 20% of patients, but frank empyema is very rare. Patchy alveolar bronchopneumonia is found in 80% of patients; the rest have segmental or lobar consolidation. Bacteremia is uncommon (15% of patients).

Diagnostic Tests

Diagnosis of meningococcal pneumonia is difficult. Isolation of *N. meningitidis* from the sputum does not distinguish a carrier from an individual with meningococcal pneumonia. Because there is contamination of expectorated material with upper respiratory tract flora, secretions must be obtained by transtracheal aspiration for culture and gram stain.

Koppes et al proposed several diagnostic criteria, including 1) a compatible clinical syndrome, 2) a chest radiograph demonstrating pulmonary infiltrates, and either 3) culture of a transtracheal aspirate yielding the organism and a consistent gram stain, or 4) isolation of *N. meningitidis* from pleural fluid or blood.

Therapy

The response of primary group Y pneumonia has been reported to be rapid to antibiotic therapy which consisted of 600,000 units of procaine penicillin G given intramuscularly every 12 hours for at least three days, followed by phenoxymethyl penicillin for a total treatment duration of 10 to 14 days. Large intravenous doses of penicillin G, 20 million units daily, (or ampicillin, 12 daily) is the antibiotic of choice for the treatment of meningococcal pneumonia in patients with meningitis or meningococcemia. Chloramphenicol is a suitable alternative for penicillin-sensitive individuals. The first or second generation cephalosporins or clindamycin should not be used to treat severe meningococcal disease, despite in vitro susceptibility, because of inadequate penetration into the cerebrospinal fluid. Respiratory isolation for a patient with suspected meningococcal pneumonia is indicated.

SELECTED READINGS

Ball JH, Young DA: Primary meningococcal pneumonia. *Am Rev Respir Dis.* 1974; 109:480.

Fletcher W: Meningococcal broncho-pneumonia in influenza. *Lancet* 1919;1:104.

Galpin JE, Chow AW, Yoshikawa TT, et al: Meningococcal pneumonia. *Am J Med Sci* 1975;269:247.

Hersh JH, Gold R, Lepow ML: Meningococcal group Y pneumonia in an adolescent female. *Pediatrics* 1979;64:222.

Irwin RS, Woelk WK, Coudon WL III: Primary meningococcal pneumonia. *Ann Interm Med* 1975;82:493–498.

Koppes GM, Ellenbogen, Gebhart RJ: Group Y meningococcal disease in United States Air Force recruits *Am J Med* 1977;62:661.

Meltzer JI, Kneeland Y Jr: Primary meningococcal lobar pneumonia without meningitis. *Ann Intern Med* 1957;46:183.

Paine TF Jr, Garrard CL Jr, Walker PJ: Meningococcal pneumonia. *Arch Intern Med* 1967;119:11.

Putsch RW, Hamilton JD, Wolinsky E: *Neisseria meningitidis*, a respiratory pathogen? *J Infect Dis* 1970;121:48.

34 *Legionella and Legionella-like Organisms*

Richard W. Gilpin

MICROBIAL CHARACTERISTICS

Morphology

Legionella and *Legionella*-like organisms (LLO) are gram-negative bacilli which have a fairly uniform width (0.3 to 0.9 μm) and length (2.5 μm). A few bacteria in some isolates are much longer. The bacteria usually are found as individual cells, but may form chains or long filaments. *Legionella* and LLO have an outer and inner membrane structure typical of gram-negative bacteria (Figure 34-1). Electron lucent cytoplasmic vacuoles, which probably contain poly-β-hydroxybutyrate, are often observed (Figure 34-1). These vacuoles appear as large bumps within *Legionella* in scanning electron micrographs. These bacteria do not form endospores and are not encapsulated. *Legionella* have a branched-chain fatty acid composition that is unusual for gram-negative bacteria and affords identification on the basis of analysis of cellular fatty acids by gas-liquid chromatography.

A single polar flagellum has been found on isolates that have been grown on media that permits rapid growth. Flagellated *Legionella* have also been observed in human lung tissue in areas that do not have a dense population of *Legionella* or do not have a heavy infiltrate of inflammatory cell debris. Pili (fimbrae), one half the diameter of the flagellum, have also been observed by electron microscopic studies of *Legionella* grown in vitro.

There are no unique morphological characteristics that can easily distinguish *Legionella* from other gram-negative rods. The cytoplasmic vacuoles, flagellum, and pili are not always observable and may be missing in some species.

Staining Characteristics

Legionella and LLO from in vitro cultures all stain gram negative. The pink color may be faint, however, unless the safranin or carbol fuchsin (preferred) counterstain is left on smears for at least one minute. *Legionella* in tissue or other clinical specimens will usually not take the gram stain. Therefore, the gram stain procedure has limited usefulness for identification of these bacteria in clinical material. *Legionella* and

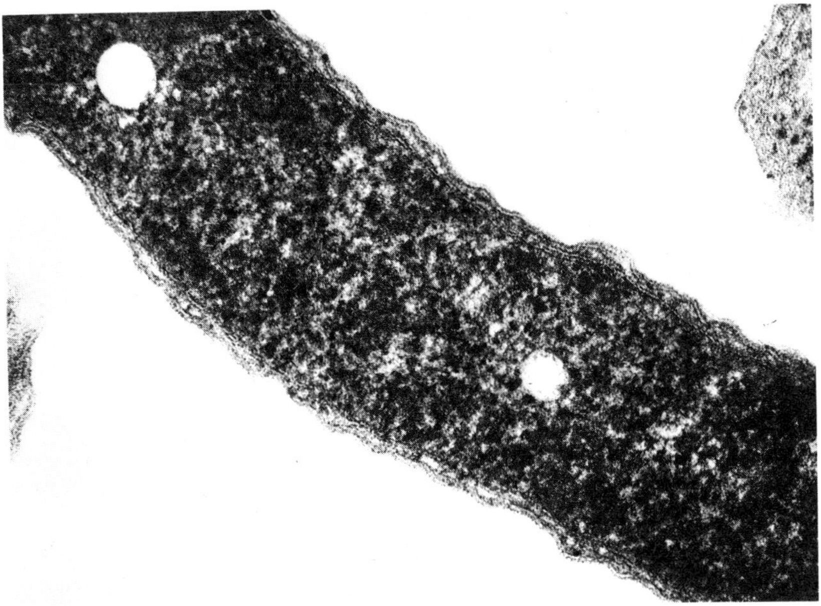

Figure 34-1 *Legionella pneumophila* structure in thin section. The *Legionella* were fixed with glutaraldehyde, followed by osmium tetroxide, dehydrated in ethanol, embedded in Epon and sectioned. Sections were stained with uranyl acetate and lead citrate. The wrinkled cell wall outer membrane and the inner cytoplasmic membrane are quite apparent. Two electron-lucent cytoplasmic inclusions can be seen. Magnification: 140,000 X.

LLO are not considered to be acid-fast.

There are two staining procedures that may identify bacteria such as *Legionella* in lung or other tissues. Various modifications of the Giemsa stain have produced variable results because of differentiating *Legionella* from a background of inflammatory cell debris. The Dieterle silver impregnation stain originally developed for staining spirochetes in tissue is useful, because the bacteria appear as dark red rods against a yellow to pink background of cellular debris. The Warthin-Starry silver impregnation method also produces satisfactory results. Other standard histological stains, including hematoxylin and eosin, are rarely useful.

Flagella may be stained by the Leifson flagellar stain but this has limited application for clinical diagnosis. β-hydroxybutyrate inclusions of *Legionella* may stain blue-black with the Sudan Black B fat stain, but this also has limited diagnostic usefulness.

Growth Characteristics

Legionella and LLO are unusual because they do not grow on the routine bacteriological media available in clinical microbiology laboratories. This includes sheep blood agar, chocolate agar, nutrient agar,

Mueller-Hinton agar, trypticase soy agar, and all of the selective/differential agar or broth media used for gram-negative enteric bacteria. There is some evidence to suggest that peroxides in the above culture media may inhibit the growth of *Legionella*. For this reason, the types of media for *Legionella* culture will be reviewed. The first in vitro culture medium to be developed utilized a Mueller-Hinton agar base, modified by the addition of 1% IsoVitalex and 1% hemoglobin. However, *Legionella* growth on this medium is slow. It was soon discovered that these bacteria grow better on a medium containing casein hydrolysate plus beef extractives or yeast extract when two filter-sterilized supplements, L-cysteine and ferric pyrophosphate-soluble were added. These media are known as Feeley-Gorman (FG) agar and charcoal (0.2% activated charcoal) yeast extract (CYE) agar, respectively. Some *Legionella* do not grow well on FG agar. Therefore, the current medium of choice is CYE agar modified by the inclusion of a buffer. The most commonly used filter sterilized broth medium is the same as CYE agar with the omission of activated charcoal and agar. Autoclaved broth medium may not support growth.

Further modifications of CYE agar have been made in order to differentiate between the various species of *Legionella* and inhibit growth of other bacteria. Buffered CYE agar medium containing glycine, α-ketoglutarate, cefamandole, polymyxin B, anisomycin, vancomycin, bromthymol blue, and bromcresol purple may permit isolation of *Legionella* from samples that contain high numbers of other bacteria. However, buffered CYE agar remains the first choice for primary isolation of *Legionella* and LLO. Stock cultures can be stored in the dark at room temperature on CYE agar slants for at least two months.

Legionella grow best on CYE medium in humid air supplemented with 2.5% CO_2 at 35°C. Primary cultures from clinical sources may require five to seven days before colonies can be seen. Unfortunately, other bacteria present in a specimen may overgrow and/or inhibit the growth of *Legionella* during this prolonged incubation period. Primary clinical or environmental samples may need to be passed through guinea pigs and/or embryonated hen eggs before *Legionella* or LLO can be isolated on CYE agar. *Legionella* and LLO are aerobic bacteria that utilize amino acids as a source of carbon and energy. However, *Legionella* may use some carbohydrates as a carbon source.

Taxonomy

Speciation of *Legionella* and LLO has moved rapidly during the last few years. There are currently nine proposed species; *L. pneumophila*, *L. micdadei*, *L. bozemanii*, *L. dumoffii*, *L. gormanii*, *L. longbeachae*, *L. wadsworthii*, *L. jordanis*, and *L. oakridgensis*. There are additional LLO isolates that have not been classified at this time. There seems to be a precedent for retaining the genus name, *Legionella*, for the isolates that have been characterized. The current literature also uses other taxonomic names, original isolate numbers or letter designations, and even different genus names. Therefore, the following tables have been compiled to show the taxonomic (Table 34-1) and physiological (Table 34-2) differences among the *Legionella* that have been investigated.

Serology

There are currently eight serogroups of *L. pneumophila* (Table 34-3). Most of the sporadic clinical cases of Legionnaires' disease studied through 1979 were caused by *L. pneumophila*, serogroup 1, followed by serogroups 2, 3 and 4. Data is incomplete on the frequency of serogroups 5 and 6 among clinical cases. There appears to be a *Legionella* common antigen, termed F-1, which is located on the surface of the bacterium.

Genetics

The genome size of *Legionella* is in the range of 2.5×10^9 daltons and the guanine plus cytosine (GC) content is between 35% and 43%, with an average content of 39%. No genetic relationship to previously known bacteria has been established by DNA hybridization studies. Plasmids have been detected in some *Legionella* isolates, but what they code for is not known.

Table 34-1
Taxonomic Classification of Legionella and LLO

Proposed Name	Original Isolate Designation*	Other Proposed Name
Legionella pneumophila	Legionnaires' disease bacillus, *Philadelphia,* OLDA	None
L. micdadei	*TATLOCK*, HEBA, Pittsburgh pneumonia agent (PPA)	*Tatlockia micdadei* *L. pittsburghensis*
L. bozemanii	*WIGA*, MI-15	*Fluoribacter bozemanae*
L. dumoffii	*NY-23*, Tex-K1	*Fluoribacter dumoffii*
L. gormanii	*LS-13*	*Fluoribacter gormanii*
L. longbeachae	*Long Beach 4*	None
L. jordanis	*BL-540*	None
L. oakridgensis	*Oak Ridge 10*	None
L. wadsworthii	*Wadsworth 81-716A*	None

*Italicized original isolate designation is the type strain for that species.

Table 34-3
Legionella pneumophila Serogroup Strains

Bacterial Isolate	Serogroup
Knoxville 1	1
Togus 1	2
Bloomington 2	3
Los Angeles 1	4
Dallas 1E	5
Chicago 2	6
Chicago 8	7
Concord 3	8

EPIDEMIOLOGY

Distribution in Nature

Legionella and LLO are distributed ubiquitously in natural aquatic environments. *Legionella* are also found in man-made aquatic environments such as shower heads, faucets, hot water tanks, heat rejection devices like cooling towers and evaporative condensers used for air conditioning, and, most recently, recreational whirlpools. There does not seem to be a human or animal reservoir. Cases of legionellosis have been found in most areas of the United States and in many countries around the world.

Epidemiologic investigations of legionellosis have been based on retrospective evaluations of patient sera and postmortem tissue. In studies of sera from adult populations, approximately 4% to 5% of the people have antibody titers to serogroup 1 *L. pneumophila* which suggests possible past infection but not necessarily disease.

A retrospective study by England et al (1981) of the first 1005 cases of documented sporadic legionellosis caused by *L. pneumophila* serogroups 1–4 produced many interesting results. Cases were reported in all states, except Alaska and South Dakota. The attack rate in 1978 was 2.4 cases per million population. Ages ranged from 16 months to 89 years with a median age of 55 years for males and 56 years for females. The relative risk for males was 2.6-fold higher than for females. Currently, 250,000 cases of legionellosis are estimated to occur each year in the United States. Sporadic cases seem to be more common than outbreaks. The epidemiological relationships to age, underlying disease, immunosuppression, smoking, travel, and exposure to recent excavations are similar for both sporadic cases and outbreaks.

Seasonality

Sporadic cases and outbreaks of legionellosis in the United States and in other countries occur more frequently during the summer months.

Table 34-2
Physiological Classification of Legionellae*

Characteristic	Legionella Species: *L. pneumophila*	*L. micdadei*	*L. bozemanii*	*L. dumoffii*	*L. gormanii*	*L. jordanis*	*L. longbeachae*	*L. oakridgensis*	*L. wadsworthii*
Growth on CYE agar	+	+	+	+	+	+	+	+	+
Growth on FG agar	+	+ adapt.†	+ adapt.	+ adapt.	−	+	+	+	ND
Growth on blood agar	−	−	−	−	−	−	−	−	−
Color on BTB + BCP agar‡	white/green	blue/gray	green	ND§	ND	ND	ND	ND	Green
Fluorescence on CYE agar	dull yellow	dull yellow	blue/white	blue/white	blue/white	dull yellow	dull yellow	dull yellow	dull yellow
Brown pigment on FG agar									
without tyrosine	±	−	−	+	+	+	+	+	−
tyrosine	+	+	+	+	ND	ND	ND	ND	−
Gram stain	negative	negative	negative	negative	negative	negative	negative	negative	negative
Acid fast	−	−	−	−	−	−	−	−	−
Flagella (Leifson stain)	+	+	+	+	+	+	+	−	+
Motility	+	ND	+	ND	ND	+	ND	−	+
Oxidase	±	+	−	−	−	+	+	−	−
Catalase	+	+	+	+	+	+	+	+	+
Urease	−	−	−	−	−	−	−	−	−
Gelatinase	+	±	+	+	+	+	+	+	+
β-lactamase	+	±	±	+	+	+	±	+	+
Hippurate hydrolysis	+	−	−	−	−	−	−	−	−
NO_3 reduction	−	−	−	−	−	−	−	−	−
Starch hydrolysis	+	±	+	+	−	ND	ND	ND	ND
Bromcresol purple spot test	−	+	−	ND	ND	ND	ND	ND	ND
Acid from carbohydrates	−	−	−	−	−	−	−	−	−

*Adapted from Morris et al, 1980; Orrison et al, 1983; and others. †Adapted to FG agar. ‡CYE agar containing bromthymol blue (BTB) and bromcresol purple (BCP). §Not determined.

Isolation of *L. pneumophila* from natural lakes or ponds in the United States is highest during the months of May, June and July. Of 1005 sporadic cases during the 1977–1979 period, 73% occurred between the months of June and October, with most cases (43%) during the months of August and September.

Transmission

Outbreaks of legionellosis have often been related to airborne transmission. The current evidence implicates the moist air exhaust of cooling towers, evaporative condensers, and other air-handling equipment as possible sources. Although *L. pneumophila* are often identified in concentrated water samples from cooling towers and evaporative condensers, the bacterium has not been isolated directly from the aerosol exhaust of air-conditioning equipment. Laboratory tests of the viability of *L. pneumophila* in aerosols indicate that the relatively short half-life of its viability is greater in humid air.

If cooling towers are a source of infective *Legionella*, there should be an increased risk for people who service or maintain the equipment. However, a serologic survey of mechanics, mechanic's helpers, and water treatment servicemen who maintain 3000 cooling towers in the New York metropolitan area failed to confirm this.

Legionella have been isolated from shower heads in hospitals and hotels. However, acquisition of legionellosis from these sources has not been proven conclusively.

PATHOGENICITY

Virulence Factors

The factor or factors responsible for the ability of *Legionella* to establish the disease state have yet to be identified. An early hypothesis involved endotoxin activity because most gram-negative rods have the lipid A-associated endotoxin in the lipopolysaccharide of their cell wall. *Legionella* do produce a strongly positive Limulus lysate test, a nonspecific in vitro test for endotoxin. However, *Legionella* do not produce significantly positive results in the more specific in vivo rabbit pyrogenicity and mouse lethality tests.

Exotoxins and/or exoenzymes have been suggested as possible virulence factors and include proteolytic, hemolytic and cytotoxic activities. Numerous other enzymes, including an enzyme that inhibits oxygen-dependent killing by phagocytic cells have been described in the literature.

Legionella do not seem to be highly infective once they have been passed several times in vitro. Passage of in vitro grown *Legionella* through hen embryonated yolk sac or guinea pigs restores a moderate level of virulence.

Investigation of the infectivity of *Legionella* aerosols for guinea pigs found that the geometric mean LD_{50} dose was approximately 3×10^4 bacteria per lung (Davis et al, 1982). The lethal dose by the intranasal or intraperitoneal routes is reportedly much greater. It is apparent from other reports that guinea pigs may be infected by a relatively low aerosol dose (100 to 200 bacteria) without developing lethal disease. Also, no cross-infection to a sentinal guinea pig placed in a cage with an infected guinea pig has been found. The infective dose for the healthy human host has not been determined. However, patients who have a compromised immune response are possibly at higher risk. Only one case of possible patient-to-patient transmission has been reported. However, the CDC recommends that known cases be placed in respiratory isolation.

Guinea pig peritoneal macrophages isolated from normal guinea pigs phagocytize yolk sac-grown Philadelphia 1 strain of *L. pneumophila* at a lower rate than do macrophages isolated from previously infected, convalescing guinea pigs. Adding immune sera increases the rate of phagocytosis by macrophages from both normal and immune guinea pigs. However, once *Legionella* are phagocytized, they begin to multiply in vacuoles and eventually kill the macrophages from both normal and convalescing guinea pigs. This is not influenced by the presence of immune sera. *Legionella* grown in vitro are also phagocytized, but they are subsequently killed by the macrophages. *Legionella* within histiocytes or macrophages in tissue from both humans and guinea pigs are often observed to be intact with no evidence of bacterial lysis. There are undoubtedly some virulence-associated factors involved in the survival and multiplication of *Legionella* within macrophages, but they remain to be elucidated.

DESCRIPTION OF CLINICAL DISEASE

Legionellosis or Legionnaires' disease, whether occurring sporadically or in an outbreak, is basically an acute bacterial bronchopneumonia. A mild, nonpneumonic disease produced by *Legionella* has also been described (Pontiac fever).

The clinical aspects of severe legionellosis have been described by many authors. The incubation period ranges from two to 10 days. Pneumonia is accompanied by a high fever (39°C–41°C); nonproductive cough which may later become productive and possibly contain blood; headache; a change in mental status; nausea; diarrhea; and vomiting. Chest roentgenograms may initially show an infiltrate, usually confined to a lower lobe, which may progress to bilateral involvement. Pulmonary cavitation has also been reported. Renal and hepatic involvement have been frequently described. *Legionella* antigen has also been found in urine. Elevated serum lactic acid dehydrogenase, SGOT, and alkaline phosphatase are frequently reported. Initial leukocyte counts among sporadic cases vary from 4700 to 28,000 with an average of 9900/mm^3. The red cell sedimentation rate may become elevated (> 55 mm/hr) in some cases.

Pathologic findings from fatal cases show a high frequency of bilateral pulmonary consolidation. There is often a dense fibropurulent pneumonia with bacteria at the edge of consolidated areas. Focal areas of hemorrhage are common. There is an acute inflammatory reaction, diffuse alveolar damage with intact *Legionella* present within alveolar macrophages. Immunocompromised patients may have a fibroserous pneumonia without much inflammation.

It is apparent that *Legionella* may spread by endobronchial, interstitial, endolymphatic, and hematogenous routes. Bacteria may spread with migrating phagocytic cells. *Legionella* have been found in hilar lymph nodes, spleen, bone marrow, kidneys, and pulmonary venules.

DIAGNOSTIC TESTS

Direct Fluorescent Antibody (DFA) Test

This test is used for the early diagnosis of legionellosis. Specific antisera are produced by immunizing rabbits with a formalinized or heat-killed vaccine without Freunds' adjuvant. The gammaglobulin fraction of the serum is conjugated with fluorescein isothiocyanate and used to idenitfy *Legionella* in specimens by means of fluorescent microscopy. Rhodamine-conjugated normal rabbit serum is used as a diluent in order to counterstain autofluorescent debris. DFA reagents for *L. pneumophila* serogroups 1–6, *L. bozemanii*, *L. dumoffi*, *L. gormanii*, *L. micdadei*, and *L. longbeachiae* are now available from commercial sources. The DFA test is more specific and sensitive than the usual histologic staining procedures. It can be done on sputum, if available, or on other respiratory secretions, such as tracheal aspirates, or pleural fluid. Liquifaction and concentration of sputum may be helpful. This test can also be performed on microscope slide imprints of fresh or formalinized lung tissue or deparaffinized lung tissue sections. False-negative DFA tests may occur as a result of inadequate numbers of *Legionella* in the specimens.

The omission of Freunds' complete adjuvant from the vaccines and the inclusion of the rhodamine counterstain have eliminated much of the nonspecific staining associated with some of the early DFA tests. A recent report suggested, however, that patients with *Bacteroides fragilis* infection may produce a positive, cross-reactive DFA test to serogroup 1 *L. pneumophila* but not to serogroups 2–4. Also, *Pseudomonas fluorescens*,

P. alcaligenes, and the *Flavobacterium-Xanthomonas* group were reported to stain positively with serogroup 1 antisera.

Preparation of specimens, examination of slides, and interpretation of DFA results are presented in the CDC Manual. Since there are very few organisms in lung exudates, observation of ≥ 5 fluorescing bacteria is considered positive. For clinical specimens, except lung exudates, ≥ 25 strongly fluorescing bacteria per smear is considered positive. If there are < 25 strongly fluorescing bacteria per smear, the actual numbers are reported. No strongly fluorescing bacteria per smear is reported as negative. Lung exudates are difficult to evaluate because of the presence of autofluorescing debris in the specimens. Therefore, familiarity with the morphology of *Legionella* and experience with fluorescent microscopy are needed for proper interpretation. Appropriate controls must be run in parallel with test samples.

Culture

It is recommended that nonformalinized specimens examined by the DFA test also be cultured on buffered CYE agar with and without additional supplements. The combination of culture plus DFA test produces results that are more diagnostically useful than when each is used alone. A survey of sporadic cases found that nearly half of DFA-positive specimens were culture positive. Blood should also be cultured since *Legionella* have been isolated from the blood of a few patients with legionellosis. A diphasic (broth/agar) CYE blood culture medium is recommended but standard aerobic blood culture medium also has been used successfully.

There are two reasons that may explain false-negative cultures in patients with legionellosis. First, viable *Legionella* may not be present in respiratory secretions unless retrograde spread of the organism has occurred in the airway. Second, human anterior pharyngeal flora contaminating specimens of respiratory secretions may inhibit the growth of *Legionella*. For example, we have found that some isolates of *Staphylococcus aureus*, *Streptococcus pneumoniae*, *Pseudomonas aeruginosa*, and some viridans streptococci inhibit the growth of *L. pneumophila* Philadelphia 1 on buffered CYE agar. Culture of clinical specimens is recommended, however, because there have been reports of occasional positive cultures from specimens that were DFA-negative.

Various modifications of the culture medium are being evaluated at this time. Some of these modifications are designed to permit differentiation between some species of *Legionella*, while others contain antibiotics and other supplements to inhibit the growth of other bacteria and fungi while permiting the growth of *Legionella*. At this time, buffered CYE agar medium is recommended for primary isolation and is commercially available.

Laboratories with suitable biological containment facilities have successfully recovered *Legionella* by intraperitoneal injection of clinical specimens into guinea pigs. Culture of guinea pig spleen homogenates or peritoneal washings after three to five days directly on CYE agar or on CYE agar after passage through the yolk sac of embryonated hen eggs has often resulted in isolation of *Legionella* when direct plating results were negative. The procedures for in vivo passage are presented in the CDC Manual.

Indirect Immunofluorescence (IFA) Test

This is a serological test for antibody to *Legionella* in patient's serum. The IFA test can be used to confirm legionellosis when paired acute (within seven days of onset) and convalescent (20 to 40 days after onset) patient sera show a fourfold or greater rise in titer to ≥ 128. When only one serum sample is available, a single or standing titer of ≥ 256 is presumptive evidence of previous or current infection.

Patients with legionellosis seroconvert to a diagnostically positive IFA titer, unless they succumb to the disease before an antibody response is elicited or they have a defective immune response to the organism. However, seroconversion may take up to three weeks. Therefore, the IFA test has limited usefulness in the early diagnosis of legionellosis. The DFA test and culture produce positive diagnosic results earlier, but they may often be negative. In this instance, early diagnosis must be based on clinical signs and symptoms and later confirmed by the IFA test.

The IFA test procedure and interpretation of results is presented in the CDC Manual. State public health laboratories are equipped to perform this test. The antigens for the IFA test are *Legionella* that are grown on CYE agar and heat-killed. The bacteria are suspended in normal chicken yolk sac fluid and fixed to a microscope slide. Various dilutions of patient's serum are incubated with the antigen. The slide is then washed and incubated with fluorescein-conjugated antihuman serum to determine whether antibodies in the patient's serum attached to the known antigen. Fluorescence intensities are graded from 0 to 4+. The highest dilution of the patient's serum that produces at least 1+, barely visible staining, is considered the end point. It is very important to include appropriate controls with all tests. As with the DFA test, some experience is required to evaluate staining intensities and background staining of yolk sac material, filamentous bacteria and other artifacts. The current commercially available IFA test kits using individual serogroup bacterial preparations seem to have a sensitivity of 85% and a specificity of 92%.

There are a variety of cross-reactions that may occur, however. Patient sera with antibody to other gram-negative bacteria may cross-react with *Legionella*. This cross-reactivity may be effectively blocked with immunoabsorbant from *Escerichia coli* strain 013:K92:H4. However, this procedure is not routinely used. No cross-reactions against *L. pneumophila* antigens have been found in sera from cases of Q fever, tularemia, or psittacosis, or in sera of patients with rheumatoid factor.

Other Diagnostic Tests

Several other tests for *Legionella* antigen and antibody have been developed and compared to the more established DFA and IFA tests. A brief description of these tests will suffice because most are not widely used. A microagglutination test has been developed for detection of IgM class antibody. A microenzyme-linked immunosorbent assay (ELISA) has been developed to detect antibodies to serogroup 1 *L. pneumophilia* and *Legionella* antigen in urine. Various agglutination tests, indirect hemagglutination, ELISA, radioimmunoassays (RIA), and counter-immunoelectrophoresis tests to detect *Legionella* antigen have been described. A guinea pig skin test reportedly can detect the presence of *Legionella* antigens when they are injected intradermally into immunized guinea pigs. Biochemical tests for the presence of *Legionella* enzyme activities are also under development.

In summary, laboratory tests are available for early diagnosis and retrospective confirmation of legionellosis. The most useful tests at this time are the DFA and IFA tests in combination with culture on buffered CYE agar directly or after passage through guinea pigs and/or chicken embryo yolk sacs. The two fluorescent antibody tests require trained laboratory personnel if test results are to be correctly interpreted. Development of more selective culture media and diagnostic tests will probably continue for some time. Therefore, it is necessary to keep abreast of the literature and information available at state or local public health laboratories, the Centers for Disease Control and current reviews.

THERAPY

There have not been controlled clinical trials, but the evidence reported in the literature indicates that erythromycin and rifampin are active against *Legionella* with in vitro assays, with in vivo models of legionellosis, and in patients. Erythromycin gluceptate alone is given intravenously in amounts ranging from 0.5 to 1.0 g every six hours. As a patient's condition stabilizes, the dosage may be reduced and erythromycin may be given orally. Antibiotic therapy is often continued for up to three weeks. The combination of erythromycin and rifampin is recommended if a patient is not responding to erythromycin alone. A considerable amount of supportive therapy must be given to patients with severe legionellosis.

In vitro antimicrobial sensitivity studies with *Legionella* often produce results that are at variance with results of tests with animal models and clinical experience. The aminoglycosides, penicillins, cephalosporins, tetracycline, and chloramphenicol, although they may be active in vitro, are not clinically effective. The ability of *Legionella* to survive and multiply within macrophages may explain why antibiotics that penetrate tissue are effective in vivo even though other antibiotics that are active in vitro are not useful clinically. Also, most *Legionella* produce a β-lactamase that is most active on the cephalosporin group of antibiotics. Clearly, more controlled clinical trials will be needed before questions concerning the efficacy of antibiotic therapy can be resolved.

PREVENTION

Although a primary mode of transmission seems to be inhalation, the source and nature of infective *Legionella* remains to be clearly established. There is a tentative relationship between legionellosis cases and aerosolized water. Therefore, preventive measures recommended at this time are adequate disinfection of aerosol-producing equipment. Cooling towers and evaporative condensers heavily contaminated with *Legionella* should be treated with effective levels of an appropriate chemical biocide. Recirculating water systems may also be treated with suitable ultraviolet light systems. Equipment heavily contaminated with organic matter may not be effectively treated by chlorination, because the organic material will neutralize the free chlorine. Therefore, free chlorine levels must be monitored during disinfection procedures when calcium hypochlorite is used.

One problem that prevents more effective preventative measures is the lack of an efficient, cost-effective method to monitor the numbers of viable *Legionella* in water samples that have a high background bacterial flora. It is usually difficult to isolate *Legionella* from such samples by direct plating on CYE agar, because the other bacteria in the sample frequently overgrow or inhibit *Legionella* growth. The guinea pig intraperitoneal injection method is currently used, but it is time consuming and rather expensive. A more efficient isolation method is clearly needed.

Other preventive measures such as vaccination are being investigated. Immunization of guinea pigs has prevented subsequent infection, but more research will be required before the suitability of a vaccine can be established.

ACKNOWLEDGMENTS

The author wishes to thank John J. Bozzola, PhD, Department of Microbiology at The Medical College of Pennsylvania, Philadelphia, for his contribution of electron micrographs to this chapter; critical reading of the manuscript by Susan B. Dillon of the same department is gratefully acknowledged. Portions of the work presented were supported in part by The Whitaker Foundation and by The Biomedical Research Support Grant Program of The Public Health Service, National Institutes of Health.

SELECTED READINGS

Davis GS, Winn WC Jr, Gump DW, et al: Legionnaires' pneumonia after aerosol exposure in guinea pigs and rats. *Am Rev Respir Dis* 1982;126:1050–1057.

England AC III, Fraser DW, Plikaytis BD, et al: Sporatic legionellosis in the United States. The first thousand cases. *Ann Intern Med* 1981;94:164–170.

Helms CM, Viner JP, Renner ED, et al: Legionnaires' disease among pneumonias in Iowa (FY 1972–1978) II. Epidemiologic and clinical features of 30 sporatic cases of *L. pneumophila* infection. *Am J Med Sci* 1981;281:2–13.

Hicklin MD, Thomason BM, Chandler FW, et al: Pathogenesis of acute Legionnaires' disease pneumonia. *Am J Clin Pathol* 1980;73:480–487.

Jones GL, Hebert GA (ed): *"Legionnaires." The Disease, the Bacterium and Methodology.* Atlanta, Georgia, Centers for Disease Control, 1979.

Katz S (ed): *Legionellosis.* Cleveland, Ohio CRC Press (in press).

Lattimer GL, Ormsbee RA, *Legionnaires' Disease.* New York, Marcel Dekker, Inc, 1981.

Morris GK, Steigerwalt A, Feeley JC, et al: *Legionella gormanii* sp. nov. *J. Clin Microbiol* 1980;12:718–721.

Orrison LH, Cherry, WB, Tyndall RL, et al: *Legionella oakridgensis*: Unusual new species isolated from cooling tower water. *Appl Environ Microbiol* 1983;45:536–545.

Reingold AL, Band JD, Legionellosis, in Easmon CSF, Jaszewicz J (eds): *Medical Microbiology*, vol 1, New York, Academic Press, 1982.

35 Other Obligate Anaerobes Including Actinomyces

Jack L. LeFrock
Abdolghader Molavi
Arnold Lentnek

Anaerobic bacteria are well recognized but frequently overlooked pathogens in pleuropulmonary infections. Until recently, there has been widespread failure to obtain appropriate specimens and to utilize optimal techniques for their transport and culture. During the past decade, proper culturing techniques have documented the importance of anaerobes in infections manifesting as pneumonitis, lung abscess, necrotizing pneumonia, and empyema.

The most frequent underlying condition for anaerobic pleuropulmonary infections is impaired consciousness or dysphagia. Altered states of consciousness due to alcoholism, cerebrovascular accident, general anesthesia, drug overdose, diabetic coma, or seizure disorder or dysphagia due to esophageal or neurologic disease, precede these infections in the majority of cases.

The second most common predisposing factor is periodontal disease or gingivitis. Other conditions associated with these infections include bronchogenic carcinoma, bronchiectasis, and subdiaphragmatic or pelvic infections.

PATHOGENESIS

The common thread in the diverse clinical settings of anaerobic pleuropulmonary infections is aspiration of the oropharyngeal secretions containing pooled bacteria from the tongue, gingiva, buccal mucosa, and pharynx (Figure 35-1). Normally, aspirated material is handled effectively by cough, ciliary action, and alveolar macrophages. If not checked by these normal host defenses, the process leads to pneumonitis in dependent pulmonary segments.

Anaerobic bacteria have the propensity to cause tissue necrosis. If treatment is delayed, simple pneumonitis may progress to lung abscess or to necrotizing pneumonia. Lung abscess is a solitary or dominant cavity, measuring at least 2 cm in diameter, which communicates with a bronchus. Necrotizing pneumonia is a pneumonitis with multiple small cavities within one or more pulmonary segments or lobes. The distinction

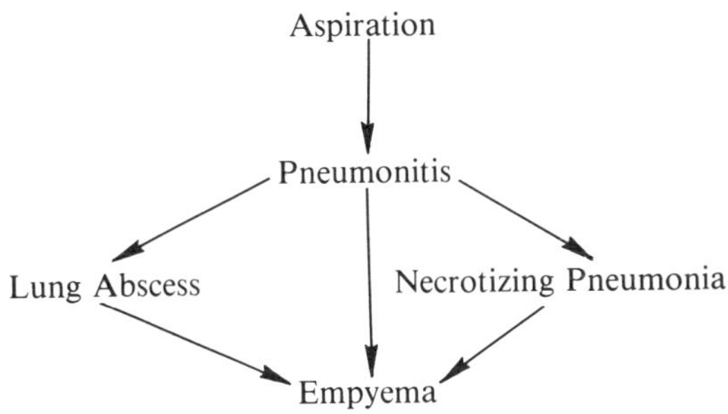

Figure 35-1 Pathogenesis of anaerobic pleuropulmonary infections after aspiration.

is somewhat arbitrary, since both types of infection are expressions of the same pathologic process. Neither the specific etiologic organisms nor the predisposing conditions determine the type of clinical disease that results. Host defense mechanisms and the size of the infecting inoculum may influence the outcome.

Parenchymal pulmonary infection may extend peripherally by contiguous spread, ultimately reaching the pleura and producing empyema. Empyema also develops if the necrotizing process establishes a communication between the bronchial lumen and the pleural space, allowing air to enter the latter, ie, a bronchopulmonary fistula. Infection of the pleural space may also follow transdiaphragmatic spread of a subphrenic infection.

Anaerobic bacteria also may arrive in the lung via the bloodstream. Bacteremia or septic emboli in such cases commonly originate in the female pelvic organs (ie, suppurative pelvic thrombophlebitis) or less commonly in the neck (ie, jugular thrombophlebitis), but prostatitis, gastrointestinal infections, and endocarditis also have been implicated as sources. The heparinase-like activity of *Bacteroides fragilis* is thought to account for the tendency of this organism to produce septic thrombophlebitis.

MICROBIOLOGY

The periodontal structures, tongue, buccal mucosa, and oropharynx each harbor a unique commensal flora composed of anaerobic as well as aerobic bacteria. In the oropharynx the anaerobes thrive primarily in the crevices around the teeth or tonsillar crypts. The anaerobic counts and the relative proportion of anaerobes to aerobes in oropharyngeal secretions increase significantly in the presence of periodontal disease and gingivitis; they decrease in persons without teeth. Saliva contains bacterial species from all these sources in counts of approximately 4×10^7

aerobic and facultative bacteria and 10^8 anaerobes per mL. The principal anaerobes are *Fusobacterium nucleatum*, *Bacteroides melaninogenicus*, *B. oralis*, *Peptostreptococcus*, *Peptococcus*, and *Veillonella*. Present in smaller numbers are *Leptotrichia buccalis*, *Eubacterium*, *Bifidobacterium*, *Actinomyces*, *Propionibacterium*, *Arachnia*, *Clostridium*, anaerobic vibrios, and spirochetes. Also present in the mouth are two recently identified *Bacteroides* species, *B. bivius* and *B. disiens*, both of which may produce disease.

Aspiration, therefore, produces contamination of the lower respiratory tract by a complex flora in which anaerobes outnumber aerobes by a significant factor. Despite aspiration of over 100 different species, there is a marked simplification so that a combination of only about four to five species (two or three anaerobes and one or two aerobes) survive in the lung to result in pneumonia.

The bacteriology of aspiration-associated pleuropulmonary infection depends upon whether it is hospital or community acquired. In community-acquired infections, anaerobes are the exclusive pathogens in 60% of cases. In the remaining cases, anaerobes are present along with aerobes, which are predominantly streptococci. By contrast, in hospital-acquired infections, anaerobes are the exclusive pathogens in only 17% of cases. In 47%, a mixture of aerobic and anaerobic organisms are found, and in 36%, aerobes are the exclusive pathogens. The predominant aerobic bacteria in hospital-acquired disease include Enterobacteriaceae and *Pseudomonas aeruginosa*. The colonization of the upper respiratory tract with these potential pathogens in hospitalized patients must be taken into account in devising therapeutic regimens.

There are over 200 different obligate anaerobic species described in laboratory manuals, but fortunately only a limited number of species are commonly encountered in clinical specimens and these usually can be readily identified by growth in relation to oxygen concentration in the atmosphere, reaction and morphology of bacteria in gram stains, and colonial and biochemical characteristics.

Anaerobic organisms vary widely in sensitivity to oxygen, ranging from relatively aerotolerant to extremely oxygen-sensitive species. Established growth of aerotolerant species (ie, colonies on an agar plate or organisms in pus) can tolerate exposure to oxygen in air for several hours, but in vitro growth is best initiated in an atmosphere of reduced oxygen tension (eg, an anaerobic "Gas Pak" jar or chamber). Extremely oxygen-sensitive species are killed within minutes of exposure to even very low concentrations of oxygen. Fortunately, most pathogenic anaerobes are relatively aerotolerant. This simplifies their isolation from clinical specimens. In addition to a low redox potential provided by exclusion of oxygen, many anaerobes require a lower redox potential for growth. This may be provided by the metabolic activity of other bacteria or by reducing agents formed by tissue breakdown due to either ischemia, trauma, neoplasm or infection with facultative organisms. In the laboratory, media used for growth of anaerobes are supplemented with tissue (eg, chopped meat, liver) or reducing agents (eg, thioglycolate) to lower the redox potential.

Two major genera of gram-positive anaerobic cocci commonly isolated from clinical specimens are *Peptostreptococcus* and *Peptococcus*. Both can look similar on gram stain; each can appear singly, in pairs, or in chains, spherical or elongated. They generally appear smaller than their aerobic counterparts. On blood agar they grow as convex, opaque, shiny or dull, gray-white colonies. *Peptostreptococcus* produces a fecal odor, but *Peptococcus* has no odor. *Streptococcus intermedius* and *S. morbillorum*, which may become aerotolerant on subculture, previously were classified as anaerobes, but are now included in a genus of facultative anaerobes. Anaerobic cocci can be differentiated in the laboratory by biochemical characteristics.

The important genera of gram-negative bacilli in anaerobic lung infections are *Fusobacterium* and *Bacteroides*. Fusobacteria consists of three major species: *F. nucleatum*, *F. mortiferum*, and *F. necrophorum*. The most frequent clinical isolate, *F. nucleatum*, can be distinguished on gram stain from other gram-negative rods by its characteristic slender, tapered morphology. On blood agar, its colonies are generally nonhemolytic and have a convex, glistening appearance. They are sensitive to bile and nonmotile. Biochemical characteristics distinguish it from other *Fusobacterium* species.

Bacteroides species are the most important clinical anaerobes. The "*B. fragilis group*" includes five separate species (*B. fragilis*, *B. thetaiotamicron*, *B. distasonis*, *B. vulgatus* and *B. ovatus*) which are part of the normal bowel flora. Organisms of the *B. fragilis* group are pleomorphic, stain weakly with gram stain, and occasionally may look like safety pins. They grow as convex, gray-white, translucent colonies, and their growth is not inhibited by bile. They produce β-lactamases, which make them resistant to many penicillins and cephalosporins. The five species can be distinguished by biochemical characteristics and DNA homology patterns. *B. fragilis* can be distinguished from the rest of the group by a species-specific capsular polysaccharide, identified by an indirect fluorescent antibody technique.

The second important *Bacteroides* group is *B. melaninogenicus*, composed of three species, *B. asaccharolyticus*, *B. melaninogenicus ss intermedius*, and *B. melaninogenicus ss melaninogenicus*. All are part of the indigenous oral flora. They are bacilli or coccobacilli that require vitamin K and hemin for growth and form black colonies after two to ten days' growth on solid media. The colonies often fluoresce red under ultraviolet light before the black pigment develops. The red fluorescence also may be noted in purulent material. Many strains are penicillin sensitive, but penicillin resistance on the basis of β-lactamase production is increasing; up to 60%of strains may now be resistant.

The lipopolysaccharides of *B. fragilis* and *B. melaninogenicus*, unlike that of *Fusobacterium*, are chemically incomplete when compared with the lipopolysaccharides (endotoxins) of aerobic bacteria, and they lack the biologic potency characteristic of endotoxin. The inactivity may explain the relative infrequency of disseminated intravascular coagulation in *Bacteroides* bacteremia. *B. fragilis* and *B. asaccharolyticus* strains have species-specific polysaccharide capsules, which are thought to be virulence factors. In an animal model of experimental intra-abdominal sepsis, an inoculum of an encapsulated *B. fragilis* strain alone has been reported to cause abscesses, but abscess formation following inoculation of unencapsulated strain required concomitant presence of an aerobe.

PLEUROPULMONARY SYNDROMES

Four distinct pleuropulmonary syndromes due to anaerobic bacterial species can be clinically recognized: pneumonitis, primary lung abscess, necrotizing pneumonia, and empyema. More than one of these commonly coexist. Their individual characteristics generally are similar to those of syndromes caused by aerobic or facultative organisms. However, considering the entire clinical picture one can usually make the diagnosis without difficulty.

Most anaerobic pleuropulmonary infections involve multiple bacterial species. In view of their common pathogenetic mechanisms, it is not surprising that similar species of bacteria are involved in all the syndromes.

Anaerobic Bacterial Pneumonitis

The role of anaerobic bacteria in pneumonitis is only occasionally suspected and rarely proved. This condition is easily overlooked because important hallmarks of anaerobic pulmonary infections (putrid sputum, tissue necrosis, and indolent course) generally are absent and expectorated sputum is not valid for anaerobic culture.

Most cases are early stages of infections that would progress to lung abscess, necrotizing pneumonia, or empyema if left untreated. However, occasionally the infection may persist for weeks with no apparent tendency towards necrosis.

Anaerobic bacterial pneumonia usually is polymicrobial. The predominant organisms recovered are *Peptostreptococcus* sp, *Fusobacterium*, *B. melanogenicus*, *Peptococcus* sp, and *B. fragilis*.

This syndrome usually is characterized by an acute course and a rapid response to proper therapy. The presenting features closely resemble those of pneumococcal pneumonia, especially with regard to fever, leukocyte count, the number of lobes involved, and the location of infiltrate. However, patients with anaerobic bacterial pneumonitis have a higher frequency of underlying bronchogenic neoplasm or associated conditions predisposing to aspiration. Shaking chills, putrid sputum and bacteremia usually are absent.

The most important clinical clue to the presence of anaerobic pneumonia is a history of aspiration or suspected aspiration. If suitable material is to be obtained for culture, percutaneous transtracheal aspiration is generally required.

The duration of fever after institution of appropriate antimicrobial treatment (about two to four days) generally is comparable to that of pneumococcal pneumonia. Some patients, however, may develop pulmonary abscesses despite such treatment. This is more likely to occur if treatment is initiated somewhat late and may be associated with a more prolonged febrile course of about seven days after initiation of therapy.

Lung Abscess

Primary lung abscess is caused mainly by anaerobic bacteria. Aspiration due to impaired consciousness or dysphagia is the usual underlying mechanism. Most patients have associated conditions—including alcoholism, epilepsy, drug overdose, general anesthesia, or neurologic disease leading to altered consciousness. Poor oral hygiene, periodontal infection, and gingivitis are also common in these patients. Primary lung abscess is rare in toothless adults; when it occurs, the underlying condition usually is bronchogenic carcinoma and not aspiration.

Aspiration of oropharyngeal secretions initially produces pneumonitis, which usually is segmental and often subpleural. As necrosis and liquefaction occur, the center of the pneumonitis evolves into an abscess, which becomes a cavity with an air-fluid level when bronchial drainage is established. The cavity generally appears about 12 days after the time of aspiration. Infection may spread to noncontiguous segments by the intrabronchial route and to the pleura. Approximately one third of lung abscesses are complicated by empyema, with or without a bronchopleural fistula.

Primary lung abscess usually is polymicrobial, with anaerobes outnumbering aerobes 4–5 to 1. One study found an average of three bacterial species per patient, averaging 2.4 anaerobic strains and 0.6 aerobic or facultative strains. In 58% of cases the infecting flora was exclusively anaerobic; in 42%, both anaerobes and aerobes were present. The predominant anaerobic isolates were *F. nucleatum*, *B. melaninogenicus*, *Peptostreptococcus* sp, *Peptococcus* sp, microaerophilic streptococci, and *B. fragilis*.

Classical lung abscess tends to be an indolent infection. Patients usually present with insidious onset of cough and fever, sometimes associated with pleuritic chest pain. Sputum is typically foul and copious. Anemia and weight loss are common. The course is chronic but with a potential for sudden, severe complications, such as brain abscess, massive hemoptysis, or rupture of the pleura and development of pyopneumothorax.

The classic appearance of primary lung abscess on a chest x-ray is a single cavity, with an air-fluid level and a thick, smooth wall, in the subpleural area of a dependent segment (Figure 35-2). The segments most commonly involved are the posterior segments of the upper lobes or the superior segments of the lower lobes (which are dependent in the recumbent position) and the basilar segments of the lower lobes (which are dependent in the upright position). The disease is suspected clinically by recognizing this classic radiologic appearance in patients with periodontal disease and/or conditions predisposing to aspiration. The diagnosis is assured by putrid sputum showing many polymorphonuclear leukocytes and a mixture of gram-negative and gram-positive bacilli and gram-positive cocci on gram stain. Failure to isolate an aerobic pathogen on culture and/or a significant qualitative and quantitative discrepancy

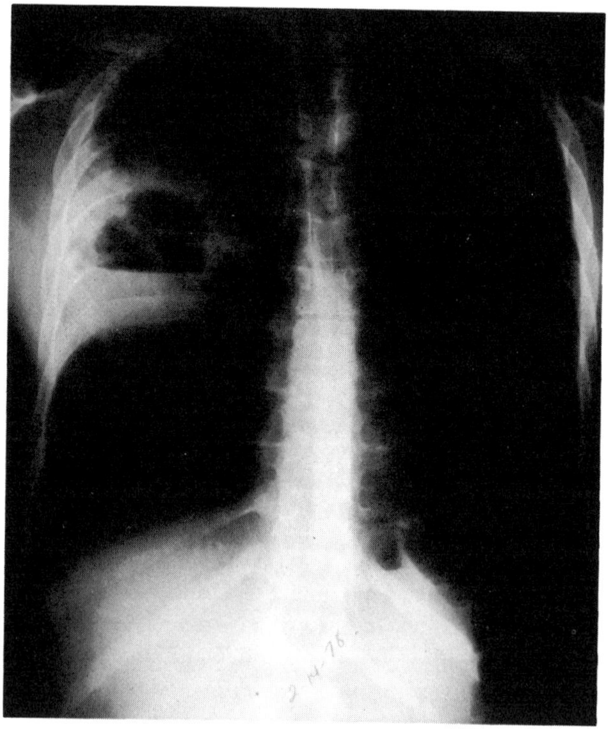

Figure 35-2 Chest radiograph of a chronic alcoholic patient with a right upper lobe anaerobic lung abscess showing an air fluid level.

between the smear and the culture lends further support to the diagnosis.

Occasionally, fungal or tuberculous infections, carcinoma, or pulmonary infarction may present with a radiologic picture similar to that of a primary lung abscess. In such cases, however, air-fluid level and the clinical features of lung abscess usually are not present. In cavitating carcinomas the cavity wall is irregular. Pulmonary abscess may also be due to organisms, including *Klebsiella*, *H. influenzae*, *S. aureus*, *S. pneumoniae* (especially Type 3), *Nocardia*, and *Aspergillus*.

In any patient with lung abscess it is important to look for associated problems, such as an obstructing foreign body, neoplasm, or tuberculosis.

The principal management of primary lung abscess is treatment with antimicrobial agents for approximately one to two months, depending on the patient's clinical and radiologic response. Postural drainage is important, together with bronchoscopy to facilitate drainage and to detect underlying obstructive lesions, such as tumors or foreign bodies. This approach cures most patients. Surgical intervention usually is not necessary even if the abscess cavity persists with no or minimal improvement after six to eight weeks of therapy. Almost all cavities eventually close. Surgical resection is indicated for massive hemoptysis.

Necrotizing Pneumonia

Necrotizing pneumonia is distinguished from lung abscess by the presence of multiple small cavities rather than a single large cavity. There are also clinical and pathologic differences. However, the underlying conditions, pathogenesis, and spectrum of pathogens are similar to those of primary lung abscess.

Aspiration of the oropharyngeal secretions initially produces anaerobic pneumonitis, which then undergoes necrosis, with the production of multiple small abscesses. Histologic studies show multiple adjacent abscesses, sometimes resulting in large sloughs of tissue ("pulmonary gangrene"). The disease usually is confined to one pulmonary segment or lobe, but it may extend to other lobes. Since the introduction of antibiotics, anaerobic necrotizing pneumonia has become less common, as the pneumonitis can be treated early, before necrosis develops.

In most patients with anaerobic necrotizing pneumonia the infection is polymicrobial, and anaerobes are the exclusive isolates. Occasionally, however, cultures also yield aerobic or facultative organisms. The anaerobes most commonly encountered are *F. nucleatum*, *B. melaninogenicus*, *Peptostreptococcus* sp, *Peptococcus* sp, and microaerophilic streptococci. *B. fragilis* is uncommon. *Clostridium* sp, including *C. perfringens*, may be recovered from patients with necrotizing pneumonia and empyema.

Patients with anaerobic necrotizing pneumonia usually are quite ill, with high fever and leukocytosis. They commonly have putrid sputum and/or empyema when first seen. Some patients have only pneumonitis on initial chest film, but cavitations typical of necrotizing pneumonia appear on subsequent x-rays.

The tempo of necrotizing pneumonia is highly variable. The infection may be quite destructive, spread rapidly, and end fatally. Not uncommonly, however, it remains localized and runs a subacute, smoldering course. The mortality rate (20%) is greater than that of other anaerobic pulmonary infections. The reasons are not clear but may include differences in the virulence of the infecting species.

Because of this high mortality, the diagnosis must be made promptly, and antimicrobial therapy must be initiated immediately. Many aerobic organisms—including *P. aeruginosa*, *S. aureus*, *Klebsiella pneumoniae*, *Proteus*, *Pasteurella*, *Nocardia*, mycobacteria, and fungi—may also produce necrotizing pneumonia. An accurate etiologic diagnosis is therefore essential. Treatment should be intensive and of sufficient duration to prevent relapse. In patients with an associated empyema, adequate drainage of the empyema fluid must be established.

Empyema

The advent of chemotherapy has produced a striking change in the bacteriologic spectrum of empyema. Today, anaerobes are the most common pathogens isolated from infected pleural fluid.

Anaerobic empyema commonly develops as a complication of a preexisting pulmonary infection. The infection may extend to the pleura by contiguous spread or by a bronchopleural fistula, which is the usual cause of an air-fluid level in the pleural space. However, anaerobes in the empyema fluid may generate sufficient gas to produce an air-fluid level without a fistula.

Anaerobic empyema also may result from transdiaphragmatic spread of subphrenic or other infradiaphragmatic infections, in which case there may be no associated pulmonary infection. In rare instances it may arise from leakage of an esophageal perforation or from septic pulmonary emboli.

The isolation rate for anaerobes in patients with empyema varies with the expertise of the laboratory. In a study at three specialized laboratories anaerobic bacteria were recovered in 76% of cases and were the exclusive isolates in 35%. In most patients the empyema fluid yielded multiple isolates. The most common anaerobes were *F. nucleatum*, *B. melaninogenicus*, *B. fragilis*, *Peptostreptococcus* sp, microaerophilic streptococci, *Peptococcus* sp, and *Clostridium* sp. Among the aerobic and facultative bacteria, *Escherichia coli* and *P. aeruginosa* predominated.

The infection of the pleural space may present acutely with pleuritic pain, particularly when it is due to septic pulmonary emboli or to rupture of a lung abscess. More commonly, patients with empyema have been sick for a least a week and usually longer before coming to the physician. Chest pain, fever, night sweats, cough, and weight loss are common complaints; anemia and leukocytosis are frequent findings.

Treatment is directed at providing adequate drainage of the empyema fluid, as well as appropriate antimicrobial therapy. Repeated needle aspiration may be adequate if the fluid is thin and free-flowing, but such cases are rare. Insertion of an intercostal tube for continuous closed drainage should not be delayed if the empyema fluid 1) is thick and purulent, 2) shows organisms on gram stain, 3) has a glucose concentration below 40 mg/100 mL, or 4) has a pH less than 7. More than one chest tube may be needed if the empyema is loculated and not free flowing. Open thoracostomy with rib resection is necessary if closed-tube drainage is ineffective. Decortication, with removal of the thick fibrous tissue covering the lung, may be required to obtain lung expansion and obliterate the empyema cavity.

Septic Pulmonary Emboli

Metastatic localization is common in anaerobic bacteremia, the lung being the most common secondary site. The pulmonary lesions may be difficult to distinguish from those that follow aspiration unless the patient is carefully examined for predisposing factors and for a primary site of infection. More commonly, however, metastatic involvement of the pulmonary parenchyma presents as localized, well-circumscribed lesions with features similar to those of metastatic staphylococcal pneumonia. The abscesses, which usually are peripheral, may be single or multiple, may involve one or more lobes, and may develop over a period of days.

Septic emboli usually develop abruptly, and there is often a latent period of about one day between the onset of pulmonary symptoms and radiologic changes. The primary source is most commonly the female pelvis, with a localized abscess or septic thrombophlebitis; but emboli may arise as a complication of prostatitis, intra-abdominal abscess, or tricuspid valve endocarditis. In addition to antimicrobial therapy, surgical intervention at the primary site of infection often is required to prevent further embolization and to cure the patient.

DIAGNOSIS

Diagnosis of anaerobic pleuropulmonary infection depends on clinical, radiologic, and bacteriologic clues (Table 35-1).

Clinical Clues

Certain clinical features herald the presence of anaerobic infec-

Table 35-1
Diagnostic Clues to Anaerobic Pleuropulmonary Infections

Clinical
Foul-smelling sputum or pleural fluid
Subacute or chronic presentation
Aspiration (confirmed or suspected) and/or periodontal disease
Radiologic
Pulmonary infection with tissue necrosis
Empyema with air-fluid level in the absence of bronchopleural fistula or prior thoracentesis
Septic embolization association with prostatic or gynecologic infection
Bacteriologic
Multiple different morphologic types of gram-positive cocci and gram-negative bacilli in sputum or pleural fluid
Failure to recover a likely pathogen on aerobic culture
Discrepancy between gram-stained smear and culture
Anaerobic bacteria isolated from pleural fluid or from transtracheal aspirate

tions. One is aspiration, which may be suspected from the history in three fourths of patients. Periodontal or gingival disease should increase suspicion that pleuropulmonary infection may be due to anaerobes. In toothless persons with confirmed anaerobic lung infection a search should be made for evidence of bronchial obstruction or subdiaphragmatic foci of infection.

Another important clinical clue is the subacute nature of the infection. Most patients report having symptoms for more than a week before seeking medical attention.

Fetid breath and sputum generally are hallmarks of anaerobic pulmonary infections, but their absence does not rule out such infections. Sputum is fetid in most patients with lung abscess or anaerobic necrotizing pneumonia, but not fetid in patients with anaerobic pneumonitis. Thus, fetid sputum tends to occur relatively late in the course of the infection, when abscesses form. The sputum odor also is influenced by the type of anaerobic bacteria involved, being absent in some pulmonary infections caused by anaerobic gram-positive cocci.

A fetid odor of sputum occasionally is misleading in patients with pulmonary infections. It may result from contamination of the expectorated sputum by fetid oropharyngeal secretions, as in patients with necrotizing gingivitis. Careful oropharyngeal examination should clarify this situation.

Radiologic Clues

Anaerobic bacteria have a well-known propensity to cause tissue necrosis. Cavity formation and air-fluid levels in a dependent, poorly aerated and drained bronchopulmonary segment are immediate clues to a possible anaerobic process. However, tissue necrosis can occur with a number of other organisms, such as *S. aureus*, *K. pneumoniae*, *P. aeruginosa*, and mycobacteria. Therefore, radiologic findings are not pathognomonic for anaerobic infections.

Pyopneumothorax, in the absence of a bronchopleural fistula or prior thoracentesis, indicates the presence of gas-forming organisms and suggests an anaerobic etiology.

Bacteriologic Clues

The gram-stained smear is the most important test for rapid assessment of the presence of anaerobes. Although bacterial morphology can on occasion be characteristic, it is often impossible to distinguish many facultative from obligate anaerobes on the basis of bacterial morphology alone. However, the polymicrobial etiology of the infection is reflected in the gram stain of purulent material by the presence of many different morphologic types. The organisms seen on gram stain may fail to be isolated because of their fastidious growth requirements.

In view of the complex anaerobic flora of the oropharyngeal secretions, expectorated sputum should not be cultured anaerobically for diagnostic purposes. Such cultures would be meaningless, since they would invariably contain normal flora acquired during passage through the oral cavity. To study the role of anaerobes in pulmonary infection it is necessary to use specimens, such as percutaneous transtracheal aspirates, empyema fluid, or direct lung aspirates, that are devoid of upper airway contamination. Transtracheal aspiration should be performed only by physicians well trained in the procedure and should be avoided with patients who are uncooperative, hypoxemic or who have bleeding disorders. Direct lung aspirate is useful for bacteriologic evaluation of selected patients with pulmonary infections. Its role in diagnosis of anaerobic infections has not been extensively studied.

ANTIMICROBIAL THERAPY

Most anaerobic pleuropulmonary infections are polymicrobial, but therapy need not be directed at all species identified in the original gram-stained smears and in culture. Significant pathogens usually are present in relatively large numbers.

Penicillin G (5 to 10 million units intravenously daily in an adult) has been the drug of choice for initial treatment of all anaerobic pleuropulmonary infections. Nearly all bacteria encountered in these infections have been sensitive to penicillin. The major exceptions are *B. fragilis* and *B. melaninogenicus. B. fragilis* generally is resistant to penicillin and cephalosporins and usually is sensitive to clindamycin, metronidazole, chloramphenicol and cefoxitin. However, no need has been established to direct therapy specifically at this species in patients with anaerobic pulmonary infection. In addition, up to 60% of *B. melaninogenicus* recently have been noted to be resistant to penicillin. The clinical significance of this is as yet unknown.

Clindamycin (300 to 600 mg orally or parenterally every six to eight hours) is an effective alternative to penicillin, and a recent study (Levison et al, 1983) suggests that clindamycin is more efficacious than penicillin G in the therapy of anaerobic lung abscess. Clindamycin should be considered for patients with rapidly progressive or fulminant infection in which *B. fragilis* is or may be present and for patients who do not respond to penicillin within five to seven days. Cefoxitin also can be used. Chloramphenicol, though effective against anaerobes, should not be routinely employed for these infections because of its rare, but fatal, hematologic toxicity. Metronidazole is highly active against many anaerobes, particularly *B. fragilis*, but has relatively poor activity against aerobic, microaerophilic or facultative bacteria. It should not be used alone for initial treatment of anaerobic pleuropulmonary infections; metronidazole failures may occur in patients in whom microaerophilic or bacteria are significant pathogens (Perlino, 1981).

For hospital-acquired aspiration pneumonia, a combination of clindamycin and an aminoglycoside is the treatment of choice. Therapy for anaerobic pneumonia must generally be prolonged to prevent relapse. For uncomplicated pneumonitis, therapy should continue until the patient has been afebrile for five to sevens days. Necrotizing pneumonia usually requires at least four weeks of therapy to prevent relapse. Lung abscess should be treated until either complete clearing or a stable residual lesion is reached. Cavity closure usually occurs within two months and clearing of infiltrate within three months.

Anaerobic pneumonia or empyema from a hematogenous source (such as pelvic thrombophlebitis) or from a contiguous source (such as subphrenic abscess) may involve *B. fragilis* as the sole or predominant pathogen. Therapy should then be directed against this species, and appropriate medical and surgical measures should be instituted against the infection at the primary site.

ACTINOMYCES SPECIES

Compared to other infectious diseases, actinomycosis (almost always caused by *Actinomyces israelii*) is quite rare. Unlike nocardiosis, its incidence has not increased during the present era of antibiotics, steroids, and malignancies. Actinomycosis occurs usually in either a cervico-facial, thoracic or abdominal form.

Microbial Characteristics

Although formerly thought to be a fungus, the organisms of the genus *Actinomyces* are bacteria. They are nonmotile, nonspore-forming, gram-positive, often beaded rods which may branch to form a Y, V, or T configuration. Unlike *Nocardia*, which they may resemble morphologically, the actinomycetes are nonacid-fast and obligately anaerobic. Colonies of actinomycetes may appear in broth cultures, pus, or tissues as hard, white-yellow granules 1 to 2 mm in diameter, called sulfur granules. These are composed of masses of tangled gram-positive filaments cemented together by a polysaccharide protein secreted by the organism. The five species (*A. bovis*, *A. israelii*, *A. naeslundii*, *A. odontolyticus*, and *A. viscosus*) can be differentiated biochemically and serologically. Except for *A. viscosus*, they do not produce catalase. The end products of their glucose fermentation are acetic, formic, lactic, and succinic acids, detected by gas-liquid chromatography.

A. israelii is the principal cause of human actinomycosis; *A. viscosus* and *A. naeslundii* are involved in caries and periodontal diseases.

Arachnia propionica, which resembles the actinomycetes culturally and morphologically, can cause disease clinically similar to actinomycosis. It is differentiated by producing propionic acid from glucose, having diaminopimelic acid in the cell wall, and being serologically distinct.

A. israelii is almost never found in pure culture in actinomycotic lesions, being accompanied by other bacteria including anaerobic cocci, *Bacteroides melaninogenicus*, *Actinobacillus actinomycetem comitans*, a microaerophilic gram-negative rod, and staphylococci.

Epidemiology

Actinomycosis is worldwide in distribution. *A. israelii* has been isolated only from humans or animals, but neither man-to-man nor animal-to-man transmission has been documented. Actinomycetes are normal commensals on the mucosal surfaces of the body, and are found wherever anaerobic conditions prevail, mainly the tonsillar crypts, gingivodental crevice, and lower intestinal tract. Since all species except *A. bovis* inhabit the human oral cavity, the source of infection is endogenous. In fluorescent antibody studies of dental plaque, two or more species of *Actinomyces* were found in all specimens. *A. israelii* were found in 96% of the specimens.

Thoracic actinomycosis appears to peak at two age periods: 11 to 20 years, and 30 to 50 years. Men are affected about twice as often as are women.

Pathogenicity

Actinomycetes produce no toxins or antiphagocytic factors and few proteolytic enzymes. The filamentous growth could aid their survival by deterring phagocytosis. The sulfur granules could be antiphagocytic and may interfere with the penetration of antibiotics.

Disease occurs when the organisms penetrate deeper into tissues through breaks in the mucosa, usually as the result of trauma, to gain access to an anaerobic environment provided by dead or devitalized tissue. Dental procedures frequently precede the development of cervico-facial actinomycosis. The often-quoted association between chewing straw and actinomycosis is probably related, not to contamination of the straw with exogenous actinomycetes, but to repeated trauma to the gums.

Once *A. israelii* proliferates within tissues, it produces a chronic inflammatory reaction characterized by suppuration, necrosis, and fibrosis. The active infection spreads across fascial planes toward the skin, forming nodular abscesses which contain only a small amount of pus and which are interconnected by fistulas. Abscesses close to the skin rupture and form chronic draining sinuses. Actinomycosis spreads mainly by direct contiguity, but occasionally the organisms invade the bloodstream, and widespread dissemination occurs.

Thoracic actinomycosis apparently arises from aspiration of sufficient quantities of *A. israelii* and/or other microorganisms to produce atelectasis. The resulting anaerobic conditions favor the development of pulmonary actinomycosis. The infection usually begins as a localized pneumonitis in one of the lower lobes, but any lobe can be involved. Less commonly, pulmonary actinomycosis occurs by direct extension from either an esophagical lesion or an intra-abdominal lesion following extension through the diaphragm.

Clinical Diseases

Initial symptoms include fever, which is typically low-grade, night sweats, weight loss, and cough, usually productive of purulent or blood-streaked sputum. As pulmonary parenchymal lesions advance to the chest wall, the fever may increase markedly. Subcutaneous abscesses, chest wall fistulas and rib involvement may occur. Although chronic draining sinuses involving the chest wall are typical, empyema or pulmonary parenchymal abscess may occur without cutaneous fistulas. Diagnosis is difficult, and the disease is often misdiagnosed as tuberculosis.

Physical examination reveals unilateral or bilateral rales, dullness to percussion, and in some cases evidence of frank consolidation. Signs of pleural fluid may be present. Even if no draining sinuses are detected, the chest wall should be examined carefully for evidence of focal or diffuse inflammation.

Actinomycosis may be present with manifestations of mediastinal

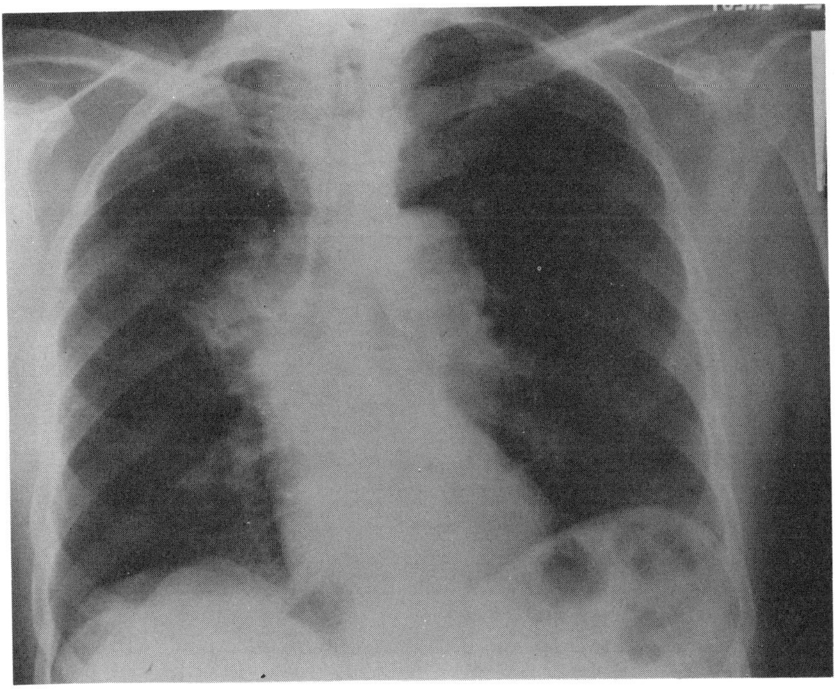

Figure 35-3 Chest radiograph revealing a right hilar mass as well as an ill-defined right upper lobe infiltrate in a patient proven to have pulmonary actinomycosis on lung biopsy.

involvement when pulmonary parenchymal disease is absent. Mediastinal actinomycosis usually is associated with abscesses that penetrate to the skin in the paravertebral regions. Thoracic actinomycosis may spread to the pericardium, heart, vertebral bodies, or through the diaphragm and involve abdominal organs. Thoracic infections also are more likely than any other form of actinomycosis to disseminate via the bloodstream to vital organs. Such patients have the poorest prognosis.

X-ray findings depend on the extent of the infection. Chest x-rays (Figure 35-3) may show focal infiltrates, areas of consolidation, abscesses, cavities, or pleural effusions. Miliary lung involvement is rare, but has been observed after hematogenous dissemination. Involvement of bones adjacent to pulmonary parenchymal lesions is common, as evidenced radiologically by osteolytic or blastic changes in the ribs or occasionally in the thoracic vertebrae.

Diagnostic Tests

Early diagnosis of actinomycosis remains a problem for most physicians. Diagnosis may be misdirected or delayed by several factors, including difficulty in recovering the organism, its presence as part of the

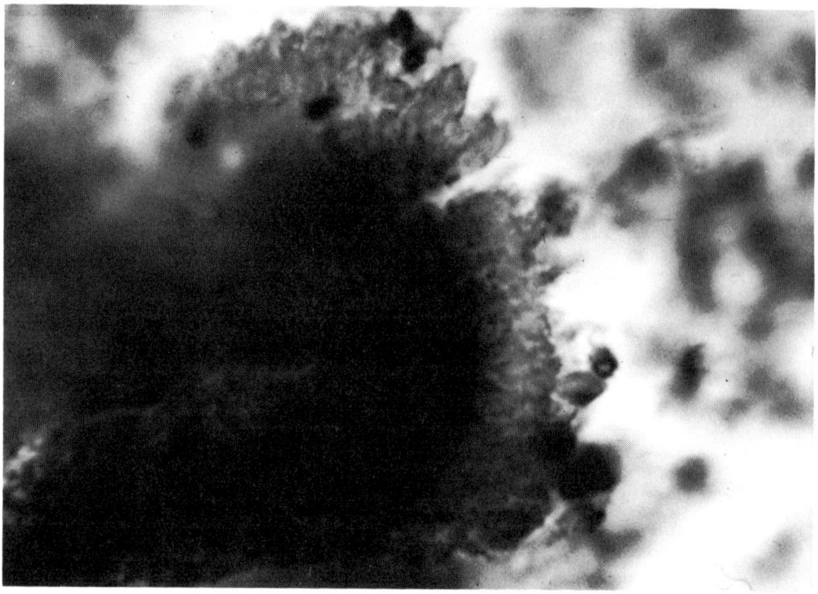

Figure 35-4 *Actinomyces* granule in tissue section; note clubbed peripheral fringe.

normal oral flora, and its special growth requirements.

The key to recognizing actinomycosis is a high index of suspicion, so that gram stains of infected material and anaerobic cultures are obtained in all possible cases. Pus from aspirates or draining sinuses and biopsied specimens of infected tissue are suitable for culture. Tissue should be stained with hematoxylin and eosin; use of the Brown and Brenn modification of the gram stain enhances recognition.

If sulfur granules are present (Figure 35-4), they can be located by diluting the tissue specimen with saline and filtering it through gauze. Such granules should be cultured because grossly similar structures may be found in other diseases, such as cutaneous nocardiosis and botryomycosis. An agar-gel double-diffusion test for serum antibodies to *Actinomyces* was recently developed, but it is not generally useful.

Therapy and Prevention

Penicillin is the drug of choice, although tetracyclines are also effective. For patients with pulmonary actinomycosis, intravenous administration of 12 to 20 million units of aqueous penicillin daily in the adult for four to six weeks is recommended, followed by six to eight months of oral penicillin. Alternate therapy in those allergic to penicillin is tetracycline 500 mg every 6 h for six to eight months. Definite abscesses or empyema require surgical drainage. Infected ribs and other foci of osteomyelitis may warrant resection. The most important way to prevent actinomycosis is to maintain a high standard of oral hygiene.

SELECTED READINGS

Bartlett JG: Anaerobic bacterial pneumonitis. *Am Rev Respir Dis* 1979;119:19–23.

Bartlett JG, Finegold SM: Anaerobic infections of the lung and the pleural space. *Am Rev Respir Dis* 1974;110:207–228.

Bartlett JG, Gorbach SL, Finegold SM: The bacteriology of aspiration pneumonia. *Am J Med* 1974;56:202–207.

Bartlett JG, Gorbach SL, Thadepalli H, et al: Bacteriology of empyema. *Lancet* 1974;1:338–340.

Bates M, Cruickshank G: Thoracic actinomycosis. *Thorax* 1957;12:99.

Brown JR: Human actinomycosis: A study of 181 subjects. *Hum Pathol* 1973; 4:319.

Estrera AS, Platt MR, Mills LJ, et al: Primary lung abscess. *J Thorac Cardiovasc Surg* 1980;79:275–282.

Flynn MW, Felson B: The roentgen manifestations of thoracic actinomycosis. *Am J Roentgenol Rad Ther Nucl Med* 1970;110:707.

Levison ME, Mangura CT, Lorber B, et al: Penicillin vs. clindamycin for the treatment of anaerobic lung abscess. *Ann Intern Med* 1983;98:466–471.

Light RW, Girard WM, Jenkinson SG, et al: Parapneumonic effusions. *Am J Med* 1980;69:507–512.

Lorber B, Swenson BM: Bacteriology of aspiration pneumonia: A prospective study of community- and hospital-acquired cases. *Ann Intern Med* 1974;81: 329–331.

Perlino CA: Metronidazole vs. clindamycin treatment of anaerobic pulmonary infection: Failure of metronidazole therapy. *Arch Intern Med* 1981;141: 1424–1427.

Robboy SJ, Vickery AL Jr: Tinctorial and morphologic properties distinguishing actinomycosis and nocardiosis. *N Engl J Med* 1970;282:593.

Slade PR, Slesser BV, Southgate J: Thoracic actinomycosis. *Thorax* 1973;28:73.

Weese WE, Smith IM: A study of 57 cases of actinomycosis over a 36 year period. *Arch Intern Med* 1975;135:1562.

36 *Mycobacteria*

Clifford G. Wlodaver
Rob Roy MacGregor

Tuberculosis is a necrotizing bacterial infection. The lungs are the most common organ involved. Infection may remain asymptomatic, or disease may develop soon after the initial exposure (primary tuberculosis). The much more common form of disease, however, is reactivation of a dormant focus months to years after the initial infection, usually presenting clinically as a state of wasting and chronic pneumonia. Since the advent of antituberculosis chemotherapy, the disease is curable in almost every case. The incidence of infection and disease has subsequently decreased dramatically. Tuberculosis, nonetheless, remains a significant health problem and deserves consideration in the differential diagnosis of most pulmonary diseases.

BACTERIOLOGY

The causative agent in tuberculosis is *Mycobacterium tuberculosis.* Other mycobacteria, referred to as nontuberculous or atypical, may rarely cause disease similar to tuberculosis. *Mycobacterium avium-intracellulare* and *M. kansasii* are the organisms most often involved in these diseases.

Microscopy

Mycobacteria are acid-fast, nonmotile, nonsporulating rods. The organism's lipid-rich, hydrophobic cell wall accounts for its characteristic staining properties: relatively resistant to staining with water-soluble dyes, requiring heat or addition of surface-active agents to facilitate uptake. Once stained, however, they are resistant to decolorization by an acid-alcohol wash, which is the origin of the term "acid-fast." The Ziehl-Neelsen procedure is the conventional acid-fast staining technique. In addition to *M. tuberculosis* and the other mycobacteria, rhodococcus, *Nocardia*, and the Pittsburgh Pneumonia Agent are also acid-fast to some degree, such that confirmation by culture is necessary.

Since the acid-fast bacilli (AFB) may be difficult to recognize and may be present in small numbers, the smear should be examined carefully for 30 minutes and compared to a positive control. Many microbiology laboratories are now using a fluorochrome procedure, using such stains as auramine and rhodamine, since it facilitates rapid screening of sputum specimens. Positive results should be confirmed by a staining technique to demonstrate the organism's acid-fast character.

Cultures

Since cultures are more sensitive and specific than smears in the detection of tuberculosis, all specimens suspected of containing *Mycobacteria* also should be cultured. The drawback of culture, however, is that it will take from three to eight weeks to become positive, the former being the usual interval, particularly if the smear were initially positive. The slow in vitro growth of this organism compared to most other bacteria helps one appreciate the chronic course of tuberculosis observed clinically.

There are two kinds of media commonly used for culture. One is a complex medium containing egg and potato extract such as the Lowenstein-Jensen medium; the other is semisynthetic and contains oleic acid and albumin, known as the Middlebrook 7H-11 agar medium. Mycobacteria are obligate aerobes, which aids in understanding why most pulmonary tuberculosis occurs in the lung apices, where the alveolar PO_2 is highest.

Identification

The colonies are cream-colored, dry and rough with irregular edges. *M. tuberculosis* can be distinguished from other mycobacteria by its slow rate of growth, failure to develop pigment, ability to produce niacin, susceptibility to INH, and tendency to grow in a serpentine fashion. The latter property, referred to as cord formation, is significant to the clinician because virulence is associated with its presence. Moreover, cording may be recognized within 10 to 21 days of incubation, thereby permitting an early, albeit presumptive diagnosis of *M. tuberculosis*. Guinea pig inoculations are no longer widely used because of their relative costliness, and the technological advantages of the biochemical methods.

Specimen Collection

The first expectorated sputum in the morning offers the best chance to recover mycobacteria. A series of at least three separate specimens should be collected on successive days, since the presence of the organisms may be intermittent. Sputa should not be collected over a long time period since this increases the risk of contamination. If expectorated specimens are unobtainable—because the patient is a child or debilitated—sputum induced by inhalation of hypertonic heated aerosols should be attempted. If this fails to yield adequate specimens, gastric aspiration can be performed, because organisms are cleared from the lung by the mucociliary blanket, and drained into the stomach. This should be done first thing in the morning before overnight gastric contents have been passed from the stomach. A smear of such a specimen is less reliable than that of sputum because of the frequency of saprophytic acid-fast bacilli in the stomach, and should be avoided.

Finally, if bacteriologic diagnosis remains in question, invasive procedures such as transtracheal aspiration, bronchoscopy with brushing, washing and transbronchial biopsy, and percutaneous needle biopsy or open lung biopsy are available options. If tuberculosis is highly suspected, however, the risks of these procedures should be weighed against those of a trial of antituberculous chemotherapy. Conversely, when a pulmonary lesion of unknown etiology is being evaluated by one of these procedures, specimens should always be sent for acid-fast smear and culture. If bronchoscopy is performed, sputum produced subsequently should be collected and examined since the yield may be higher than that obtained at the time of bronchoscopy.

PATHOGENESIS (Figure 36-1)

Tuberculosis is not highly infectious. A fairly prolonged or frequent association with an infectious person generally is required for infection to be transmitted.

Transmission

Transmission occurs through the airborne route, such that the greatest risk is to persons who share an enclosed environment with someone who has the disease. Such a person forms an aerosol of saliva, mucus

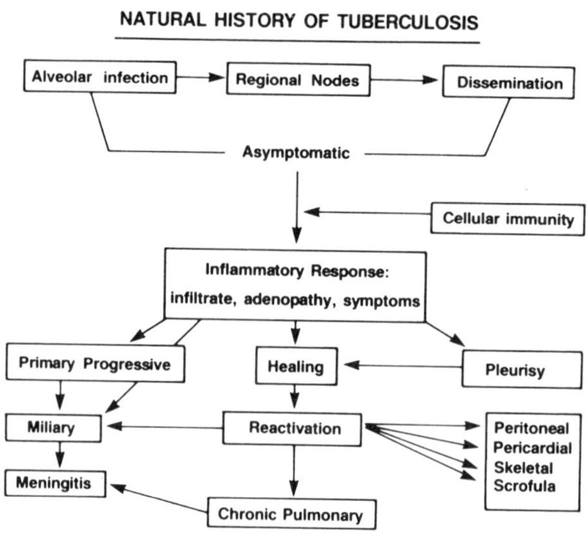

Figure 36-1

and organisms by coughing, sneezing, singing or perhaps merely by breathing and talking. Most droplets are heavy and fall quickly to the floor. Through the evaporation of water, however, the dried residue of some of the smaller particles may remain suspended in air for prolonged periods of time, and these so-called *droplet nuclei* may be inhaled. If sufficiently small, they may find their way to the respiratory bronchioles and alveoli where removal is difficult and bacteriological multiplication can begin. Fomites, such as dishes and eating utensils, and clothes and bedding are of virtually no importance in the spread of infection.

The transmission and pathogenesis of infection with mycobacteria other than *M. tuberculosis* and *M. bovis* are not understood. Many of these bacteria can be found in the environment (soil, water, food, etc), and can be grown occasionally from the upper respiratory tract of healthy persons, as well as from the bronchial secretions of individuals with chronic lung diseases. These organisms cause disease less often than *M. tuberculosis*. Immunocompromised hosts are particularly vulnerable.

Initial Infection and Dissemination

Initially, the proliferating organisms cause very little tissue reaction and, for the first few weeks after infection, the previously unexposed host has no specific immune defense against the multiplication of the mycobacteria. They gain access to the lymphatics, regional and hilar nodes, and disseminate widely via the lymphohematogenous route, setting up foci which then have the potential to cause disease at any subsequent time. The initial infection and dissemination are asymptomatic. But, during this time the patient's cellular immune system becomes activated, reacting to the antigenic challenge presented by tuberculoprotein on the cell wall of the mycobacteria. Activated T-lymphocytes and macrophages subsequently surround organisms containing this protein and kill most of them. In some instances, particularly when there is a large inoculum of organisms, the lymphocytes may elaborate cytotoxins that cause cellular necrosis, called *caseation*, because of its cheeselike appearance. Macrophages differentiate into epithelioid cells and fibroblasts to form multinucleated giant cells. The aggregation of acid-fast bacilli, mononuclear cell infiltration, multinuclear giant cells and caseation form a tuberculous granuloma (Figure 36-2). Fibrosis and calcification occur as the lesion ages.

Development of Cell-Mediated Immunity and Skin Test Reactivity

Cell-mediated immunity develops in two to 10 weeks after initial infection with *M. tuberculosis*. It is responsible for skin test reactivity to tuberculoprotein. The infected person's lymphocytes have become sensitized for life and will react to any subsequent challenge with this

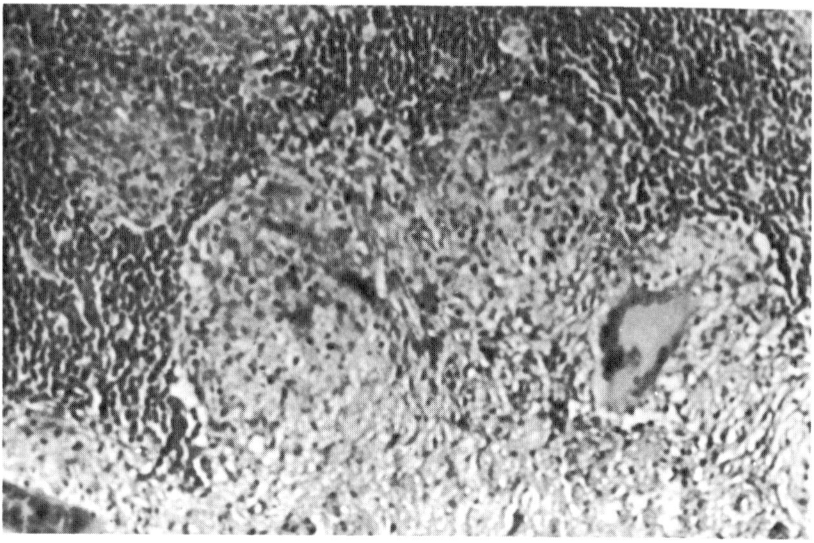

Figure 36-2 Tuberculous granuloma of a lymph node, with a multinucleate giant cell. The acid-fast stain of this specimen was positive (40 X).

protein.

Development of the inflammatory response is associated with an infiltrate at the site of primary infection and regional adenopathy, and occasionally is accompanied by "flu-like" symptoms of myalgia and fever. Whether or not the infection will progress to disease depends on the initial efficacy and ultimate integrity of the cellular immune response. If circumstances are unfavorable for multiplication of the organisms, they may remain dormant for several years, persisting in the fibrous tissue.

Development of Tuberculous Disease

A small percentage of the initial infections will progress directly to disease, presenting clinically as pneumonia, pleurisy or disseminated disease. In primary tuberculous pneumonia, the initial inoculum proliferates and spreads endobronchially before containment can take place, resulting in an acute pneumonia. Another manifestation of primary tuberculosis occurs when organisms spill into the pleural cavity, resulting in a large antigenic stimulus and subsequent inflammation and pleural effusion. A pleural effusion also may occur at any time after the initial infection. Finally, if the dissemination of organisms entirely overwhelms and outpaces its inhibition by cell-mediated immunity, disseminated disease will develop, known as miliary tuberculosis, because of the millet seed-sized lesions it produces. Miliary tuberculosis also can occur following recrudescence of an old lesion with subsequent hematogenous dissemination.

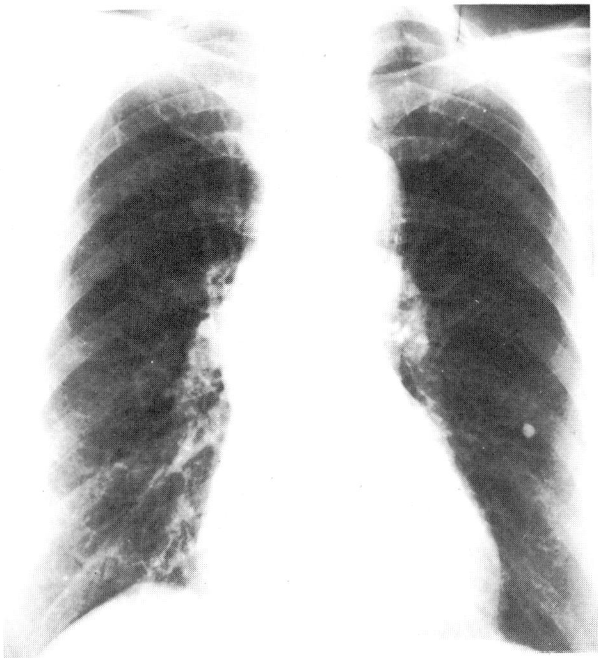

Figure 36-3 Ghon complex.

More commonly, however, the host-parasite relationship is such that the organisms become sealed off and disease does not occur. The patient never realizes that he has been infected with tuberculosis. The telltale signs that infection has occurred are the skin test reactivity to tuberculoprotein, and perhaps the calcified initial pulmonary lesion and regional lymph node seen on chest x-ray, known as a Ghon complex (Figure 36-3).

At some later date, if the host-parasite balance breaks down to favor the latter, reactivation of the infection may proceed to disease. Although this may occur at any site of primary dissemination, the majority of cases involve the lung, in particular the apices, where the PO_2 is highest. When reactivation occurs, cavitation may ensue (Figure 36-4), breaking down mechanical barriers and liberating organisms for further spread via the bronchial tree, and becoming the source of infection to others.

The clinical manifestations of these lesions are discussed in the section on clinical syndromes.

Factors Predisposing to Reactivation

Several situations that predispose to reactivation tuberculosis are listed in Table 36-1. Most of these can be understood mechanistically by their depressive effect on cell-mediated immunity. The importance of

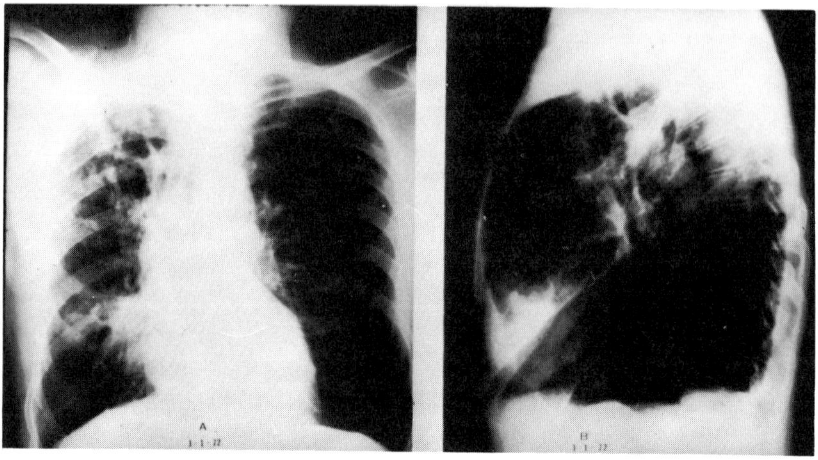

Figure 36-4 Chronic tuberculosis with cavitation.

local factors walling off infection is illustrated by the development of disease associated with destructive lung lesions, such as neoplasia, trauma and surgery. Similarly, destructive infections such as lung abscess can erode into an old tuberculosis focus, thereby releasing organisms.

CLINICAL SYNDROMES

Skin Test Reactivity

The standard skin test reagent for *M. tuberculosis* is known as *purified protein derivative* (PPD), which comes in strengths of 1, 5, and 250 tuberculin units (TU). The intracutaneous injection of 0.1 mL of the 5-TU PPD is known as the Mantoux test. Applied and interpreted correctly (Table 36-2), the reaction to this test defines whether or not the patient's cell-mediated immune system has ever become sensitized to PPD (via primary infection), as discussed in the section on cell-mediated im-

Table 36-1
Factors that Predispose to Reactivation of an Old Tuberculous Focus

Cytotoxic therapy	Gastric resection
Corticosteroid therapy	Malnutrition
Radiation therapy	Old age
Malignancy (especially pulmonary and lymphoproliferative disorders)	Sarcoidosis
Diabetes	Anthracosis/silicosis
Severe viral disease (eg, influenza)	Thoracic surgery and trauma
Alcoholism	Destructive infections of lung (eg, abscess, histoplasmosis)

Table 36-2
Principles of Skin-Testing

1. Use Tween—stabilized tuberculin (5 units - PPD)
2. Mantoux intradermal injection
3. Read induration at 48 hours; valid up to 96 hours
4. Read two perpendicular diameters by light touch
5. Record millimeters of induration, not negative or positive
6. > 5 mm is a positive reaction

   5–10 mm, probable atypical mycobacteria cross-reaction

   > 10 mm, "significantly positive," indicates *M. tuberculosis* infection

munity. Whereas infected persons so defined do not have tuberculous *disease*, they represent the population in which reactivation disease can develop. Five percent to 15% of persons who develop a positive skin reaction will progress to active disease within five years. Of those remaining well for five years, a further 3% to 5% will develop disease at some later time, such that the total morbidity of persons infected with *M. tuberculosis* ranges from 8% to 20%. The relative risks of reactivation of an old tuberculous focus are shown in Table 36-3.

There are several clinical situations in which the interpretation of the skin reaction is uncertain. False-negative reactions may occur because of improper techniques, and when cell-mediated immunity is immature, depressed, or overwhelmed by disseminated disease (Table 36-4). Up to 15% of patients with active pulmonary tuberculosis will be 5-TU PPD-negative. In individuals who do not react to tuberculin but are suspect for tuberculosis, skin tests to which virtually all persons react, such as dermatophyton, mumps, streptokinase-streptodornase, and *Candida*

Table 36-3
Relative Risk of Reactivation of Old Tuberculous Focus

Recent converter (infection)	1/30 in first year after infection
Household contacts	1/37 during 10-year observation
Old active disease, untreated	1/70 per year
"Scars" on x-ray, no known active disease	1/125 per year
Rx with drugs that suppress cell-mediated immunity (steroids, cytotoxins)	–
Diseases of impaired CMI (sarcoid, leukemia, lymphoma)	–
Chronic debilitating disease (diabetes, COPD, cancer, etc)	–
Strongly positive reaction	– (> 30 mm 3 × rate for 10 mm)

albicans, should be applied to test the integrity of the patient's cellular immune system. This group of skin tests is known collectively as an anergy panel.

False-positive reactions may occur because of cross-reactivity between *M. tuberculosis* and the nontuberculous mycobacteria. These reactions usually are in the 5 to 10 mm range, and are especially common in the southeastern United States where sensitivity to other mycobacteria is common. Skin tests for the nontuberculous mycobacteria are not commonly available. Moreover, their interpretation is difficult, such that ultimate differentiation from *M. tuberculosis* requires bacteriologic identification. Previous exposure to the antituberculosis vaccine, BCG, may also cause tuberculin sensitivity without indicating infection. Since there is no way of differentiating tuberculous infection from reactivity to BCG, the United States Public Health Service recommends disregarding a history of BCG in evaluating a positive PPD.

Table 36-4
False-Negative Tuberculin Skin Tests

I. Technical
   A. Improper amount of tuberculin given
      1. Dilutions or amount incorrect
      2. Loss of potency
      3. Adsorption on syringes
      4. Subcutaneous injection
   B. Incorrect reading

II. Nonspecific Decrease In Immunity
   A. Intercurrent infections (eg, CMV, measles, infectious mononucleosis)
   B. Cachexia
   C. Hypothyroidism
   D. Dehydration

III. Decrease in Delayed Hypersensitivity
   A. Hormonal
      1. Late pregnancy and puerperium
      2. During steroid therapy
   B. Nonhormonal
      1. Sarcoidosis
      2. After viral immunization
      3. With diseases of the lymphoid system
      4. With irradiation
      5. With immunosuppressive therapy

IV. Undeveloped Hypersensitivity
   A. Early in tuberculosis

V. Immunologic Blockade
   A. Miliary or far advanced tuberculosis

VI. Loss of Reactivity
   A. Associated with old age

Repeated tuberculin skin testing of an uninfected individual is not sensitizing and does not result in a positive reaction. In contrast, in a person with an established mycobacterial infection, sequential testing—as might occur in annual routine screening of hospital employees—can result in an increase in size of the skin reaction. This is known as the *booster phenomenon*, and carries considerable clinical significance since it can be mistaken for a recent conversion and the implications therein. The phenomenon is noted to occur as soon as one week after the initial test, and may persist for a year, or longer. It may occur at any age, but is noted more frequently in the elderly, for two reasons. First, from an epidemiologic standpoint, this group is more likely to harbor tuberculosis. Second, skin test reactivity wanes over time, such that the initial PPD in an elderly person with quiescent infection is more likely to be smaller than that in a younger person with a comparable stage of infection. When sequential testing is employed, the American Thoracic Society recommends an initial two-stage skin test to eliminate the possibility of a booster phenomenon being interpreted as a recent conversion. If the first test is < 10 mm, a second should be given one to two weeks later. If the second test is also < 10 mm, this indicates no infection. In this case, a significant reaction on subsequent testing will indicate recent conversion. If the second test is > 10 mm, this indicates a remote infection and the booster phenomenon.

Since the definition of tuberculous infection is a positive 5-TU PPD, the usefulness of 1 and 250-TU, multiple puncture tests and antigens prepared from other mycobacteria is controversial and has led to considerable confusion. Use of the 1-TU PPD has been proposed when there is the possibility of a very strong reaction that might cause a large and angry local inflammation. The 250-TU PPD is recommended when the 5-TU is negative and tuberculosis is still suspected. A negative reaction to the 250-TU makes the diagnosis of tuberculosis unlikely. A positive reaction means that the diagnosis of active tuberculosis cannot be dismissed, although it may also represent a falsely positive reaction secondary to cross-reactivity with the nontuberculous mycobacteria. There are several multiple puncture skin tests commercially available. Although they are easier to perform and generally more convenient than the Mantoux test, interpretation is less well defined. These tests are recommended by some as good for screening out nonreactors since the dose usually is high. As a consequence, however, positive reactions may be secondary to nontuberculous mycobacteria and require confirmation with the Mantoux test. False-negative results also occur occasionally, usually because application of these tests is difficult to standardize. Antigens prepared from the nontuberculous mycobacteria exist, but reactions to these agents lack specificity such that their use is mainly for epidemiologic surveys, and limited when attempting to identify which mycobacteria is causing disease in an individual patient.

Table 36-5
Indications for INH Prophylaxis

1. Recent conversion to positive PPD
2. Household contact of active case
3. Old Tb, never treated
4. Positive PPD or anergy in patients to be treated with steroid or cytotoxic therapy
5. Positive PPD in patient with cancer or debilitating disease

Both the early and late appearance of tuberculous disease can be prevented in 70% to 80% of infected individuals if prompt therapy with isoniazid (INH) is given when conversion is discovered. Accordingly, it would seem reasonable to treat all persons who are tuberculin-positive. This approach is not totally acceptable, however, because INH causes liver disease in some individuals. Table 36-5 lists the recommendations formulated by the American Thoracic Society and the Centers for Disease Control regarding which PPD-positive individuals should receive INH, weighing the relative risks of reactivation of an old focus of tuberculosis (Table 36-3) against the age-related risk of developing INH-associated hepatitis (Table 36-6). Since recent converters, household contacts, individuals with a history of old active tuberculosis that has not been treated, and individuals with scarring on chest x-ray are all at significant risk of reactivation, they should receive INH regardless of age. Likewise, previously untreated persons who are particularly predisposed to reactivation of an old tuberculous focus (Table 36-1), regardless of age, should be considered good candidates for INH. Finally, any PPD-positive individual less than 35 years old should receive INH.

Whereas the complication of INH-related liver disease is well described, there remains some controversy regarding the most judicious approach to its management. No one would argue that symptoms of hepatitis and marked elevations of hepatic enzymes necessitate immediate discontinuation of the drug. Less clear, however, is what to do about the mild elevations in hepatic enzymes that occur in many patients during the first few months of therapy. Arbitrary limits for discontinuing the drug when the SGOT increases three- to five-times normal have been proposed.

Table 36-6
Age-Related Risk of INH Hepatitis

Age	Risk
under 20	rare
20–34	up to 0.3%
35–49	up to 1.2%
over 50	up to 2.3%

Since these elevations are transient and not accompanied by any symptoms, an alternative and perhaps more rational approach would be to advise patients regarding the symptoms and signs of hepatitis and to discontinue the INH at once should symptoms develop. Such a plan would obviate any systematic evaluation of hepatic enzymes.

Primary Tuberculosis

Primary tuberculosis occurs when the initial focus evolves into an acute infiltrate. The symptoms and signs are those of acute bacterial pneumonia. Formerly, this disease occurred mainly in children. As the prevalence of tuberculosis decreases, however, there are an increasing number of tuberculin-negative persons entering adulthood. When these adults first become infected, they may develop a disease that is atypical for adult tuberculosis and difficult to recognize. It differs from chronic, reactivation disease in that hilar adenopathy is prominent. The middle and lower lobes are commonly involved as opposed to apical disease in chronic tuberculosis. The initial PPD may be negative. Diagnosis depends on recovery of the organism.

Tuberculous Pleural Disease

If a parenchymal tuberculous lesion extends to the pleura, tuberculous pleurisy develops. This usually occurs as a manifestation of primary disease. Although self-limited, 65% of untreated patients will develop active pulmonary tuberculosis within five years.

Approximately two thirds of the cases present with an acute disease similar to bacterial pneumonitis, with cough and pleuritic chest pain as the major symptoms. The disease is insidious in onset in the remainder of cases. Temperature may be normal at the onset, and friction rubs are not common. The initial PPD is negative in almost one third of cases, but ultimately becomes positive on repeat testing. The chest x-ray shows a pleural effusion that is most often unilateral. Active parenchymal lesions are seen in approximately one third of the cases. Pleural fluid is characterized by a predominance of lymphocytes, although early cases may show predominantly polymorphonuclear cells. Mesothelial cells usually are absent. There is an elevated protein and LDH. The glucose usually is >50 mg%. Diagnosis is based on recovery of the organism by pleural biopsy culture and histologic exam, and pleural fluid culture. Although culture of pleural fluid is positive in $<30\%$ of cases, pleural biopsy culture and histologic exam are each positive in more than two thirds of patients. If a patient is PPD-positive and has an unexplained pleural effusion, empiric treatment for active tuberculosis is recommended.

Reactivation Pulmonary Tuberculosis

Chronic pulmonary tuberculosis develops from reactivation of an old focus of infection. Epidemiologically, advanced age, non-white race, and urban environment are associated with this disease, as are conditions that depress cell-mediated immunity and disrupt mechanical barriers (Table 36-1).

The disease is initially asymptomatic, and small apical infiltrates can persist for months to years, in tenuous balance with host defenses, undergoing minor regressions and extensions. When the host defenses are depressed and the balance is tipped in favor of the mycobacteria, proliferation ensues and stimulates increased inflammatory reaction in the lung. Symptoms usually develop insidiously and progress slowly. The most common symptoms are weight loss and fatigue. Although fever frequently is present, this may not be recognized by the patient. Night sweats may occur, along with cough and sputum production. Chest pain may occur if the lesion extends to the pleural surface, although effusions usually do not develop (dry pleurisy). Hemoptysis may occur secondary to ulceration of the bronchial mucosa and usually is minor. Severe hemoptysis occurs uncommonly and is discussed below.

The disease progresses by direct extension and is characterized by slow deterioration attributed to the chronic inflammatory reaction induced in this host-parasite relationship. If a cavity develops, endobronchial extension of disease ensues and the patient can rapidly become more ill.

On physical examination, it is important to appreciate that the patient may not appear ill (Table 36-7). Wasting and fever may be present, but their absence is still consistent with active disease. Signs of pulmonary infiltration are often subtle or altogether absent. When present, they include rales, especially when inspiration is preceded by full expiration and a small cough (posttussive rales), bronchial breath sounds, whispered pectoriloquy, dullness to percussion, and increased tactile fremitus. If a cavity is present, a hollow breath sound may be heard, and is referred to as amphoric breathing since it resembles the sound made when blowing across the mouth of a jar (amphora). Fibrosis may cause decreased and asymmetric ventilatory excursion of the chest wall, deviation of the trachea, and apical dullness. Early infiltrates and cavities may be undetectable by physical exam, emphasizing the importance of the chest x-ray if tuberculosis is suspected.

The chest x-ray is critical for diagnosis, determination of extent of disease, and evaluation of response to therapy. The characteristic findings for tuberculosis are a patchy infiltrate, with or without cavitation, in the apical and posterior segments of the upper lobes, although other areas can be involved (Figure 36-4). Tomograms occasionally reveal cavities not seen on standard films.

Epidemiologic surveys have generated data from which statistical probabilities regarding PPD reactivity are based. A reaction of 5 mm or more is considered significant if the individual is suspected of having

Table 36-7
Pulmonary Tb: History and Physical Examination Data from the Hospital of the University of Pennsylvania Tb Review

History	No. of Patients Evaluated	No. Positive	Percent Positive
Cough	36	29	81
Anorexial, weight loss (Average—22 pounds)	36	27	75
Sweats, chills	34	21	62
Fatigue, malaise	29	17	59
Fever	34	15	44
Hemoptysis	29	7	24
Active tuberculosis in the past	21	4 (definite) 3 (possible)	33
Physical finding			
Fever (100° F)	41	6	15
Wasting	34	12	35
Pulmonary rales	36	10	28
Dullness	37	10	27
Hepatomegaly	36	7	15
Splenomegaly	36	2	6

Reprinted with permission from MacGregor RR: A year's experience with tuberculosis in a private urban teaching hospital in the post-sanitorium era. *Am J Med* 1975;58:221.

tuberculosis or is a close contact of a person with tuberculosis. A reaction of 10 mm or more is considered significant when screening populations.

Although the clinical history, chest x-ray and tuberculin reactivity may be suggestive of tuberculosis, the diagnosis of active tuberculosis depends on demonstration of the organism. Smears for acid-fast bacteria should be done on sputum, and if positive, will lend strong support to the diagnosis. Since some patients shed mycobacteria irregularly and in small numbers, several specimens should be submitted if the diagnosis is strongly suspected. Confirmation by culture is required for the definitive diagnosis. For smear-positive patients, chemotherapy for seven to 10 days does not substantially reduce the potential for obtaining a positive culture. However, in smear-negative patients who have a smaller number of organisms, chemotherapy may result in negative cultures such that all specimens should be submitted before therapy is begun. The strategy for evaluation of suspect tuberculosis is shown in Figure 36-5. A patient is isolated and treated on the suspicion of tuberculosis, before proof has been documented. Moreover, a negative smear does not argue against the diagnosis of tuberculosis, since up to 60% of smears may be negative while the culture is positive. However, a negative smear does indicate that the number of tuberculous organisms potentially present in the

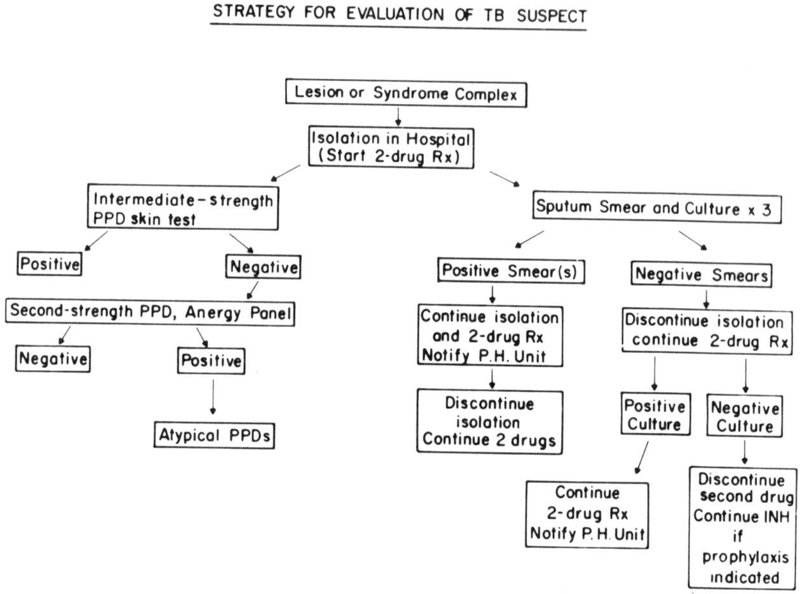

Figure 36-5

sputum is small, such that the potential for transmission is low and isolation not indicated. Practically, suspected cases are isolated until a total of three smears are negative. If smear-positive, isolation should be continued for two weeks. Treatment is begun empirically with two drugs. If cultures are negative at six weeks, the second drug is discontinued. Continuation or discontinuation of INH is predicated on skin test reactivity and risk factors.

Tuberculosis may cause nonspecific but severe abnormalities in the body's chemistry. A marked normochromic normocytic anemia may develop. The white blood cell county usually is normal, but occasionally reveals a monocytosis of 8% to 15%. The serum albumin may be decreased, and the globulins and erythrocyte sedimentation rate increased. The serum sodium may be decreased secondary to the syndrome of inappropriate secretion of antidiuretic hormone (SIADH).

There are several diseases that resemble tuberculosis and must be included in the differential diagnosis. These are listed in Table 36-8, many of which are discussed in other chapters of this book. Confusion is sometimes caused by the systemic effects of tuberculosis when other aspects of the clinical syndrome are lacking. It is remarkable how often tuberculosis does not present "classically" and is misdiagnosed. In a recent study, only 55% of cases were suspected clinically. As the incidence of tuberculosis decreases, our index of suspicion for its diagnosis decreases, resulting in an increased number of missed diagnoses. To prevent this, it seems wise to rule out the possibility of tuberculosis in all patients over 40 years old who are undergoing evaluation for pulmonary disease of undetermined etiology. In general, disease produced by other mycobacteria is indistinguishable from tuberculosis, and culture is required to make the differentiation.

Cavitation of a tuberculous infiltrate is the most common complication of disease. It is significant to the patient because it accelerates spread of disease by dissemination through the endobronchial tree. Moreover, cavitation has important epidemiologic consequences since it greatly increases the number of organisms liberated into the environment.

Hemoptysis usually is minor, but may be copious if an artery ruptures in the wall of a cavtity (Rasmussin's aneurysm). Significant hemoptysis can also occur from an aspergilloma growing in an old tuberculosis cavity. No therapy other than rest and antituberculous antibiotics is recommended unless the bleeding is massive ($>$ 400 mL in 30 minutes), which requires emergency pulmonary resection.

Tuberculous pneumonia, which can develop from primary as well as reactivation disease, is a syndrome characterized by acute onset, fever, chills, productive cough, chest pain, and leukocytosis, resembling in most every way acute bacterial pneumonia. This manifestation of tuberculosis usually occurs in blacks, diabetics, children and the elderly, and other populations with depressed cellular immunity.

Bronchopleural fistula with empyema is a complication of tuberculosis that occurs infrequently. It is seen particularly in old patients previously treated for tuberculosis with pneumothorax and no chemotherapy. It is characterized on chest x-ray by changing air-fluid

Table 36-8
Diseases That Should Be Considered in the Differential Diagnosis of Tuberculosis

Lung cancer
Mycotic infections (histoplasmosis, coccidiomycosis, aspergillosis, blastomycosis, cryptococcosis, sporotrichosis)
Actinomycosis, nocardiosis
Sarcoidosis
Aspiration pneumonia
Lung abscess
Acute bacterial and atypical pneumonias
Pneumoconiosis
Bronchiectasis
Nontuberculous mycobacterial disease, *M. kansasii* and *M. avium-intracellulare*

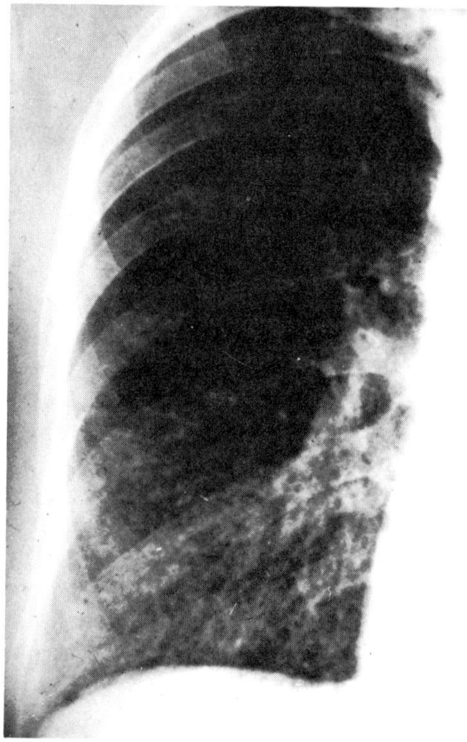

Figure 36-6 Miliary tuberculosis.

levels. In addition to chemotherapy, drainage and surgical repair are also necessary.

Miliary Tuberculosis

When tuberculosis proliferates diffusely in the lungs and other organs, the term miliary tuberculosis is applied, referring to the millet seed-sized lesions that characterize this disease. It may develop both from primary disease or from reactivation of a latent focus with subsequent dissemination.

The clinical presentation is nonspecific, the main symptoms being weakness, anorexia, weight loss, fever, cough and perhaps dyspnea. The onset is insidious, and several weeks usually pass between the initial symptoms and hospitalization.

Physical examination is remarkable for fever, rapid respirations and pulse, and wasting. Adventitious pulmonary sounds, hepatosplenomegaly and lymphadenopathy also are relatively common. The PPD usually is positive, but may be negative if the disease overwhelms the patient's immune system. Accordingly, tests for anergy should be performed when the PPD is negative and tuberculosis is still suspected. The chest x-ray classically shows miliary tubercles (Figure 36-6). However, these may not be visible for the first few weeks of disease, such that initially negative chest x-rays do not rule out this diagnosis.

The diagnostic evaluation should include a sputum smear, which is positive in approximately one third of cases, and sputum culture, which is positive in two thirds of cases. If the sputum is negative, acid-fast bacilli may be found in extrapulmonary sites. Biopsies of liver, lymph nodes, bone marrow and skin lesions, and cultures of urine and cerebrospinal fluid generally are indicated, particularly if there is any clinical evidence that these sites are involved. The alkaline phosphatase is elevated in one third of cases. The PO_2 is often decreased, and the adult respiratory distress syndrome (ARDS) may develop. The hematopoietic system shows a wide spectrum of changes, ranging from pancytopenia to a leukemoid reaction, with mild to severe leukocytosis. Most commonly, the total white blood cell count is normal, but with a relative increase in the number of band forms.

Miliary tuberculosis should be considered in the differential diagnosis of any fever of unknown origin. It may resemble a rapidly progressive lymphoma, since the disease is ultimately fatal if left untreated, and the diagnosis may remain obscure because of its nonspecific clinical presentation and the difficulty in demonstrating the organism. A therapeutic trial with antituberculosis chemotherapy may be indicated if the patient is failing and no other diagnosis has been confirmed. The temperature will often begin to decrease within three to four days of treatment.

TREATMENT AND PREVENTION

In the preantibiotic era, management of tuberculosis was limited to bedrest and surgery. The objective of bedrest, which was strict and recommended for two to four years, was to swing the tenuous balance between the patient's immune defenses and the proliferating organisms in favor of the host. This approach was often successful, especially in cases of minimally active disease. Various surgical procedures, such as induced pneumothorax and thoracoplasty, were aimed at collapsing the affected lung segment (collapse therapy), thereby decreasing the PO_2 again in an attempt to tip the balance to the host's advantage. Surgical excision of the tuberculous lesion was also attempted on occasion. These modalities were marginally effective and carried a significant risk of spread of the infection.

Conventional Chemotherapy

There was a dramatic change in the treatment and course of tuberculosis with the introduction of streptomycin in 1948, para-aminosalicylic acid (PAS) in 1950, and isoniazid (INH) in 1951. We now had the ability to eradicate infection rather than merely modifying the host-parasite relationship. INH, in combination with either streptomycin or PAS, resulted in a cure rate of at least 90%.

The principles of antituberculosis chemotherapy are listed in Table 36-9. Multiple drugs are used to decrease the development of resistance, since a certain number of naturally occurring mutants will be present and resistant to any one drug. For example, one in 100,000 and one in one million tubercle bacilli are resistant to INH and streptomycin, respectively. When streptomycin is used alone, there is a dramatic improvement initially, but ultimately 50% of patients will relapse with resistant forms. Mutants resistant to two drugs, however, are very unlikely, and so the independent activity of each drug against the small number of organisms resistant to the other prevents emergence of a group of resistant organisms. Therefore, recommendations for antituberculous therapy include the use of two bactericidal drugs, or one bactericidal drug, and one or two static drugs, to insure that the resistant mutants will not be allowed to multiply. Some regimens divide therapy into two phases: a short intensive phase with three or even four drugs to halt multiplication and rapidly reduce the number of bacilli in the body; and a prolonged maintenance phase with two drugs to eliminate the smaller number of persistant organisms.

There are presently 10 drugs approved in the U.S. for antituberculous therapy. Based on their varying degrees of effectiveness and toxicities, they are classified as primary, secondary or tertiary. INH and rifampin are the most effective and least toxic, and form the basis of most treatment regimens. Ethambutol, para-aminosalicylic acid (PAS), pyrazinamide and streptomycin are less effective and more toxic, and used as companions to the primary drugs to help prevent resistance. Tertiary drugs are the least effective and most toxic, used only when the other drugs are unacceptable becasue of toxicity or resistance. A detailed description of each drug is beyond the scope of this chapter. A list of the

Table 36-9
Principles of Antituberculosis Chemotherapy

1. Use multiple drugs to which the organism is sensitive.
2. Give drugs daily in morning before breakfast. Single peak concentration of drug preferable to maintaining constant blood levels.
3. Advise patient regarding side effects, eg, INH hepatitis, rifampin-induced orange urine.
4. Develop surveillance systems to assure compliance.
5. Always add at least two new drugs if present regimen is failing. Never add one drug.

major qualities of each drug is shown in Table 36-10. Discussion of the major therapeutic options follows, and are shown in Table 36-11.

INH and ethambutol daily for 18 months, with the addition of streptomycin initially when the number of organisms is judged to be high, has been shown to be highly effective, with cure rates greater than 95%.

Table 36-10
Drugs for Tuberculosis and Their Major Side Effects and Toxicities

Drug	Side Effects
Primary	
Isoniazid (INH)	Gastrointestinal intolerance
	Hepatitis
	Peripheral neuritis
	CNS reactions
	Interaction with phenytoin
Rifampin	Hepatitis
	Colors secretions orange
	Flu-like syndrome
	Thrombocytopenia
	Hemolysis
	Drug interactions (warfarin, oral hypoglycemics, oral contraceptives, corticosteroids, methadone)
Secondary	
Ethambutol	Optic neuritis
	Accumulation if renal insufficiency
Para-amino salicylic acid (PAS)	Gastrointestinal intolerance
Pyrazinamide	Hyperuricemia
	Hepatitis
Streptomycin	Eighth nerve damage
	Nephrotoxicity
	Accumulation if renal insufficiency
Tertiary	
Capreomycin	Eighth nerve damage
	Nephrotoxicity
	Accumulation if renal insufficiency
Cycloserine	CNS effects (psychopathy, seizures)
Ethionamide	Gastrointestinal intolerance
	Hepatitis
Kanamycin	Eighth nerve damage
	Nephrotoxicity
	Accumulation if renal insufficiency

Adapted from Addington WW: The treatment of pulmonary tuberculosis. Current options. *Arch Intern Med* 1970;130:1391.

Table 36-11
Current Options for Antituberculosis Chemotherapy (Recommendations from the Pennsylvania Department of Health)

1. Short course chemotherapy: INH 300 mg and rifampin 600 mg daily for nine months.
2. Intermittent, supervised regimen: INH 300 mg and rifampin 600 mg daily for two to four weeks, then INH 15 mg/kg, pyridoxine 100 mg, and rifampin 600 mg twice weekly for total of nine months.
3. If rifampin unacceptable: INH 300 mg and ethambutol 15 mg/kg daily for 18 months.
4. If INH unacceptable: rifampin 600 mg and ethambutol 15 mg/kg daily for 18 months.

INH is bactericidal, relatively nontoxic, and well tolerated. It acts through interference with DNA synthesis. It is acetylated in the liver and excreted by the kidney. The dose is 5 mg/kg/day given once daily. In children, 10 to 15 mg/kg/day is recommended because of more rapid excretion and decreased incidence of toxicity. The drug usually is administered orally, but parenteral forms exist and may be used when necessary. Although some people inactivate INH more rapidly than others, this appears to have little clinical significance. The most common side effects are gastrointestinal irritation resulting in nausea, vomiting and diarrhea.

The most important side effect of INH is hepatitis. This usually occurs within the first three months of therapy, but may occur at any time. It resembles viral hepatitis clinically, biochemically, and histologically. It usually is completely reversible when the drug is discontinued, although if the drug is continued a prolonged reaction can lead to cirrhosis or death from fulminant hepatitis. Its frequency increases with age (Table 36-6). There is some controversy regarding the best way to monitor a patient for the development of INH-induced hepatitis. The systematic monitoring of hepatic enzymes has shown that approximately 20% of patients will initially develop a slight rise in transaminases, which is self-limited. Some authors have arbitrarily recommended discontinuing the drug when the SGOT increases to three- to five-times normal. An alternative and perhaps more rational approach is to advise the patient on INH of the symptoms and signs of hepatitis, and to see him or her at monthly intervals. If nausea, vomiting, malaise, fever, dark urine, light stools or jaundice develops, the drug should be discontinued and the patient should consult his or her physician. Liver function tests, while not being performed routinely, would be done at this time to confirm the diagnosis. The literature is also somewhat controversial regarding whether or not underlying liver disease predisposes to INH-induced hepatitis. It is clear, however, that the presence of unrelated liver disease complicates the picture of INH hepatitis, making detection more difficult, and adding insult to an already compromised liver.

There are some other less common side effects of INH that deserve mention. A peripheral neuropathy may develop, especially in the undernourished. This usually can be prevented by taking pyridoxine in a dose of 10 mg per day, and treated with a dose of 50 to 100 mg per day. In the well-nourished patient, however, pyridoxine is probably not necessary. Several uncommon and reversible central nervous system aberrations may also occur secondary to INH, including dizziness, muscle twitching, convulsions, and a feeling of excitement that occurs approximately eight hours after taking a 300 mg dose. The latter can be alleviated by dividing the doses, eg, 100 mg every eight hours. Allergic reactions such as rash and fever develop infrequently. Finally, it should be noted that INH decreases the metabolism of phenytoin, such that simultaneous administration of these drugs may lead to a phenytoin overdosage.

Ethambutol (EMB) is a bacteriostatic antituberculous drug that acts by inhibiting RNA synthesis. The usual dosage is 15 mg/kg/day, although doses up to 25 mg/kg/day are often given initially. The most important side effect of EMB is retrobulbar neuritis, resulting in blurred vision, decreased visual acuity, central scotoma, and impaired ability to see red and green. These effects are dose-related, occurring only when the high dose of 25 mg/kg/day is continued beyond two months. Subjective symptoms of altered vision often occur before tests for visual acuity show objective changes. Initial red-green color discrimination and visual acuity testing is recommended as baseline, but no further testing is considered necessary unless symptoms develop or the patient is taking more than 15 mg/kg/day for several months. The lesions cannot be detected by ophthalmoscopy.

Streptomycin is an aminoglycoside, and acts by inhibiting protein synthesis. The dose for adults is 1 g/day, given intramuscularly. Its major toxicities are to the kidneys and eighth nerve; thus renal function, audiograms, and vestibular function should be serially evaluated. Since this drug is eliminated by the kidneys, dose modification is necessary in patients with renal failure. Rarely, neuromuscular blockade may occur if the patient receives a neuromuscular relaxant or has myasthenia gravis.

Short-Course Chemotherapy

Although INH, EMB, and streptomycin are highly effective antituberculosis therapy, treatment must be continued for 18 months. As a consequence, noncompliance with therapy may occur, and is the main cause of relapse. Accordingly, a regimen that would be equally effective, nontoxic, and tolerable as the traditional regimens, but requiring a shorter duration, would be desirable. The advent of rifampin has made such a regimen possible. Since its introduction into antituberculosis therapy, several short-course regimens with INH and rifampin have been tested and shown to be effective and nontoxic. A review of these studies has culminated in the following recommendations endorsed by the Centers for Disease Control and the American Thoracic Society.

1. A "core" of INH and rifampin, taken for a minimum of nine months' duration, is an acceptable alternative to the longer term treatment schedules used in the past. Daily doses should be 300 mg for INH and 600 mg for rifampin. Ethambutol at 15 mg/kg/day should be added when there is concern over drug resistance.
2. Following an intial phase of daily treatment (two weeks to two months), treatment should be continued with INH and rifampin either daily (if self-administered) or twice weekly (if supervised).
3. Treatment should continue for at least nine months, or longer if necessary, for a total of six months' duration after sputum culture has become negative. Because over 90% of patients taking INH-rifampin become culture-negative after three months' treatment, total duration of treatment should be nine months in most instances. Longer treatment is justified for patients suspected of not taking their treatment regularly, for those with disseminated disease, and for those with complicating medical conditions (eg, patients being treated with corticosteroids).
4. Patients should remain under surveillance for 12 months after completing therapy. This is recommended until sufficient information has been obtained about the efficacy of short-course treatment under field conditions in the United States.

Short-course chemotherapy is gradually becoming accepted as the treatment of choice for pulmonary tuberculosis by many authorities, who no longer consider it merely as an alternative to the conventional regimens.

The efficacy of these regimens stems from the simultaneous use of two bactericidal drugs, INH and rifampin. It is important to note that "short-course therapy" does not imply a shorter course of previously employed regimens such as INH and ethambutol, the latter being a static drug, therefore, requiring 18 months of therapy if relapses are to be prevented.

Rifampin acts through the inhibition of RNA polymerase and is bactericidal against *M. tuberculosis* as well as several other microorganisms. Its broad-spectrum activity distinguishes it from most of the other antituberculous drugs. It is taken orally in a single daily dose of 10 mg/kg for adults, and 15 mg/kg in children. Emergence of resistance is rapid when used alone. Rifampin is a potent inducer of drug metabolism by causing proliferation of hepatic enzymes. This effect becomes clinically relevant in patients taking warfarin anticoagulants, in whom the requirements increase. Conversely, discontinuation of rifampin may lead to overanticoagulation. Levels of oral hypoclycemic drugs, corticosteroids, methadone and oral contraceptives may also be reduced. The latter may result in symptoms of methadone withdrawal and pregnancy, respectively. A flu-like syndrome has been noted when dosage is increased and taken intermittently. Rifampin colors body secretions orange-red, particularly the urine. Contact lenses may also become colored. The patient should be informed of this in advance and reassured. This is not a reason to discontinue the drug. Thrombocytopenia may develop secondary to absorption of antirifampin antibodies onto platelets, with the subsequent fixation of complement causing platelet damage. Finally, rifampin may cause hepatitis. However, it does not increase the risk of INH hepatotoxicity. The effect is additive, not synergistic, to that of INH hepatitis. The question of preexisting liver disease predisposing to rifampin-hepatitis remains unsettled.

Treatment of Resistance

Drug resistance may be primary, occurring naturally without any previous exposure to the drug, or secondary, developing after an abortive initial period of therapy. The rates for primary resistance vary among the different drugs and with geographical origin. Asian and Hispanic immigrants have particularly high rates. When primary resistance is suspected, or when there is initial drug failure on standard regimens, treatment with INH, rifampin, streptomycin and pyrazinamide should be initiated until sensitivity tests are available. INH and rifampin, and the combination of streptomycin and pyrazinamide, are bactericidal. When the initial treatment is correct, late relapse is rare. If it does occur, the organisms usually are still sensitive to the original regimen and retreatment with those same antibiotics is appropriate.

Secondary resistance usually develops as a consequence of noncompliance and manifests clinically as early relapse. Treatment should be guided by susceptibility testing. Since this takes several weeks to months, initial retreatment must be empiric. The principle is to use at least two drugs to which the patient has never been exposed. Adding one new agent can cause additional resistance to develop and should never be done. When sensitivities become available, treatment is adjusted accordingly. A drug previously used may be used again if the organism is sensitive. INH is used regardless of resistance since some of the organisms may remain sensitive.

Therapeutic Trial

Tuberculosis is a relatively common cause of fever of unknown origin. If a patient's clinical course is deteriorating with a febrile, wasting disease and the diagnosis remains in question, a trial with INH and EMB may be diagnostic and therapeutic. Rifampin should not be used since this antibiotic is active against several other bacteria and a response to it would not be specific for tuberculosis.

Corticosteroids

As adjunct therapy to specific antituberculous chemotherapy, corticosteroids have been shown to accelerate the clinical improvement of severely ill patients. In addition to improving the toxicity associated with severe disease, accelerated x-ray clearing and cavity control also have been demonstrated. The beneficial effects are secondary to the steroid-associated decrease in exudation, fibrosis and tissue destruction. When used, a period of four to six weeks is sufficient. Moreover, some will give two weeks of daily therapy, then switch to an alternate-day regimen, thereby reducing the likelihood of secondary infection.

Special Situations

There are a few special situations regarding antituberculous therapy that deserve comment. In pregnant women, INH and ethambutol are well tolerated by mother and fetus. Experience is limited with rifampin. Streptomycin can cause fetal toxicity. Ethionamide may be teratogenic. INH, rifampin and streptomycin are secreted into milk.

In patients with renal insufficiency, certain precautions must be taken. The levels of INH and rifampin are not affected and the usual doses are given. In the particular situation of severe renal insufficiency in a slow acetylator, the dose of INH should be reduced. Ethambutol is excreted almost entirely by the kidneys and should probably be avoided, especially since blood levels are not readily measurable. Similarly, streptomycin and other aminoglycosides are excreted by the kidneys, and will accumulate when there is renal insufficiency. INH, ethambutol and the aminoglycosides are dialyzable. Treatment with these drugs can be simplified if they are given immediately following a period of dialysis. If ethambutol must be used, the dose should be decreased. As yet there is little data on the dialyzability of rifampin.

Hepatic disease presents a particular concern when antituberculous therapy is necessary, since INH and rifampin, the most effective antituberculous drugs, are potentially hepatotoxic. Although the hepatotoxicities of INH and rifampin are probably idiosyncratic, it intuitively makes sense to design the least hepatotoxic regimen in a patient whose baseline liver function is abnormal. Alternatively, if INH and rifampin are to be used together, particular attention should be paid to their potential hepatotoxicity. In severe hepatic disease, the dose of INH and rifampin should be decreased. Finally, the interaction of rifampin with many other commonly used drugs and the property of INH to interfere with the excretion of phenytoin, must be recognized and dealt with.

Secondary Management Measures

Although antituberculous chemotherapy is the definitive treatment for tuberculosis, secondary measures in managing the disease, such as hospitalization, isolation, assuring compliance, and follow-up, also deserve comment. There is no a priori reason for hospitalization, and most patients will do well at home. Hospitalization of newly diagnosed cases to prevent spread of infection is not necessary, since a patient's contacts have little or no risk of becoming infected after effective chemotherapy is begun. A case can be made, however, for a short admission to obtain cultures, educate the patient regarding his disease, and initiate therapy. Severe illness, hemoptysis and treatment failure necessitate the facilities offered by in-hospital care.

As discussed in the section on pathogenesis, tuberculosis is spread via the airborne route. Accordingly, measures to control cough and reduce the inoculum of droplet nuclei in the environment form the basis of isolation techniques. The patient should be instructed to cover his mouth when coughing or sneezing. Masks can be used when this is not possible. Rooms equipped with negative-pressure ventilatory systems rapidly dilute any aerosolized particles, and prevent infectious aerosol from moving out of the patient's room.

Isolation is necessary only for smear-positive patients since the risk of contagion is minimal if the patient is smear-negative. Once chemotherapy is initiated, infectiousness decreases rapidly. Accordingly, isolation for a period of two weeks is recommended, although sputum may remain smear-positive for several weeks and culture positive for three to four months. Added precautions should be considered for persons working with children and immunocompromised hosts.

Poor compliance is the main cause of relapse, which may occur with resistant organisms. Therefore, concerted effort should be directed at promoting compliance. The severity and curability of tuberculosis should be explained to the patient. Mechanisms to survey and assure compliance are essential. Once a patient has successfully completed the treatment regimen, relapse is so unlikely that long-term follow-up is not recommended.

PREVENTION

Since tuberculosis is preventable with INH, much attention is directed toward management of those persons who are potentially infected and liable to develop disease. If a normal, healthy individual is found to have a 5-TU PPD of 10 mm or more, he has infection, albeit subclinical. Use of INH in this situation is treatment of infection, strictly speaking, although it is commonly referred to as INH chemoprophylaxis, meaning prophylaxis against the development of disease. The guidelines for management of conversion of PPD status are discussed in an earlier section, and are shown in Table 36-5.

A second form of INH prophylaxis is the treatment of close contacts of a patient with active tuberculosis before it is known whether or not they have become infected (ie, develop a positive PPD skin test). Such therapy is recommended for children less than 4 years old and for immunocompromised hosts because of the increased severity of tuberculosis in these populations, and for household contacts because of their increased likelihood of contracting the infection. If untreated, 2.5% of household contacts will develop active tuberculosis within the next year. For less intimate exposure to an individual with active tuberculosis, a logical approach is to skin test initially, and repeat skin test in two to three months. If the repeat test is negative, no treatment is necessary. The management of patients exposed to INH-resistant organisms is uncertain.

In the United States, prophylaxis against tuberculosis is based on skin test reactivity and INH, as discussed above. It should be noted, however, that a vaccine exists and is used in some parts of the world where tuberculosis is more prevalent. The vaccine, known as *BCG* (Bacillus of Calmette-Guerin) is an attenuated strain of bovine tubercule bacilli. It has been shown to prevent the development of serious disease in up to 80% of those effectively immunized (ie, who develop a positive tuberculin test following inoculation). Its efficacy in preventing natural infection is more controversial. The United States Public Health Service and the American Thoracic Society recommended that BCG be considered in 1) persons with negative tuberculin tests and repeated exposure to untreated sputum-positive patients, and 2) in well-defined communities or groups where an excessive rate of new infections can be demonstrated and the usual skin test surveillance and treatment programs have failed or are inapplicable. Vaccination with BCG, when effective, causes conversion of skin test reactivity to PPD, thereby complicating the use of the skin test in the diagnosis of tuberculosis.

SELECTED READINGS

American Thoracic Society: Diagnostic standards and classification of tuberculosis and other mycobacterial diseases (14th edition). *Am Rev Respir Dis* 1981; 123:343–358.

American Thoracic Society and Center for Disease Control: Guidelines for short-course tuberculosis chemotherapy. *Morbid Mortal Weekly Rep* 1980;29: 97–105.

Berger HW, Mejia E: Tuberculosis pleurisy. *Chest* 1973;63:88–92.
Dandoy S: Current status of general hospital use for patients with tuberculosis in the United States. *Am Rev Respir Dis* 1982;126:270–273.
Dutt AK, Stead WW: Chemotherapy of tuberculosis for the 1980's. *Clin Chest Med* 1980;1:243–252.
Fox W: Whither short-course chemotherapy? *Br J Dis Chest* 1981;75:331–357.
Glaseroth J, Robins AG, Snider DE: Tuberculosis in the 1980's. *N Engl J Med* 1980;302:1441–1450.
Harris HW: Mycobacterial infections, in Grieco MH (ed): *Infections in the Abnormal Host.* Yorke Medical Books. 1980, pp 360–381.
Johnston RF, Wildrich KH: "State of the art" review. The impact of chemotherapy on the care of patients with tuberculosis. *Am Rev Respir Dis* 1974;109: 636–664.
Khan MA, Kovnat DM, Bachus B, et al: Clinical and roentgenographic spectrum of pulmonary tuberculosis in the adult. *Am J Med* 1977;62:31–38.
Kopanoff DE, Snider DE Jr, Caras GJ: Isoniazid-related hepatitis: A U.S. Public Health Service Cooperative Surveillance Study. *Am Rev Respir Dis* 1978;117:99–1001.
MacGregor RR: A year's experience with tuberculosis in a private urban teaching hospital in the post-sanitorium era. *Am J Med* 1975;58:221.
Mayock RL, MacGregor RR: Diagnosis, prevention and early therapy of tuberculosis. *DM* May 1976.
Reichman LB: Tuberculin skin testing. The state of the art. *Chest* 1979;76:764–770.
Stead WW, Kerby GR, Schlueter DP, et al: The clinical spectrum of primary tuberculosis in adults. Confusion with reinfection in the pathogenesis of chronic tuberculosis. *Ann Intern Med* 1968;68:731–745.

37 *Mycoplasma pneumoniae*

Richard Snepar

Mycoplasma pneumoniae, the "Eaton Agent," produces illness in man ranging from mild upper respiratory tract infection to severe bronchitis and pneumonia.

Microbial Characteristics

Mycoplasma pneumoniae is one of seven members of the genus *Mycoplasma* recovered from the respiratory tract of man. Initially identified as the organisms responsible for bovine pleuropneumonia, *Mycoplasma* were called pleuropneumonia-like organisms. These agents are the smallest free-living organisms. Unlike other bacteria, *Mycoplasma* do not have a rigid cell wall, but instead are bounded by a triple-layered cell membrane. Cell wall-active antibiotics are therefore ineffective against these organisms.

On agar, growth of *Mycoplasma pneumoniae* produces a homogeneously granular appearance in contrast to the "fried egg" appearance of other mycoplasmas. Yeast extract and supplementary serum are required for optimum growth. Growth is best under aerobic conditions, but nonetheless is so slow that visible colony formation may require up to three weeks. In the presence of sheep or guinea pig red cells, β (clear) hemolysis is produced. Growth is inhibited by erythromycin, tetracycline and specific antisera to a lipid extract of *M. pneumoniae* membrane.

Epidemiology

M. pneumoniae is transmitted mainly by means of aerosols. *Mycoplasma pneumoniae* infections occur in many countries and are found throughout the year. Transmission of infection requires prolonged close contact, as occurs in the family, college campuses and the military. Spread of disease is slow, even in the family setting; although once the organism is introduced, a high percentage of susceptible contacts will become infected. In populations of military recruits or college students, 10% to 50% of pneumonias are due to this agent.

Illness with *M. pneumoniae* is greatest in the age range from 5 to 25 years and is uncommon after age 50, although people at any age can become infected.

Pathogenicity

Shedding of *Mycoplasma pneumoniae* occurs two to eight days preceding the onset of symptoms and can last for ten to 14 weeks despite antibiotic therapy. The organism attaches to the respiratory mucosa at a cell membrane receptor consisting of neuraminic acid. Although extracellular throughout infection, the agent causes metabolic impairment of the mucosal cells and interferes with ciliary motion. Bronchiolar thickening with edema and congestion and peribronchiolar infiltration with lymphocytes and plasma cells is seen.

The mild nature of disease, its rare association with pneumonia in young children and its increasing severity with age, suggest that pulmonary infiltrates are the result of immunologic responses to reinfection. Although *M. pneumoniae* generally is thought to be restricted to the respiratory tract, in rare instances, *M. pneumoniae* has been isolated from blood, pericardial fluid, pleural fluid, cerebrospinal fluid, vesicular skin lesions and middle ear fluid.

Recovery from infection depends on the development of antibody. Resistance to infection is related to the magnitude of antibody response. The duration of immunity is unknown, however, and reinfections can occur.

Clinical Manifestations

Infection with *M. pneumoniae* results in pharyngitis, tracheobronchitis, myringitis and pneumonia. Tracheobronchitis is the most common clinical syndrome, and pharyngitis or myringitis also may be seen as isolated manifestations of this disease. Pneumonia occurs in only 10% to 30% of those infected during endemic disease.

Pneumonia follows an incubation period of two to three weeks. The onset usually is gradual. A prominent headache and fever ranging from 38°C to greater than 40°C usually are present. A severe, nonproductive or mildly productive, hacking cough becomes the dominant respiratory symptom. Earache is also common. The patient may have upper respiratory symptoms that precede or accompany the pneumonic manifestations, and family members may also have had recent respiratory illness. On physical examination, myringitis (which can on occasion be bullous), pharyngitis, cervical lymphadenopathy, and rales may be present. However, the symptoms may be more impressive than the physical findings. Significant pleural effusions are unusual. The chest roentgenogram reveals a localized bronchopneumonia of a lower lobe and less often bilateral infiltrates. The chest radiographic findings alone are not diagnostic of *M. pneumoniae.* Gram stain of sputum usually reveals polymorphonuclear leukocytes with no predominant organism. *Mycoplasma* pneumonia may become severe in patients with sickle cell anemia, preexisting cardiopulmonary disease and immunodeficiencies. Death from respiratory insufficiency is unusual.

Nonrespiratory manifestations of infection with *M. pneumoniae* may occur and include cold agglutinin-induced hemolytic anemia, arthralgias and polyarthritis, skin rashes, Stevens-Johnson syndrome, transverse myelitis, meningoencephalitis and myocarditis.

Diagnostic Tests

The diagnosis of *M. pneumoniae* infection may be made either by isolation of the organism or by demonstration of a rise in specific antibody. The specimen of choice for isolation of *M. pneumoniae* is either sputum or a throat washing, although a throat swab may suffice. Isolation of the organism is best accomplished in a diphasic medium of agar and a liquid phase that contains glucose and a pH indicator.

The demonstration of complement-fixing antibodies is the most useful serologic test. A fourfold or greater rise in antibody titer in acute and convalescent sera is considered diagnostic. A single convalescent titer of 1:64 or greater is suggestive of disease with *M. pneumoniae.*

Cold agglutinins, which are IgM antibodies that bind to the erythrocyte I antigen, in titers of 1:32 or greater are present in over 50% of patients with *Mycoplasma* pneumonia. The titer correlates directly with the severity of pulmonary involvement. Titers are higher during the second and third week of illness when hemolysis may follow lowering of body temperature. The presence of cold agglutinins is not diagnostic for *M. pneumoniae* and can be seen with other viral infections and dysproteinemias. Occasionally, nonspecific serologic tests for syphilis (VDRL) may be falsely positive.

Therapy

Treatment of *M. pneumoniae* pneumonia has been shown to shorten the duration of fever, rales and cough and hasten the resolution of radiographic abnormalities. Tetracycline or erythromycin, 500 mg every six hours taken orally should be instituted in patients with presumed *M. pneumoniae* pneumonia. A two to three week course of therapy is recommended since relapse has occurred with shorter antibiotic courses. Therapy for tracheobronchitis and pharyngitis is not warranted since these are mild, self-limited illnesses.

Prevention

There is no known method to prevent *M. pneumoniae* infection. Vaccines with both killed and alive attenuated agents have thus far been ineffective. Attempts at limiting close contact with infected persons should be made. Transmission of infection is not altered by antimicrobials.

SELECTED READINGS

Balassanian N, Robbins F: *Mycoplasma pneumoniae* infection in families. *N Eng J Med* 1967;277:719.

Chanock RM: Mycoplasma infections of man. *N Engl J Med* 1965;273:1199.

Couch RB: *Mycoplasma pneumoniae*, in Mandell GL, Douglas RG, Bennett JE (eds): *Principles and Practice of Infectious Diseases.* New York, Wiley and Sons, 1979, p.1484.

Denny FW, Clyde WA Jr, Glenzen WP: *Mycoplasma pneumoniae* disease: Clinical spectrum, pathophysiology, epidemiology and control. *J Infect Dis* 1971;123:74.

George RB, Weill H, Rasch JR, et al: Roentgenographic appearance of viral and mycoplasmal pneumonias. *Am Rev Respir Dis* 1967;96:1144.

Levine DP, Lerner MA: The spectrum of *Mycoplasma pneumoniae* infections. *Med Clin North Am* 1978;62:961.

Murray HW, Masur H, Senterfit LB, et al: The protean manifestations of *Mycoplasma pneumoniae* infection in adults. *Am J Med* 1975;58:229.

38 *Branhamella catarrhalis*

Matthew E. Levison

Branhamella catarrhalis (formerly *Neisseria catarrhalis*) is a gram-negative diplococcus which occurs as a commensal in the upper respiratory tract. This organism can, however, be pathogenic. It has been implicated as an infrequent cause of self-limited infections such as acute bronchitis, exacerbations of chronic bronchitis, acute maxillary sinusitis, otitis media in children and perhaps acute laryngitis. Also, cases of meningitis, endocarditis and bacteremia have been described.

There have been a few reports of pneumonia due to *Branhamella*, based on sputum gram stain revealing predominance of gram-negative diplococci (Figure 38-1), and cultures of sputum or transtracheal aspirate that yield "pure" or predominant growth of *B. catarrhalis*, together with suggestive chest radiographic and clinical signs. Almost all the patients were immunocompromised or had underlying lung disease. Rarely has

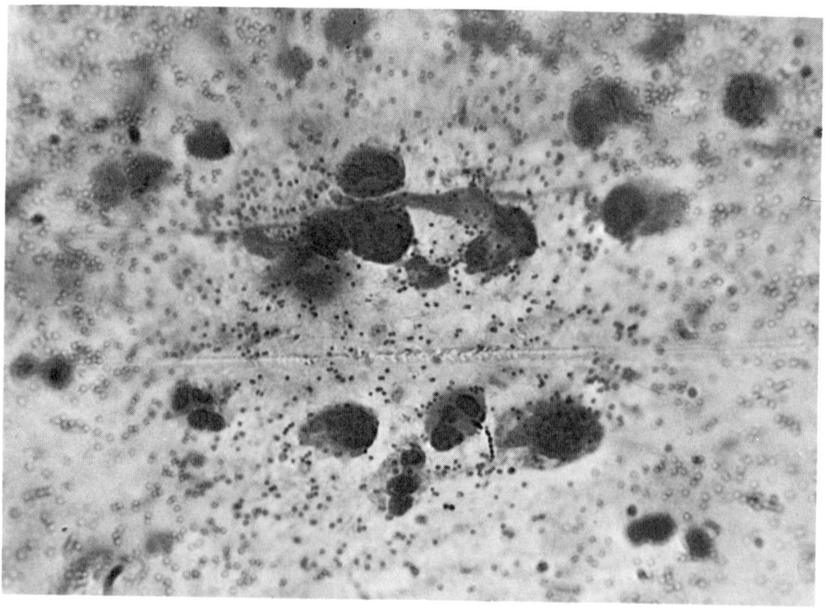

Figure 38-1 Gram stain of sputum from a patient with *B. catarrhalis* pneumonia which demonstrates predominance of gram-negative diplococci. Other pathogens to be considered when confronted with such a gram stain are the meningococcus, *Acinetobacter*, and *Hemophilus influenzae*.

Branhamella been implicated as a cause of pneumonia in a previously healthy patient. Many strains produce β-lactamase which is apparently more active against penicillinase-sensitive penicillins than cephalosporins. Therefore, either a β-lactamase-resistant cephalosporin, tetracycline, erythromycin or trimethoprim-sulfamethoxazole is probably the best initial therapy for these infections.

SELECTED READINGS

Johnson MA, Drew WL, Roberts M: *Branhamella (Neisseria) catarrhalis*—A lower respiratory tract pathogen? *J Clin Microbiol* 1981;13:1066–1069.

Srinivasan G, Raff MJ, Templeton WC, et al: *Branhamella catarrhalis* pneumonia: Report of two cases and review of the literature. *Am Rev Respir Dis* 1981;123:553–555.

39 *Chlamydiae*

George A. Poporad

Chlamydia causes two clinically distinct infections of the lower respiratory tract: psittacosis caused by *Chlamydia psittaci*, and infant pneumonia caused by *Chlamydia trachomatis*. There is some evidence to suggest that *C. trachomatis* might also cause pneumonia in the immunosuppressed adult host.

ETIOLOGY

Chlamydia are small (200 to 1000 nm) nonmotile bacteria that are obligate intracellular parasites. There are two species within the genus *Chlamydia*, *C. psittaci* and *C. trachomatis*. *C. psittaci* is a ubiquitous organism in nature whose many diverse serotypes cause disease in birds and mammals. Man becomes secondarily infected from an animal reservoir. Serotyping *C. psittaci* strains is not currently feasible because of lack of sensitivity of the techniques and the difficulty in performing them. *C. trachomatis* has man as its only natural host, and causes infection involving the eye (trachoma, inclusion conjunctivitis), genital tract (lymphogranuloma venereum, nongonococcal urethritis, salpingitis) and lung (infant pneumonia). *C. trachomatis* includes 15 serotypes distinguished by immunofluorescense. Types A, B, Ba, and C are associated with trachoma, D through K with genital tract infection other than lymphogranuloma venereum, and L_1, L_2, L_3 with lymphogranuloma venereum. Infant pneumonia is associated with the genital strains of *C. trachomatis* (D–K).

Chlamydia induce their own phagocytosis into a susceptible host cell, where they divide by binary fission within the phagosome. Although *Chlamydia* possess DNA and RNA, they are dependent upon the host cell to provide specific amino acids and ATP for energy. As the organisms replicate within the cytoplasm of the host cell, they form characteristic inclusions. *C. trachomatis* forms a single inclusion that displaces the nucleus. The inclusion contains glycogen which can be stained with iodine, and thus is easily identified in cell culture (Figure 39-1). *C. psittaci* forms inclusions that rupture early and distribute themselves around the nucleus without displacing it. These inclusions do not contain glycogen and they can be identified by Giemsa stain.

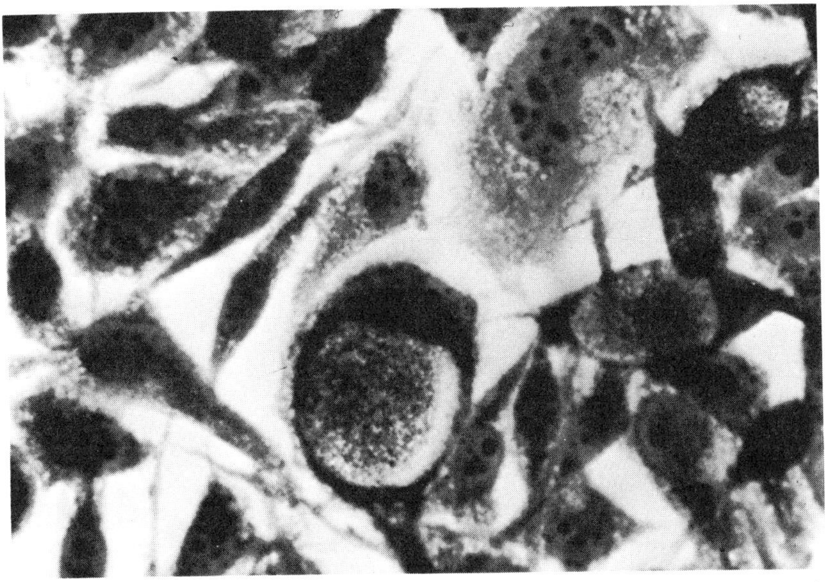

Figure 39-1 *Chlamydia trachomatis* inclusion bodies in cycloheximide-treated McCoy cells (Giemsa stain). (Courtesy of Christine Forrer and Kenneth Sabasinski of The Children's Hospital of Philadelphia, Departments of Infectious Disease and Pathology.)

C. psittaci

C. psittaci causes psittacosis, a disease of birds transmitted to man. Psittacine birds (parrots, parakeets) were originally described as the vectors for the illness. The term "ornithosis," preferred by some, reflects the recognition that a broad range of bird species may act as a reservoir for the organism, but "psittacosis" remains the more commonly accepted term.

Epidemiology The distribution of *C. psittaci* is worldwide in birds and certain mammals. Psittacine birds are considered the major reservoir. They have a relatively low infection rate but the crowding and stress involved in capture and shipping cause the rate to increase. The organism is also found in canaries, finches, pigeons and poultry (turkeys, chickens, ducks, and pheasants). The avian disease is characterized by diarrhea, conjunctivitis, and wasting, and can be fatal. Illness, however, can be mild or asymptomatic. *C. psittaci* can be isolated from the feathers, feces, blood, or tissues (liver, spleen) of infected birds and the organism may be shed intermittently or continuously for months.

Transmission to man occurs with bird handling or during contact with bird tissues, feces, cage dust or feathers, or in feeding mouth to beak. Rarely does disease occur through bird bites. Close or prolonged contact is not needed. In fact, 20% of infected people do not recall any prior contact with birds. People at occupational risk include pet shop owners, workers on poultry farms or in processing plants, zoo workers, and veterinarians. Disease usually is sporadic, although isolated epidemics have been reported, mostly in association with the slaughter of turkeys in processing plants. Man-to-man transmission has occurred, reflected in outbreaks of hospital-acquired infection. These secondary cases appear more severe than cases involving bird-to-man acquisition. Immunity after a first infection is not complete and second attacks of illness have been reported.

Pathogenesis and pathology Man is infected through airborne transmission of *C. psittaci* with the respiratory tract as the portal of entry. From the respiratory tract, organisms pass to the reticuloendothelial system of the liver and spleen where they replicate. Organisms then spread hematogenously to lung and other organs. This two-stage process involved in infection accounts for the long incubation period (10 to 14 days) before presentation of clinical illness. In the lung, infection is reflected by a lobular interstitial pneumonia. A lymphocytic inflammatory response is elicited, with subsequent edema of alveolar walls and interstitial spaces. The presence of macrophages with cytoplasmic inclusions are characteristic of the infection. Congestion and thrombosis of capillaries occur, producing necrosis of alveolar walls. Small hemorrhages may develop accounting for the occasional hemoptysis seen clinically. Bronchial and bronchiolar changes are minimal. There may be enlargement of hilar lymph nodes, spleen, and liver with focal necrosis found in the latter two organs.

Clinical manifestations Psittacosis has a varied presentation and clinical course. Following an incubation period averaging 10 days (range four to 15 days), there is sudden onset of high fever (up to 104°F), rigors, backache and photophobia. It is not uncommon, however, to have early symptoms extend over two to four days, with a gradual increase of fever, malaise, and anorexia. At the height of illness, severe headache and myalgias are prominent. The patient may complain of a mild sore throat. A persistent nonproductive cough usually is present from the onset or develops several days into the illness. Occasionally, hemoptysis is present. Cough may be absent or minimal in some patients. When pulmonary involvement is extensive, the patient may be dyspneic or cyanotic. Pleuritic pain is rare. Changes in mental status may occur toward the end of the first week and usually are associated with hypoxia. The patient may become lethargic, confused or delirious with progression to stupor and coma. Symptoms suggestive of meningoencephalitis have been described but the CSF exam usually is normal.

Gastrointestinal complaints are rare, but occasionally patients may complain of nausea, vomiting, diarrhea and abdominal distention. Jaundice is seen only in very severe cases. A pale macular rash reminiscent of "rose spots" seen in typhoid fever may appear, and erythema nodosum has been described.

Physical exam may reveal a relative bradycardia compared to the height of fever. Auscultatory findings in the lung usually are minimal. Fine crepitant rales may be heard over localized areas in the lower lung fields but signs of consolidation are absent. Pleural effusions, and pleural and pericardial friction rubs have been described. Examination of the abdomen may frequently reveal nontender hepatomegaly or, in 10% to 70% of cases, splenomegaly.

Laboratory studies reveal a leukocyte count that usually is normal, although there may be a modest leukopenia or leukocytosis. Anemia may develop during the illness. Examination of the sputum shows few leukocytes and no bacterial pathogens. Liver function studies usually are normal. Proteinuria may be present during the acute illness.

The chest radiographic findings can be varied. There may be soft patchy infiltrates radiating out from the hilum toward the lower lung fields. There may also be a miliary or nodular pattern, or lobar consolidation. Very often, the x-ray findings reflect more extensive lung involvement than anticipated by physical exam.

Diagnosis *C. psittaci* may be isolated from throat washings, sputum, and blood during the first two weeks of illness. *Chlamydia* can be grown in the yolk sac of embryonated eggs or tissue culture, with the subsequent demonstration of typical intracytoplasmic inclusions by appropriate stain (Giemsa or iodine). Extraordinary care is needed to avoid laboratory spread of the organism, and only specialized laboratories perform these cultures. The usual method of diagnosis is by serology. A fourfold or greater rise in complement-fixing antibody titers to group antigen is diagnostic. Antibody titers generally rise as early as four days after onset of illness, but it is important to remember that antibiotic treatment may delay antibody appearance for three to five weeks. A single titer of 1:16 in a patient with a compatible clinical history is suggestive.

A clinical clue to the diagnosis of psittacosis is the presence of splenomegaly in a patient presenting with an atypical pneumonia syndrome. A differential diagnosis should include *Mycoplasma* pneumonia, Legionnaires' disease, and viral pneumonia. Usual bacterial etiologies should also be considered when the onset of illness is abrupt and chest x-ray shows lobar consolidation.

Therapy Tetracycline, 2 to 3 g/day, in divided doses is the antibiotic of choice for treatment. Response to therapy may occur in two to three days or it may be delayed. Clearing of chest radiographic findings may take weeks. Relapses may occur, and it is recommended to continue therapy 10 to 14 days after defervescence. The prognosis is good with a 1% mortality caused by pulmonary insufficiency or toxemia. Chloramphenicol is an alternative antibiotic.

Prevention The most obvious way to prevent illness is to avoid contact with birds. Transmission to man has been reduced by the requirement that birds imported from countries other than Canada be quarantined for 30 days and be treated prophylactically with tetracycline in their feed. A patient suffering from psittacosis should be placed in respiratory isolation. Articles contaminated with secretions must be disinfected, as well as the patient's room after discharge. Cases of psittacosis must be reported to public health officials to allow investigation into the source of exposure and possible contacts.

C. trachomatis

C. trachomatis is primarily an oculo-genital colonist and pathogen. In 1977, Beam and Saxton described a distinctive subacute pneumonia syndrome in infants 1 to 6 months of age associated with the isolation of *C. trachomatis* from nasopharyngeal cultures and high serum chlamydial antibody titers. Other investigative evidence, including the isolation of this organism from open lung biopsies, has confirmed the clinical association of this syndrome with *C. trachomatis* respiratory tract infection.

Epidemiology It is believed that disease is transmitted from a mother with cervical infection to the infant during birth. Contamination of the infant's conjunctiva and/or nasopharynx appears to precede subsequent spread to the lower respiratory tract. All newborns are susceptible to infection. One study recorded an infant pneumonia attack rate of 20% in those infants born to mothers with *Chlamydia* cervical infection. Given a 4% cervical infection rate (higher in some studies) in pregnant women, infant pneumonia can be expected to develop in eight of 1000 new births. Compared to other perinatal infections (one per 6000 live births for herpes simplex, three per 1000 live births for group B streptococcal infection), *Chlamydia* lung infection is a major health problem in infants.

There are no reports of nosocomial spread of disease, and there is no evidence for recurrent illness.

Pathology Data is very limited and restricted to lung biopsy material. There can be a diffuse interstitial and alveolar infiltration with both monocytes and neutrophils. Alveolar destruction may occur. A widespread necrotizing bronchiolitis has been reported.

Clinical manifestations and laboratory The majority of symptoms begin at less than 8 weeks of age with a peak at 1 to 3 months. No cases have been reported beyond 6 months of age. Onset is gradual with nasal obstruction and discharge, tachypnea, and the development of a distinctive cough. The cough is paroxysmal, closely spaced, and stacatto in character. The infant usually is afebrile and does not appear acutely ill or toxic. The illness has not proven to be fatal, but it can be marked by severe respiratory distress and episodes of apnea. Lung exam reveals diffuse, fine sticky rales on inspiration and, rarely, wheezing on expiration. Up to 50% of infants may have concurrent conjunctivitis by exam or history. Otitis media can be seen in up to one half of cases.

White counts usually are normal or only slightly elevated. Approximately 70% of cases will have absolute eosinophil counts of $>300/mm^3$. Chest x-ray usually reveals bilateral symmetric interstitial infiltrates and hyperexpansion of the lungs. Areas of atelectasis and alveolar infiltration can be present. Serum IgA, IgM, and IgG levels are two to three times normal.

Diagnosis Clinical criteria for diagnosis includes presentation at 1 to 3 months of age, a history of cough and congestion for greater than one week's duration, a chest x-ray showing interstitial pneumonia and hyperinflation, eosinophilia, and increased serum gammaglobulin levels. The presence of conjunctivitis can be a reliable indicator of *Chlamydia* infection, but its absence does not rule it out. Included in the differential diagnosis are bacterial pneumonias, especially pertussis which presents with a spasmatic cough and a distinctive whoop in inspiration not present in *Chlamydia* infant pneumonia, and viral pneumonias such as cytomegalovirus and respiratory syncytial virus.

C. trachomatis can be isolated from the nasopharynx or conjunctiva (Figure 39-1). An aspirate of the nasopharynx is slightly more sensitive than a swab. Specimens should be collected in a special transport medium that selectively inhibits other bacteria, and they should be refrigerated if processed within 24 hours or frozen at $-60°C$ if time to processing is longer.

Antibody to *C. trachomatis* (microimmunofluorescence method) found in tears, nasopharyngeal secretions, and serum in an infant with a typical presentation is highly associated with infection. Infants shedding *Chlamydia* who have the pneumonia syndrome have higher serum antibody titers than those who are asymptomatic or who only have conjunctivitis. Serum antibody titers $>1{:}32$ suggest infection.

Treatment and prevention There are no well-controlled therapeutic trials, but clinical improvement has been observed and *Chlamydia* shedding teminated after appropriate antimicrobial therapy. Recommended regimens include sulfisoxazole 15 mg/kg/24 h or erythromycin 50 mg/kg/24 h for two to three weeks. Symptoms usually improve by the fifth day of therapy, cultures are negative by nine days, and the chest x-ray usually clears by three weeks. Untreated, rales and chest x-ray abnormalities persist for months.

Preventive measures include treating *Chlamydia* genital tract infections. The question of whether to screen for *Chlamydia* infection during pregnancy and subsequently treat infected mothers has not been answered as to efficacy and cost. It is important to note that the policy of routine treatment of infants with silver nitrate eye drops is not effective in eliminating *Chlamydia* from the conjunctiva.

C. trachomatis has been recently isolated from the lower respiratory tract of six adults with illness ranging from chronic bronchitis to severe diffuse interstitial pneumonia. All patients were either elderly and suffering from chronic diseases (diabetes, COPD), or were immunosuppressed (renal transplant, acute lymphatic leukemia). The severity of lung involvement seemed to correlate with the degree of immunosuppression. In three of these six patients cytomegalovirus was isolated concurrently. Therapy directed against *C. trachomatis* resulted in prompt clinical improvement in three patients (one patient with bronchitis, two with pneumonia). The true significance of this organism in causing pneumonia in immunosuppressed adults remains to be defined.

SELECTED READINGS

Beem MD, Saxon EM: Respiratory-tract colonization and a distinctive pneumonia syndrome in infants infected with *Chlamydia trachomatis. N Engl J Med* 1977;296:306.

Gregg MB, White PF: Psittacosis and chlamydial pneumonia of infancy, in Wehrle PF, Top FK (eds): *Communicable and Infectious Disease.* St Louis, CV Mosby, 1981.

Harrison HR, English MG, Lee CK, et al: *Chlamydia trachomatis* infant pneumonitis: Comparison with matched controls and other infant pneumonitis. *N Engl J Med* 1978; 298:702.

Schachter J: Chlamydial infections. *N Engl J Med* 1978;298:428–435, 540–549.

Schachter J, Holt J, Goodner E, et al: Prospective study of chlamydial infection in neonates. *Lancet* 1979;2:377.

Schaffer W, Drutz DJ, Duncan GW, et al: The clinical spectrum of endemic psittacosis. *Arch Intern Med* 1967;119:433.

Seibert RH, Jordan WS, Dingle JH: Clinical variations in the diagnosis of psittacosis. *N Engl J Med* 1956;254:925.

Tack KJ, Rasp FL, Hanto D, et al: Isolation of *Chlamydia trachomatis* from the lower respiratory tract of adults. *Lancet* 1980;1:116.

Tipple MA, Beem MO, Saxon EM: Clinical characteristics of the afebrile pneumonia associated with *Chlamydia trachomatis* infection in infants less than six months of age. *Pediatrics* 1979;63:192.

40 *Coxiella burnetii (Q Fever)*

George A. Poporad

Q fever, caused by the *Rickettsia Coxiella burnetii*, is a systemic illness principally manifested in its acute form by fever and variable involvement of the lung and liver. A chronic form of the illness presents as subacute bacterial endocarditis.

Organism

Rickettsiae are highly fastidious bacteria and are obligate intracellular parasites. They are small, pleomorphic coccobacilli that stain very poorly with Gram's stain, but can be seen using Giemsa or Gimenez stains. The agent of Q fever is placed in a different genus, *Coxiella*, than other *Rickettsia* because of the following distinguishing characteristics: 1) *C. burnetii* does not elicit agglutinins against *Proteus vulgaris* X strains which are responsible for the Weil-Felix reaction; 2) it is very resistant to drying and other harmful environmental factors; 3) it does not require an arthropod vector for transmission; and 4) it does not cause rash in man. *C. burnetii* grows in the cytoplasm of endothelial and serosal cells, and grows well in the yolk sac of chick embryos.

Epidemiology

C. burnetii is a zoonotic parasite, ubiquitous in nature and found worldwide including most every state in the United States. There is a high frequency of asymptomic infection in domestic animals such as cattle, sheep and goats as well as many wild animals and ticks. Arthropod vectors appear important in maintaining the infection in nature, but they are not responsible for human disease.

Apparently healthy infected animals shed a large number of organisms in milk, urine, feces, and especially in products of conception. Placenta from infected animals can contain as many as 10^9 infective doses per gram of tissue. Man typically becomes infected by contact with aerosolized organisms from infected livestock, particularly at parturition. *C. burnetii* is very resistant to desiccation and can persist for months in soil and straw and on a variety of objects such as clothing, farm machinery, and trucks. Once aerosolized, organisms can be found in the air for up to 12 days, and studies suggest that the inhalation of a single organism can cause disease in man. Outbreaks have occurred among workers in wool and felt plants, in tanneries, as well as in dairies, slaughterhouses, and sheep-shearing camps. Because of widespread dissemination by air currents of hardy aerosolized organisms, the association between man and livestock, however, need not be a direct one for human infection. Cases have been traced to contaminated clothing, dusty straw, and soil contaminated by animal excreta. *C burnetii* is commonly found in unpasteurized milk of infected cows and it appears that ingestion of infected raw milk can cause asymptomatic infection.

There has been an increased prevalence of *C. burnetii* infection in domestic animals in recent decades, but the diagnosis of cases in man remains sporadic. This possibly can be attributed to underdiagnosis of clinical illness, movement away from farm living and exposure, milk pasteurization, and the probable existence of a large population of people who have asymptomatic infection.

Pathogenesis and Pathology

Available evidence suggests that *C. burnetii* can enter the body through small abrasions in the skin, through the conjunctiva, or by ingestion of raw milk. The majority of cases, however, are associated with inhalation of aerosols of the organism. Q fever often is regarded primarily as a respiratory disease, but it is actually a systemic illness as suggested by its long incubation period (three weeks), documented bacteremia (blood inoculated into guinea pigs), and the variable occurrence of pneumonia (4% to 90% of cases). Hepatitis, and rarely pleuropericarditis, encephalitis and subacute endocarditis can be part of the illness.

As most cases of acute Q fever are not fatal, pathology reports of lung involvement are scarce. In most fatal cases, death is due to lobar pneumonia. Gross appearance of the lung has shown consolidation resembling pneumococcal pneumonia, but the histologic picture more closely resembles that seen in pneumonias caused by *Chlamydia* or viruses. Findings are those of a severe intra-alveolar, focal necrotizing and hemorrhagic process, with a predominance of macrophages in the alveolar exudate. Neutrophils are conspicuously absent. There can be an associated necrotizing bronchitis and bronchiolitis.

Clinical Features

Acute illness occurs after an incubation period ranging from two to four weeks and initially presents as a flu-like syndrome. There is a sudden onset of fever up to 104°F, shaking chills, severe sweating, myalgias, backache, chest pain which may be pleuritic, and anorexia. A severe frontal headache usually is present, and is one of the most prominent symptoms. Photophobia and retro-orbital pain are commonly present. Disorientation and confusion occur in a few patients. There may be mild coryza and sore throat. A slight dry cough can appear about the fifth day after onset, and in a minority of patients sputum may develop and become blood tinged. Clinical signs include a relative bradycardia, conjunctival suffusion, a slightly inflamed pharynx, and an enlarged liver and/or spleen. Physical findings in the chest usually are minimal or absent even in the presence of a pneumonic process.

Chest x-ray abnormalities when present are sufficiently distinctive to suggest the diagnosis. Most cases reveal multiple round, segmental opacities. The opacities are ground glass in appearance, from one to seven in number and are usually found in the lower lobes. Linear atelectasis may also be present. Lobar consolidation, typical of a bacterial pneumonia, is seen in some cases. Pleural reaction and small amounts of pleural fluid may accompany consolidation.

Hepatitis, reflected in abnormal liver function studies, is commonly present. Headache, photophobia, neck pain, and disorientation can be severe enough to suggest meningoencephalitis, but examination of the cerebral spinal fluid is usually normal. Other reported complications of infection include myocarditis and pericarditis, and subacute endocarditis that may appear months to years after an acute attack.

Untreated, fever typically is remittent and persists for an average of two weeks before rapid lysis. The duration of fever tends to increase with age and may last as long as 57 days. Complications are not common and mortality is rare, but convalescence may be protracted over several months with persistence of weakness and fatigue. Resolution of the chest x-ray occurs over 10 to 70 days, with most patients clearing after 30 days.

Diagnosis

Q fever probably is underdiagnosed because of its sporadic occurrence, its varied and sometimes nonspecific manifestations, and the inability to easily culture the organism. In the acute illness, without lung involvement, a differential diagnosis should include influenza, brucellosis (an illness also likely to occur in farming communities), mononucleosis, typhoid fever, and leptospirosis. With pneumonitis and a nondiagnostic sputum gram stain or culture, pneumonia caused by *Mycoplasma, C. psittaci, Legionella*, or viruses should be considered.

A firm diagnosis can only be made with laboratory assistance. In acute illness, organisms can be cultured from blood and urine by intraperitoneal inoculation into mice, hamster, and guinea pigs, or yolk sacs of embryonated chicken eggs. However, isolation procedures present a real hazard of infection to laboratory workers and should only be performed in special laboratories.

The more usual, simpler and safer method of diagnosis is through documenting a rise in complement-fixing antibody titers. Interpretation of serology requires an understanding of antigenic phase variation in strains of *C. burnetii.* Strains newly isolated from animals and ticks are phase I organisms and react only with convalescent serum. Phase I strains are converted to antigenic phase II strains by serial passage through embryonated chicken eggs. Phase II strains react with early as well as convalescent sera. Complement-fixing antibodies against phase II strains are present in 90% of infected individuals by four weeks. Antibodies to phase I strains are found in patients with chronic disease, ie, endocarditis.

More sensitive agglutinating antibody tests are available in reference laboratories.

Treatment and Prevention

Q fever is not as responsive to antibiotic therapy as other rickettsial illnesses. Tetracycline, 500 mg orally every six hours in the adult for about one week, can be effective in decreasing the duration of fever if given within the first three days of acute illness. In the average case, however, antibiotic administration appears to make little difference on the course of the illness. Chloramphenicol can be chosen as an alternate antibiotic but, as with tetracycline, response to therapy is variable.

Human vaccines prepared from either killed or live attenuated organisms appear effective in providing protection, but at present are associated with a high incidence of local reactions and there are questions as to their safety. Vaccines are being evaluated for use in cattle, but as disease in livestock is asymptomatic, there is no economic impetus on farmers to effect disease control.

SELECTED READINGS

Brown GL: Clinical aspects of Q fever. *Postgrad Med J* 1973;49:539.

Derrick EH: The course of infection with *Coxiella burnetii. Med J Aust* 1973;1:1051.

Leedom JM: Q fever: An update, in Remington JS, Swartz MN (eds): *Current Clinical Topics in Infectious Diseases I.* New York, McGraw-Hill, 1980, p 304.

Ormsbee RA: Q fever *Rickettsia*, in Horstall FL, Tamm I (eds): *Viral and Rickettsial Infections of Man*, ed 4. Philadelphia, JB Lippincott, 1965, p 1144.

41 *Respiratory Syncytial Virus*

Richard Snepar

Respiratory syncytial virus (RSV) is responsible for a spectrum of clinical syndromes ranging from mild upper respiratory disease to bronchiolitis and bronchopneumonia. The virus, initially designated "Chimpanzee Coryza Agent" for its role in respiratory disease in chimpanzees, was later found to be a cause of respiratory disease in infants. It is now recognized to be the principal cause of lower respiratory disease in infants and young children.

Microbiologic Characteristics

Respiratory syncytial virus is an enveloped RNA virus belonging to the family Paramyxoviridae. Its RNA helix is surrounded by an envelope with glycoprotein spikes. Following adsorption onto cell lines, the virus is found in the cytoplasm within seven to ten hours and matures at the cytoplasmic membrane. The virus grows well in human cell lines and its presence in cell cultures is detected by its characteristic syncytial cytopathic effect.

Epidemiology

Natural infection with respiratory syncytial virus is limited to man and chimpanzees. The virus has wide geographic distribution. Epidemics occur yearly usually between mid-winter and spring. A rise in hospital admissions for pediatric pneumonia and bronchiolitis heralds the presence of RSV in the community. Most children have serologic evidence of prior infection by 5 years of age, but reinfection is not unusual. During an epidemic, a large proportion of the population may experience infection. When present, RSV usually is the sole infecting virus in the community. This phenomenon of "interference" is also seen with many parainfluenzae viruses and influenza.

Although RSV causes disease at all ages, most lower respiratory infections due to RSV occur in patients under 2 years of age, with the majority under 6 months despite presence of maternal antibody. RSV accounts for 60% to 90% of bronchiolitis and up to 40% of pneumonia cases in infants and young children. Infection with RSV appears to be more severe in males and in those of lower socioeconomic status.

Respiratory syncytial virus has the ability to survive in the environment at room temperature. The virus can be obtained from counter tops for up to six hours, from cloth gowns and paper tissue for up to 45 minutes, and from skin for up to 20 minutes. This factor is important in the transmission of RSV.

Pathogenesis

The portals of entry are the eye and nose, and less frequently the mouth. Infection progresses from the upper respiratory tract to involve the lower respiratory tract. Inflammation of the respiratory mucosa occurs, which may progress to necrotizing bronchiolitis, bronchiolar obstruction and pneumonia. Sloughed epithelium and mucous secretions compromise the lumen of small airways with resulting impedence to air flow, particularly in expiration. Hyperinflation results and with complete obstruction, atelectasis occurs.

RSV infection occurs in the presence of specific antibody against virus. It is unclear whether hypersensitivity, exaggerated cell-mediated responses or absence of local antibody plays a role in the pathogenesis of severe disease in infants. The titer of RSV-specific IgE in nasopharyngeal secretions has been found to correlate with severity of illness and wheezing in infants infected with RSV. Acquired immunity to RSV is incomplete and repeated infections are common but generally less severe than the initial infection.

Clinical Diseases

The incubation period of RSV infection is about five days. Initially, nasal congestion, pharyngitis and occasionally otitis media are present. Fever of 38°C to 40°C is common. The risk of lower respiratory tract infection is high in infants and young children (those with primary infections). In this instance, cough is present and may be paroxysmal or persistent. Dyspnea associated with the findings of tachypnea, prolonged expiration, wheezing, rales and intercostal retractions suggests bronchiolitis or pneumonia.

The chest radiographic findings may range from normal to extensive pneumonia. Diffuse interstitial infiltration is the most frequent finding in hospitalized patients. Hyperaeration, indicative of obstructive emphysema, commonly occurs with or without patchy areas of consolidation, representing atelectasis or alveolar pneumonia, and is suggestive of infection with RSV.

In adults RSV infection usually is a mild illness. It presents as an upper respiratory tract illness or tracheobronchitis, often accompanied by low grade fever. Severe infections (influenza-like syndrome, bronchopneumonia and exacerbations of asthma and chronic bronchitis) do occur, especially in the hospitalized and chronically ill.

Diagnostic Tests

The diagnosis of RSV infection is best made clinically in the proper epidemiologic setting. The virus can be recovered from nasal wash secretions promptly inoculated onto a human cell line if specimens are handled appropriately.

Indirect immunofluorescence has been used successfully to detect RSV antigen but is not widely available. Retrospective diagnoses may be made with neutralization or complement fixation tests, although antibody rises may not be detectable in the infant under 6 months of age.

Treatment

No specific therapy is available for RSV infections. Good supportive care with particular attention to respiration and improvement of hypoxemia is crucial in the treatment of the severely ill infant.

Prevention

Prevention of RSV infection depends on the interruption of spread from personal contacts and contaminated environmental surfaces. This is of limited usefulness in the community. Nosocomial spread to susceptible patients and house staff is common. Hand washing is effective, and infected infants should be isolated from other infants on the ward. Disposable gowns may prevent contamination of clothes. Vaccines have not yet been shown to be protective for RSV infections despite their ability to produce adequate antibody responses.

SELECTED READINGS

Glezen WP, Denny FW: Epidemiology of acute lower respiratory disease in children. *N Engl J Med* 1973;288:498.

Hall CB: Respiratory syncytial virus, in Mandell GL, Douglas RG, Bennett JE (eds): *Principles and Practice of Infectious Diseases*. New York, Wiley and Sons, 1979, p 1186.

Hall CB, Douglas RG, Geiman JM: Possible transmission by fomites of respiratory syncytial virus. *J Infect Dis* 1980;141:98.

McClelland L, Hilleman MR, Hamparian VV, et al: Studies of acute respiratory illness caused by respiratory syncytial virus. *N Engl J Med* 1961;264:1169.

Mufson M, Krause H, Mocega H, et al: Viruses, *Mycoplasma pneumoniae* and bacteria associated with lower respiratory disease among infants. *Am J Epidemiol* 1970;91:192.

Reilly CH, Stokes J Jr, McClelland L, et al: Studies of acute respiratory illness caused by respiratory syncytial virus. *N Engl J Med* 1961;264:1176.

Rice RP, Loda F: A roentgenographic analysis of respiratory syncytial virus pneumonia in infants. *Radiography* 1966;87:1021.

Welliver RC, Wong DT, Sun M, et al: The development of respiratory syncytial virus-specific IgE and the release of histamine in nasopharyngeal secretions after infection. *N Engl J Med* 1981;305:841.

42 *Rhinovirus*

Richard Snepar

Rhinoviruses are the major cause of the common cold, and may play a role in acute sinus infections and asthma. They include a large group of antigenically distinct viruses with common biologic properties.

Microbial Characteristics

Rhinoviruses are members of the picornavirus group. They are small viruses, with single-stranded RNA as their genetic core surrounded by a capsid. The virus is acid labile, which distinguishes it from enteroviruses. Optimum growth occurs at 33°C to 35°C, which corresponds to the temperature found at the nasal mucosa.

Rhinoviruses infect cells by adsorption to specific receptors on the cell surface. Virus synthesis and maturation occurs in the cytoplasm. The virus grows well in human diploid cell lines and can be recognized by its typical cytopathic effects in two to 10 days. Over 100 types of rhinoviruses have been identified based on type-specific surface antigens. It is uncertain whether there exists a gradual antigenic drift or a large number of stable antigenic types.

Epidemiology

Rhinoviruses are ubiquitous and man is the sole host. Infections first occur early in childhood and appear throughout life, although the peak acquisition of antibodies appears in young adults. They are responsible for the annual autumn epidemic of colds, coincident with school opening, and a large proportion of summer colds. Infection rates diminish in winter but rise again in the spring.

Transmission occurs in situations of close contact. The home and school are major epidemiologic settings. The school child is the usual source with secondary attack rates ranging from 20% to 75%. Hand-to-hand transmission of infected nasal secretions, followed by autoinoculation of nasal and conjuctival mucosa, is an efficient means of spread and may be more important than transmission via aerosols. The virus can survive on skin and environmental surfaces for a few hours after contamination of these sites.

Pathogenicity

Rhinoviruses can be recovered in nasal secretions 24 hours after inoculation, and clinical illness appears on the second to fourth days. Infection produces a rise in IgA-neutralizing antibodies in serum and nasal secretions. It is unclear whether serum or nasal antibodies represent the most important immune mechanism. Immunity appears to last for years, although reinfections do occur.

Clinical Disease

Rhinoviruses produce the constellation of symptoms and signs associated with the common cold. Nasal discharge and upper airway obstruction are predominant symptoms and may be associated with malaise, sore throat and cough. Fever usually is low grade or absent. The physical exam reveals inflamed nasal mucosa, and mild pharyngeal erythema is often seen. The illness usually lasts for approximately one week. Acute viral sinusitis and otitis media may complicate a small proportion of cases.

Rhinoviruses are associated with an increased number of respiratory infections in asthmatics, ie, "wheezy bronchitis" or "infectious" asthma, and has been shown to complicate chronic bronchitis.

Rhinovirus, as a cause of croup, bronchitis, bronchiolitis and pneumonia in children as well as atypical pneumonia in adults, has been reported, and while these syndromes do occur, the exact incidence remains unclear.

Diagnostic Tests

The diagnosis of rhinovirus can be made through virus isolation from nasal wash specimens or demonstrations of neutralizing antibody in serum. Unfortunately, the large number of rhinovirus immunotypes makes serodiagnosis difficult.

Therapy

Therapy is symptomatic. Colds are best treated with rest, hydration and nasal decongestants. Aspirin is useful for constitutional symptoms.

Prevention

Hand washing and avoidance of autoinoculation appears to be the optimal method of prevention. No vaccine is available, but experimental vaccines have been effective against a single antigen type. The large number of serotypes remains an obstacle to an effective vaccine.

SELECTED READINGS

Dick EC, Chesney PJ: Rhinovirus, in Feigen RD, Cherry JD (eds): *Textbook of Pediatric Infectious Diseases*. New York, WB Saunders, 1981, P 1167.

Gwaltney J Jr: Rhinovirus, in Mandell GL, Douglas RG, Bennett JE (eds): *Principles and Practice of Infectious Diseases*. New York, Wiley and Sons, 1979, p 1124.

Gwaltney JM Jr, Jordan WS Jr: Rhinovirus and respiratory disease. *Bacteriol Rev* 1964;28:409.

Gwaltney J Jr, Moskalsky PB, Hendley JO: Hand to hand transmission of rhinovirus colds. *Ann Intern Med* 1978;88:463.

Jackson GG, Muldoon RL: Viruses causing common respiratory infections in man. Rhinoviruses. *J Infect Dis* 1973;127:328.

Stott EJ, Killington RA: Rhinoviruses. *Annu Rev Microbiol* 1972;26:503.

43 *Measles*

Richard Snepar

Measles virus produces a highly communicable disease consisting of rash, high fever, cough, coryza and conjunctivitis in its classical form. The pattern of infections with measles has changed dramatically over the last two decades.

Mircrobial Characteristics

Measles virus is a member of the family Paramyxoviridae, and shares the genus *Morbillivirus* with two other antigenically similar viruses: canine distemper and rinderpest. Unlike other paramyxoviruses, these three viruses do not have any virion-associated neuraminidase activity and do not adsorb to neuraminic acid-containing cellular receptors. Measles virus exhibits hemagglutination, while the other members of its genus do not.

Measles virions consist of two structures: a nucleocapsid and an envelope. The inner nucleocapsid consists of a coiled helix of protein and single-stranded RNA. This is surrounded by an envelope of lipids and glycoproteins that contains short projections or spikes. The hemagglutinating, hemolytic and cell fusion properties of the virion reside in the surface of the envelope. The hemagglutinin agglutinates Old World Monkey red blood cells, and is the basis for the major serologic test for measuring antibody to measles virus, hemagglutination inhibition. The hemolysin is believed to facilitate entry of measles virus into cells. The virus was first isolated in vitro in human and simian kidney cells, although it subsequently has been cultivated in other cell lines.

Measles virus infection produces two characteristic cytopathological effects. Multinucleated giant cells (syncytia) occur from the fusion of infected cells. This is dependent on the presence of a virus-specific protein or "fusion factor," and is seen with wild measles virus infection. The second cytopathological effect, spindle cell formation, is typical of vaccine strains and consists of spindle-shaped cells that have long cytoplasmic processes.

The measles virions attach to the cellular receptors by means of the spikes on the virus envelope and enter the cell by either fusion or phagocytosis. The nucleocapsids are then released into the cytoplasm. Viral RNA synthesis takes place predominantly in the cytoplasm, and is followed by the development of the envelope antigens that accumulate in the cytoplasmic membrane. Once intracytoplasmic inclusion bodies of nucleocapsid filaments appear, the cell membrane becomes altered and begins to resemble the virus envelope. Finally, the membrane buds to form young infectious virions.

Epidemiology

Man is the only natural host for measles virus. The disease is seen throughout the world, although incidences vary. In the United States, since the licensure of live measles virus vaccine, the incidence of measles has decreased 90%.

The introduction of the live virus vaccine in 1963 also has altered the age distribution of measles in the United States. Prior to immunization programs, surveys showed that at least 95% of Americans had measles by the age of 15. However, in recent years an increased incidence of infection has become apparent in older adolescents and adults.

Measles may occur at any time of the year, but most outbreaks occur in the late winter and early spring. It is one of the most contagious of all infectious diseases. Spread occurs from direct contact with droplets of respiratory secretions of infected persons, and patients are most infectious when cough and coryza are at their peak.

Pathogenicity

Measles virus most likely invades the respiratory epithelium, where local multiplication causes a primary viremia with localization to the reticuloendothelial system. Necrosis subsequently occurs in these cells, and the virus reinvades leukocytes causing a secondary viremia. After this phase, the respiratory mucosa again becomes involved, with the clinical findings of cough and coryza and often bronchiolitis and pneumonia. Invasion of T-lymphocytes has been postulated to cause the depression of cell-mediated immunity characteristically seen with this disease.

Clinical Diseases

Classical measles develops nine to 11 days following exposure, with the onset of high fever, malaise and conjunctivitis. Respiratory tract involvement is manifest by rhinitis and cough. These prodromal symptoms are followed by a maculopapular rash. It appears first on the forehead, spreads to the face, neck, and trunk and then to the extremities. The rash usually lasts for about five days. Koplik's spots, blue-gray lesions mounted on a red base which appear opposite the molars on the buccal mucosa, can be seen one to two days prior to rash and are a diagnostic finding. The uncomplicated illness lasts seven to 10 days.

Measles may be complicated by measles pneumonia, with or without secondary bacterial pneumonia, bacterial otitis media and encephalitis. Pneumonia has been reported to occur in about 3% of 50% of patients, the frequency probably varying with the thoroughness in which this complication is sought. Pneumonia is the most common cause of death in patients with measles, especially in younger children and the malnourished. However, pneumonia in adolescents, even when clinically severe, is reported to have a good prognosis. Secondary bacterial pneumonia is usually due to *Streptococcus pneumoniae*, *Staphylococcus aureus* or *Hemophilus influenzae*. Its presence is suggested by worsening of respiratory symptoms, persistent high fever and leukocytosis. Radiographic findings of measles pneumonia are not distinctive and may be similar to the findings in measles pneumonia complicated by bacterial superinfection. A fine reticulonodular infiltrate most commonly is found. Usually, it is multilobular, with the lower lobes predominating. The course of the pulmonary findings generally parallels the cutaneous findings.

In the patient with deficient cellular immunity or leukemia, a severe, often fatal, interstitial pneumonia (Hecht's) may occur. It is characterized by the presence of multinuclear giant cells and intranuclear and intracytoplasmic inclusion bodies. Rash may be absent. Prolonged persistence of measles virus in the lung is common and a decreased production of specific antibodies is seen in these patients. Tuberculosis is exacerbated by measles infection, and infection or measles vaccine can cause temporary tuberculin anergy.

Over the last decade, the syndrome of atypical measles has been recognized. This occurs primarily in patients who received killed measles vaccine prior to the introduction of live virus vaccines. Because the introduction of killed vaccine took place in the mid-1960s, these patients are generally adolescents or young adults. Unlike classical measles, following a similar prodrome, the rash begins peripherally involving the palms and soles, progresses to the proximal extremities and trunk and frequently has a petechial or purpuric component. The face is often spared. Pulmonary involvement is a prominent finding. Over 75% of patients have abnormal chest roentgenograms, ranging from hilar adenopathy to nodular or patchy diffuse or lobar infiltrates. Pleural effusions may occur. The illness may be prolonged but fatalities are unusual. This syndrome is thought to represent hypersensitivity to measles virus in a partially immune host. Absence of antibody to F-protein, a surface glycoprotein, which is responsible for cell-to-cell spread of the measles virus, is found in some of these patients. This may be responsible for the failure of the killed vaccine to prevent measles infection.

Diagnostic Tests

The diagnosis of measles can often be made clinically. The differential diagnosis includes rubella, scarlet fever, infectious mononucleosis, enterovirus infection and drug allergy. Atypical measles may be confused with rocky mountain spotted fever or meningococcemia. Isolation of virus from throat washings, blood or urine is difficult and not utilized routinely. Detection of measles antigen by indirect immunofluorescence is possible but not widely available. The most commonly utilized laboratory method for the diagnosis of measles is the hemagglutination inhibition test. A fourfold rise in antibody titer in acute and convalescent serum is considered diagnostic.

Treatment

The therapy for uncomplicated measles is symptomatic. Bacterial superinfection may be difficult to distinguish from primary measles pneumonia, but when suspected should be treated with the proper antibiotics; however, antimicrobial prophylaxis is not indicated.

Prevention

Infection with measles can be effectively prevented with the live virus vaccine. It is usually given near 15 months of age. Vaccine failure occurs if the vaccine is given prior to 12 months of age when the serologic response may be inadequate. Children, adolescents and young adults who have not had measles and were not vaccinated with live measles vaccine should be immunized. Live vaccine is contraindicated in pregnant women, or patients with impaired cell-mediated immunity. Passive immunization with human immune serum globulin (0.25 mL/kg) intramuscularly is recommended as soon as possible following measles exposure to prevent or modify measles in susceptible people (a child between 6 and 15 months of age, or an older child who has never been vaccinated and has not had measles previously). Unless measles occurs, this should be followed in three months by immunization with live virus measles vaccine. In immunocompromised children following measles exposure, a larger dose of immune serum globulin is recommended (0.5 mL/kg, maximum dose 15 mL).

SELECTED READINGS

Annunziato D, Kaplan NH, Hull WW, et al: Atypical measles syndrome: Pathologic and serologic findings. *Pediatrics* 1982;70:203.

Cherry JD: The "new" epidemiology of measles and rubella. *Hosp Pract* 1980;15:49.

Gershon A: Measles (Rubeola) virus, in Mandell GL, Douglas RG, Bennett JE (eds): *Principles and Practice of Infectious Diseases.* New York, Wiley and Sons, 1979, p 1203.

Gremillion DH, Crawford GE: Measles pneumonia in young adults. *Am J Med* 1981;71:539.

Margolin FB, Gandy TK: Pneumonia of atypical measles. *Radiology* 1979; 131:653.

Martin DB, Weiner L, Nieburg P, et al: Atypical measles in adolescents and young adults. *Ann Intern Med* 1979;90:877.

Morgan EM, Rapp F: Measles virus and its associated diseases. *Bacteriol Rev* 1977;41:636.

44 *Coxsackievirus*

George A. Poporad

Coxsackievirus infection usually is asymptomatic, but relatively familiar clinical manifestations include aseptic meningitis, epidemic pleurodynia, pericarditis, and exanthems. A few serotypes have been identified as the cause of a small percentage of acute respiratory illnesses, principally in children and military populations.

Viral Characteristics

Coxsackievirus is classified as an enterovirus, a subgroup of the family Picornaviridae. The viruses in this family are characterized by their small size (20 to 30 nm in diameter), single-stranded RNA core, and a surrounding protein shell or capsid that exhibits icosahedral symmetry. Coxsackievirus is divided into groups A and B depending on antigenicity, pathologic expression of disease in animals, and the sensitivities of various tissue culture systems to infection. There are 23 serotypes of group A and six of group B.

Epidemiology

Coxsackievirus circulates widely in man, especially among infants and children. As with most enteroviruses, there is a seasonal periodicity to its prevalence, summer and autumn months being associated with higher isolation rates and concomitant illness. Respiratory illnesses associated with the virus usually are sporadic, but a particular strain, Type A21, can be the cause of epidemic illness among military recruits.

Pathogenesis and Pathology

Transmission of virus occurs through aerosolized droplets. Development of clinical infection appears to be directly related to inoculum size and the previous antibody status of the host. Preexisting antibody protects against infection.

Respiratory tract infection caused by coxsackievirus rarely is fatal, so pathologic descriptions of the disease are rare. In the few patients who have died (infants), the alveolar walls are thickened and edematous and are infiltrated with mononuclear cells. Alveoli are filled with an exudate of protein, mononuclear cells and red blood cells. A hyaline membrane may form along the smaller air passages and alveoli.

Clinical Illness

After an incubation period of several days, infection of the respiratory tract can express itself as an afebrile "common cold" syndrome (nasal obstruction, rhinitis), a "flu-like" syndrome (fever, myalgias, chills, sore throat, cough), or, very rarely, as pneumonia. There is nothing pathognomonic in its presentation to help differentiate it from the more common causes of viral upper respiratory infections or pneumonitis (such as influenza, rhinovirus, or adenovirus). The pneumonia presents with fever, nonproductive cough, rales, normal to slightly elevated leukocyte count, and an x-ray pattern ranging from diffuse patchy infiltrates to localized bronchopneumonia. Usually, the illness is self-limited, with symptoms and signs resolving in three to four days, but, rarely, deaths secondary to fulminant pneumonia have been reported.

Diagnosis

Coxsackievirus may be isolated from throat swabs, or less commonly, from feces, but it can be very difficult assessing the etiologic significance of the isolate. If the illness occurs in late summer or fall, or in a community or population (military recruits) where similar illnesses are accompanied by virus isolation, the possibility of coxsackievirus causing the infection increases.

Acute infection is associated with fourfold rises in neutralizing and hemagglutination-inhibiting antibody titer. However, testing against 29 serotypes is impractical unless a specific serotype is suspected, such as Type A21 in a military outbreak of illness.

Therapy and Prevention

Therapy is sypmtomatic. Although specific antibody against a serotype appears protective, the usually benign course of the disease and the infrequency of illness make vaccine development impractical.

SELECTED READINGS

Couch RB, Cate TR, Gerone PJ, et al: Production of illness with a small-particle aerosol of coxsackie A-21. *J Clin Invest* 1965;44:535.

Couch RB, Douglas RG, Lindgren KM, et al: Airborne transmission of respiratory infection with coxsackievirus A Type 21. *Am J Epidemiol* 1970;91:78.

Flewett TH: Histologic study of two cases of coxsackie B virus pneumonia in children. *J Clin Pathol* 1965;18:743.

Johnson KM, Bloom HH, Mufson MA, et al: Acute respiratory disease associated with coxsackie A-21 virus infection. I. Incidence in military personnel: Observations in a recruit population. *JAMA* 1962;179:112.

Knight V: *Coxsackievirus and Echovirus. Viral and Mycoplasmal Infections of the Respiratory Tract.* Philadelphia, Lea and Febiger, 1973.

45 *Varicella-Zoster*

George A. Poporad

Varicella-zoster virus (VZV) is a herpesvirus and as such shares with the family's other members (herpes simplex virus, Epstein-Barr virus, cytomegalovirus) the properties of latency and reactivation. Primary infection with VZV in normal hosts presents as a generalized vesicular rash and accompanying systemic manifestations whose severity varies directly with the patient's age (varicella). After primary infection, the virus can persist in dorsal nerve root ganglions. Reactivation of this latent infection is characterized by a unilateral vesicular eruption in a dermatomal distribution (zoster). The primary infection (varicella) has the potential to cause pneumonia, both in normal and immunocompromised hosts, and zoster, in only immunocompromised hosts.

Viral Characteristics

VZV is indistinguishable morphologically from other members of the herpesvirus group. It contains a nucleic acid core of double-stranded DNA enclosed in an icosahedral protein capsid consisting of 162 capsomers. An envelope of lipids and glycoproteins surrounds the nucleocapsid. The overall diameter of the virion is approximately 200 nm.

Epidemiology

Varicella is a highly contagious disease primarily involving children. Its occurrence is seasonal with most cases appearing in late winter or spring. Eighty-five percent of cases occur in children before 9 years of age and most of the remaining cases occur during the teenage years. Following introduction of infection into a household, 88% of susceptible children will develop the illness within two weeks and 96% can be expected to become ill within two incubation periods (approximately one month) of the index case. Few people escape infection until adulthood.

The development of pneumonia during primary VZV infection varies with age and immune status. In the normal host, pneumonia complicates varicella in about 10% to 15% of patients, although accurate data is difficult to obtain because lung involvement can be minimal and associated with a paucity of physical findings. Most cases of varicella pneumonia occur in adults. Ninety percent of those with documented varicella pneumonia are older than 19 years of age, and 75% of cases occur in the third through fifth decades. When pneumonia does present in a normal child with varicella, it usually has a bacterial etiology, and *Hemophilus influenzae*, *Streptococcus pneumoniae*, and *Streptococcus pyogenes* are the usual pathogens. Varicella pneumonia in the normal host usually is a self-limited illness, but mortality can approach 10% to 30% usually in the immunocompromised patient.

Varicella pneumonia in younger age groups occurs most often in immunocompromised hosts. In the neonate, there are reported cases of "varicella neonatorum" which presents as disseminated visceral disease, including pneumonia, in neonates born to mothers who develop varicella in the peripartum period. In children receiving anticancer therapy, varicella can disseminate in approximately 30% of infected patients, with pneumonia affecting about 78% of those who do disseminate. Mortality from varicella in these children is approximately 7% compared to less than one in 100,000 for varicella in the general population. Pulmonary and central nervous system involvement are determinants for a fatal outcome.

Herpes zoster occurs exclusively in those individuals who have had previous infection with VZV. Because it represents reactivation from previous infection, there is no seasonal predilection. It occurs in people of all ages with the frequency increasing directly with age. The frequency of zoster in the general population is reported to be approximately 5.4%, with the rate increasing to a high of 16% in patients in the ninth decade of life. There is an increased frequency and severity of infection in patients with malignancies, particularly lymphomas. Frequency of illness ranges from 4% to 25% in patients suffering from Hodgkin's disease. Dissemination occurs in less than 2% of cases of zoster in the general population, usually in the elderly, but in immunocompromised hosts, particularly those with Hodgkin's disease, the frequency of dissemination increases to 6% to 25%. Pneumonia is a rare occurrence in disseminated illness. Zoster rarely is life threatening and there is a low mortality (< 5%) associated with dissemination.

Pathogenesis and Pathology

Man is the only known host for VZV. The virus is spread from person to person by contact with vesicular skin lesions and possibly by the respiratory route, although the latter has not been confirmed. Normal hosts appear to be contagious prior to onset of the rash (implying a respiratory route mode of spread) and for only a few days after the onset of skin lesions, this corresponding with the ability to isolate virus from vesicular fluid. Susceptible individuals exposed to zoster can develop varicella, although zoster appears to be a less contagious illness than varicella. Infectivity and the ability to isolate virus decreases in both types of infection as vesicular lesions dry and begin to crust.

Varicella virus has a particular affinity for epithelial tissues. Infected cells develop intranuclear inclusions and undergo ballooning degeneration. As they disintegrate, small fluid-filled spaces develop, forming the vesicle. Accompanying the vesicle formation, there is disordered cell division creating multinucleated giant cells. With disseminated disease, vesicles similar to those found on the skin occur on pleural surfaces, in the tracheobronchial tree, on surfaces of the liver and spleen, and on the mucosa of the gastrointestinal tract. In the lung, there are areas of focal neurosis. Microscopic examination shows interstitial pneumonitis with edema, septal cell proliferation, and invasion of the septal walls with mononuclear cells. The bronchioles are filled with an exudate, and the alveoli and bronchioles may be lined with a hyaline membrane composed of red cells, fibrin and mononuclear cells. Typical eosinophilic intranuclear inclusions are found in mononuclear cells in the exudate, septal cells, epithelial cells of the tracheobronchial tree, and capillary endothelium.

Clinical Manifestations

The incubation period for varicella ranges from three to 21 days, with an average of 14 days. The illness is characterized by a generalized papulovesicular skin eruption with few systemic manifestations in children. The temperature can be elevated to 100° to 102°F for a few days during the evolution of the rash. The exanthem usually begins on the scalp or trunk and subsequently spreads centrifically, with lesions appearing in different stages of evolution. Mucous membranes of the mouth and conjunctiva may be involved. In the usual uncomplicated case, no new lesions develop after approximately four days and the child goes on to crusting and healing of the vesicles. Rare complications of the illness include encephalitis, aseptic meningitis, acute cerebellitis, Guillain-Barré syndrome, Reye's syndrome, arthritis and purpura fulminans.

The illness typically is more severe in normal adults and immunocompromised children. In the normal adult, systemic manifestations consisting of chills, high fever, myalgia and arthralgia are common. The rash can be quite severe, becoming confluent and hemorrhagic and involving the mucous membranes of the mouth and throat. Pneumonia in the adult can range from mild asymptomatic lung involvement discovered only on routine chest x-ray to severe fulminant illness. Symptomatic pneumonia usually develops in the face of severe skin involvement and symptoms become most pronounced at the height of the rash. Pneumonia typically occurs early in the course of the illness, one to six days after the onset of rash. Cardinal symptoms include cough, dyspnea, tachypnea, hemoptysis, and chest pain reflecting pleural involvement. High fever usually is present, but examination of the chest can be unimpressive. Laboratory data is significant for a normal to slightly increased leukocyte count with a leftward shift in the differential, and hypoxia in

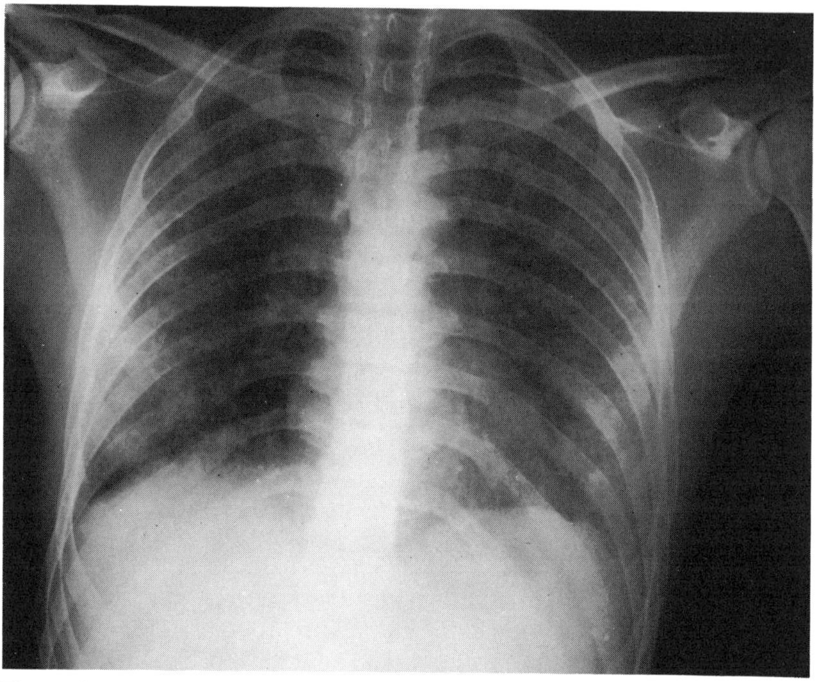

Figure 45-1 A previously healthy 36-year-old adult acquired varicella from household contact and developed severe cutaneous varicella rash and varicella pneumonia. Note diffuse, widespread nodular infiltrate in both lung fields.

severe cases. The chest x-ray picture is characteristic (Figure 45-1). There are diffuse, ill-defined, coarse nodular infiltrates throughout both lung fields that tend to coalesce at the bases. Pleural effusions are rare. The disease can be fatal within three days, but varicella pneumonia in the adult usually is self-limited and recovery correlates with the clearing of skin lesions, within seven to 14 days. X-ray changes may persist for up to two and one-half months, and nodular calcifications can develop, probably in areas of focal lung necrosis. Residual lung damage reflected in an abnormal diffusion capacity can persist for years.

In children on anticancer therapy, skin lesions developing for longer than five days from the onset of the initial eruption together with prolonged fever should raise the suspicion of visceral dissemination. This can involve the liver, central nervous system, and lung. Pneumonia, as stated earlier, prognosticates a higher mortality. Those who survive follow a similar course to recovery as the adult.

Zoster manifests itself as radicular pain occurring several days before the onset of a vesicular eruption in a dermatomal distribution. One to three dermatomes may be involved and the exanthem occurs most commonly in the thoracic area. The evolution of individual lesions is identical to varicella. New lesions develop for three to four days, occasionally as long as seven days.

In the elderly and immunocompromised patient, zoster may disseminate outside its original dermatomal distribution to involve other areas of the skin and visceral organs. With cutaneous dissemination, new lesions will appear in a generalized distribution, usually about one week after the onset of the localized eruption. Some of these patients will develop visceral involvement with dissemination to the lung, central nervous system, liver, pancreas and gastrointestinal tract. Pulmonary involvement is relatively infrequent. However, mortality in disseminated zoster, although low, most commonly occurs as a consequence of severe lung involvement.

Diagnosis

A clinical diagnosis is not difficult to make with the presence of the typical skin eruption. The chest x-ray picture described, although classic, is nonspecific and can be seen in such diseases as sarcoidosis, carcinomatosis, and miliary tuberculosis. Pneumonia in a normal child with varicella is commonly of bacterial etiology. Clues to a bacterial cause include pneumonia first appearing after defervescence from the varicella, an abrupt onset of symptoms with a rapid secondary rise in temperature, elevated peripheral leukocyte count, lobar consolidation on chest x-ray, and sputum gram stain and culture revealing pathogenic bacteria, usually *H. influenzae, S. pneumoniae* or *S. pyogenes.*

The laboratory rarely is needed to help in diagnosis. Virus can be isolated from vesicular lesions in both varicella and zoster during the first days of the rash. Serology by complement fixation can demonstrate a rise in antibody titer over a two- to four-week period, later in immunocompromised patients. There is a report of intranuclear inclusions being demonstrable in sputum.

Therapy and Prevention

Antiviral therapy is playing an expanding role in VZV infections involving those patients at high risk for complications, ie, immunosuppressed hosts. Vidarabine (adenine arabinoside) has proven useful in treating immunosuppressed patients with varicella. In one study, vidarabine at a dose of 10 mg/kg/day for five days accelerated cessation of new vesicle formation, decreased the median daily lesion count, lowered fever more rapidly, and decreased complications (pneumonitis, hepatitis, death) compared to placebo. Vidarabine produced a similar reduction in zoster-related visceral complications when used in immunocompromised patients. Recently, acyclovir (at a dose of 500 mg/m^2 of body surface area per dose, three times daily for seven days) has been shown to prevent cutaneous and visceral dissemination of zoster in immunocompromised adults. Experts in the field would recommend either acyclovir or vidarabine therapy in immunocompromised patients who develop varicella or who are moderately to severely ill with zoster. Although the usefulness of antiviral therapy has not been determined in established visceral disease, these drugs can be recommended in the treatment of severe visceral complications, including pneumonia in normal hosts.

Passive immunization with varicella-zoster immune globulin (VZIG) has been shown effective in reducing the severity of varicella in immunocompromised children. This preparation is made available for protection of such patients (≤ 15 years old) after significant exposure to varicella or zoster and in newborn infants of women who develop a varicella rash from five days before until two days after delivery. VZIG should be given as soon after exposure as possible. It is more likely to be effective if given within 72 hours; after 96 hours it is of uncertain value. Recommended dosage is based on body weight, with one complete vial (125 units) given for each 10 kg, up to a maximum of five vials for children weighing over 50 kg.

Control of infection requires the realization that varicella is highly contagious. Immunocompromised hosts should be protected from exposure. To prevent spread of infection in a hospital setting, children who are suspected of incubating the illness should be discharged or not admitted, if possible. Likewise, children who develop the illness during hospitalization should be sent home. Strict isolation is needed for those patients who require hospital care, and only those personnel who have had a previous history of varicella should care for the patient. Similar isolation is recommended for those patients with zoster, even though it is considered less contagious than varicella.

SELECTED READINGS

Balfour HH, Bean B, Laskin OL, et al: Acyclovir halts progression of herpes zoster in immunocompromised patients. *N Engl J Med* 1983;308:1448.

Dolin R, Reichman RC, Mazur MH, et al: Herpes zoster-varicella infections in immunosuppressed patients. *Ann Intern Med* 1978;89:375.

Feldman S, Hughes, WT, Daniel CB: Varicella in children with cancer: Seventy-seven cases. *Pediatrics* 1975;56:388.

Oppenheimer EH: Congenital chickenpox with disseminated visceral lesions. *Bull John Hopkins Hosp* 1944;74:240.

Triebwasser JH, Harris RE, Bryant RE, et al: Varicella pneumonia in adults. *Medicine* 1967;46:409.

Weinstein L, Meade RH: Respiratory manifestations of chicken pox. *Arch Intern Med* 1956;98:91.

Whitley RJ, Hilty M, Haynes R, et al: Vidarabine therapy of varicella in immunosuppressed patients. *J Pediatrics* 1982;101:125.

Whitley RJ, Soong S, Dolin R, et al: Early vidarabine therapy to control the complications of herpes zoster in immunosuppressed patients. *N Engl J Med* 1982;307:971.

46 *Herpes Simplex*

George A. Poporad

HERPES SIMPLEX VIRUS PNEUMONIA

Herpes simplex virus (HSV) is a member of the Herpetoviridae family and as such shares with the families' other members (varicella-zoster virus, Epstein-Barr virus, cytomegalovirus) the properties of latency and reactivation. After primary infection, HSV can lie dormant in nerve tissue for a variable period of time, and then be reactivated by a broad range of stimuli. Both the primary infection and reactivation infections may be asymptomatic or be associated with clinical disease. Type 1 herpes simplex virus (HSV-1) is responsible for skin, oral, ocular, and CNS infection (encephalitis). Type 2 (HSV-2) causes genital and neonatal infections. Both types have the potential to disseminate in the neonate and compromised host, involving multiple organs including the lung.

Viral Characteristics

HSV contains a nucleic acid core of double-stranded DNA enclosed in an icosahedral protein capsid consisting of 162 capsomers. This nucleocapsid is surrounded by an envelope of lipids and glycoproteins. The virion has an overall diameter of 150 to 200 nm (Figure 46-1). The two types, HSV-1 and HSV-2, have differences in their clinical and epidemiologic patterns of disease (Table 46-1), as well as possessing different biochemical and biologic characteristics such as pock size on chick embryo chorioallantoic membranes, the ability to form plaques in chick embryo cultures, and base composition of their DNA.

Epidemiology

HSV has man as its only natural reservoir. Infection is caused by direct inoculation of skin or mucous membranes with infected secretions from symptomatic or asymptomatic excretors. Transmission may occur through sexual, skin-to-skin, or mouth-to-skin contact. Approximately 0.65% to 15% of adults may be excreting HSV-1 or HSV-2 at any given time depending on the population studied.

In neonatal disease, exposure to the virus can occur in utero through transplacental spread or by ascension of the virus from an infected genital tract when fetal membranes are prematurely ruptured. The neonate also may acquire infection by passing through an infected birth canal. There is a 40% risk of neonatal infection if virus is present in the

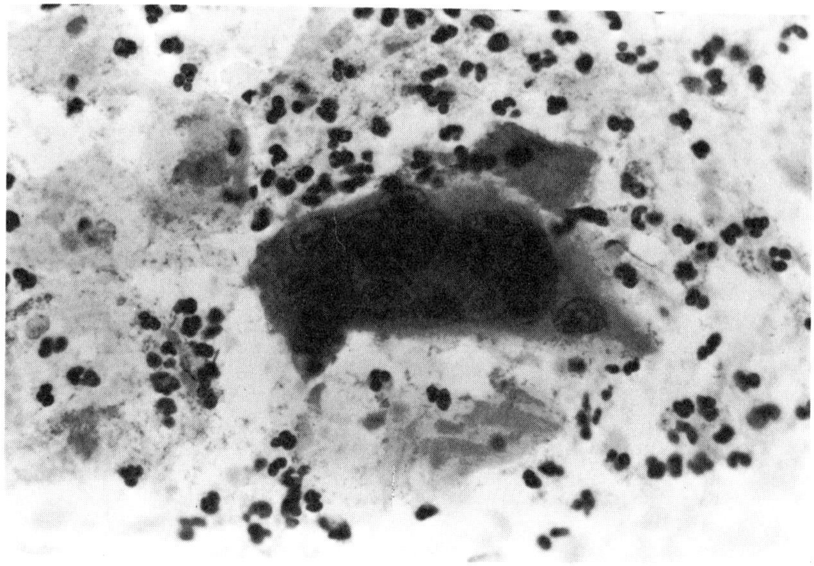

Figure 46-1 Herpes virus electronmicrograph of outer viral envelope enclosing the central nucleocapsid. Courtesy of John J. Bozzola, PhD, Department of Microbiology, Medical College of Pennsylvania.

mother's genital tract at delivery. Postdelivery acquisition can occur through contact with infected hospital personnel or family members. Neonatal herpetic disease is most commonly caused by HSV-2 because of genital tract exposure during delivery, but HSV-1 can be responsible for up to 30% of the illnesses.

There is an increased incidence of HSV infection with increasing age that is also related to socioeconomic status. In lower socioeconomic groups there is a rapid rise in HSV-1 antibodies during early childhood, with 80% to 100% of this subgroup having serologic evidence of infection by adulthood. This compares with 30% to 50% in those groups with

Table 46-1
Clinical and Epidemiologic Differences Between Herpes Simplex Virus 1 and 2

	HSV-1	HSV-2
Type of Infection	Found primarily in oral secretions with infection of nongenital sites (oral, eye, skin above waist); encephalitis	Found primarily in genital secretions with infection of primarily genital sites (genital tract, skin below the waist)
Transmission	Nonvenereal; oral to other body site	Venereal; mother to neonate

a higher standard of living. HSV-2 antibodies generally do not appear until after puberty and are directly correlated with sexual activity. Again, lower socioeconomic groups have a higher incidence of infection, with 20% to 60% infected compared to 10% in higher socioeconomic groups.

Usually, symptomatic infection with the virus is localized clinically to a specific area, ie, HSV-1 causing infection of the mucocutaneous area of the mouth and skin above the waist, and HSV-2 causing genital lesions and infection of the skin below the waist. Both viruses have the potential to disseminate in compromised hosts. These compromised hosts include neonates, and children or adults who are malnourished, who have loss of skin integrity (diffuse burns or eczema), or who are immunosuppressed (children with measles, transplant recipients, patients with lymphomas or leukemia, and patients receiving cancer chemotherapy and corticosteroids).

Recently, disseminated herpes simplex virus infections have been described in the acquired immune deficiency syndrome (AIDS). AIDS is a syndrome characterized by a marked suppression of T-cell immunity with resultant opportunistic infection. To date, the illness has affected previously healthy young homosexual men, parenteral drug abusers, steady female sexual partners of IV drug abusers or bisexual men, children of mothers with AIDS or who belong to high-risk groups for AIDS, Haitians, and hemophiliacs. The opportunistic infections include *Pneumocystis carinii* pneumonia, cryptosporidiosis, and disseminated atypical mycobacterial and fungal, as well as viral disease. The immune deficiency is thought to be due to the host's response to an infectious agent, possibly viral, acquired during sexual contact or through the parenteral use of drugs or blood products.

Pathogenesis and Pathology

Primary infection with the virus involves viral contact with skin and mucous membranes and then invasion of epithelial cells. Viral replication causes cell death and an accompanying inflammatory response causes vesicle formation. Viral replication occurs locally and spreads cell to cell. Lymphatics and lymph nodes draining the primary site are involved and can be sites of viral replication.

After the primary infection, the virus travels proximally via neuronal axons to sensory ganglions where it remains dormant until reactivated by diverse stimuli such as fever, sunlight exposure, emotional stress, or trauma. The virus has been isolated from trigeminal, sacral, superior cervical, and vagus ganglions. The mechanism of viral reactivation is unknown. Cytotoxic and neutralizing antibodies do not prevent recurrent illness or fatal disease. The role of cell-mediated immunity is not defined, but its importance is suggested by the increase in severity of infection in patients with compromised cellular immune function.

In a newborn or immunocompromised host, and infrequently in an apparently normal host, infection can spread contiguously from the oral cavity to involve the esophagus, tracheobronchial tree or lung. Local trauma such as endotracheal intubation or nasogastric tube placement is a major inciting factor. The virus also has the potential of disseminating hematogenously from a local infection to visceral organs such as liver, lung, adrenal gland, and brain. Viremia has been documented in newborns and the immunosuppressed host.

The pathology of herpetic involvelment of the tracheobronchial tree is characterized by ulceration and necrosis of epithelium. Epithelial cells undergo ballooning degeneration, form giant cells, and develop typical eosinophilic intranuclear inclusions (Figure 46-2). Cells can separate and desquamate into the bronchial lumen. In the lung, alveolar lining cells undergo similar degeneration with giant cell and intranuclear inclusion formation. The alveolar walls are necrosed and the alveoli are filled with a proteinaceous exudate that can be hemorrhagic. Neutrophilic infiltration is sparse. There can be evidence of severe bacterial or fungal superinfection.

Clinical Course

Primary herpetic infection becomes clinically apparent from two to

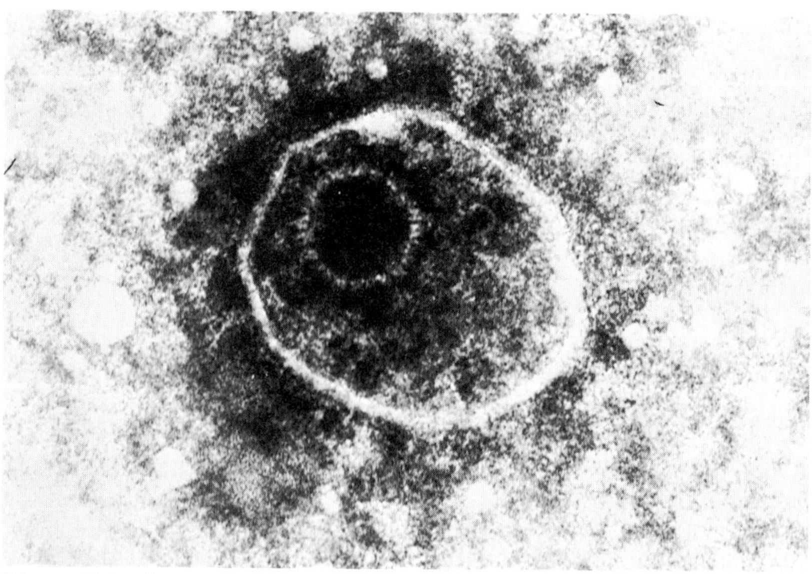

Figure 46-2 A characteristic multinucleated cell of herpetic infection with intranuclear inclusions. Note the ground-glass appearance of the nuclei with condensation of chromatin near nuclear membranes. Polymorphonuclear cells and bacteria are present in the background. (Papanicolaou stain × 160). Courtesy of Donna Eckardt, BSCT (ASCP), Department of Pathology, Medical College of Pennsylvania.

20 days after exposure. In the neonate, signs of infection may present as early as the first day of birth or as late as three weeks after birth. Infection in the newborn can present in several ways: as localized vesicles and ulcerations of the skin, conjunctiva, and/or mouth; as localized CNS disease (meningoencephalitis) with or without localized skin, eye and/or mouth involvement; and as disseminated disease involving the lung (pneumonia), the liver (hepatitis), or the bone marrow (pancytopenia). Accompanying signs and symptoms of dissemination can be nonspecific and include fever, anorexia, lethargy, vomiting and jaundice. The hallmark of the disease when present is skin vesicles, but about 20% of newborns with HSV infection never have skin involvement. Progression of disease from localized skin vesicles to involvement of other sites can occur in up to 70% of newborns. Mortality approaches 80% with CNS disease, pneumonia, or disseminated intravascular coagulation. All newborns with skin vesicles have recurrent skin lesions during the first year of life, and a significant number continue to have recurrent lesions after the first year. Recurrent skin infections after 1 month of age, however, are not associated with further progression of disease.

In the immunocompetent host over the age of 1 month, symptomatic primary infection with HSV-1 manifests itself as a gingivostomatitis, pharyngitis, or tonsillitis. Small vesicles form on the pharyngeal and oral mucosa that ulcerate and increase in number. Pain, fever, and cervical adenopathy accompany the illness. Autoinoculation to other sites (ie, fingers) is not uncommon especially in children.

Primary infection of the eye (usually HSV-1) presents as a unilateral follicular conjunctivitis with regional adenopathy, or as a blepharitis with vesicles on the lid margin.

Primary genital infection, common in adolescents and young adults, is usually caused by HSV-2. In the male, vesicular lesions on an erythematous base occur on the glans penis or penile shaft. In the female, lesions may involve the vulva, perineum, buttocks, cervix or vagina. Infection usually is associated with fever, malaise, anorexia and bilateral tender inguinal adenopathy. Involvement of the anal areas and rectum is being recognized with increased frequency in male homosexual populations due to mouth-anal or genital-anal contact.

Recurrent herpetic infection tends to be much less severe with less fever, constitutional symptoms and adenopathy, and with less extensive lesions than primary infection. Recurrent oral infection usually presents as "herpes labialis" with vesicular formation and pain at the vermillion border of the lip. Ocular infection can recur as keratitis, blepharitis, or keratoconjunctivitis. Recurrent genital infections in females can present only on the cervix and be asymptomatic.

As discussed previously, in the immunocompromised child or adult, primary or secondary herpetic infection can reach the tracheobronchial tree and lung from local contiguous spread or through hematogenous dissemination. With hematogenous dissemination, mortality approaches 100%. Lung involvement usually presents as dyspnea, cough and fever, with associated hypoxemia. The typical x-ray picture is a diffuse interstitial pneumonia, although focal and multifocal infiltrates can be present. The interstitial pneumonia pattern suggests a hematogenous origin, whereas focal pneumonitis suggests contiguous spread from the upper respiratory tract.

Diagnosis

The diagnosis of a pneumonia caused by HSV can be suspected when typical vesicular lesions are found on the lips, mucous membranes of the oral cavity, skin, or genitals in a neonate or immunocompromised patient with an interstitial pulmonary infiltrate. The presence or absence of skin lesions, however, does not confirm or negate pulmonary involvement. Likewise, culturing herpes simplex from the oropharynx or sputum does not necessarily imply HSV lung infection.

Serology is of little value in the diagnosis of acute illness except in neonates. Antibodies appear from one to four weeks after primary infection and are most commonly detected by neutralization or complement fixation techniques. IgM found in the serum of newborns offers good evidence of perinatal infection. Primary infection in the child or adult can only be diagnosed serologically in retrospect by demonstrating a fourfold rise in antibody titer. Serologic diagnosis is, however, complicated by the fact that HSV-1 and HSV-2 share common antigens, and it is difficult to differentiate between the serum antibodies of a specific viral type, particularly in the serum of individuals who have antibodies to both types. A primary infection with HSV-1 would be difficult to detect in the face of previous HSV-2 infection and vice versa. Also, it appears that IgG and IgM persist in recurrent illness with little titer change. Therefore, recurrent infection cannot be differentiated from primary infection.

The most sensitive method of diagnosis of HSV pneumonia is lung biopsy. Typical intranuclear inclusions separated from the nuclear membrane by a nonstaining halo can be demonstrated (Figure 46-2). The virus can be isolated in tissue culture and the cytopathic changes develop so rapidly that a tentative diagnosis can be provided in 24 to 48 hours and confirmed by indirect immunofluorescent antibody staining. The virus also can be demonstrated in biopsy specimens by direct immunofluorescence and electron microscopy. HSV, cytomegalovirus and varicella-zoster virus produce similar intranuclear inclusions, but can be distinguished, one from the other, by indirect immunofluorescent antibody staining of virus-infected cells. Also, clinically, varicella-zoster infection is associated with characteristic skin lesions.

Therapy and Prevention

At present, there is no proven effective therapy to prevent or treat HSV dissemination and involvement of the lung. As neutralizing antibodies are not protective against viral recurrence or dissemination, gammaglobulin administration is not considered useful. Similarly, vaccine administration would not be effective against recurrent disease, and producing an effective vaccine to protect against primary infection is hampered by concerns about the potential for latency and recurrence of a live vaccine virus.

Antiviral chemotherapy plays a limited but expanding role in therapy. In neonatal disease vidarabine (adenosine arabinoside) has been shown to reduce mortality in newborns with disseminated disease, including pneumonia, and localized CNS involvement, but the effect of therapy on morbidity is less impressive. Vidarabine may prevent progression of localized involvement of skin, eye or mouth to more serious forms of HSV infection, if given sufficiently early in the course of illness. The recommended dosage of vidarabine in the neonate is 15 mg/kg daily IV, given over 12 hours for 10 days. In children and adults, parenteral acyclovir has proven useful in treating mucocutaneous herpes simplex infection in immunocompromised patients. There is insufficient clinical data to unequivocally recommend the use of either vidarabine or acyclovir, for other forms of HSV infection, ie, HSV pneumonia and/or disseminated disease, but experts in the field, nevertheless, would use parenteral acyclovir therapy in those children or adults with life-threatening disseminated HSV infection because of its increased in vitro activity against HSV and demonstrated efficacy in less serious illness due to herpes simplex virus.

Prevention of HSV infection depends on avoiding contact with infected lesions. Patients with herpetic lesions should be kept away from newborns, children with eczema or burns, or from immunosuppressed patients. Medical and dental personnel should wear gloves when examining patients with potentially infectious lesions. Genital herpes in late pregnancy is potentially dangerous to the neonate, and cesarean section is recommended to avoid neonatal exposure if cervical infection is present clinically at parturition or if virus is isolated near the time of delivery.

SELECTED READINGS

Arvin AM, Yeager AS, Bruhn FW, et al: Neonatal herpes simplex infection in the absence of mucocutaneous lesions. *J Pediatr* 1982;100:715.

Becker WB, Kipps H, McKenzie D: Disseminated herpes simplex virus infection. *Am J Dis Child* 1968;115:1.

Douglas RG, Anderson S, Weg JG, et al: Herpes simplex pneumonia. *JAMA* 1969;210:902.

Herout V, Vortel V, Vondrackova A: Herpes simplex involvement of the lower respiratory tract. *Am J Clin Pathol* 1966;46:411.

Honig PJ, Brown D: Congenital herpes simplex virus infection initially resembling epidermolysis bullosa. *J Pediatr* 1982;101:958.

Mildvan D, Mathur U, Enlow RW, et al: Opportunistic infections and immune deficiency in homosexual men. *Ann Intern Med* 1982;96:700.

Nahmias AJ, Roizman B: Infection with herpes simplex virus I and II. *N Engl J Med* 1973;289:667–672, 781–789.

Nash G, Major MC, Foley FD: Herpetic infection of the middle and lower respiratory tract. *Am J Clin Pathol* 1970;54:858.

Ramsey PG, Fife KH, Hackman RC, et al: Herpes simplex virus pneumonia. *Ann Intern Med* 1982;97:813–820.

Wade JC, Newton B, McLarin C, et al: Intravenous acyclovir to treat mucocutaneous herpes simplex virus infection after marrow transplantation. *Ann Intern Med* 1982;96:265.

Whitley RJ, Nahmias AJ, Soong S, et al: Vidarabine therapy of neonatal herpes simplex virus infection. *Pediatrics* 1980;66:495.

Whitley RJ, Nahmias AJ, Visintine AM, et al: The natural history of herpes simplex virus infection of mother and newborn. *Pediatrics* 1980;66:489.

47 *Epstein-Barr Virus*

George A. Poporad

Epstein-Barr Virus (EBV) commonly causes a benign, self-limited lymphoproliferative illness manifested as fever, pharyngitis, and adenopathy (infectious mononucleosis). Nonlymphoid tissues may be involved, presenting clinically as hepatitis, encephalitis and, rarely, pneumonia.

Organism

EBV is a herpesvirus and as such shares common morphologic properties with the other human herpesviruses (herpes simplex virus, varicella-zoster virus, and cytomegalovirus). EBV contains a nucleic acid core of double-stranded DNA enclosed in an icosahedral protein capsid consisting of 162 capsomers. An envelope of lipids and glycoproteins surrounds the nucleocapsid. The overall diameter of the virion is approximately 200 nm.

Epidemiology

The prevalence of EBV infection as determined by seroconversion depends on age and socioeconomic status. Most infections occur in children before the age of 5 years, followed by another surge during the second decade of life. By adulthood, 90% to 100% of most populations studied have antibodies. Lower socioeconomic groups more frequently have EBV antibody prevalence than age-matched controls of a higher economic status. Infectious mononucleosis (IM) occurs most frequently in populations in which primary EBV exposure is delayed until adolescence and young adulthood. Its peak incidence in the United States is in the 10- to 30-year age group. It is uncommon to occur after age 30 and rare after 40 years of age. College and military populations experience the highest morbidity.

Low titers of EBV are present in throat washings of those suffering from IM, and EBV can persist in the oropharynx for up to 18 months after clinical recovery. Also, virus can be cultured from throat washings in 10% to 20% of healthy adults. Not surprisingly, the majority of people who develop IM recall no previous contact with another case. The degree of contagion is low, and intimate contact between a susceptible host and a shedder of EBV appears necessary to pass the infection.

It appears that EBV can cause persistent latent infection as evidenced by the fact that a small percentage of lymphocytes continue to carry EBV in the blood of all seropositive individuals. Also, immunocompromised individuals (renal transplant recipients, patients with lymphoma, patients receiving immunosuppressive therapy) have an increased frequency of EBV excretion in the oropharynx (ranging from 16% to 60%), suggesting reactivation without clinical illness.

EBV, unlike the other members of the herpes group of viruses, has not been documented to be a major threat to the immunocompromised patient. At present there have been no distinct clinical syndromes attributed to EBV in immunocompromised hosts.

Several large series report a 3% to 5% prevalence of pneumonia associated with IM. There are also isolated cases in the literature reporting atypical pneumonia and pleural effusions associated with IM or with evidence of primary EBV infection determined by specific serology. It must be pointed out, however, that in many reports the diagnosis of IM was made before the etiologic role of EBV had been defined, and in some cases depended on varying methods and criteria of determining the presence of heterophile antibodies in significant titer. Also, in some cases, other etiologic agents that are known to cause the "atypical pneumonia syndrome" were not excluded.

Pathogenesis and Pathology

The host range of EBV appears rather limited. Cells known to be susceptible to infection are B-lymphocytes of humans, lymphoid cells of higher primates, and epithelial cells obtained from biopsies of nasopharyngeal carcinoma. Susceptible cells possess surface receptor sites specific for EBV.

Knowledge of EBV replication within an infected cell is incomplete because there is no host cell that permits completion of viral replication in vitro. With viral infection, B-lymphocytes can be transformed from cells with limited in vitro growth potential to lymphoid cells capable of rapid and persistent multiplication, and capable of continuous in vitro cultivation. There is the belief that a proportion of infected lymphoid cells produce viral progeny and subsequently die, but there is no specific information available on how EBV virus is assembled or released.

After viral entry into a susceptible cell, Epstein-Barr nuclear antigen (EBNA) is demonstrable in nuclei of infected cells. With viral synthesis, viral capsid antigen (VCA) is expressed, but only in those few cell lines that are capable of synthesizing virus (producer cells). Most cells infected with EBV are not capable of expressing the antigen (nonproducer cells). In certain infected cell lines, an early antigen (EA) can be induced by chemical manipulation or by superinfecting a nonproducer cell line with EBV. The expression of EA under these conditions probably represents a derepression of EA-producing genes. Early antigen may be diffuse (EA-D) and be seen in the nucleus and cytoplasm of the cell, or restricted (EA-R) and seen as discrete masses in the cytoplasm.

On the basis of available evidence, infection with EBV probably occurs through the oropharynx. Presumably, infected lymphoid cells in the oropharynx are transformed and proliferate. Some undoubtedly permit virus growth, die and release EBV progeny. During the incubation period which lasts from 30 to 50 days, EBV and EBV-transformed B-lymphocytes are thought to proliferate and disseminate to distant lymphoid tissues and to certain nonlymphoid organs.

With human infection, there are several viral-specific and nonspecific antibodies produced. Specific antibodies are made against the previously mentioned viral antigens. Nonspecific heterophile antibodies, which are IgM, are directed against antigens found on sheep, horse and beef red cells. Heterophile antibodies do not cross-react with EBV-specific antibodies.

In early human EBV infection, non-EBV-specific cell-mediated immunity is depressed as reflected by cutaneous anergy and a decreased proliferative response of T-cells to mitogens. There is, however, an intense lymphocytosis with the appearance of atypical lymphocytes in the peripheral blood. It is hypothesized that the atypical lymphocyte is an activated cell produced in response to the virus-infected B-lymphocytes.

The basic pathologic abnormality reported in EBV infection is intense proliferation of lymphoid tissues. This is maximal in the lymphoid organs such as lymph nodes, spleen, and tonsils, but other organs such as liver, brain, lung, kidney, heart and testes may be involved to a varying extent. In those few cases with lung involvement that have come to autopsy, lung pathology typically reveals an interstitial pneumonia with mononuclear infiltration of perivascular and peribronchial tissue and intra-alveolar septa. There may be evidence of a superimposed bacterial infection.

Clinical Manifestations

Acute infection with EBV causes a spectrum of illnesses ranging from asymptomatic disease to the specific mononucleosis syndrome. In children, primary EBV infection often is asymptomatic and heterophile negative. With increasing age up to adolescence and young adulthood, infection more frequently is clinically apparent and 90% of cases demonstrate heterophile antibodies.

In symptomatic illness, after an incubation period that ranges from 30 to 50 days, there is a prodrome lasting several days which includes malaise, anorexia, retro-orbital headaches, chills, and feverishness. Most patients go on to develop the mononucleosis syndrome of severe sore throat, fever that can be as high as 104°F, and adenopathy, but some may only experience prolonged fever with malaise and/or lymphadenopathy. A rash may develop in about 5% of patients that can be macular, scarlatiniform, petechial, urticarial or erythema multiforme-like. Ampicillin administration can induce a skin eruption in 90% to 100% of patients receiving the drug. The rash is thought to be due to antibodies produced during IM interacting with the drug to form immune complexes. Pharyngitis can range from mild injection to follicular tonsillitis or exudative pharyngitis. Palatal petechiae can be found in up to 60% of patients. Cervical adenopathy is present in 80% to 90% of patients and involves the posterior as well as submandibular and anterior nodes. Axillary and inquinal adenopathy may also occur. Nodes are minimally tender, freely movable and range from pea to walnut size. Hepatomegaly is present in 10% to 15% and splenomegaly in about 50% of cases.

Lung involvement can be manifested by a paroxysmal nonproductive cough and radiographic changes compatible with an interstitial pneumonia. Paratracheal and hilar adenopathy and, rarely, pleural effusions also have been reported.

The most significant laboratory manifestation of the illness is a lymphocytosis that peaks to a high of 50% to 70% of the total leukocyte count during the second or third week of illness. Total leukocyte counts usually are in the 15–20,000/mm³ range but may be > 50,000/mm³. Many of the lymphocytes (> 20%) are atypical, being larger than a mature lymphocyte and possessing an irregular vacuolated cytoplasm. Nuclei often are lobulated and eccentrically placed.

Liver function tests are abnormal in most cases of IM. Hepatocellular enzymes are most commonly elevated at two to three times normal and bilirubin may be high enough to cause jaundice in about 8% of cases.

The great majority of patients with IM recover uneventfully over a two- to three-week period. Malaise may persist for several weeks to months. Complications can occur and include upper airway obstruction, splenic rupture, autoimmune hemolytic anemia and thrombocytopenia, meningoencephalitis, Guillain-Barré syndrome, transverse myelitis, hepatic failure, myocarditis, and pericarditis. Death, although rare, is most commonly caused by splenic rupture, neurologic involvement, or airway obstruction.

Diagnosis

The clinical manifestations of sore throat, fever and lymphadenopathy together with an atypical lymphocytosis should raise clinical suspicion and prompt the ordering of appropriate serologic tests. In most cases (90%), peak titers of heterophile antibodies appear between two and three weeks into the illness. Sheep and horse erythrocyte agglutinins as well as beef erythrocyte hemolysins are demonstrable. Horse red cell agglutination is most sensitive. The classic heterophile antibody titer is reported as the highest serum dilution at which sheep erythrocytes are agglutinated after absorption of test serum with guinea pig kidney to eliminate other hemagglutinins. A titer of ≥ 40 with a compatible clinical picture establishes the diagnosis. Titer height does not correlate with severity of illness. Heterophile antibody titers drop or disappear within months to a year after infection. Commercially available kits that are both sensitive and specific also can be used to demonstrate heterophile antibodies.

In approximately 10% of cases of clinically diagnosed mononucleosis the heterophile test will be negative. Heterophile negative mononucleosis can be seen in children and in cases of a mononucleosis syndrome caused by cytomegalovirus or toxoplasmosis. For heterophile negative cases, and for diagnosis in atypical presentations, determination of specific EBV antibodies can confirm EBV infection. Patients in the acute phase of illness have high peak titers of IgM and IgG antibodies to VCA. The IgM antibodies disappear between one and two months, but IgG antibodies only decline to lower but persistent levels. Antibodies to EBNA usually are absent (< 1:2) in the acute phase but rise several weeks or months after the onset of illness and remain detectable for life. Most patients (> 80%) also develop a transient anti-EA-D response in acute illness. Serodiagnosis can be established by demonstrating the presence of high IgM and IgG titers against VCA, the presence of anti-EA-D, and the absence of anti-EBNA. A follow-up titer showing a decrease or loss of IgM anti-VCA and anti-EA-D and the emergence of anti-EBNA confirms the diagnosis.

The chest x-ray picture with lung involvement is nonspecific and there is nothing to distinguish it from interstitial patterns seen with other atypical pneumonias.

Treatment and Prevention

Therapy for mononucleosis is largely symptomatic and supportive. Because of the danger of splenic rupture, contact sports or heavy lifting must be avoided. As the spread of virus requires intimate contact, isolation procedures are not necessary.

Corticosteroids have been shown effective in shortening the duration of fever and reducing the severity of sore throat. Their use can be recommended in severe pharyngeal involvement with encroachment of the airway and in complications such as severe thrombocytopenia, hemolytic anemia, myocarditis, pericarditis and probably severe lung involvement. Recommended dosage is 50 to 80 mg prednisone per day with tapering dosage over a one- to two-week period. Symptomatic response usually is rapid. At present, specific antiviral chemotherapy or vaccines are not available.

SELECTED READINGS

Andiman WA, McCarthy P, Markowitz RI, et al: Clinical, virologic, and serologic evidence of Epstein-Barr virus infection in association with childhood pneumonia. *J Pediatrics* 1981;99:880–886.

Arendt J: The roentgenological aspect of infectious mononucleosis. *Am J Roentgenol* 1950;64:950–958.
Chang RS: *Infectious Mononucleosis.* Boston, GK Hall, 1980.
Custer RP, Smith EB: The pathology of infectious mononucleosis. *Blood* 1948;3: 830–857.
Eaton OM, Little PF, Silver HM: Infectious mononucleosis with pleural effusion. *Arch Intern Med* 1965;115:87–89.
Evans A: Infectious mononucleosis in University of Wisconsin students. *Am J Hygiene* 1960;71:342–362.
Fermaglich DR: Pulmonary involvement in infectious mononucleosis. *J Pediatrics* 1975;86:93–95.
Grose C, Henle W, Horwitz MS: Primary Epstein-Barr virus infection in a renal transplant recipient. *South Med J* 1977;70:1276–1278.
McCort JJ: Infectious mononucleosis: With special reference to roentgenologic manifestations. *Am J Roentgenol* 1949;62:645–654.
Mundy GR: Infectious mononucleosis with pulmonary parenchymal involvement. *Br Med J* 1972;1:219–220.
Wechsler HF, Rosenblum AH, Sills CT: Infectious mononucleosis: Report of an epidemic in an army post. *Ann Intern Med* 1946;25:113–133.

48 *Adenovirus*

Richard Snepar

Adenoviruses are important causes of upper and lower respiratory tract infections in children and adults. They were discovered by Rowe in 1953 who noted their presence in a majority of surgically removed adenoidal and tonsillar tissue.

Microbial Characteristics

Adenoviruses have double stranded DNA as their genetic material. The DNA is associated with a number of internal proteins. This is surrounded by a capsid, or protein coat, containing 252 subunits (capsomers) arranged in an icosahedral structure. These subunits consist of hexons (which are hollow six-sided structures) and pentons (hollow five-sided structures). Fibers project from the pentons. The hexons, pentons and fibers differ from one another immunologically. The hexons and pentons carry the complement-fixing antigens, which are common to all human adenoviruses and are useful in the serologic diagnosis of adenovirus infection. Type-specific antibodies binding to fibers inhibit hemagglutination and those binding to hexons neutralize infection. These type-specific determinants on fibers and hexons allow serotypes to be distinguished.

Adenoviruses are propagated readily in human epithelial cell lines such as HeLa. Their presence is noted by their characteristic cytopathologic effect: densely granular, rounded cells, tightly clumped or fused together. They are resistant to lipid solvents, such as bile salts, which probably allows the organism to survive in the bowel. Adenoviruses are resistant to agents, such as adenine arabinoside or cytosine arabinoside, which are active against some other DNA viruses.

The virus infects tissue by adsorption onto the cell surface. Penetration occurs and, once intracellular, the virus loses its protein coat. The virus replicates in the nucleus of the infected cell.

There are 35 immunologically distinct adenoviruses of human origin at present. Certain serotypes are responsible for characteristic syndromes. For example, Types 3 and 7 cause pharyngoconjunctival fever, while Types 1, 2, 4–6 cause upper respiratory disease in children.

Epidemiology

Human adenovirus infections occur in all parts of the world. The highest incidence is in the winter and spring months, although pharyngoconjunctival fever is seen in the summer.

Most infants have maternally derived neutralizing antibody to one or more of the common adenoviral types and this appears to be protective during the first six months of life. However, when adenoviral infection occurs in the neonate, it tends to be severe. By age 5, 70% to 80% of children have neutralizing antibody to several common types of adenovirus, such as Types 1, 2 and 5.

Adenoviruses cause about 5% to 10% of lower respiratory tract infections (pneumonia, croup bronchitis and bronchiolitis) in children. Adenoviral infections are common until adolescence when the frequency begins to diminish. Adenoviruses rarely produce pneumonia in civilian adults. However, epidemics of adenoviral upper and lower respiratory tract infections occur in military recruits.

The virus is excreted in respiratory or eye secretions during and for up to three weeks after the acute illness. The virus may remain latent in tonsillar and adenoidal tissue. Many asymptomatic patients excrete adenovirus in the stool for years after initial infection. Transmission of infection occurs by the fecal-oral route, person-to-person contact and via aerosols or contaminated fomites. The frequency of infection is greater in crowded populations, ie, among military recruits.

Pathogenicity

Adenovirus may infect the respiratory, intestinal and urinary tracts and conjunctiva, and is capable of three interactions with cells. The first is lytic infection, in which the virus replicates and causes cell death with the release of numerous viral progeny. The second is latent infection. The third is oncogenic transformation in which the virus is integrated into host DNA but no infectious virions are produced. Although oncogenicity has been reported in experimental animals, there has been no evidence of this phenomenon in man. Immunity is due to the presence of type-specific neutralizing antibody.

Clinical Disease

Adenoviruses are responsible for a number of clinical syndromes involving the respiratory tract. Febrile pharyngitis (fever, pharyngeal exudate and cervical adenopathy) usually is seen in children and may be associated with laryngotracheitis, bronchitis or pneumonia. The usual adenoviral types incriminated are 1–5 and 7. An epidemic febrile respiratory disease (so-called acute respiratory disease or ARD) is seen in military recruit populations and consists of constitutional symptoms, conjunctivitis, pharyngitis, laryngitis and tracheitis. The disease usually is caused by adenovirus Types 4 and 7. Peak seasons of illness are winter and spring. In epidemics, wheezing may be seen in two thirds of patients.

Pneumonia can occur, and chest radiographs reveal patchy interstitial infiltrates primarily in the lower lung fields. Pneumonia due to adenovirus must be differentiated from *Mycoplasma*, parainfluenza and influenza infection. The illness lasts from one to four weeks and has a favorable prognosis; although fatalities have occurred rarely.

Adenoviruses do not cause pneumonia in children as frequently as respiratory syncytial virus or parainfluenza, but may cause a severe and occasionally fatal infection, especially when it occurs in children under 18 months of age. It is an acute illness with fever and cough associated with the physical findings of tachypnea, wheezes and rales. This occurs as a consequence of a progressive necrotizing bronchiolitis and hemorrhagic bronchopneumonia. Extrapulmonary manifestations are common (encephalopathy, hepatitis, nephritis, bleeding tendency and exanthems). The chest radiographs reveal diffuse infiltrates often with hyperaeration and atelectasis. Permanent pulmonary sequelae (bronchiectasis, bronchitis obliterans and unilateral hyperlucent lung) have been documented in surviving children. Severe systemic infection with adenovirus (hepatic necrosis, pericarditis and bilateral pneumonia) also has been documented in immunocompromised patients.

Pharyngoconjunctival fever is a summertime illness that occurs in small epidemics and consists of fever, uni- or bilateral conjunctivitis and pharyngitis. Epidemic keratoconjunctivitis occurs in adults from contaminated ophthalmic instruments and eye solutions and hand-to-eye contact by medical personnel or among family members. It is an insidious bilateral conjunctivitis and keratitis due to adenovirus Type 8 that may produce visual disturbances for months.

Diagnostic Tests

The diagnosis of adenovirus infection often can be made on clinical grounds in the proper setting. Definitive diagnosis is dependent on viral isolation, antigen detection, or demonstration of a fourfold rise in serum antibodies. The virus can be cultured from pharynx, sputum, conjunctival scrapings, urine or stool. Indirect inmmunofluorescence appears to be a reliable method for viral antigen detection in exfoliated cells. Complement fixation is the most convenient method of serodiagnosis, but is not useful in establishing the specific adenovirus type; whereas, the neutralization and hemagglutination inhibition tests are utilized to detect type specific antibodies.

Therapy

Therapy is supportive and serious sequelae are unusual.

Prevention

Oral vaccines have been developed for use in the military that contain live enteric-coated Types 4 and 7. This has been proven to be effective in reducing rates of acute respiratory disease in military recruits. Commercial use of these vaccines is not recommended because of the sporadic occurrence of these serotypes in civilians.

SELECTED READINGS

Baum SG: Adenovirus, in Mandell GL, Douglas RG, Bennett JE (eds): *Principles and Practice of Infectious Diseases.* New York, John Wiley and Sons, 1979, p 1353.

Duddy BA, Top FH, et al: Acute respiratory disease in military trainees. *Am J Epidemiol* 1973;97:187.

Huebner RJ, Rowe WP, Ward TG, et al: Adenoidal-pharyngeal-conjunctival agents. *N Engl J Med* 1954;251:1077.

Jackson GG: Adenoviral infections, in Beeson PB, McDermott W, Wyngarden JB (eds): *Cecil Textbook of Medicine.* New York, WB Saunders, 1979, p 236.

Jackson GG, Muldoon RL: Viruses causing common respiratory infections in man. Adenoviruses. *J Infect Dis* 1973;127:834.

Spencer MJ, Cherry JD: Adenovirus, in Feigen RD, Cherry JD (eds): *Textbook of Pediatric Infectious Diseases.* New York, WB Saunders, 1981, p 1279.

Zafnadnik J, Spencer M, Porter D: Adenovirus infection in the immunocompromised patient. *Am J Med* 1980;68:725.

49 *Cytomegalovirus*

Clifford G. Wlodaver
Harvey M. Friedman

Microbial Characteristics

Cytomegalovirus belongs to the human Herpes family of viruses. Other members include herpes simplex types I and II, Epstein-Barr, and varicella-zoster viruses. The morphology of these viruses are similar. They contain an outer envelope 180 to 250 nm in diameter and a dense inner core 100 to 110 nm in diameter. CMV is a double-stranded DNA virus with icosahedral symmetry, consisting of 162 capsomers.

Growth of human CMV is species specific. The virus will not grow in laboratory animals, but will replicate in certain human tissue culture systems, particularly human diploid fibroblast strains derived from embryonic lung or foreskin.

The number of different serotypes of CMV has not yet been defined. By neutralization tests, strain differences can be readily detected. However, strains also share common antigens. Therefore, the use of one strain in serologic tests enables detection of antibody titer rises caused by most, if not all, CMV strains.

Epidemiology

Infection with CMV is frequent and the prevalence increases with age. In North America, by age 50, approximately 50% have been infected, as measured by antibody in sera of the general population. In countries where living conditions are crowded, infection occurs at a much earlier age. Following infection, the virus may remain latent in the body for life. The site of latency has not been clearly established, and perhaps multiple tissues are involved.

The routes of transmission have been defined for some forms of CMV infection. Congenital CMV infection develops following transplacental transmission of the virus. Perinatal CMV infection occurs following passage of the baby through an infected birth canal (cervical excretions), or contact of the infant with infected breast milk. Venereal spread has been reported and is particularly common among male homosexuals. Organ transplantations and transfusions containing white blood cells from CMV seropositive donors are also risk factors. The virus is introduced within the transplanted tissues or transfused blood in a latent state. Reactivation of the latent virus subsequently occurs, sometimes leading to clinical disease in recipients of these tissues.

Clinical Disease

Most CMV infections are asymptomatic. When disease develops, however, the manifestations are varied. Transplacental infection of the fetus can produce severe central nervous system disorders, including mental retardation, impaired motor development and hearing loss. Pneumonitis, chorioretinitis, hepatosplenomegaly, and thrombocytopenia also occur. Presently, CMV is the leading cause of birth defects from an infectious agent in North America. In young adults the most common manifestation of CMV is a mononucleosis-like syndrome. Prolonged fever, fatigue, and atypical lymphocytosis are common features. Pharyngitis and adenopathy are less prevalent than during Epstein-Barr virus (EBV) infection and the heterophil or "mono-spot" test is negative. Approximately 10% of all mononucleosis-like illnesses are caused by CMV, while most of the remainder are caused by EBV.

Disease caused by CMV plagues the immunocompromised host, including patients receiving chemotherapy for malignancy and transplant recipients. CMV infection in transplantation has been studied extensively. Approximately 30% of kindey recipients and 50% of bone marrow patients develop overt CMV disease. Reactivation of latent CMV infection can occur following immunosuppression. Generally, this form of infection leads to mild disease or is asymptomatic. In contrast, primary infection, that is, newly introduced infection occurring in a previously susceptible immunocompromised recipient, is often more severe.

CMV disease generally occurs one to three months after renal or bone marrow transplantation. It is characterized by prolonged fever, myalgias, arthralgias, leukopenia, and thrombocytopenia. Visceral involvement occurs in severe cases and includes hepatitis, gastrointestinal ulcerations and hemorrhage, encephalitis and pneumonitis.

CMV pneumonia is the single most common cause of pulmonary infection in the renal and bone marrow transplant population. The pneumonia is remarkable for the paucity of specific symptoms and signs. The patients may complain of shortness of breath and a nonproductive cough. Auscultation may be normal or reveal rales. Hypoxia is often present. The chest x-ray can take many forms, most commonly a diffuse interstitial infiltrate. Other patterns include a diffuse alveolar infiltrate, focal consolidation, or rarely, nodular lesions. Pneumonia develops or progresses despite broad-spectrum antibiotics, a sequence which suggests a viral etiology.

CMV involvement of the lung may be associated simultaneously with other infections. In particular, *Pneumocystis carinii* and CMV are common copathogens. In addition, immunocompromised hosts are susceptible to a wide variety of other opportunistic organisms. CMV itself is immunosuppressive which may predispose patients to infection with other agents. Recently, an acquired immunodeficiency syndrome (AIDS) has been recognized in male homosexuals, drug addicts, Haitians and hemophiliacs. Many of these patients have CMV infection. Some of the patients have Kaposi's sarcoma. What role, if any, CMV has in the etiology of AIDS or Kaposi's sarcoma remains to be established.

Less frequently described features of CMV disease in normal or compromised hosts include Guillian-Barré syndrome, myocarditis, pancreatitis, arthritis, and urinary retention.

Diagnosis

Diagnosis of CMV infection is based on demonstrating a fourfold or greater rise in antibody titer, isolation of virus from blood, urine, throat washings, bronchial washings or biopsy specimens, detection of viral inclusions in cells by histology or cytology, or identification of the virus by electron microscopy.

CMV infection must be distinguished from CMV disease, however, since many immunocompromised patients will develop asymptomatic shedding of reactivated virus. A diagnosis of CMV *disease* requires a clinical syndrome consistent with that caused by CMV at a time when CMV *infection* is documented by laboratory testing.

Treatment and Prevention

At present, there is no specific treatment for CMV. During serious infection, immunosuppressive therapy should be decreased or discontinued, including corticosteroids and antithymocyte globulin, since evidence suggests that such therapies worsen the outcome in CMV-infected patients. Although vidarabine (ara-A, arabinoside A) is effective against other herpes viruses, ie, herpes simplex and varicella-zoster, it has not proven useful for CMV. Likewise, acyclovir, a new antiviral agent, lacks clinical efficacy for CMV.

For prevention, administration of high-titered immune serum to bone marrow transplant recipients modifies the incidence and severity of infection. Avoiding transfusions of blood products from CMV sero-positive individuals also decreases the incidence of infection. This strategy is particularly important in premature infants born to CMV sero-negative mothers and in bone marrow transplant patients.

Among renal transplanted recipients, most cases of severe CMV illness occur in recipients of kidneys from CMV sero-positive donors. Some centers have adapted a strategy of avoiding transplantation of CMV sero-positive kidneys, particularly if the recipient is CMV sero-negative (ie, nonimmune). This approach is successful in reducing the incidence of severe CMV disease, but also markedly limits the number of donors available for transplantation. In a setting in which demand already exceeds supply, the value of this approach remains to be determined.

Vaccination trials with live, attenuated CMV and interferon prophylactic studies are currently in progress. Conclusions regarding efficacy and safety of these approaches must await results of these studies.

SELECTED READINGS

Cheeseman SH, Rubin RH, Stewart JA, et al: Controlled clinical trial of prophylactic human-leukocyte interferon in renal transplantation: Effects on cytomegalovirus and herpes simplex infections. *N Engl J Med* 1979;300: 1345–1349.

Fleisher GR, Starr SE, Friedman, HM, et al: Vaccination of pediatric nurses with live attentuated cytomegalovirus. *Am J Dis Child* 1982;136:294–296.

Ho M: Cytomegalovirus, in Mandell GL, Douglas RG, Bennett JE (eds): *Principles and Practices of Infectious Diseases.* New York, John Wiley and Sons, 1979, pp 1307–1323.

Ho M: *Cytomegalovirus. Biology and Infection.* New York, Plenum Publishing Corp, 1982.

Jordan MD, Rousslau WE, Stewart JA, et al: Spontaneous cytomegalovirus mononucleosis. *Ann Intern Med* 1973;79:153–160.

Myers JD, Leszczynski J, Zaia JA, et al: Prevention of cytomegalovirus infection by cytomegalovirus immune globulin after marrow transplantation. *Ann Intern Med* 1983;98:442–446.

Peterson PK, Balfour HH, Marker SC, et al: Cytomegalovirus disease in renal allograft recipients: A prospective study of the clinical features, risk factors and impact on renal transplantation. *Medicine* 1980;59:283–300.

Ramsey PG, Rubin RH, Tolkoff-Rubin NE, et al: The renal transplant patient with fever and pulmonary infiltrates: Etiology, clinical manifestations, and management. *Medicine* 1980;59:206–222.

Stagno S, Pass RF, Myer E, et al: Congenital cytomegalovirus infection: The relative importance of primary and recurrent maternal infection. *N Engl J Med* 1982;306:945–949.

Winston DJ, Ho WG, Howell CL, et al: Cytomegalovirus infections associated with leukocyte transfusions. *Ann Intern Med* 1980;93:671–675.

50 *Influenza*

George A. Poporad

Influenza is an acute febrile viral illness of epidemic nature characterized by headache, myalgias and cough. Its usual benign, self-limited course can be complicated by primary viral or secondary bacterial pneumonias that may be associated with high mortality rates.

Etiology

Influenza virus belongs to the family Orthomyxoviridae. The virus is of medium size (80 to 100 nm), possesses an RNA genome, and is enclosed by a lipid envelope. Spike-like projections composed of glycoprotein extend from the viral surface. The virion can be either spherical or elongated in shape (Figure 50-1). The nucleocapsid, or viral core, consists of eight separate segments, each containing single-stranded RNA, an associated nucleoprotein (NP) and polypeptides possessing polymerase activity. The separate RNA segments afford opportunities for frequent genetic reassortment or recombination, and the antigenicity of the NP protein determines the influenza virus serotypes, Types A, B, and C. The viral core is surrounded by an inner protein membrane (M protein) that provides structural stability to the virion. The outer lipid envelope is partially formed from the plasma membrane of the host cell in which the virion was assembled. The two glycoproteins projecting from the viral surface have either hemagglutinating (HA) or neuraminidase (NA) activity and are important determinants of infectivity and virulence. The hemagglutinin spike is involved in viral attachment to host cell. Specific antibody to it prevents initiation of infection. The neuraminidase spike is thought to facilitate release of newly formed virus particles from infected cells. Antibody to neuraminidase is only partially protective.

Epidemiology

The influenza viruses, especially Type A, have a remarkable ability to undergo antigenic changes in the HA and NA surface proteins. Genetic recombination of the RNA genome among different influenza viruses or possibly between human and animal strains can cause major changes in one or both surface proteins producing viral subtypes containing HA or NA proteins antigenically distinct from those subtypes previously circulating in a population. This phenomenon of major antigenic variability is called “antigenic shift.” It has been recognized only

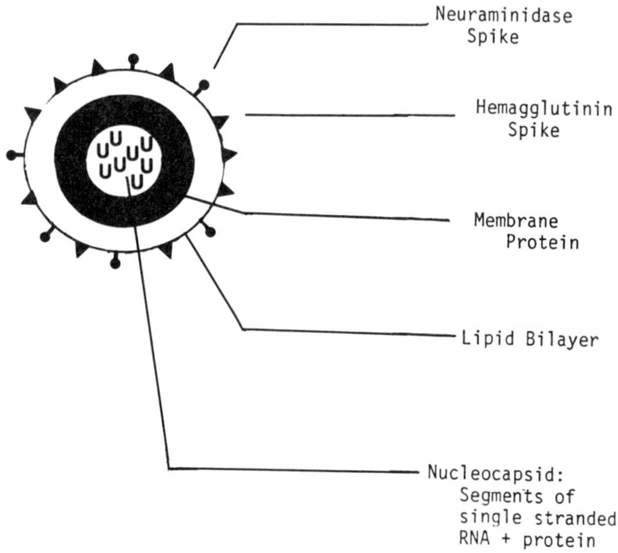

Figure 50-1 Schematic representation of influenza virus.

in Type A virus. It involves HA more frequently than NA and occurs at intervals of 10 to 30 years.

Antigenic shift is associated with the appearance of pandemic influenza because it introduces into a population a viral subtype against which little or no immunity exists, either from previous natural exposures or from vaccination. To date, five HA and two NA antigenic variants have been recognized for Type A virus, and they are identified as H_0, H_1, H_2, H_3, H_{SW1}, and N_1 and N_2, respectively. H_{SW1} was discovered in an influenza epidemic at Fort Dix, New Jersey in January, 1976. It is antigenically similar to both an influenza virus isolated from swine in 1931 (thus the "SW" designation) and the virus believed to have caused the 1918 pandemic. Antigenic shifts responsible for pandemic disease occurred in 1918 ($H_{SW1}N_1$), 1929 (H_0N_1), 1946 (H_1N_1), 1957 (H_2N_2), 1968 (H_3N_2), and 1977 (H_1N_1). The antigenic shift of both glycoproteins in 1957 resulted in severe illness. This contrasted with a shift in both proteins in 1977 which resulted in relatively mild disease, possibly because of lingering immunity from the previous H_1N_1 era (1946–1957) and decreased virulence of the virus.

Relatively minor alterations in the surface glycoproteins may also occur through point mutations of the RNA genome. These minor changes, called "antigenic drifts," occur frequently (every one to three years for Type A, less frequently for Type B) and produce viral strains within a subtype that have minor antigenic differences. Each new strain is identified by site and year of isolation. Thus, influenza A England/72

H_3N_2 indicates an influenza Type A virus of the H_3N_2 subtype isolated in England in 1972. Examples of strains of the same subtype that have develped through antigenic drift are A/Port Chalmers/73 H_3N_2 and A/Scotland/74 H_3N_2. Antigenic drifts are associated with yearly winter influenza epidemics since the level of immunity to a new viral strain is less than the prior strain. Presumably, after circulating in a population for 10 to 30 years, these viral strains possessing minor antigenic variations induce a high level of immunity and a new subtype then emerges through antigenic shift as described above.

Influenza pandemics may begin at any season of the year. They appear to arise from a single focus, with illness spreading from one area or country to another along major routes of travel. Attack rates are high and all age groups are affected. Following the initial spread of illness, secondary and tertiary waves may occur over a period of one or two years, usually in the winter.

Influenza epidemics usually occur during the winter months, October to April in the Northern Hemisphere and May through September in the Southern Hemisphere. They are characterized by their abrupt beginning, reaching a peak in two to three weeks, and continuing for five to six weeks. There is rapid but irregular spread of illness through a region or community. Some communities experience no activity while others have major outbreaks, and those regions escaping illness one winter might be affected the following winter. Children usually are the first to experience illness which spreads to working adults and then to the elderly in institutions. An epidemic in a region or community is reflected in increased school and work absenteeism, increased hospitalizations due to pneumonia and exacerbations of underlying chronic cardiopulmonary disease, and increased mortality rates from pneumonia and influenza. Average overall attack rates during epidemics approximate 10% to 20%, but this is variable depending on the selected population and age group.

As discussed, influenza A virus is capable of a high degree of antigenic variability, and is responsible for epidemic and pandemic disease through antigenic drift and shift. Influenza B virus, in contrast, is more stable antigenically. It has thus far not undergone antigenic shift associated with pandemic disease, and antigenic drift occurs less frequently compared to Type A virus. Therefore, although Type B virus produces a similar illness, its overall impact on a population is usually less severe compared to Type A virus. Type C virus has not been associated with any large scale outbreaks and produces only a mild, uncomplicated upper respiratory tract illness.

Pathogenesis and Pathology

Influenza virus is spread from person to person by respiratory secretions. Viral shedding from an infected individual is present within 24 hours of onset of illness and is maximal for one to two days thereafter. Aerosolized droplets containing virus are deposited in the respiratory tract and penetrate columnar epithelial cells in susceptible hosts. The infection results in necrosis and denudation of the ciliated epithelium of the tracheobronchial tree. Submucosal hyperemia and hemorrhage may result. Involvement of the lung can produce intra-alveolar hemorrhage and thickening of the alveolar septae with hyaline membrane formation. Involved alveoli contain an exudate of fibrin and a paucity of polymorphonuclear leukocytes. Denudation of the tracheobronchial tree cripples the respiratory tract's defense mechanisms, allowing secondary bacterial invaders to reach the lung and produce bacterial pneumonia. In this case, pathologic lung changes are consistent with bacterial pneumonia in addition to the tracheobronchial tree findings of influenza.

Clinical Findings

After an incubation period of one to two days, the abrupt onset of systemic symptoms begins. These include a fever that may reach 104°F, chilliness or rigors, malaise, myalgias, frontal or orbital headaches, and anorexia. There usually is an associated prominent dry cough and nasal discharge. There may be complaints of photophobia or burning eye pain. The patient appears toxic with a flushed face, hot moist skin, and watery reddened eyes. Lung examination may reveal unilateral crepitant rales with no infiltrate seen on chest x-ray, suggesting bronchial or bronchiolar involvement. In the uncomplicated case, systemic symptoms generally abate in approximately three days. As the systemic symptoms disappear, pharyngitis and nasal obstruction may develop and persist along with cough for several days. A convalescent period may follow lasting one to three weeks, in which cough and malaise are frequent complaints before the patient fully recovers. Pulmonary function abnormalities may occur and persist in patients without obvious pneumonic involvement, suggesting that lower respiratory tract invasion may occur in uncomplicated influenza.

A potentially lethal complication of influenza infection is pneumonia, which may be either primary viral, secondary bacterial, or mixed viral and bacterial (Table 50-1). The clinical spectrum of primary viral pneumonia can range from relatively asymptomatic lung involvement to life-threatening pulmonary failure. Patients have been described presenting with a mild segmental pneumonia that runs a benign course. In patients with severe illness, following the typical onset of influenza, there is a rapid progression of cough and fever to dyspnea and cyanosis. Physical examination reveals bilateral rales and rhonchi without signs of consolidation, and the chest x-ray usually shows diffuse bilateral pulmonary infiltrates. Laboratory studies reveal a significant leukocytosis and severe hypoxia. Sputum examination and culture reveal no bacterial

Table 50-1
Pneumonias Complicating Influenza

	Viral Pneumonia	Bacterial Pneumonia	Mixed Viral, Bacterial
Onset	Coexistence with and progression from typical influenza syndrome	Patient improves following normal course of influenza, then relapses	Variable, may reflect features of both viral and bacterial
Clinical Findings	Bilateral rales without consolidation	Consolidation	Variable
Laboratory	X-ray: bilateral lung involvement Leukocytosis Sputum negative for bacterial pathogens	X-ray: localized infiltrate Leukocytosis Sputum exam and culture suggests bacterial etiology	X-ray: variable Leukocytosis Sputum may suggest bacterial component to etiology

Adapted from Douglas (1977).

pathogens, and there is no response to antibiotics. Very often, the patient dies of a fulminant hemorrhagic pneumonia. Those few who survive develop diffuse pulmonary fibrosis. The risk for developing severe influenza viral pneumonia seems to be greater in those patients with heart disease (especially mitral stenosis), in patients with other chronic illnesses, and in women during the last trimester of pregnancy.

Secondary bacterial pneumonia occurs as a complication typically three or more days after an influenza illness as the patient is experiencing a period of clinical improvement. There is a recurrence of fever and cough with purulent sputum production. Areas of consolidation are found on auscultation of the lungs, and the chest x-ray usually shows a localized pulmonary infiltrate. Sputum gram stain and culture generally reveals a bacterial pathogen, usually *Streptococcus pneumoniae*, *Staphylococcus aureas*, or *Hemophilus influenzae*. There should be a response to specific antibiotic therapy. Patients who develop secondary bacterial pneumonias are most often elderly with chronic cardiopulmonary or metabolic diseases.

Other potential complications of influenza infection include Reye's syndrome in children and rhabdomyolysis. Reye's syndrome is associated more commonly with Type B virus infection.

Diagnosis

Diagnosis can be suggested on epidemiologic grounds. Patients who present with a typical syndrome in a community where influenza virus infection is documented most likely have influenza. The virus can be isolated from sputum, throat and nasal swabs, or nasal washes during the first two days of illness. Specimens should be transported in appropriate medium to the laboratory as soon as possible for inoculation into cell cultures. Two-thirds of positive cultures can be detected within three days of inoculation and the remainder in five to seven days.

Serologic diagnosis can be made retrospectively by complement fixation or hemagglutination inhibiting antibody tests. Acute and convalescent serum obtained 2 to 3 weeks later should be tested. A fourfold or greater rise or fall in titer is considered diagnostic of infection.

Treatment

Treatment for influenza pneumonia is primarily supportive. It includes fluid and electrolyte management and supplemental oxygen. Intubation and tracheostomy with assisted ventilatory support and positive end expiratory pressure (PEEP) may become necessary. There is an association between salicylate use and the development of Reye's syndrome. Therefore, it may be prudent to avoid the use of aspirin or aspirin-containing compounds in children (less than 16 years old) for the treatment of fever or other symptoms.

Amantadine has been shown to reduce the duration of signs and symptoms in uncomplicated influenza A infection and to reverse an associated increase in small airways resistance documented in some patients. Whether this data can be extrapolated to the treatment of influenza Type A viral pneumonia is unknown. At present, there are no controlled studies supporting the use of antiviral agents in the treatment of influenza viral pneumonia.

Proven or suspected secondary bacterial pneumonia should be treated with appropriate antibiotics. If a specific bacterial pathogen cannot be found on sputum gram stain or culture, antibiotics selected should have activity against *S. pneumoniae*, *S. aureus*, and *H. influenzae.* Cefamandole 12 g/day IV in divided doses may be a reasonable choice since it has in vitro activity against all three organisms. Alternatives include nafcillin 12 g/day IV in divided doses (for *S. aureus*) plus ampicillin (for *S. pneumoniae*, *H. influenzae*) at a similar dose. Chloramphenicol 4 g/day in divided doses (for *S. pneumoniae*, *H. influenzae*) can be substituted for ampicillin if *H. influenzae* resistance to ampicillin is suspected. In the penicillin allergic patient, vancomycin can be substituted for nafcillin and chloramphenicol used in place of ampicillin. Any suggestion of pneumonia due to a gram-negative rod other than *H. influenzae* would necessitate the addition of an aminoglycoside.

Prevention

Prevention therapy relies on use of an inactivated viral vaccine. Vaccines generally contain Types A and B virus of the sub-types and strains isolated from the previous winter's influenza season. For example, vaccine for 1981 through 1983 seasons has consisted of A/Brazil/78 H_1N_1, A/Bangkok/79 H_3N_2 and B/Singapore/79. Efficacy rates in preventing outbreaks vary from 67% to 92%. The vaccine is recommended for people at increased risk of mortality from the pulmonary complications of influenza. This includes people of all ages with chronic cardiopulmonary and kidney disease, people with malignancies or on immunosuppressive therapy, and people suffering from severe chronic anemias such as sickle cell disease and from metabolic diseases such as diabetes mellitus. Evaluating a pregnant woman's need for immunization should be done on the same basis used for other persons, ie, vaccinating pregnant women with any of the above underlying high risk conditions. Vaccination is also recommended for people above the age of 65. Consideration should be given to the vaccination of persons under the age of 65 who provide essential community services (policemen, firemen, hospital workers). The only contraindication to vaccination is a history of hypersensitivity to eggs. When vaccine is to be given to pregnant women, it is recommended to wait until the second or third trimester, even though there is no evidence to suggest any risk to the mother or fetus. Reactions to vaccine administration include local effects at the site of administration (pain, erythema, and swelling) and occasionally systemic effects manifested as myalgias and fever.

During the 1976 National Immunization Program against swine influenza virus, the occurrence of the Guillain-Barré syndrome gained significant notoriety. During that program, in which approximately 20% of the nation's population was vaccinated, the risk of developing Guillain-Barré was estimated at 1/100,000 vaccinations with an associated mortality of 5% (or 1/2,000,000 vaccinations). Data collected during the following three influenza seasons have shown no clear association between influenza vaccination and the Guillain-Barré syndrome. Available evidence suggests that the risk of developing the Guillain-Barré syndrome is far lower than the risks associated with influenza in persons for whom the vaccine is indicated.

Amantadine can be used for influenza prophylaxis. Its level of efficacy is reported to approximate 70% against influenza caused by Type A virus. Amantadine should be given at the start of a confirmed outbreak of influenza A in the community, and continue through the duration of the outbreak (ie, 200 mg/daily po for five to six weeks). Amantadine is not recommended for general use because of the length of treatment required and the associated side effects of the drug. Side effects involve the central nervous system and include insomnia, light-headedness, nervousness, difficulty in concentration, and drowsiness. The teratogenic risk of amantadine is unknown and it should not be used in pregnant women.

SELECTED READINGS

Amantadine: Does it have a role in the prevention and treatment of influenza? A National Institutes of Health consensus development conference. *Ann Intern Med* 1980;92(part 1):256.

Baine WB, Luby JP, Martin SM, et al: Severe illness with influenza B. *Am J Med* 1980;68:181.

Douglas R: Influenza: The disease and its complications. From Status Report On influenza. *Hosp Practice* 1977.

Influenza vaccine 1981-82. *Morbid Mortal Weekly Rep* 1981;30:279.

Jones SR: Potential complications of influenza A infections. *West J Med* 1976;125:341.

Kaye D, Rosenbluth M, Hook EW, et al: Endemic influenza. II: The nature of the disease in the post pandemic period. *Am Rev Respir Dis* 1962;85:9.

Louria DB, Blumenfeld HL, Ellis JT, et al: Studies on influenza in the pandemic of 1957-58. II: Pulmonarycomplications of influenza. *J Clin Invest* 1959;38:212.

Langmuir AD, Schoenbaum SD: The epidemiology of influenza. From Status Report On Influenza. *Hosp Practice* 1977.

Winterbauer RH, Ludwig WR, Hammar SP: Clinical course, management, and long term sequelae of respiratory failure due to influenza pneumonia. *Johns Hopkins Med J* 1977;141:148.

51 *Aspergillus*

George H. Talbot

MICROBIOLOGICAL CHARACTERISTICS

Members of the genus *Aspergillus* produce a broad spectrum of illness by virtue of their activity as either primary pathogens or secondary invaders. These filamentous fungi belong to the Deuteromycotina, a subdivision of the Fungi Imperfecti (those not possessing sexual forms); within this subdivision are two major classes, the *Blastomycetes* and the *Hyphomycetes*. The latter, which contains the aspergilli, is characterized by the presence of well-developed mycelia, with conidia (spores) either absent, adherent directly to the hyphae, or present on conidiophores (specialized hyphal branches capable of bearing vegetative spores). By contrast, the *Blastomycetes*, of which *Candida* is a representative genus, reproduce solely by cell budding.

Aspergilli grow well when cultured on Sabouraud's agar, a commercially available dextrose-and-peptone-based medium to which antibiotic supplements may be added for selective inhibition of bacterial contaminants. Czapek-Dox agar is also useful. The addition of 20% sucrose to either medium may facilitiate isolation of those aspergilli growing well only when competition is reduced by high osmotic pressures. Growth on Sabouraud's may appear within several days or be delayed as long as three to four weeks.

Like all molds, aspergilli in culture form fluffy, cottony or velvety, colonies whose macroscopic appearance derives from aerial growth above the medium. This distinguishes them from yeasts, which possess a smoother, creamy or pasty quality.

Although, on occasion, the pathologist can speciate *Aspergillus* directly from clinical specimens if typical conidiophores have formed within tissue, in general, species determination must be made by the microbiologist following laboratory isolation. Major macroscopic and microscopic features aiding identification are listed in Table 51-1. Table 51-2 summarizes the more important characteristics of medically significant *Aspergillus* species.

Patient material may be examined in either 20% potassium hydroxide or equal parts of 40% potassium hydroxide and blue-black indelible ink. Staining highlights hyphal walls, but not rapidly growing hyphal tips. In unstained preparations these tips contain refractile, still viable cytoplasmic contents, whereas the nonviable hyphae appear empty. *Aspergillus* organisms usually are septated. The regularly spaced septae are not edged by constriction of the mycelial wall. The 2.5 to 8μm wide hyphae characteristically branch at a 45-degree angle. On histopathologic examination, this virtually pathognomonic architecture is best observed with the silver methenamine stain (Figure 51-1). Periodic acid-Schiff and hematoxylin-eosin stains also may demonstrate organisms. The latter stain usually is of lesser sensitivity. Gram stain is not reliable: aspergilli appear gram-negative, if they are visible at all. Finally, direct immunofluorescent techniques have been useful in some laboratories.

Table 51-1
Distinguishing Features of Aspergillus Species

1. Colony color (surface, and on plate reverse)
2. Colony texture and growth rate
3. Conidiophore morphology, especially
   a) length
   b) size of the vesicle (the swollen apex of the conidiophore)
   c) number of rows of sterigmata (oblong outgrowths from the vesicle, from which spores are formed)
4. Conidial arrangement, size and color

Table 51-2
Identification of Aspergillus Species Grown on Czapek-Dox/Medium

Species	Colony Color		Maximum Vesicle Diameter (μm)	Rows of Sterigmata	Conidia (μm)
	Surface	*Reverse*			
A. fumigatus	dark blue-green	brown	30	1	2.5–3.5
A. niger	brown to black	yellow	100	2	5.5–8.0
A. flavus	yellow to dark green	red-brown	65	1–2	3.5–4.5
A. terreus	cinnamon-brown	brown	16	2	1.8–2.4
A. versicolor	yellow to blue-green	wine red	16	2	2.0–3.0
A. clavatus	pale blue- or gray-green	brown	50–180	1	3.5–4.5 × 2.4–3.0
A. nidulans	dark green	purplish red	10	2	3.0–3.5

Adapted with permission from Austwick PKC: Medically important *Aspergillus* species (Chapter 60) in Lennette EH, Balows A, Hausler WJ, et al (eds): *Manual of Clinical Microbiology,* ed 3. Washington, DC, American Society of Microbiology, 1980.

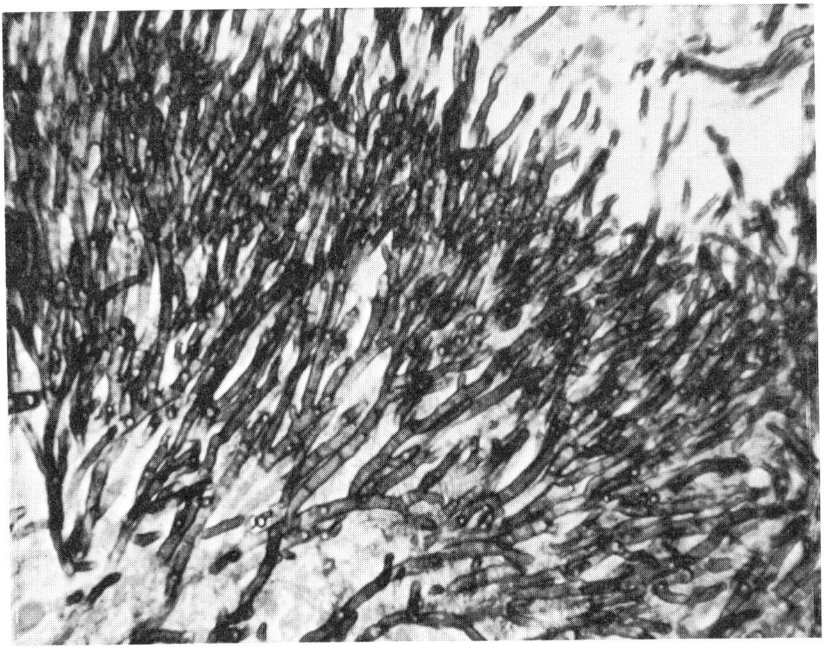

Figure 51-1 Methenamine silver nitrate stain of aspergilli in tissue showing septated hyphae with branching at acute angles.

EPIDEMIOLOGY

Aspergillus species are widely distributed in nature, especially where dead and decaying vegetable matter exists as a suitable substrate for growth. Spores are resistant to relative extremes of temperature and pH. This hardiness, plus the modest conditions of moisture required for germination, explain the organism's ubiquitous character and regular appearance as an uninvited guest on refrigerated foodstuffs.

Outdoor spore counts show seasonal variation; as might be expected, greater numbers of spores can be demonstrated during the late summer and early fall. Counts may range as high as 50 or more spores per 100 cubic feet of air. Although *Aspergillus niger* is the species most commonly recovered from outside air, *A. fumigatus* and *A. flavus* have been reported to be frequent inside hospital buildings. Hospital air filtration systems appear to decrease total counts significantly.

Pulmonary disease due to *Aspergillus* species is acquired by the inhalation route; sporular diameter is sufficiently small to allow penetration into the distal airways and alveoli. Patients have ample opportunity for exposure to spores both inside and outside the hospital environment. Only those individuals housed in laminar air flow units escape such exposure.

Temporal and spatial clustering of cases of invasive pulmonary aspergillosis (vide infra) has been described. These "outbreaks" have often been attributed to point sources such as contaminated ventilation systems, nearby construction or demolition, and even hospital fireproofing materials. Despite the occasional finding of spore-bearing conidiophores in vivo, person-to-person transmission of aspergilli has not been conclusively documented.

PATHOGENICITY

Aspergillus species cause clinically evident disease in three distinct ways:

1. *Hypersensitivity*, induced by inhaled spores or colonizing organisms acting as allergens. This will be discussed further below.
2. *Toxin production.* Aflatoxin, the best known of these mycotoxins, is a potent hepatotoxin and carcinogen. Both acute hepatitis and hepatocellular carcinoma have been associated with ingestion of aflatoxin-contaminated foodstuffs (especially grain). Expression of illness depends on the magnitude and duration of exposure. Unfortunately, the role of mycotoxins in *Aspergillus*-induced pulmonary disease, if any, is ill-defined.
3. *Tissue invasion*, potentially the most lethal form of illness, usually occurs in the immunocompromised host, although on occasion apparently normal individuals may be afflicted. Important predisposing factors include a) qualitative and especially quantitative granulocyte abnormalities, and b) the presence of devitalized tissue. Animal studies suggest, in addition, an important role for corticosteroid therapy. Such treatment also has been implicated in the pathogenesis of human aspergillosis, as has the administration of cytotoxic drugs and broad-spectrum antibiotics. Other factors, including inoculum size, appear important in selected cases.

Postmortem examination of compromised patients with invasive pulmonary aspergillosis usually reveals infarction, necrotizing pneumonitis, or a combination of these two lesions. Much of the pathologic and the clinical expression of *Aspergillus* disease results from the organism's pronounced tendency to invade blood vessels, with consequent thrombosis and often widespread infarction. In addition, invasive bronchitis, consolidation, and abscess formation may occur. Microscopically, masses of hyphae cluster towards the center of the suppurative parenchymal lesions, which are surrounded by a peripheral zone of organizing pneumonia and variable numbers of granulocytes, plasma cells, and eosinophils. In some patients, suppuration is less prominent and thrombosis with infarction predominates. This process may mimic an ordinary pulmonary infarct due to thromboembolism; the microscopic finding of hyphal vascular invasion reveals the true pathogenetic mechanism.

CLINICAL SYNDROMES

The clinical manifestations of pulmonary aspergillosis classically have been divided into three major syndromes: 1) hypersensitivity reactions, 2) the fungus ball, or aspergilloma, and 3) invasive disease. Recently, authors have reported overlap syndromes wherein patients' clinical courses demonstrated features characteristic of more than one classic syndrome. Evidence supporting the hypothesis that pulmonary aspergillosis is best understood as a spectrum of disease will be reviewed below. For the purposes of initial discussion, the three classic syndromes will be considered as distinct entities.

Hypersensitivity Lung Disease

Allergic bronchopulmonary aspergillosis Allergic bronchopulmonary aspergillosis (ABPA), the best known hypersensitivity lung disease due to *Aspergillus*, was first described in 1952. Patients with this disorder are usually young (average age at diagnosis, 25.5 years) and present with intermittent episodes of wheezing, transient pulmonary infiltrates, and blood and sputum eosinophilia. Fever, pleuritic chest pain, and expectoration of brown plugs or flecks may occur. Examination of sputum often shows characteristic hyphal elements or, if cultured, *A. fumigatus.* Further evaluation reveals elevation of serum IgE, immediate skin test reactivity (Type I hypersensitivity) to *Aspergillus* antigen, and serum IgG *Aspergillus* precipitating antibodies (found in 80% to 90% of patients). On occasion, Arthus skin test reactivity (Type III hypersensitivity, ie, reaction to antigen-antibody complexes) to *Aspergillus* antigen occurs. Plain chest films (Figure 51-2) showing hilar enlargement mimicking adenopathy and so-called "tramline," "gloved finger," or "toothpaste" shadows may suggest the presence of bronchiectasis, which should be evaluated by bronchography if possible. Central bronchiectasis is pathognomonic of ABPA. Table 51-3 summarizes diagnostic criteria for ABPA. The presence of the first six of the primary criteria makes ABPA very likely; when all seven are documented, the diagnosis is virtually certain.

Long-term follow-up of patients with ABPA sometimes may reveal irreversible deterioration in pulmonary function, especially in the absence of treatment. However, the frequency and magnitude of these

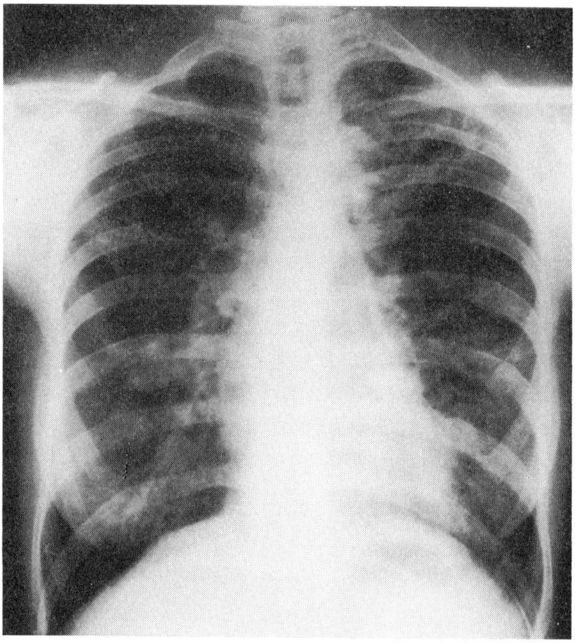

A

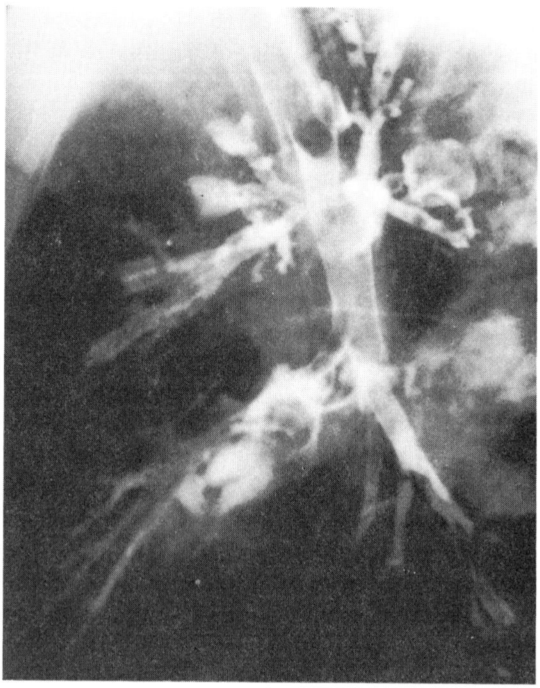

B

Figure 51-2 Chest radiograph of a patient with allergic bronchopulmonary aspergillosis **A**, and the bronchogram **B**, which demonstrate central bronchiectasis.

Table 51-3
Diagnostic Criteria for Allergic Bronchopulmonary Aspergillosis

Primary
Episodic asthma
Transient or chronic pumonary infiltrates
Eosinophilia (blood)
Elevated IgE
Aspergillus precipitins
Immediate skin test reactivity to *Aspergillus* antigen
Central bronchiectasis
Secondary
Aspergillus fumigatus in sputum (or repeated microscopic documentation of characteristic hyphae)
Expectoration of brown plugs or flecks
Arthus reactivity to *Aspergillus* antigen

Reproduced with permission from Rosenberg M, Patterson R, Mintzer R, et al: Clinical and immunological criteria for the diagnosis of allergic bronchopulmonary aspergillosis. *Ann Intern Med* 1977;86:405–414.

alterations are debated, and some authors suggest that major progression is relatively unusual. In contrast, acute exacerbations of disease may be accompanied by significant reduction in total lung capacity, vital capacity, forced expiratory volume at one second, and carbon monoxide diffusing capacity. Elevation of serum IgE levels is an indicator of a forthcoming episode of pulmonary functional deterioration. Both the immunoglobulin and the pulmonary physiologic abnormalities resolve after treatment.

The pathophysiology of ABPA has not been fully elucidated. As noted, current evidence suggests a role for both Type I and Type III immunologic reactions to the *Aspergillus* organisms colonizing the bronchial tree. Delayed (Type IV) hypersensitivity also has been implicated in the pathogenesis of disease.

Corticosteroids are the mainstay of therapy for ABPA. Prednisone in doses of 0.5 mg/kg/day, with reduction after one week to 0.5 mg/kg on alternate days, usually is effective in controlling the clinical and laboratory manifestations of disease. The appropriate use of bronchodilators aids attempts at reduction of corticosteroids to the minimum necessary maintenance dose. Beclomethasone diproprionate is of uncertain benefit, but may be useful for selected individuals. Although some exacerbations may be accompanied by full-blown clinical symptoms and signs, others may be relatively asymptomatic with predominantly laboratory manifestations such as an abnormal chest x-ray and elevated serum IgE. Many patients may require long-term, in some instances lifetime, therapy.

Extrinsic allergic alveolitis In contrast to ABPA, in which *Aspergillus* colonizes the endobronchial tree and releases antigens in vivo, *Aspergillus*-induced extrinsic allergic alveolitis and extrinsic asthma are expressions of hypersensitivity lung disease due to inhalation of *Aspergillus* antigens.

Extrinsic allergic alveolitis is caused by continuing exposure to a variety of organic substances, including the familiar thermophilic actinomycetes. In some instances, aspergilli are at fault. "Malt-worker's lung" is produced by inhalation of *Aspergillus* organisms (usually *A. clavatus*) growing on barley. "Farmer's lung" may result from repeated challenge with a number of different allergens, aspergilli among them.

The affected individual develops symptoms up to six hours after inhalation of organisms. Bronchospasm is rare since the airways are spared. Cough, dyspnea and, on occasion, fever and chills, dominate the clinical picture. Diffuse interstitial infiltrates are noted on chest x-ray. Eosinophilia is lacking. Pulmonary function and radiographic abnormalities disappear on cessation of exposure, but recurrent challenge over months to years can lead to irreversible pulmonary fibrosis.

Elevation of IgG precipitins to *Aspergillus* occurs as it does in ABPA. Skin testing, however, inconsistently reveals a Type I reaction; a Type III reaction is invariably expected. Type IV hypersensitivity (ie, delayed-type or cell-mediated hypersensitivity) may also play a role.

Treatment of extrinsic allergic alveolitis is best accomplished by eliminating the offending allergen from the patient's environment, or by removing the individual from the situation in which exposure occurs. When neither solution is economically feasible, exposure can be minimized by use of a mask, or symptoms ameliorated with corticosteroid therapy.

Extrinsic asthma Extrinsic asthma due to inhalation of *Aspergillus* spores represents a third manifestation of *Aspergillus* hypersensitivity lung disease. Affected individuals demonstrate acute bronchospasm, but characteristically lack fever and pneumonitis; their presentation is nonspecific and does not differentiate them from persons reacting to other environmental allergens. In contradistinction to extrinsic allergic alveolitis, irreversible lung damage does not occur.

Aspergilloma

Although *Mucor* and *Pseudoallescheria boydii* or other fungi are sometimes responsible for pulmonary "fungus balls," or mycetomas, *Aspergillus* species, especially *A. fumigatus*, are the most common cause. Aspergillomas are saprophytic growths of *Aspergillus* developing within areas of previously abnormal, cavitated lung. They have been associated with a multitude of underlying chronic cavitary pulmonary disorders, including tuberculosis (perhaps most common), sarcoidosis, histoplasmosis, and ankylosing spondylitis. Presumably, any disease capable of causing cavitation can provide the appropriate milieu.

Although some aspergillomas are discovered fortuitously during a patient's evaluation for extrapulmonary complaints, most are diagnosed because of fever, cough, hemoptysis, or weight loss. Hemoptysis, scanty or profuse, is the most common symptom, occuring in 50% to 90% of patients. Other complaints occur less frequently.

The diagnosis of aspergilloma is suggested by the characteristic radiographic findings and by the presence of an appropriate underlying pulmonary illness. The chest x-ray reveals an upper lobe cavity that is partially filled by a rounded soft-tissue density rimmed by a crescent of air (Figure 51-3). Lower lobe mycetomas are also encountered. Decubitus films (to detect fungus ball movement within the cavity) and tomography may prove helpful radiologically. *Aspergillus* precipitins are detected with high frequency (80% or greater). Organisms can often be cultured from expectorated sputa or from specimens obtained by bronchoscopy or percutaneous needle aspiration. The radiologic, serologic, and microbiologic findings usually are sufficient to allow a confident diagnosis prior to, or in the absence of, surgical resection.

The natural history of aspergillomas is variable. Some may enlarge or produce major hemoptysis, while others remain stable; as many as 7% to 10% lyse spontaneously. Because of this variable clinical course, the considerable controversy that exists about optimal management of these lesions is likely to continue until a controlled trial of therapeutic alternatives is reported. At present, most authorities agree that systemic antifungal therapy is not helpful. Conflicting data exist regarding the utility of intracavitary instillation of amphotericin B. The surgical literature suggests that resection should always be attempted if the patient is otherwise a surgical candidate; medical authorities are considerably less sanguine about this approach. Until controlled data are available, therapy must depend upon individual preference. Intracavitary amphotericin B instillation may improve symptoms in selected patients. Resection should be considered for the patient with severe constitutional symptoms, acute massive hemoptysis (more than 600 mL in 24 hours), or persistent hemoptysis of moderate degree.

Invasive Aspergillosis

Although frequently limited to the pulmonary parenchyma alone, invasive aspergillosis may simultaneously affect other areas of the respiratory tract (bronchi, nose, sinuses) and also may produce disseminated disease with involvement of the brain, thyroid, heart, and gastrointestinal and genitourinary tracts. *Aspergillus fumigatus* usually is the offender, but other species are encountered. *A. flavus*, a particularly troublesome organism for some cancer centers, has a poorly understood proclivity for producing sinopulmonary disease.

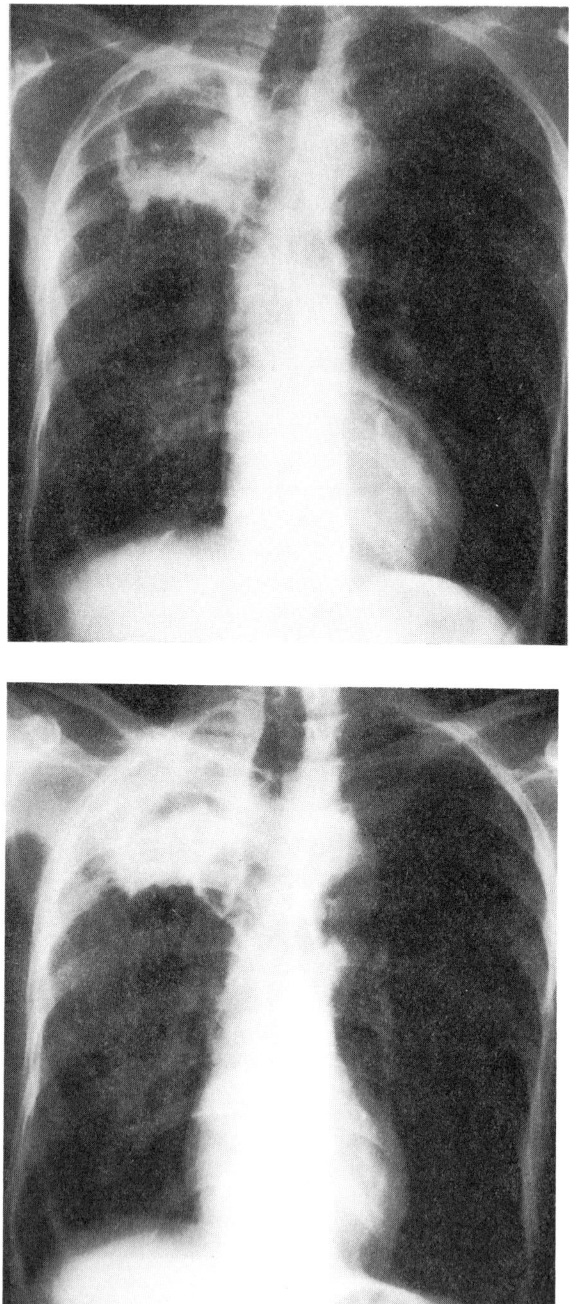

A

B

Figure 51-3 Chest radiograph of a patient with a chronic right upper lobe pulmonary cavity before **A**, and after **B**, the development of an aspergilloma within the cavity.

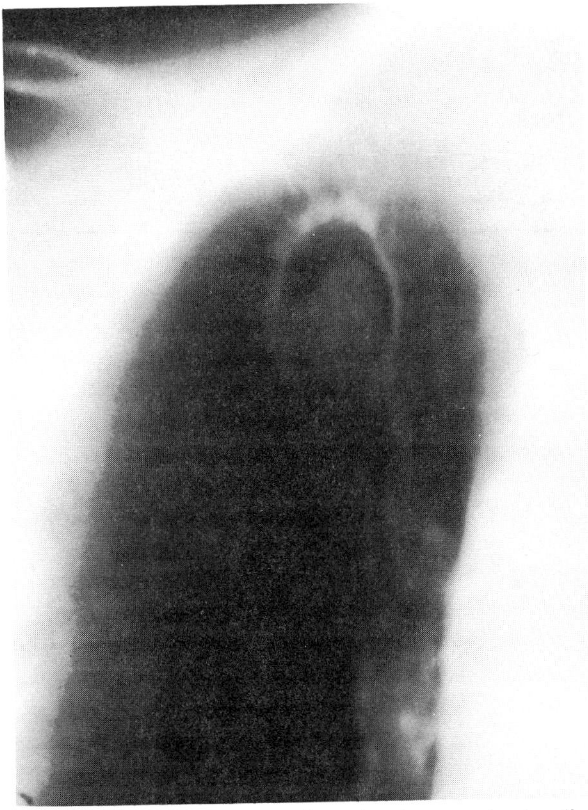

Figure 51-3C Radiograph demonstrating the improved visualization of a mycetoma by tomography.

The majority of cases of invasive pulmonary aspergillosis occur in severely immunocompromised hosts, especially patients with acute leukemia or chronic myelogenous leukemia in blast crisis. Renal transplant recipients and individuals with lymphoma or solid tumors are less commonly affected. Proposed risk factors include severe granulocytopenia (< 500 neutrophils per mm^3) and therapy with corticosteroids, cytotoxic agents, and broad-spectrum antibiotics. Qualitative granulocyte defects, notably chronic granulomatous disease of childhood and variant adult forms, also have been implicated. Apparently normal individuals occasionally develop invasive disease. Exposure to an overwhelming inoculum of *Aspergillus* spores or subtle local or systemic host defense deficiencies may account for these cases.

In the patient with one or more risk factors, persistent fever, pleuritic chest pain, or cough with or without hemoptysis should raise the possibility of invasive aspergillosis, even in the absence of a pulmonary infiltrate. The appearance of pneumonitis, especially an area nodular in

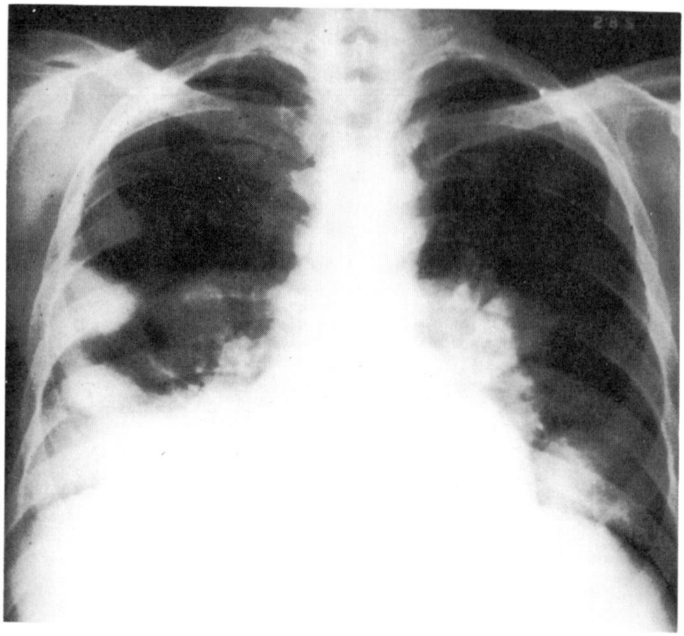

Figure 51-4 Chest radiograph of a patient with invasive aspergillosis showing multiple nodules.

form, is highly suggestive. Multiple nodules, patchy infiltrates, and lobar pneumonia also are observed (Figure 51-4). These lesions may not only cavitate, but may also develop the radiographic appearance of a fungus ball (Figure 51-5). This process is to be distinguished from the true aspergilloma, which occurs in a preexisting cavity. Pleural effusion and *Aspergillus* empyema are infrequent complications.

The diagnosis of invasive pulmonary aspergillosis can be difficult to establish. An awareness of its possibility in the appropriate clinical and epidemiologic setting is perhaps the most important step. KOH examination of expectorated sputum first may suggest the diagnosis. Although the recovery of *Aspergillus* species on culture of respiratory secretions is often disregarded or presumed due to laboratory contamination, isolation of *A. flavus* or *A. fumigatus* from even a single specimen should be considered suggestive of invasive disease, given the appropriate setting. Multiple isolations increase this likelihood. Usually, the clinician will wish to establish an unequivocal diagnosis. Percutaneous needle aspiration of the lung or bronchoscopy with washings and transbronchial biopsy are variably successful. Open lung biopsy may be required for demonstration of characteristic tissue invasion, but this too may be falsely negative.

In patients with *Aspergillus flavus* infection, careful examination of the nose and paranasal sinuses may be rewarding. A nasal erosion, ulcer,

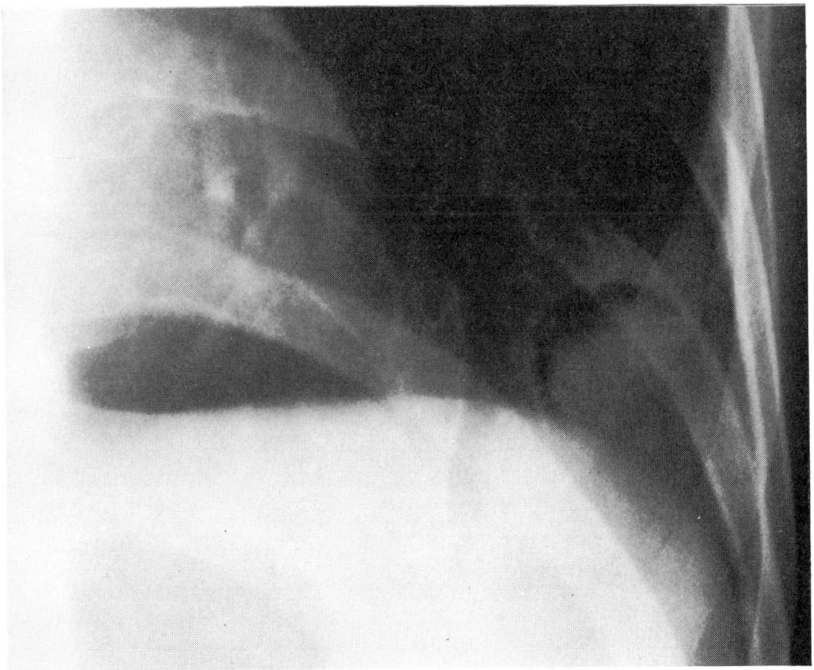

Figure 51-5 Chest radiograph of a patient who had a focal infiltrate in the left lower lobe which cavitated, resulting in the appearance of a "fungus ball."

or eschar that reveals organisms by culture or histology is highly predictive of concomitant or future invasive pulmonary aspergillosis.

Serologic diagnostic techniques have had largely disappointing results to date. Precipitins are found in only a minority of patients. When positive, they often appear late in the course of disease, well after the patient's fate is decided. Recently, favorable experience with detection of circulating antigen has been reported. Further development of this procedure hopefully will result in greater accuracy of noninvasive diagnostic techniques.

Treatment of invasive pulmonary aspergillosis is often frustrating. The ultimate outcome usually depends on the early institution of antibiotic therapy and on the course of the underlying disease. Those patients whose underlying disease is controlled have a more favorable prognosis, especially if their peripheral granulocyte counts recover to $> 1000/mm^3$.

Parenteral amphotericin B is the drug of choice. Although dosage recommendations may vary among experts, a dose of 0.6 to 0.7 mg/kg per day for a total dose of 2 to 2.5 g is reasonable. Miconazole and ketoconazole do not appear to be reliably efficacious. Combination therapy, consisting of amphotericin B plus either 5-fluorocytosine or rifampin, has been employed in selected situations, but controlled data on their efficacy compared to amphotericin B alone are lacking. The role of white blood cell tranfusions, if any, also has not been defined. Resection of areas showing persistent chest roentgenographic abnormalities has been suggested, but in the author's opinion, this approach should be viewed with caution since the disease is most likely multicentric, even though not necessarily radiographically apparent. Surgical intervention is probably best reserved for patients with life-threatening hemoptysis or invasive nasal and sinus disease.

Prevention of invasive pulmonary aspergillosis is difficult. Avoidance of large inhaled inocula such as might occur by smoking contaminated marijuana is a rational but unproven measure that could be important for the immunocompromised host. Filtering hospital air has been shown to decrease spore counts; an association with decreased disease incidence has been suggested. Strict control of air quality by laminar air flow techniques may be particularly effective. However, at present the most important method of disease prevention is prompt, effective treatment of predisposing illnesses and, possibly, judicious avoidance of overuse of corticosteroids and broad-spectrum antibiotics.

Overlap Syndromes

The classification of pulmonary aspergillosis into three distinct syndromes is undoubtedly an oversimplification masking its true nature as a spectrum of disease. Patients with aspergilloma or ABPA on occasion develop full-blown invasive aspergillosis. Contrarily, those with the invasive form or an aspergilloma sometimes develop hypersensitivity symptoms such as bronchospasm. Binder and colleagues (1982) have redescribed yet another type of pulmonary aspergillosis which they term "chronic necrotizing pulmonary aspergillosis." This illness is characterized by the indolent progression of fungal invasion, accompanied by cavitation and often by mycetoma formation. In this instance, a mycetoma develops de novo from an area of infiltration; an antecedent chronic cavity is not present. Widespread pulmonary invasion and visceral dissemination do not occur, presumably because the affected individual is only moderately compromised. Intravenous amphotericin B appears to be the treatment of choice. Gefter et al (1981) have described a similar illness in a series of five patients.

It is clear, then, that the manifestations of pulmonary aspergillosis depend upon both the nature of the infecting organism and the immune status of the host. The consequent clinical syndrome results from the interactions of these two factors.

SELECTED READINGS

General

Campbell MC, Stewart JC: *The Medical Mycology Handbook.* New York, John Wiley and Sons, 1980.

Lennette EH, Balows A, Hausler WJ, et al (eds): *Manual of Clinical Microbiology*, ed 3. Washington, DC, American Society of Microbiology, 1980.

Rosen PP: Opportunistic fungal infections in patients with neoplastic diseases. *Pathol Annu* 1976;11:255–315.

Aspergillosis

Aisner J, Murillo J, Schimpff SC, et al: Invasive aspergillosis in acute leukemia: Correlation with nose cultures and antibiotic use. *Ann Intern Med* 1979;90:4–9.

Binder RE, Faling LJ, Pugatch RD, et al: Chronic necrotizing pulmonary aspergillosis: A discrete clinical entity. *Medicine* 1982;61:109–124.

Gefter WB, Weingrad TR, Epstein DM, et al: "Semi-invasive" pulmonary aspergillosis. A new look at the spectrum of *Aspergillus* infections of the lung. *Radiology* 1981;140:313–321.

Glimp RA, Bayer AS: Pulmonary aspergilloma. Diagnostic and therapeutic considerations. *Arch Intern Med* 1983;143:303–308.

Meyer RD, Young LS, Armstrong D, et al: Aspergillosis complicating neoplastic disease. *Am J Med* 1973;54:6–15.

Nalesnik MA, Myerowitz RL, Jenkins R, et al: Significance of *Aspergillus* species isolated from respiratory secretions in the diagnosis of invasive pulmonary aspergillosis. *J Clin Microbiol* 1980;11:370–376.

Nichols D, Dopico GA, Braun S, et al: Acute and chronic pulmonary function changes in allergic bronchopulmonary aspergillosis. *Am J Med* 1979;67:613–637.

Pennington JE: *Aspergillus* lung disease. *Med Clin North Am* 1980;64:475–490.

Rosenberg M, Patterson R, Mintzer R, et al: Clinical and immunologic criteria for the diagnosis of allergic bronchopulmonary aspergillosis. *Ann Intern Med* 1977;86:405–414.

Varkey B, Rose HD: Pulmonary aspergilloma. A rational approach to treatment. *Am J Med* 1967;61:626–631.

Wang JF, Patterson R, Robert M, et al: The management of allergic bronchopulmonary aspergillosis. *Am Rev Respir Dis* 1979;120:87–92.

Weiner MH, Talbot GH, Gerson SL, et al: Antigen detection in the diagnosis of invasive aspergillosis: Utility in controlled, blinded trials. *Ann Intern Med* (in press).

Young RC, Bennett JE, Vogel CL, et al: Aspergillosis. The spectrum of disease in 98 patients. *Medicine* 1970;49:147–173

52 *Mucorales*

George H. Talbot

Microbiologic Characteristics

The potentially confusing nomenclature describing the agents of mucormycosis is best understood by reference to the accompanying figure (Figure 52-1). The Zygomycotina comprise one of four subdivisions of the Perfect Fungi (those fungi reproducing sexually). The major class within this subdivision is the *Zygomycetes*, which in turn is divided into three orders. Species of the order Entomophthorales are relatively rare causes of human disease. Members of the order Mucorales, and in particular those genera within the family *Mucoraceae*, have much greater medical significance. Although the term "mucormycosis" is used to describe illness caused by any organism in the order Mucorales, most cases result from infection with one of three genera of the *Mucoraceae*: *Rhizopus*, *Absidia*, and *Mucor*.

The Mucorales are characterized by relatively broad, coenocytic (containing many nuclei and few septae) hyphae that branch at right angles. Family, genus, and species distinctions are based in large part upon morphological differences observed during the asexual cycle. Physiologic characteristics, as well as details of sexual reproduction, also

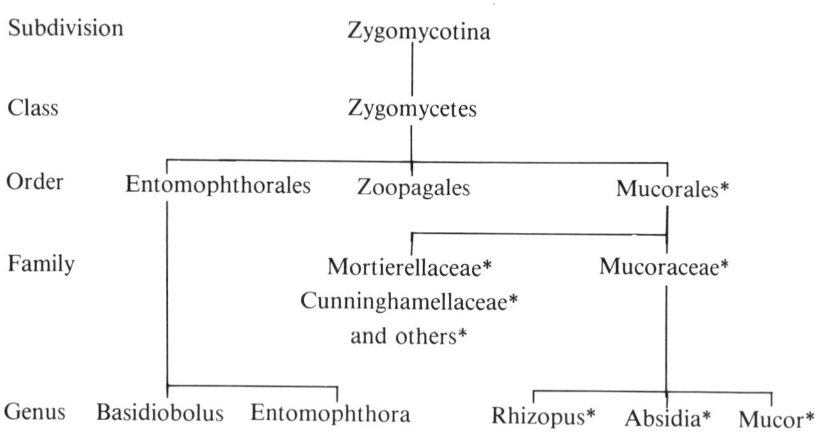

*Agents of mucormycosis.

Figure 52-1 Classification of the agents of mucormycosis.

are useful. For a detailed discussion of classification, the interested reader is referred to the general references cited in Chapter 51.

Under proper conditions, the agents of mucormycosis grow well on Sabouraud's agar, providing that cyclohexamide (a known growth inhibitor) is not employed in the medium. Plating a sufficient inoculum is also important. Growth occurs in two to five days, then rapidly blossoms to fill the container with grayish white colonies.

Clinical specimens may be examined directly with the aid of a KOH preparation, thereby revealing the characteristic 15 to 25 μm diameter nonseptate hyphae (Figure 52-2). Biopsy or autopsy material is best stained with either hematoxylin and eosin or methenamine silver. Gram stain and the PAS reaction are not as reliable. In tissue sections, hyphal arrangement tends to be less orderly than that seen with the aspergilli, which often appear in radial or parallel array. Histopathologic identification of the organisms is often critical, since even appropriately handled clinical material may not produce growth on culture. Additional features that may be helpful in distinguishing the *Zygomycetes* include the type of tissue invasion and the nature of the inflammatory response. Mucormycosis is characterized by extensive necrosis, edema, and vascular invasion with diffuse infiltrations of polymorphs (in the nongranulocytopenic host). By contrast, the Entomophthorales, the agents of subcutaneous mycosis, produce a granulomatous response.

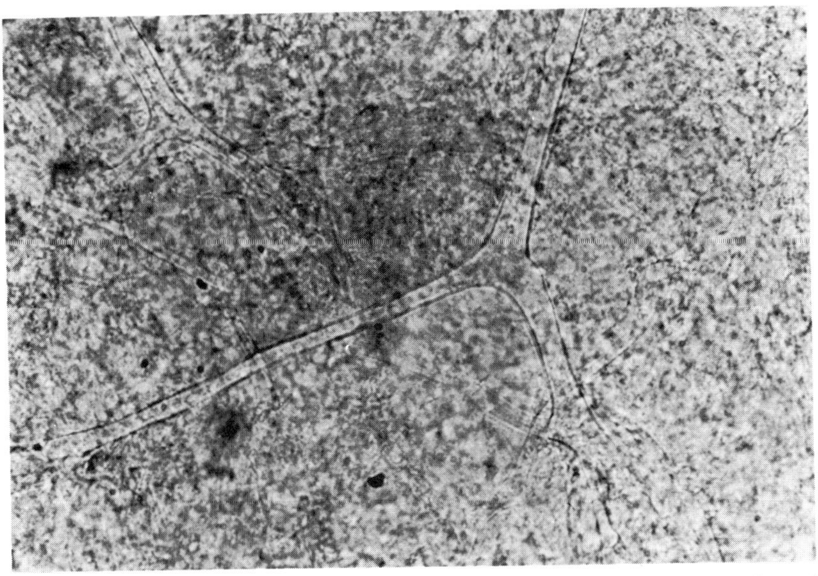

Figure 52-2 *Rhizopus* sp. Nonseptate hyphae in unstained wet mount of nasal scrapings from a patient with diabetic ketoacidosis and rhinocerebral zygomycosis. (Photomicrograph courtesy of David M. Wright, MD.)

Epidemiology

Like the aspergilli, the Mucorales are ubiquitous environmental inhabitants with a worldwide distribution. Illness occurs when a susceptible individual inhales a sufficient inoculum of these universally present spores; in general, this type of exposure is neither predictable nor apparent. Recently, a number of cases of cutaneous *Rhizopus* disease have been linked to contaminated adhesive bandages. Person-to-person transmission is not thought to occur.

Pathogenicity

As noted, mucormycosis is the consequence of host defense defects as well as of exposure to the pathogen. The first step in the production of disease is germination; the local milieu, including the presence of humoral facilitators or inhibitors of germination, may be a critical determinant of eventual outcome. The type and degree of cellular reaction is also important; the granulocyte plays a central role. Patients with illnesses causing quantitative and qualitative polymorphonuclear functional abnormalities (eg, acute leukemia and diabetic ketoacidosis, respectively) are particularly susceptible to mucormycosis, although the exact manifestations of infection may differ. Corticosteroid therapy also has been implicated in disease pathogenesis.

Clinical Syndromes

Mucormycosis produces diverse clinical syndromes, categorized according to the organ system(s) affected: rhinocerebral, pulmonary gastrointestinal, cutaneous, and disseminated. Vascular invasion with consequent infarction is the hallmark of mucormycotic infection, whatever its anatomic localization.

Pulmonary mucormycosis usually mimics invasive pulmonary aspergillosis in its presentation. Patients with leukemia or lymphoma are most often afflicted, although occasionally uncontrolled diabetes mellitus, burns, or renal failure provide appropriate predisposing conditions. Normal individuals are rarely affected.

Clinical signs and symptoms, roentgenographic abnormalities, and complications (including massive hemoptysis and widespread dissemination) are identical to those noted for invasive pulmonary aspergillosis. Although it usually pursues a fulminant course, pulmonary mucormycosis occasionally will produce more indolent disease, such as a solitary pulmonary nodule. Other persons, commonly diabetics, have developed evidence of endobronchial obstruction following localized bronchial infection. Death has occurred from massive hemoptysis. This latter group of patients might be described more precisely as having zygomycosis, since in those cases reported, differentiation of Mucorales from Entomophthorales was not accomplished.

Diagnostic Tests

The microbiologic and histologic characteristics of the Mucorales are described above. Cultural confirmation of histologically demonstrated organisms is desirable, but not always possible. Antemortem diagnosis of mucormycosis may be aided in the future by serologic assays for detection of either circulating antibody or antigen. Initial experience with the former technique is encouraging; routine testing for antigenemia is not yet feasible, although monoclonal antibody technology may produce improved results.

Therapy

Successful therapy of pulmonary mucormycosis is rarely accomplished. Cure usually results from various combinations of the three currently available therapeutic modalities: antifungal chemotherapy, treatment of underlying disease, and surgical intervention.

The mainstay of antifungal chemotherapy of mucormycosis is amphotericin B, which appears useful despite observations of high-level resistance of Mucorales organisms. The dose of amphotericin is similar to that recommended for aspergillosis (Chapter 51). Methodologic inadequacies in susceptibility testing may account for the apparent contradiction of in vivo response despite in vitro resistance. As with invasive pulmonary aspergillosis, improvement in the underlying disorder, usually leukemia or lymphoma, is a critical variable. Selected patients, particularly those with life-threatening hemoptysis, may benefit from resection of involved lobes or segments.

Prevention

Possible preventive measures are at best inferred from an analysis of the risk factors discussed above. Avoidance of unnecessary corticosteroid therapy, control of diabetes mellitus, and effective therapy of malignancy represent reasonable goals. Conceivably, effective filtration of hospital air might reduce the number of spores available for inhalation and therefore decrease the number of nosocomial infections with these organisms, but of course, the community-acquired infection rate would not be altered.

SELECTED READING

Lehrer RI (moderator): Mucormycosis. *Ann Intern Med* 1980;93:93–108.

53 *Candida*

George H. Talbot

Microbial Characteristics

Members of the genus *Candida* are classified within the class *Blastomyces,* family *Cryptococcaceae*. When cultured, they grow well aerobically on routine media, including blood agar, at 25°C to 37°C, becoming visible within two to five days. Selective media, such as Sabouraud's agar, also readily support growth. Usually a stark white at first, colonies then develop the smooth, moist, creamy whiteness common to yeasts.

Microscopically, these organisms are observed to produce rounded or oval budding cells occurring singly or in chains and clusters. By budding, cells also form pseudohyphae, which can be distinguished from true hyphae by close inspection for characteristic "pinching" at the site of the apparent septation. A number of microscopic features are useful in speciation. One particularly useful for the presumptive identification of *C. albicans* is the formation of germ tubes (fingerlike extensions of cytoplasm) when organisms are incubated in serum for several hours.

Candida species may be differentiated not only by the use of morphologic criteria, but also by a variety of biochemical reactions, including patterns of carbohydrate utilization, nitrate assimilation, and urease production. Additional medically important *Candida* species include *C. tropicalis*, *C. krusei*, and *C. parapsilosis*; *C. stellatoidea*, *C. guillermondii*, and *C. pseudotropicalis* are occasionally encountered. Members of the genus *Torulopsis* recently have been reclassified as *Candida* organisms.

Potassium hydroxide preparations of scrapings, sputum, or other clinical material confirm the presence of organisms and provide reasonable clues as to their type. Gram stain can be helpful, especially in the evaluation of urinary sediment; *Candida* species appear intensely gram positive. Biopsy or autopsy specimens readily reveal organisms when stained by the H and E, PAS, Gram, or methenamine silver method. Fluorescent antibody techniques using species-specific antisera have been useful in some hands when yeasts are seen in tissue sections but cultures are negative.

Epidemiology

Candida species are normal inhabitants of the human gastrointestinal tract from mouth through large intestine in 20% to 40% of individuals. The organism occurs in smaller numbers than does the resident bacterial flora. *Candida* also are found in the vagina and on the skin.

Pathogenicity

Because of the frequency with which *Candida* species are colonizers, simple isolation of them from a clinical specimen is not necessarily at all suggestive of disease, unless the site sampled is normally sterile (eg, blood). Even then, *Candida* may be a contaminant, rather than a pathogen, so that the physician's assessment must weigh both microbiologic and clinical data. Compounding this problem is the similarity of factors favoring *Candida*-induced illness with those favoring candidal overgrowth. The diagnosis of disease due to *Candida* infection is established with certainty only when histopathologic demonstration of tissue invasion and recovery of the organism on culture accompany a compatible clinical syndrome.

The major host defenses against candidal invasion are as follows: 1) an intact mucocutaneous barrier, 2) the presence of normal gastrointestinal and cutaneous microflora, 3) qualitatively and quantitatively normal granulocytes and macrophages, 4) intact cell-mediated immunity, and 5) certain humoral factors, including serum opsonins and transferrin. Deficiences in any of these systems may allow transformation of this normally benign commensal into a lethal pathogen.

Hospitalized patients are particularly likely to have significant alterations in their immune status. Invasive diagnostic and therapeutic procedures, broad-spectrum antibiotic therapy, and the administration of corticosteroids and cytotoxic drugs often devastate local and systemic defenses, providing ample opportunity for fungal overgrowth and subsequent invasion.

Pathological examination of the lower respiratory tracts of patients succumbing to pulmonary candidiasis reveals one of two patterns. If spread to the lungs has occurred from the oropharynx, aspirated debris and *Candida* organisms may be seen inside the tracheobronchial tree, with ulceration and/or transmucosal fungal invasion into the parenchyma itself. An extensive neutrophilic reaction is present in those patients having sufficient granulocyte reserves. In contrast, when *Candida* has reached the lungs hematogenously, multiple parenchymal abscesses are observed. Grossly these may mimic miliary granulomatous disease or diffusely metastatic carcinoma. Cavitation is rare, and significant vasculitis is not universal, in contrast to the situation seen with invasive aspergillosis or mucormycosis. Here, too, a granulocytic response is expected.

Clinical Syndromes

The only universally accepted manifestation of *Candida*-induced pulmonary disease is invasive pneumonitis. This entity is relatively rare, occurring almost exclusively in severely immunocompromised, hospitalized individuals.

As noted above, the mere isolation (or visualization) of *Candida* organisms from the respiratory secretions of a patient does not establish the diagnosis of pulmonary candidiasis, even when an infiltrate is present. Rather, histopathologic evidence of tissue invasion must be obtained. This fact is often forgotten or never learned, resulting in significant overdiagnosis of this syndrome.

The clinician typically encounters true *Candida* pneumonia in the desperately ill, granulocytopenic patient with underlying malignancy who has been treated with corticosteroids, immunosuppressive drugs, and broad-spectrum antibiotics. Indwelling vascular or urinary catheters or gastrointestinal tract ulceration may provide a portal of entry for hematogenous spread to the lungs and elsewhere. Recurrent aspiration, often clinically inapparent, seems more likely to result in candidiasis restricted to the lower respiratory tract, although occasionally further dissemination may occur from that site.

Pulmonary candidiasis should be suspected in the immunocompromised patient with an undiagnosed pulmonary infiltrate who develops objective evidence suggestive of disseminated candidal infection, including endophthalmitis, characteristic macronodular skin lesions, or culture-proven candidemia. Diagnosis is difficult and may only be established at postmortem examination. Closed or open lung biopsy may provide an antemortem diagnosis.

A positive assay for *Candida* precipitins may substantiate, but not prove, the physician's clinical impressions. A significant rate of false-positive and false-negative results limits the utility of currently available techniques. However, newer methods show more promise.

Treatment and Prevention

Amphotericin B is the drug of choice for invasive pulmonary candidiasis. Although dosage recommendations may vary among experts, a dose of 0.4 to 0.5 mg of amphotericin/kg per day for a total dose of about 1.5 to 2 g is reasonable. Some patients may benefit from the concomitant administration of 5-fluorocytosine, which frequently produces snyergistic in vitro killing or inhibition of *Candida* sp simultaneously exposed to amphotericin B. 5-fluorocytosine should not be used alone since rapid emergence of resistance is a common problem. These two drugs remain the mainstays of anticandidal treatment. Experience to date with newer agents such a miconazole and ketoconazole does not suggest that either should replace amphotericin B, with or without 5-FC, in the treatment of invasive pulmonary candidiasis. Prevention of *Candida* pneumonia is challenging at best. Successful therapy of predisposing illnesses and avoidance of potential risk factors such as antibiotic and corticosteroid therapy are suggested with ease but often accomplished only with great difficulty.

SELECTED READINGS

Edwards JE Jr (moderator): Severe candidal infections. Clinical perspective, immune defense mechanisms, and current concepts of therapy. *Ann Intern Med* 1978;89:91–106.

Masur H, Rosen PP, Armstrong D: Pulmonary disease caused by *Candida* species. *Am J Med* 1977;63:914–925.

Rose HD, Sheth NK: Pulmonary candidiosis. A clinical and pathological correlation. *Arch Intern Med* 1978;138:964–965.

54 *Histoplasma capsulatum*

Jaime Carrizosa

Histoplasma capsulatum has two morphologic forms, yeast and mycelial. The yeast are small, oval and thin-walled (2 to 4 μm in diameter), and are found in infected tissues and in growth on blood agar at 37°C after five days. The mycelial form is found in the soil contaminated by bird or bat droppings and in growth on solid media at room temperature. On Sabouraud agar at room temperature, the fungus grows as brown to white fluffy colonies that contain branching septate hyphae-bearing spores, which allow rapid identification of the fungus because of its characteristic appearance.

The histoplasmin skin test antigen, obtained from a mycelial culture filtrate, is commercially available for skin testing. The yeast phase antigen is present in a suspension of merthiolate-treated, intact yeast cells.

Epidemiology

The fungus is most common in warm and temperate climates along large river valleys. The Mississippi and Ohio river valleys are the highest areas of endemicity in the United States. *H. capsulatum* infection is rare in Australia and Europe. In West Africa a different Histoplasma, *H. capsulatum* var. *duboisii*, is responsible for most of the reported infections.

Pathogenesis

When contaminated soils are disturbed, heavy concentrations of spores become airborne. Inhalation of the spores, which are sufficiently small to reach the alveoli, is followed by intraalveolar transformation to budding yeast forms. Macrophages engulf the organisms and a granulomatous reaction is rapidly evident with formation of multinucleated giant cells, central caseous necrosis and surrounding fibrosis in the lung and adjacent lymph nodes. This reaction may eventually calcify, leading to the characteristic scattered calcifications seen in radiographic studies in the lung, lymph nodes, liver and spleen. Humoral and cellular immunity develops about two to four weeks after infection. When host defense mechanisms are impaired, little inflammatory reaction is seen around the proliferating yeast forms within macrophages and lymphohematogenous spread leads to widespread dissemination. Human-to-human transmission of histoplasmosis does not occur.

Clinical Manifestations

The large majority of primary pulmonary infections are asymptomatic or present as a mild, self-limited influenza-like illness. In cases of heavy spore inhalation, acute onset of chills, fever, headache, myalgias, nonproductive cough, dyspnea, pleuritic chest pain, and substernal discomfort may develop seven to 21 days after exposure. Erythema nodosum or erythema multiforme may occur, as in coccidioidomycosis. Chest roentgenograms show multiple patchy areas of pneumonitis, primarily involving the lower lobes, associated with hilar and peritracheal lymphadenopathy. Diffuse miliary lesions may occur. Compression of airways by enlarged nodes may lead to atelectasis or obstructive pneumonitis. Pleural effusion is uncommon. The clinical syndrome resolves spontaneously within several weeks and chest radiograph generally returns to normal. Some residual abnormalities have been described and consist of pulmonary nodules (histoplasmomas) which may grow slowly over 10 to 20 years with further layers of fibrotic tissue and this develops concentric rings of calcification to reach 3 to 4 cm in diameter. Other abnormalities include calcified mediastinal lymph nodes and the classical buck shot calcifications scattered over both lung fields, indicative of healed histoplasma lesions. Calcified mediastinal lymph nodes may erode into a large bronchi and result in broncholithiasis. Chronic mediastinal node infection may also initiate a progressive inflammatory reaction, believed to be associated with an increased hypersensitivity response, resulting in fibrosing mediastinitis. This process invades and obstructs all mediastinal structures and results in: 1) tracheobronchial stricture, causing dyspnea and substernal pain; 2) esophageal obstruction, causing dysphagia and odynophagia; 3) superior vena cava obstruction; 4) pericardial invasion with progressive constriction and tamponade; and 5) narrowing of the pulmonary arteries with pulmonary hypertension, hemorrhage and pulmonary infarction.

Rarely, a chronic progressive disseminated form of histoplasmosis presents with fever, sweating, weight loss, hepatosplenomegaly, Addison's disease, anemia, leukopenia and thrombocytopenia. Ulceration may be found in the mouth in this form of illness. An acute form of this disease may be seen in infants and immunosuppressed adults.

Chronic fibrocavitary histoplasmosis is seen primarily in patients with chronic obstructive lung disease, usually white males over 50 years of age. The host's inability to clear local infection leads to progressive destruction, enlarging cavities and fibrosis. The process, which generally affects the upper lobes, resembles tuberculosis clinically and radiographically, and is accompanied by fibrosis in the lower lobes, possibly secondary to bronchogenic spread. Hemoptysis, pulmonary hypertension and progressive pulmonary insufficiency are the most important complications.

Diagnosis

The laboratory diagnosis of histoplasmosis is made: 1) by the demonstration of the fungus in cultures of sputum, blood, bone marrow, cerebrospinal fluid, mucosal lesions, urine, lymph nodes, liver and lung; 2) by the identification of the organism in histologic sections; or 3) by the demonstration of an antibody response in sera obtained in the acute, convalescent and recovery phases of the infection. Sputum cultures are rarely positive in acute pulmonary histoplasmosis, but usually are positive in chronic cavity and disseminated forms of the disease on repeated examination. Cultures usually are negative in forms of the disease that result from an excessive host inflammatory response, namely histoplasmoma and fibrosing mediastinitis, although organisms can be visualized histologically. The complement-fixing antibodies to histoplasmin or yeast phase antigens, develop within three to four weeks after exposure, remain elevated for two to three months, and then slowly fall. In chronic, active pulmonary histoplasmosis, histoplasmin titers may remain elevated. Titers of ≥ 1:8 with either antigen are considered positive. Cross-reaction may occur with sera from patients with blastomycosis, coccidioidomycosis and other fungal diseases. In such instances, titers usually are between 1:8 and 1:32 and occur mainly with the yeast phase antigen. Relatively lower titers by complement fixation may be seen in disseminated histoplasmosis or immunosuppressed patients. The immunodiffusion test results in several precipitin bands which may correlate with the clinical condition of the patient; both the H and M bands are associated with active infection, while the M band also may be associated with inactive disease or recent positive histoplasmin skin test reaction.

In histopathologic specimens, the yeast is stained with PAS (red) or silver methenamine (black). In sputum or air-dried secretions stained with Giemsa or Wright stains, the organism is seen as small inclusions, 2 to 5 μm in diameter, within macrophages. Visible growth of *Histoplasma capsulatum* on Sabouraud's agar with or without antibiotics at room temperature occurs after seven to 10 days of incubation, but complete identification may require several weeks.

The histoplasmin antigen also is used for the preparation of a skin test; it consists of an intradermal injection of 0.1 mL of a 1:100 dilution of the antigen. The skin test can identify individuals previously infected in endemic areas, but has no diagnostic value. Conversion of a positive skin test to negative may occur in cases of disseminated disease, and culture-positive cases of chronic histoplasmosis can have negative skin tests. Skin testing may also interfere with both the complement fixation and immunodiffusion serologic assays.

Therapy

Primary infection usually is a self-limited disease and requires no therapy. Careful observation is required in children, debilitated patients and cases of heavy infection. When there is evidence of progressive or disseminated disease or chronic cavitary pulmonary histoplasmosis, amphotericin B in doses of 0.5 to 0.6 mg/kg every day or 1.0 to 1.2 mg/kg every other day for 10 weeks for a total dose of 1.5 to 2.5 g is the therapy of choice. Prolonged follow-up is required for one year or more since relapses can occur. Ketoconazole, a new oral antifungal agent, has been used successfully in the therapy of nonlife-threatening histoplasmosis (progressive primary pulmonary disease, chronic cavitary pulmonary disease and chronic disseminated disease). It is given in doses of 200 to 600 mg daily for at least six months, ie, one to three months after resolution of all clinical, serologic, radiologic and microbiologic signs of active disease. The true value of this drug in the therapy of histoplasmosis, however, awaits further experience.

Specific methods of prevention do not exist. A method of immunization is not available at the present time. In areas of high endemic infection, face masks to decrease inhalation of large amounts of spores should be advised when cleaning or digging in areas heavily contaminated by bird droppings or when exploring caves.

SELECTED READINGS

Brodsky AL, Gregg MB, Loewenstein MS, et al: Outbreak of histoplasmosis associated with the 1970 earth day activities. *Am J Med* 1973;54:333–342.

Cox F, Hughes WT: Disseminated histoplasmosis and childhood leukemia. *Cancer* 1974;33:1127–1133.

Goodwin RA Jr, Des Prez RM: Pathogenesis and clinical spectrum of histoplasmosis. *South Med J* 1973;66:13–25.

Goodwin RA, Loyd JE, Des Prez RM: Histoplasmosis in normal hosts. *Medicine* 1981;60:231–266.

Wheat LJ, Slama TG, Eitzen HE, et al: A large urban outbreak of histoplasmosis: Clinical features. *Ann Intern Med* 1981;94:331–337.

55 *Blastomyces dermatitidis*

Jaime Carrizosa

Blastomycosis is an infection that can involve the lungs, and is associated with dissemination to the skin, bone and other organs (liver, kidney, and spleen) due to *Blastomyces dermatitidis*.

Microbial Characteristics

This organism, a dimorphic fungus, exists in a yeast phase at 37°C both in vitro and in vivo, and in a mycelial phase on agar at room temperature. The characteristic morphology of the mature sporulating fungus requires seven to 10 day's growth on Sabouraud's agar. The yeast is 10 to 16 μm in diameter and has a thick, refractile, double layered cell wall and a single bud connected to the parent cell by a wide neck (Figure 55-1). Single budding distinguishes *B. dermatitidis* from *Paracoccidioides brasiliensis*, the cause of South American blastomycosis, whose parasitic phase has multiple buds.

Epidemiology

The fungus is widely distributed in nature, but there are specific areas of higher endemicity such as the Ohio and Mississippi river valleys but also in some areas of Canada, Mexico and Central and South America and Africa. Soil appears to be the source of the fungus that is inhaled presumably as aerosols of conidia. Man-to-man transmission has been rarely documented. Men are affected more frequently than women, usually in the third to fifth decades of life.

Pathogenesis

The presence of the organism in tissues elicits a significant inflammatory response, with formation of mixed reaction of granulomas and centrally located polymorphonuclear leukocytes. Most infections are subclinical, being rapidly controlled by normal host defense mechanisms. Heavy infection may lead to more severe disease and lympho-hematogenous dissemination. In patients with alteration of the host defense mechanisms the disease may rapidly disseminate. Chronic infection with progressive fibrotic changes can also occur, but calcification of the lesions is not a feature of blastomycosis.

Clinical Manifestations

Pulmonary blastomycosis is seen rarely as a benign influenza-like illness, associated with cough, fever, arthralgias, myalgias and sweating. The chest roentgenogram shows diffuse nodular infiltrates. Occasionally, pleuritic chest pain is a major part of the syndrome, but pleural effusions are infrequent. This acute presentation of the disease usually is self-limited and requires no treatment.

Much more commonly, the progressive form of pulmonary blastomycosis is seen which has a more chronic course of several weeks' to months' duration with fever, night sweats, weight loss, dyspnea, chest pain, productive cough, and occasionally hemoptysis. Physical findings may be suggestive of a pneumonic process and chest roentgenogram shows diffuse fibronodular infiltrates, a miliary pattern, cavitation and mediastinal node enlargement. Solitary nodules are rare. Almost all of these patients have systemic dissemination, frequently to the skin, bone or genitourinary tract. Central nervous system infection is unusual and gastrointestinal tract involvement rare.

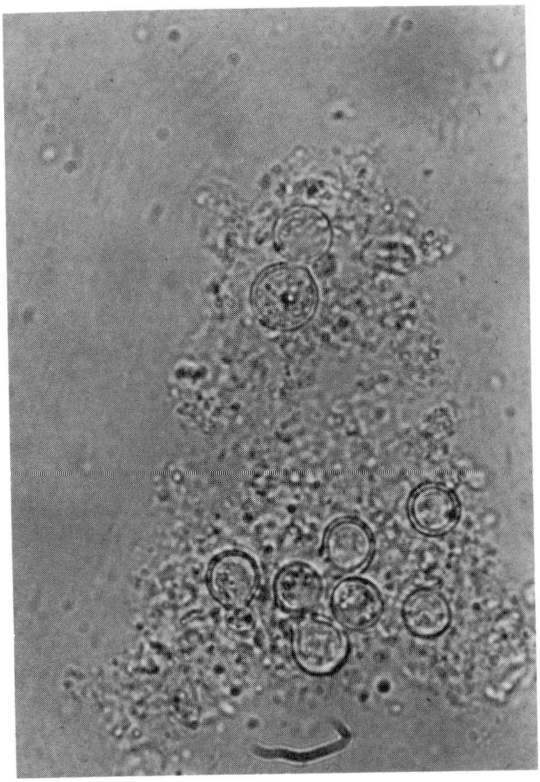

Figure 55-1 Sputum specimen obtained from a patient with active cavitary pulmonary blastomycosis. KOH preparation of sputum reveals multiple budding yeast. Note the broad base of the daughter buds and the double contour of yeast walls.

Diagnosis

The diagnosis is made by isolation or identification of the fungus in specimens of blood, sputum, urine, expressed prostate secretions, or tissue obtained by biopsy. Yeast cells of *B. dermatitidis* in pus or sputum are readily seen in wet preparations (Figure 55-1). If a presumptive diagnosis cannot be readily made from biopsies of skin or other involved tissues or wet preparations, the isolation and identification of the organism from cultures may take up to one to two months. The blastomycin skin test has no diagnostic value. Serologic studies for complement-fixing antibodies against *B. dermatitidis* lack sensitivity and specificity, and frequent cross-reactions with other fungi have been reported.

Treatment

Amphotericin B is the therapy of choice for the disease. Doses of 0.3 to 0.6 mg/kg/day or 0.7 to 0.8 mg/kg every other day for six to eight weeks are required for a total dose of 1 to 2 g, depending on the severity of disease. 2-Hydroxystilbamidine has also been used with some success in treatment of blastomycosis; doses of 225 mg/day for four to six weeks for a total dose of 8 g has been recommended. Relapse after amphotericin treatment may occur in up to 10% of patients; thus patients should be followed for several years after completion of therapy.

SELECTED READINGS

Baum GL, Lerner PI: Primary pulmonary blastomycosis: A laboratory-acquired infection. *Ann Intern Med* 1970;73:263–265.

Berger R, Kraman S: Acute miliary blastomycosis after "short-course" corticosteroid treatment. *Arch Intern Med* 1981;141:1223–1225.

Kitchen MS, Reiber CD, Eastin GB: An urban epidemic of North American blastomycosis. *Am Rev Respir Dis* 1977;115:1063–1066.

Sarosi GA, Hammerman KJ, Tosh FE, et al: Clinical features of acute pulmonary blastomycosis. *N Engl J Med* 1974;290:540–543.

Tosh FE, Hammerman KJ, Weeks RJ, et al: A common source epidemic of North American blastomycosis. *Am Rev Respir Dis* 1974;109:525–529.

56 *Cryptococcus neoformans*

Jaime Carrizosa

Microbial Characteristics

Of the several species in the genus *Cryptococcus*, *Cryptococcus neoformans* and, rarely, *C. albidus* have been reported to cause human infection. *C. neoformans*, unlike other fungi that cause deep infections, is not dimorphic. *C. neoformans* in both infected tissues and in culture are budding yeasts about 4 to 6 μm in diameter surrounded by a capsule that might vary up to 30 μm in diameter. The bud appears to be attached to the mother cell by a narrow neck. Four types have been differentiated on the basis of antigenic specificity of capsular polysaccharide. No specific relation between capsular type and clinical manifestations has been established.

Epidemiology

C. neoformans is a ubiquitous organism that is frequently found in pigeon droppings and debris from places inhabited by pigeons. The organism does not affect the pigeon and is present in its excreta where it may survive up to two years. Cryptococcosis is presumably acquired by inhalation of the aerosolized organism. Neither man-to-man nor animal-to-man spread has been documented. However, unlike the other aerosol-borne mycoses, histoplasmosis and coccidioidomycosis, cryptococcosis rarely occurs in clusters and there is no occupational predisposition.

Pathogenesis

In the alveoli and in other sites outside the central nervous system, cryptococci elicit a granulomatous inflammatory reaction. Phagocytic cells ingest and kill the yeast. Activation of the complement system and anticryptococcal antibody may be necessary for ingestion by some phagocytic cells. In the brain, cystic clusters of fungi occur with no inflammatory response.

Clinical Manifestations

The clinical manifestations of cryptococcal pulmonary infection are not prominent. Cough scmetimes productive of blood-streaked sputum, and occasionally chest pain, may occur. Pulmonary cryptococcosis usually occurs without involvement of extrapulmonary sites, and if meningeal cryptococcosis occurs, pulmonary involvement is usually no longer detectable. Chest radiographs reveal usually single or multiple masses or nodules, without mediastinal lymphadenopathy, and less frequently segmental pneumonia, cavities, pleural effusion or miliary disease. The pulmonary disease is most often self-limited. A progressive pulmonary process or systemic dissemination rarely occurs. Systemic spread may involve the central nervous system (ie, meningitis or cryptococcomas), adrenal glands, prostate, liver, kidney, bone, eye and skin.

Laboratory

The organism can be identified by its distinctive capsule in an India ink preparation. On culture, the organism is not fastidious, and grows well at 37°C, unlike nonpathogenic cryptococci, with visible growth occurring as early as 48 hours. Specific identification procedures include tests of biochemical characteristics and mouse pathogenicity. Also, colonies of *C. neoformans* develop a characteristic brown pigment on a differential medium commonly called "bird seed agar." The organism is sensitive to cycloheximide present in some selective media used for isolation of fungi and, therefore, attempts at isolation should be done on nonselective media or media that do not contain cycloheximide. The serologic diagnosis of cryptococcus is based on the detection of capsular antigen or antibodies against capsular antigens. The presence of capsular antigen in serum, urine or spinal fluid can be determined by a latex agglutination test using a hyperimmune rabbit serum coating a suspension of latex particles; appropriate controls for rheumatoid factor are necessary. The latex agglutination test for capsular antigen is considered to have high specificity, but false-negative reaction occasionally have been reported, especially in patients with localized pulmonary cryptococcosis.

Cryptococci may be visualized in histologic sections of biopsied tissue by periodic acid-Schiff and silver methenamine stains. Hematoxylin and eosin stains fail to delineate the organism. Mucicarmine stains the capsule red, and does not stain other yeast-like fungi and artifacts that may otherwise have similar morphologic features.

Diagnosis

Sputum cultures may fail to grow *C. neoformans* in patients when cryptococcal pulmonary disease is present, and conversely may grow the organism when only saprophytic colonization is present. Capsular antigen usually is not detected in body fluids of patients with pulmonary cryptococcosis. Therefore, demonstration of the organism in the lung biopsy or needle aspiration is necessary for diagnosis. Skin lesions, when present, contain cryptococci in large numbers and biopsy of these accessible lesions offer the best opportunity for a rapid diagnosis.

Treatment

The majority of cases of pulmonary cryptococcal infection are self-limited infections and do not require antibiotic therapy. Therefore, observation of the pulmonary lesion for two to three months for progression is advised. However, because of radiographic resemblance to tumor, diagnosis frequently is made only after the mass is surgically excised to exclude malignancy. Total excision is curative. Treatment with a combination of amphotericin B 0.3 to 0.6 mg/kg/day and 5-flucytosine 150 mg/kg/day is indicated for therapy of pulmonary cryptococcosis when the lesions are progressive, when there is evidence of extrapulmonary dissemination, and in patients predisposed to dissemination, ie, those on corticosteroids or with a lymphoreticular disorder. Surgical excision of a solitary lesion to exclude malignancy is curative and does not require therapy as long as the cerebrospinal fluid is normal, because the risk of cryptococcal meningitis as a postoperative complication is low.

SELECTED READINGS

Diamond RD, Bennett JE: Prognostic factors in cryptococcal meningitis. *Ann Intern Med* 1974;80:176–181.

Hammerman KG, Powell KE, Christianson CS, et al: Pulmonary cryptococcosis: Clinical forms and treatment. *Am Rev Respir Dis* 1973;108:1116–1123.

Houk VN, Moser KM: Pulmonary cryptococcis—Must all receive amphotericin B? *Ann Intern Med* 1965;63:583–596.

Kerkering TM, Duma RJ, Shadomy S: The evolution of pulmonary cryptococcosis. *Ann Intern Med* 1981;94:611–616.

57 *Coccidioides immitis*

Jaime Carrizosa

Coccidioides immitis is a fungus found in the soil, particularly in hot arid areas which include the San Joaquin Valley of California, Arizona, New Mexico, Texas, Mexico, and Central and South America. Human infection is acquired by inhalation of *C. immitis* arthrospores. This fungus produces primarily pulmonary infection, which may regress spontaneously, progress locally or disseminate systemically.

Microbial Characteristics

C. immitis is a diphasis fungus, ie, it grows in a mycelial form in soil and on solid media at 30°C and 37°C and in a yeast form in human tissues. In the mycelial phase, barrel-shaped cells (arthrospores) form along the filamentous septate hyphae which fragment, releasing the arthrospores. The arthrospores survive extreme conditions for prolonged periods of time. Aerosols created by disturbances of contaminated soil, such as windstorms, construction or farming, disseminate the organism. When airborne arthrospores are inhaled, they form thick-walled spherical structures, 30 to 60 μm in diameter, called spherules in the infected tissues. Up to several hundred internal spores, called endospores, 2 to 5 μm in diameter, can develop within a spherule. The endospores, released on rupture of the spherule, can in turn develop into new spherules in tissues. Once outside the body, the endospores from exudates can form mycelia and infectious arthrospores in casts, bandages or soil.

Pathogenesis

Inhalation of just a few spores will cause infection in a normal host. No man-to-man or animal-to-man spread has been demonstrated. Once the organisms reach the alveoli, the cellular response resembles closely the granulomatous lesion of tuberculosis, except for the neutrophilic response to endospores. In some patients, especially in the immunocompromised patient, the rapid proliferation of fungi eventually may result in lympho-hematogenous dissemination with multisystem involvement.

Clinical Manifestations

In about 60% of adults, primary infection is asymptomatic; in the rest, symptoms such as an influenza-like illness (cough, fever and chest pain) develop one to four weeks after exposure. Chest pain may be severe. Arthralgias and skin lesions resembling erythema nodosum or erythema multiforme occasionally develops, usually in women and coincident with acquisition of delayed-type hypersensitivity to coccidioidin. This symptom complex has been called "valley fever" or "desert rheumatism".

Chest roentgenograms may show infiltrates, peripherally located cavities, hilar adenopathy and pleural effusion. In most patients, recovery occurs after several weeks. Persistent thin-walled cavities or nodules (coccidioidomas) occur in about 5%. Chronic pulmonary coccidioidomycosis progressing slowly over several years may present as fibronodular or cavitary disease very similar to tuberculosis. The disease may disseminate to the skin, bone, central nervous system, liver and spleen. Dissemination is most common in men, blacks, Hispanics and Filipinos, and is particularly severe in the immunocompromised host and when infection is acquired during pregnancy. One of the most serious complications is coccidioidal meningitis. If meningitis occurs, it usually does so within six months of the primary infection.

Diagnosis

The organism grows well on Sabouraud's agar, with visible growth in three to five days and production of spores in about two weeks. Examination of the cultures is performed only after killing the organism with formaldehyde, because of the hazard of working with viable *C. immitis* cultures. The identification of spherules in exudates or in biopsied tissues, utilizing special fungal stains (periodic acid-Schiff and silver methenamine) is diagnostic. The large size of the spherules and the presence of endospores facilitate its identification.

Immunology

The coccidioidin skin test is useful as a screening test in the diagnosis and in epidemiologic studies of the disease. A positive, delayed hypersensitivity response develops within three weeks after the onset of symptoms, thus a positive skin test means past or present infection. A conversion from negative to positive is diagnostic of recent infection. As in histoplasmosis, the skin test is known to become negative when dissemination occurs. The development of anergy is an unfavorable prognostic sign. There is little skin test cross-reactivity with other mycoses that produce a similar clinical syndrome (histoplasmosis), and the skin test does not stimulate anticoccidioidal antibody, as does the histoplasmin skin test. Complement-fixing antibodies are present in more than 90% of patients eight weeks after onset of symptoms. The titers are elevated in proportion to the severity of the disease; they are higher and sustained in disseminated disease and fall with improvement, but may be negative in many patients with chronic cavitary coccidioidomycosis or coccidioidomas. Although complement fixation titers of ≥ 1:16 generally are associated with dissemination, no specific titer can be said to discriminate between disseminated and nondisseminated disease, in part because of variation of results from laboratory to laboratory.

Treatment

No therapy is required for patients with uncomplicated primary infection, or stable asymptomatic chronic cavities or fibrocavitary disease. Amphotericin is indicated in severe or prolonged primary coccidioidomycosis, overt disseminated disease, and when there is an increased likelihood of incipient or occult dissemination, ie, infancy, pregnancy, immunocompromised state, racial group predisposed to dissemination, high or rising complement-fixing antibody titers and negative skin test. Amphotericin B is given in doses of 1.0 to 1.5 mg/kg/day three times a week for a total dose of 0.5 to 1.5 g, or more, depending upon the response of the patient. Surgery is considered in cases of rapidly enlarging cavities that are at risk of imminent rupture, bronchopleural fistula, serious and persistent hemoptysis and for diagnosis when nodular lesions are suspected to be malignant. Perioperative use of amphotericin has been suggested for a total dose of about 0.1 to 1 g. Amphotericin is not recommended in patients following pulmonary resection of asymptomatic coccidioidomycosis first discovered postoperatively. Preliminary data suggest that ketoconazole may be an effective, relatively nontoxic agent for the treatment of nonmeningeal coccidioidomycosis in doses of at least 400 mg daily for a minimum of six months. Ketoconazole in doses of 200 to 400 mg daily is not effective in coccidioidal meningitis. However, further data with this agent are required to adequately judge its efficacy.

Prevention

No specific methods of prevention are available. As in histoplasmosis, prevention is based on avoidance of exposure to soils that harbor the arthrospores. No immunization is available currently, but it is under investigation.

SELECTED READINGS

Bayer AS: Fungal pneumonias: Pulmonary coccidioidal syndromes (part 1). Primary and progressive primary coccidioidal pneumonias—Diagnostic, therapeutic, and prognostic considerations. *Chest* 1981;79:575–583.

Bayer AS: Fungal pneumonias: Pulmonary coccidioidal syndromes (part 2). Miliary, nodular, and cavitary pulmonary coccidioidomycosis—Chemotherapeutic and surgical considerations. *Chest* 1981;79:686–691.

Drutz DJ, Catanzaro A: Coccidioidomycosis, part 1. *Am Rev Respir Dis* 1978; 11:559–585.

Drutz DJ, Cantanzaro A: Coccidioidomycosis, part 2. *Am Rev Respir Dis* 1978; 11:727–771.

Drutz DJ: Urban coccidioidomycosis and histoplasmosis. *N Engl J Med* 1979; 301:381–382.

Graybill JR, Lundberg D, Donovan W, et al: Treatment of coccidioidomycosis with ketoconazole: Clinical and laboratory studies in 18 patients. *Rev Infect Dis* 1980;2:661–673.

Greendyke WH, Resnick DL, Harvey WC: The varied roentgen manifestations of primary coccidioidomycosis. *Am J Roentgenol Rad Ther Nucl Med* 1970; 109:491–499.

58 *Paracoccidioides brasiliensis*

Matthew E. Levison

Paracoccidioidomycosis, or South American blastomycosis, is a systemic mycosis caused by *Paracoccidioides brasiliensis.* Although indigenous to South and Central America, paracoccidioidomycosis can be seen among immigrants to the United States, three to 20 years after leaving these endemic areas.

Microbial Characteristics

P. brasiliensis is a dimorphic fungus that appears: 1) as a thick-walled yeast, 6 to 40 μm in diameter that reproduces by multiple budding in tissues and exudates as well as in cultures at 37° C or 2) as a mold both in cultures incubated at room temperature and probably also in nature. Colonies on agar appear in 10 days when incubated at 37° C, but need 20 to 30 days of incubation at room temperature to develop.

Epidemiology

Paracoccidioidomycosis occurs in most countries of Latin America, including Mexico, but is seen most frequently in Brazil, followed by Columbia and Venezuela. Men over 30 years of age usually are affected. The frequent occurrence in farmers suggests that the disease is acquired through contact with soil, but many cases have occurred in urban settings. Neither man-to-man nor animal-to-man transmission has been reported.

Pathogenesis

Although the pathogenesis is unclear, the respiratory tract is believed to be a portal of entry and the lung, the site of the primary lesions. The fungus disseminates to other viscera, skin and mucous membranes by the hematogenous route.

Clinical Manifestations

There are five clinical forms of paracoccidioidomycosis: 1) respiratory (acute benign primary pulmonary or chronic progressive pulmonary disease, 2) cutaneous, 3) mucosal, 4) lymphatic, and 5) other visceral (eg, adrenals, bowel, testes, central nervous system).

Although a few self-limited cases of primary pulmonary infection have been documented in the literature, usually pulmonary paracoccidioidomycosis is a chronic progressive disease manifested by dyspnea, cough productive of blood-tinged or purulent sputum, malaise, fever and weight loss. Chest radiographs reveal patchy or confluent nodular infiltrates that rarely cavitate and mostly spare the apices. Pleural effusions, calcifications, and hilar adenopathy are not common. Progressive pulmonary fibrosis may result in cor pulmonale. Infiltrated, ulcerated or nodular lesions may appear on the oral mucosa (and extend to the larynx or pharynx) or on the skin, usually of the face. Lymph nodes, most commonly those of the neck, supraclavicular or axillary regions, may become massively enlarged, with subsequent formation of abscess and draining sinuses. The spleen and liver may be enlarged.

Diagnosis

Diagnosis can be established by microscopic examination of wet preparations of sputum or exudates from mucosal or cutaneous lesions, or histologic study of biopsied tissue for large, multiple budding yeast cells. Several specimens may be necessary.

The paracoccidioidin skin test is not reliable for diagnosis since the patient can be anergic when the disease is most active. The development of skin test reactivity may be associated with a favorable response to therapy. A nonquantitative immunodiffusion assay for antibodies is specific, but cannot be used to judge activity of the disease. Quantitation of the complement fixation test allows this test to be used to judge activity: the greater the complement fixation titers, the more severe is the disease process.

Treatment

Paracoccidioidomycosis is the only fungal disease susceptible to sulfonamides. Sulfadiazine (4 to 6 g/day for adults) is given for several weeks to months until improvement is apparent, and then half this dose is given for three to five years or more to avoid relapses that may occur in up to 40% of cases. Resistant organisms may develop in about 10% of cases. Amphotericin, 2 to 4 g, depending upon the extent of disease, given over 30 to 90 days, also has been used successfully and is indicated for those patients who either fail to respond to sulfonamides, who relapse, who have advanced disease, or who have allergy to sulfonamides. If possible, chronic maintenance therapy with sulfonamides, following a course of amphotericin has been recommended. Recent clinical trials suggest that ketoconazole may become an alternate drug for paracoccidioidomycosis. Most patients improve within two to three months when given 200 to 400 mg of ketoconazole per day and this therapy is continued for up to 18 months. Pulmonary lesions respond slowly and heal by fibrosis.

SELECTED READINGS

Agia GA, Hurst DJ, Rogers WA: Paracoccidioidomycosis presenting as a cavitating pulmonary mass. *Chest* 1980;78:650–652.

Londero AT, Ramos CD: Paracoccidioidomycosis. A clinical and mycologic study of forty-one cases observed in Santa Maria, RS, Brazil. *Am J Med* 1972;52:771–775.

Murray HW, Littman ML, Roberts RB: Disseminated paracoccidioidomycosis (South American blastomycosis) in the United States. *Am J Med* 1974;56:209–220.

Negroni R, Robles AM, Arechavala A, et al: Ketoconazole in the treatment of paracoccidioidomycosis and histoplasmosis. *Rev Infect Dis* 1980;2:643–649.

59 *Protozoa and Helminths*

Donald Kaye

The parasites that may cause pulmonary infection include protozoa, nematodes, trematodes and cestodes. Table 59-1 lists these organisms, the parts of the world where these infections occur, and the types of pulmonary manifestations that result.

PROTOZOA

Pneumocystis carinii

Pneumocystis is an uncommon cause of pneumonia which occurs almost only in debilitated infants and immunocompromised patients.

Microbial characteristics *P. carinii* is classified as a protozoan in the class Sporozoa. In tissue the microorganisms appear as cysts that are 4 to 6 μm in diameter. On electron microscopy, each cyst contains up to eight dense bodies ("daughter bodies" or sporozoites), each 1 to 2 μm in diameter. After the sporozoites have developed, the cyst ruptures, releasing the extracystic forms of the parasite which are called trophozoites and are 2 to 5 μm in diameter. Trophozoites also can apparently divide directly. *P. carinii* stains poorly with hematoxylin and eosin stain and is stained best by the Gomori silver methenamine method which stains the cyst wall black. Toluidine blue stains the cyst wall purple. Neither stains the trophozoite. Giemsa, Wright, Gram-Weigert and methylene blue stain the organism but not the cyst wall. *P. carinii* can be cultivated in vitro in certain tissue culture cell lines. Serological tests have been developed but are of questionable value for diagnosis.

Epidemiology *Pneumocystis* is found worldwide in humans and in animals such as guinea pigs, mice, dogs, rabbits and cats. However, there may be species specificity. No reservoirs of the organism outside of living mammals have been demonstrated. Acquisition of the parasite is probably by inhalation of droplet sprays from the respiratory tracts of infected patients. Subclinical infection is common. The organism is thought to be frequently present in lung tissue from previous infection in a latent form and then become activated at the time of decrease of immune defenses.

Clinical manifestations are most likely to occur in debilitated infants and in people whose immune status has been compromised. The infants are often premature or malnourished, and outbreaks with apparent infant-to-infant spread may occur. Onset of disease often occurs when the maternally deprived IgG levels fall. Children and adults who develop *Pneumocystis* pneumonia usually have depressed cellular immunity (T-lymphocyte function) and/or humoral immunity (B-lymphocyte function) from: 1) a congenital disease of immunity, 2) a lymphoma (especially Hodgkin's disease and lymphosarcoma), 3) drugs (corticosteroids, anti-

Table 59-1
Parasites That May Cause Pulmonary Infection

Parasite	Location	Pulmonary Process
Protozoa		
Pneumocystis carinii	Worldwide	Interstitial pneumonia
Plasmodium falciparum	Tropical and subtropical areas	Pulmonary edema, pleural effusion
Entamoeba histolytica	Worldwide	Empyema or abscess
Toxoplasma gondii	Worldwide	Interstitial pneumonia
Leishmania donovani	Worldwide	Parasitism of reticuloendothelial cells
Nematodes		
Ascaris lumbricoides	Worldwide	Pneumonia
Toxocara canis or *cati*	Worldwide	Pneumonia
Necator americanus and *Ancylostoma duodenale*	Tropical and subtropical areas	Pneumonia
Ancylostoma braziliense	Worldwide	Pneumonia
Strongyloides stercoralis	Tropical, subtropical, and occasionally temperate areas	Pneumonia
Wuchereria and *Brugia* of animal species	Asia, Africa, South America and the Far East	Pulmonary nodules
Dirofilaria immitis	Worldwide	Coin lesions
Trematodes		
Schistosoma mansoni	Africa, South America and the Caribbean Islands	Pulmonary artery, hypertension, focal consolidation, coin lesions
Schistosoma haematobium	Africa	
Schistosoma japonicum	Far East	
Paragonimus westermani, P. uterobilateralis and *P. africanus*	Far East, West Africa, and Central and South America	Nodules, cysts, abscesses, bronchiectatic cavities
Cestodes		
Echinococcus granulosus	Worldwide	Cysts
Echinococcus multilocularis	Canada, Alaska, Russia	Cysts

metabolites or radiomimetic agents) or radiotherapy used as antitumor treatment, or 4) agents used for immunosuppression in association with tissue transplantation. The infection frequently becomes clinically apparent at the time of tapering or discontinuing of corticosteroids.

Recently, a syndrome, AIDS (acquired immunodeficiency syndrome), has been described in which many opportunistic infections occur including *Pneumocystis carinii* pneumonia. T cell function is decreased with reversal of the T helper to T suppressor cell ratio. The disease affects primarily male homosexuals but also intravenous drug abusers, mates of male homosexuals, infants born to affected females, people who have received blood transfusions and certain other blood products, and Haitians.

Pathology Lesions are found almost exclusively in the lungs which show evidence of interstitial pneumonia and desquamative alveolitis. The infiltrate contains many lymphocytes, plasma cells and macrophages. Eosinophils also may be numerous. The alveoli are filled with foamy, amorphous contents which contain *P. carinii*. The organisms can be seen when stained by the silver methenamine method. The alveolar material also may contain phagocytic cells containing *P. carinii*, alveolar epithelial cells and hyaline membranes.

Clinical course The pneumonia in infants occurs between 2 and 6 months of age and usually is manifested by insidious onset and progression over one to four weeks of a nonproductive cough (which may be minimal), dyspnea and cyanosis. In the immunosuppressed the onset usually is acute, with fever and cough followed by cyanosis. The course from onset to death usually is one to three weeks. Cough may be absent. Following cure, diffuse interstitial fibrosis may occur. Physical findings on examination of the lungs usually are minimal.

Laboratory findings The chest roentgenogram demonstrates bilateral interstitial-type infiltrates. Cavitation and pleural effusions rarely, if ever, occur. The diagnosis depends upon microscopic demonstration of the parasite. Sputum smears and even smears of transtracheal aspirates usually are negative. Therefore, bronchoscopic brush biopsy and, if negative, transbronchial or percutaneous needle biopsy of the lung should be performed. If these are negative, open lung biopsy will be necessary for diagnosis. Stains that reveal *P. carinii* must be used; silver methenamine and toluidine blue stains are preferred. Early biopsy is critical for prompt diagnosis and therapy. The earlier the onset of therapy, the better the prognosis. Serological studies are currently not useful.

Differential diagnosis The appearance of a bilateral interstitial pneumonia in an immunocompromised patient should raise the suspicion of *Pneumocystis* pneumonia. After ruling out acute bacterial pneumonia, the differential diagnosis consists of viral pneumonia (eg, cytomegalovirus), fungal pneumonia, *Mycoplasma* pneumonia, pneumonias caused by *Legionella pneumophila* and similar organisms, tuberculosis, drug reaction, and pulmonary infiltration caused by the underlying disease.

Therapy The therapy of choice is trimethoprim-sulfamethoxazole in a dose of 20 mg/kg/day of trimethoprim and 100 mg/kg/day of sulfamethoxazole orally or intravenously, given in divided doses every six hours for 14 days. Presumptive prompt therapy is indicated even on only suspicion of the diagnosis as the therapy is relatively nontoxic and waiting worsens the prognosis. Alternate therapy is pentamidine isethionate 4 mg/kg/day intramuscularly for 14 days. However, pentamidine is hepatotoxic and nephrotoxic and has other toxicities. In addition a reduction of the doses of corticosteroids should be attempted.

Prognosis Untreated, the mortality rate is 50% in infants and almost 100% in the immunoincompetent child or adult. With treatment, mortality rates are 25% or less. An improved prognosis is directly related to early diagnosis and prompt onset of therapy.

Prevention Maintenance of good nutrition in infants is an important preventive measure. Chemoprophylaxis has been highly effective in certain high-risk groups such as children being treated for leukemia. The prophylactic regimen is 5 mg trimethoprim and 25 mg of sulfamethoxazole per kg body weight each day and has been continued for as long as two years. Isolation of patients with *P. carinii* pneumonia from malnourished infants and immunocompromised patients is advisable.

Plasmodium falciparum

Malaria is caused by *Plasmodium vivax*, *Plasmodium falciparum*, *Plasmodium malariae*, or *Plasmodium ovale*. However, only *P. falciparum* is associated with pulmonary disease, a rare complication, usually manifested as pulmonary edema and/or pleural effusion.

Epidemiology *P. falciparum* is endemic in most tropical and semitropical parts of the world and is transmitted by the female *Anopheles* mosquito. It occasionally is transmitted by blood transfusion or shared needles in temperate areas such as the United States.

With the bite of the mosquito, sporozoites are injected, resulting in transient parasitemia. The *P. falciparum* parasites then enter and multiply in hepatic cells. After a period of time (usually five to seven days), merozoites leave the hepatic cells and infect circulating erythrocytes. The hepatic cells subsequently remain free of infection and only erythrocytes are parasitized. The trophozoite in the red cell goes through a ring form and then develops into a multinucleated schizont. When the red cell ruptures, multiple merozoites are released to infect more red cells. Fever accompanies the rupture of red cells. The process from infection of the red cell to rupture takes 48 hours. Although synchronous rupture of red cells may occur every 48 hours with a paroxysm of fever at that time, in *P.*

falciparum malaria, rupture often remains disynchronous. Some of the merozoites that enter red cells become gametocytes which can be ingested by mosquitoes to complete the cycle. The gametocytes of *P. falciparum* are banana-shaped and are easily recognized.

The parasitized red cells beyond the ring form become sticky and adhere to capillary endothelium (and may occlude the capillaries), resulting in anoxia of the tissue with functional impairment (particularly in brain and kidneys).

The pulmonary manifestations have been attributed to plugging of the microcirculation by parasitized red cells or by microthrombi, to increased capillary permeability and/or to circulatory overload. Increased capillary permeability seems to be the major pathogenetic defect.

Pathology In severe cases of malaria caused by *P. falciparum*, the brain is edematous and has areas of necrosis and hemorrhage. The kidney may show ischemia of the renal cortex and tubular necrosis. The liver may show centrolobular degeneration and necrosis. In the lungs there may be microvascular congestion with or without thrombus formation, interstitial edema, hemorrhage and hyaline membrane formation.

Clinical course Unlike other forms of malaria, in *P. falciparum* malaria the levels of red cell parasitism may be very high (below 2% in other forms and frequently well over 5% in *P. falciparum* malaria). As many as 90% of erythrocytes may be infected. Because of the very high parasitemia and because of the tendency for forms beyong the ring stage to stick to endothelium of blood vessels, a number of complications may occur. There may be rapidly progressive and severe hemolytic anemia, disturbances of mentation including coma, renal failure and acute pulmonary edema.

The clinical manifestations of *P. falciparum* malaria are fever, anemia from hemolysis, and hepatosplenomegaly with or without manifestations of anoxia, hemorrhage and/or edema in brain, kidney, gastrointestinal tract or lungs. Although the temperature usually remains elevated in *P. falciparum* malaria, there may be paroxysms of chills, fever and sweats every 48 hours. With a paroxysm there is a shaking chill, a rise in temperature to 40 °C or more for several hours associated with headache and myalgias, and then profuse sweats during which the temperature returns to normal. The illness may begin with nonspecific symptoms such as malaise, anorexia, nausea, and cough.

Cerebral malaria is the term used for the cerebral dysfunction leading to coma and frequently death. Blackwater fever refers to massive hemolysis, hemoglobinuria and acute renal failure. In some patients quinine may play a role in precipitating blackwater fever.

Pleural effusion and/or pulmonary edema may occur but are uncommon. Although, in some patients, the pulmonary manifestations may be related to excessive fluid administration, other factors seem more important. A diffuse alveolar injury has been postulated. The major manifestations are related to increased capillary permeability and resultant pulmonary edema. Dyspnea and bloody sputum may be observed and the physical findings reflect the pleural effusion or pulmonary edema.

Disseminated intravascular coagulation may occur and add to the complicated clinical picture, but usually does not play a major role in the syndromes caused by *P. falciparum.*

Laboratory findings Examination of the peripheral smear (both thin and thick smears) is critical in diagnosis of malaria. White blood counts and smears interpreted by automated methods will not detect parasites. Typical of *P. falciparum* are: the rings are small; multiple rings are found in single erythrocytes; there are many rings but no schizonts in smears; parasitism may be over 5%; and the typical banana-shaped gametocyte may be seen. Serological tests for malaria are available and are useful for detecting infected blood donors and for doing epidemiological studies, but are of no value in making a diagnosis in a patient with malaria.

A nomocytic normochromic anemia usually is present. Leukocytosis or, more often, leukopenia may be observed. Eosinophilia is absent. Thrombocytopenia is common. The urinary sediment may reflect acute tubular necrosis. The chest x-ray may show pleural effusion, an interstitial infiltrate, or frank pulmonary edema (Figure 59-1).

Differential diagnosis In any traveler returning from a country where malaria is endemic and in drug addicts or people receiving blood transfusions, development of fever (with or without chills or sweats) should suggest the possibility of *P. falciparum* malaria. Hepatosplenomegaly may be absent early. The development of cerebral dysfunction in a febrile patient who has been in a malarious area strongly suggests the possibility of *P. falciparum* malaria.

Therapy Chloroquine has classically been the drug used for treatment of malaria caused by *P. falciparum* and is the drug of choice when the parasite is susceptible to chloroquine. However, strains of *P. falciparum* resistant to chloroquine but sensitive to quinine have been observed in many parts of the world. A notable exception is West Africa where chloroquine resistance has not been reported. The Centers for Disease Control in Atlanta, Georgia have available updated information on the location of chloroquine-resistant *P. falciparum.* Some experts still recommend chloroquine for initial therapy of a strain of unknown sensitivity provided that the patient is not seriously ill. Clearly, when the infection is life threatening, when response of parasitemia to chloroquine does not occur after 24 to 48 hours of therapy, or when infection has occurred despite proper prophylaxis with chloroquine, quinine is the agent that must be used for therapy, usually along with pyrimethamine and sulfadiazine. Many experts recommend quinine as initial therapy for all *P. falciparum* malaria in which there is a possibility of chloroquine resistance.

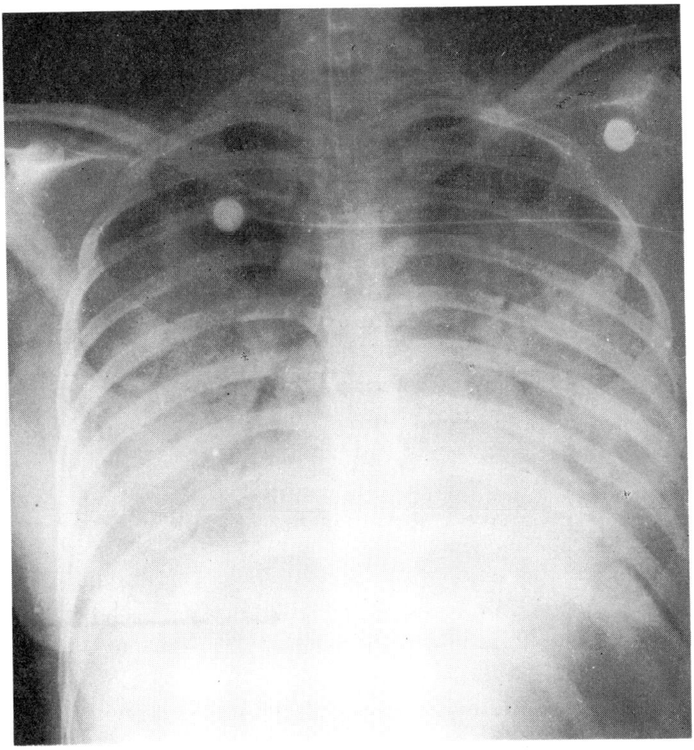

Figure 59-1 Chest x-ray in a woman with pulmonary edema from *P. falciparum* malaria.

The dose of chloroquine is 1 g chloroquine phosphate orally, followed by 500 mg in six hours and then 500 mg each day for two days. Quinine is given as quinine sulfate, 650 mg orally three times a day for 10 days or, when parenteral dosage is necessary, as quinine dihydrochloride, 600 mg IV every eight hours. Pyrimethamine is given orally at a dose of 25 mg twice a day for three days and sulfadiazine at a dose of 0.5 g four times a day for five days.

Fluid replacement is handled carefully to avoid precipitating pulmonary edema. If pulmonary edema results, intubation and assisted ventilation with positive end expiratory pressure breathing may be useful. Plasma oncotic pressure should be maintained by infusion of crystalloid solutions with careful monitoring of the pulmonary wedge pressure. Diuretic therapy is useful only if there is evidence of fluid overload as determined by pulmonary wedge pressure measurements. Heparin may be useful in patients with evidence of severe disseminated intravascular coagulation.

Prognosis *P. falciparum* malaria can be a life-threatening disease. Prompt therapy is indicated once the diagnosis is made, as the disease can become rapidly progressive. Patients who present in coma or with pulmonary edema or vascular collapse have a very poor prognosis.

Prevention Avoidance of mosquito bites by use of netting, insecticides and repellents and use of chemoprophylaxis are the major methods of avoiding malaria. Chloroquine (as 300 mg base), taken orally once a week on the same day each week, starting two weeks before entering the malarious area and continuing while in the area and for six weeks after leaving the area, will prevent malaria caused by *P. falciparum* sensitive to chloroquine. Fansidar (pyrimethamine, 25 mg, plus sulfadoxine, 500 mg), taken orally once a week as detailed above for chloroquine is effective in preventing malaria caused by *P. falciparum* resitant to chloroquine. Chloroquine is given with the Fansidar because of its superiority in preventing other forms of malaria.

Entamoeba histolytica

E. histolytica infection of the lung or pleural space occurs mainly as a complication of amebic abscess of the liver.

Microbial characteristics *E. histolytica* belong to the subphylum Sarcodina. *E. histolytica* occurs as the trophozoite (which is the invasive form) in tissue and in the intestine and as the cyst which must be ingested to produce infection. The invasive trophozoite is up to 50 μm in diameter, feeds by phagocytosis and moves by ameboid movement. It actively ingests red blood cells. There are noninvasive trophozoites that live in the intestine; they are 10 to 20 μm in diameter and are nonpathogenic. It is likely that the two types of trophozoites are related and which forms develop depends on environmental factors. Some patients carry only the noninvasive type. The trophozoites have one nucleus and are recognizable on iron hematoxylin stain in tissue and in fresh stool. The cyst form has four or less nuclei and is recognizable on iron hematoxylin or 1% to 2% iodine stain in the stool. They stain well with periodic acid-Schiff stain, but poorly with hematoxylin and eosin.

Pathogenesis The organism is acquired by ingestion of food or water contaminated with human feces containing cysts of *E. histolytica.* Trophozoites are fragile, do not survive well outside of the body, and will not withstand gastric acid and intestinal enzymes. On reaching the small intestine, trophozoites emerge from the cysts and then multiply and live in the colon. They may encyst and be passed in the stool with the person remaining asymptomatic (ie, a cyst passer). Alternatively, the trophozoites may penetrate the mucosa, form ulcerations, and multiply in the submucosa of the colon. Diarrhea with blood and pus in the stools may result. Bacteria must be present along with a low redox potential for tissue invasion of the *E. histolytica* to occur in the colon.

From the colonic site, spread to the liver may occur via the portal vein, with necrosis of liver and formation of a liver abscess(es) usually in the right lobe. Most patients who develop liver abscesses have had subclinical bowel disease. In about 10% of patients with liver abscesses, pulmonary involvement may occur.

Pulmonary involvement with *E. histolytica* may be restricted to a sympathetic serous pleural effusion above the liver abscess. Lung abscess may follow adherence of the base of the lung to the involved pleurae, and spread of disease from the liver to the lung may occur directly or via lymphatics. The hepatic abscess may also rupture into the pleural cavity with formation of empyema. A lung abscess may rupture into a bronchus with dissemination throughout the lungs. *E. histolytica* may rarely spread to the lung through the bloodstream. When abscesses result from direct penetration through the diaphragm, they are found at the bases of the lung. With hematogenous spread, the abscess may be in any part of the lung.

Epidemiology *E. histolytica*, for practical purposes, infects only man. Although fecal excretors of *E. histolytica* are found in all climates, clinical cases of amebiasis occur most often in patients living in or returning from tropical and subtropical areas with poor sanitation; up to 40% of the population in these areas may have positive stools. In the United States the prevalence of fecal carriers is about 3%. The lower socioeconomic classes are most apt to develop clinical infection. While there is no clear explanation for the higher clinical infection rate in tropical areas or in lower socioeconomic classes other than poor sanitation, some have postulated strain differences in *E. histolytica*, differences in bacterial flora related to diet (differences in bacterial flora could influence invasiveness of *E. histolytica* as well as local immunity), malnutrition increasing susceptibility, and increased genetic susceptibility in some populations. In homosexual males the infection rate is high because of fecal-oral contact.

Pleuropulmonary amebiasis occurs most commonly in males (10 males to one female) between 20 and 40 years of age, usually on the right side.

Pathology The empyema or lung abscess material is a red-brown "anchovy paste"-like liquid. The inner surface of the lining wall is red-brown, shaggy and vascular. Microscopically, the liquid consists mainly of necrotic cells with varying numbers of polymorphonuclear leukocytes, eosinophils, lymphocytes, macrophages, and *E. histolytica.* The number of inflammatory cells may be minimal. The wall of the abscess consists of lung or pleural tissue with fibrosis infiltrated with inflammatory cells. The *E. histolytica* usually are found in the peripheral part of the abscess at the boundary of the necrotic material and the wall of the abscess. They are best recognized by the nuclear chromatin pattern on iron hematoxylin stains and especially if they contain ingested red blood cells.

Clinical course The symptoms of the pulmonary disease may be overshadowed by the hepatic abscess which is almost always present.

Patients have fever and right upper quadrant abdominal pain which may radiate to the right shoulder. The liver is enlarged and tender.

With empyema, there are physical findings of pleural effusion. When lung abscess occurs, the physical findings are those of abscess. There is production of copious amounts of sputum which may be purulent, bloody, or red-brown, depending on whether or not rupture of the abscess has occurred into a bronchus. A bronchobiliary fistula may occur resulting in bile-stained sputum. Shock may result at the time of rupture of an abscess into the pleural space.

Laboratory findings The chest roentgenogram may show an elevated right diaphragm (from the liver abscess) with a right pleural effusion. With pulmonary parenchymal involvement, consolidation or an abscess may be seen. A liver abscess can be demonstrated by a liver–spleen scan and by computed axial tomography. Leukocytosis (without eosinophilia) essentially is always present. Abnormal liver chemistries, most often an elevated serum alkaline phosphatase, frequently are present.

Serologic studies demonstrating high titers of serum antibodies against *E. histolytica* are suggestive of active tissue invasion, but definitive diagnosis depends on demonstration of the microorganism. Observation of the protozoan in sputum, in empyema fluid or in an aspirate of a lung or liver abscess is diagnostic. Immunofluorescent stains are very sensitive in identifying *E. histolytica.* It is important to realize that stool examinations for *E. histolytica* are often negative by the time patients have developed liver or pulmonary amebiasis.

Differential diagnosis The major differential diagnosis is pyogenic liver abscess with involvement of the pleural space or lung. This is a difficult differential as some amebic abscesses become secondarily infected. In all liver abscesses, amebiasis must be ruled out, usually by means of serological studies.

Therapy The antiamebic therapy of choice for hepatic and pulmonary amebiasis (adult doses) is metronidazole, 750 mg three times a day for 10 days. Aspiration of empyema fluid is an important part of therapy. Needle drainage of liver or lung abscesses rarely is necessary except for diagnosis; open drainage should be avoided. Therapy should be started promptly, with a high suspicion of amebiasis as the therapy is relatively nontoxic. If high fever persists or there is any reason to suspect bacterial superinfection, needle drainage of the lung or liver and appropriate antibiotic therapy should be added.

Some physicians add parenteral emetine for the first few days or chloroquine for two to three weeks; however, this author does not. If stools are positive, diiodohydroxyquin, 650 mg three times a day for 21 days, should be added to eliminate cyst excretion.

Prognosis There are no data on mortality in pulmonary amebiasis.

However, with recognition of the disease and prompt therapy, the prognosis should be relatively good.

Prevention Prevention of amebiasis depends on sanitary disposal of feces and avoidance of ingestion of food or water that is potentially contaminated with human feces. *E. histolytica* are not completely killed by chlorination or iodination. Filtration will remove the ameba from water supplies, and boiling water for at least 10 minutes will kill the microorganisms.

Toxoplasma gondii

Toxoplasma infection of the lung is very rare and occurs as a complication of disseminated toxoplasmosis.

Microbial characteristics *T. gondii* is a protozoan in the subphylum Sporozoa. It is an obligate intracellular parasite. Trophozoites that are 3 × 7 μm are the rapidly proliferating forms that can invade mammalian cells. Once inside a cell, the trophozoites multiply by endodyogeny until the cell lyses, releasing more trophozoites. Trophozoites can develop into cysts that are up to 200 μm in diameter. The cysts have thick walls and contain up to 3000 organisms which have also reproduced by endodyogeny. Cysts can remain infectious in tissues for many years and can reactivate to cause active infection. Oocysts that are 10 to 12 μm in diameter are found only in the intestinal epithelial cells and feces of cats following ingestion of tissue cysts or oocysts. The oocysts can survive in the ground for up to one year.

Pathogenicity *T. gondii* is an organism of low pathogenicity except in the immunocompromised host and in the fetus. In the normal adult or child, while infection is common, severe disease is extremely uncommon.

Epidemiology *Toxoplasma gondii* is found worldwide in both animals and man. Infection can be acquired by ingesting infected cat feces (the cat is the only species that excretes the organism in the stool), or more commonly by ingesting poorly cooked meat that contains cysts. Infection occasionally may be acquired from blood transfusion, organ transplantation, or ingesting contaminated milk or eggs. Toxoplasmosis is extremely common (at least 25% of the normal adult population has been infected), with the chances of infection increasing with age. The infection rate is lower in vegetarians and higher in those who eat rare meat and those who have exposure to cats. In general, infection is less common in cold climates.

The most important type of toxoplasmosis is infection in the newborn, either from maternal infection and penetration of the placenta (usually during the later stages of pregnancy) or perhaps occasionally from infection of the newborn at time of birth.

After ingesting a cyst, trophozoites are released, and invade and multiply in intestinal epithelial cells. Some trophozoites gain access to the vascular system and are distributed throughout the body where they invade cells. Multiplication of trophozoites in cells causes cell lysis and an acute inflammatory process. As immunity develops, *Toxoplasma* start to encyst and tissue damage stops. Clinical manifestations may be due to newly acquired infection, or may be caused by reactivation of cysts.

Pathology The pulmonary lesions in infants are scattered areas of consolidation with subpleural petechiae. Microscopically, the alveoli are filled with alveolar epithelial cells and macrophages that contain *Toxoplasma.* The alveolar walls are infiltrated with plasma cells and lymphocytes. In the adult, interstitial pneumonia rarely may be seen. *T. gondii* as trophozoites and often as cysts are present in the macrophages and in the alveoli.

Clinical course Toxoplasmosis usually is asymptomatic in children and adults or produces a self-limited illness with fever and/or lymphadenopathy. Rash, hepatosplenomegaly, and chorioretinitis may occur. Occasionally, severe disseminated infection results usually in those who are immunocompromised (eg, from Hodgkin's disease or from immunosuppressive therapy), and is probably due to reactivation of latent infection. There is widespread involvement of organs (eg, encephalitis and myocarditis) and the lung also may be involved. The pulmonary involvement usually is an x-ray or autopsy finding and not of clinical significance.

Congenitally acquired generalized toxoplasmosis may occur, usually resulting in death or severe disease. Pneumonia occasionally may occur as a part of the generalized infection in infants. However, most neonatal toxoplasmosis that is clinically apparent causes central nervous system damage as the major manifestation (hydrocephalus, microcephalus, chorioretinitis).

Laboratory findings Pulmonary involvement in disseminated toxoplasmosis is rare and is a minor part of the illness. The diagnosis is suspected because of roentgenographic findings of pneumonia in a patient with disseminated toxoplasmosis. The histology of lymph node involvement may be sufficiently characteristic to be highly suggestive of toxoplasmosis. However, the diagnosis of toxoplasmosis usually is made serologically by demonstrating a rise in serum antibody titer (by indirect immunofluorescent or Sabin-Feldman dye test methods). Rises in antibody titers usually take one to two weeks to occur. High titers are reached in one to two months and then decline over months to years. Therefore, a single high titer may be related to past inactive infection unless it can be demonstrated to be IgM antibody (which indicates active infection).

Tissue obtained surgically or at autopsy can be inoculated intraperitoneally into mice for subsequent demonstration of *T. gondii* in peritoneal fluid from the mice. Tissue cultures also can be used for isolation. Trophozoites may be seen in tissue with Giemsa stain but are difficult to visualize. Immunofluorescent antibody techniques are more useful. Periodic acid-Schiff stains will demonstrate cysts. However, presence of cysts only indicates past infection and does not necessarily mean active infection.

Differential diagnosis Congenital toxoplasmosis resembles congenital syphilis, rubella, cytomegalovirus infection, and herpes simplex. All can cause chorioretinitis. Toxoplasmosis, cytomegalovirus and rubella can cause hydrocephalus, microcephaly and cerebral calcifications. Toxoplasmosis with fever or adenopathy in the adult or child can resemble infectious mononucleosis, cytomegalovirus infection or other viral illnesses, lymphoma, sarcoid, and tuberculosis.

Severe disseminated disease must be differentiated from other disseminated infections and tumors that can cause encephalitis, myocarditis, pneumonitis and other organ involvement.

Therapy The treatment of choice (adult doses) is pyrimethamine, 50 mg daily for three days, followed by one-half the dose for one month in combination with sulfadiazine or triple sulfonamide, 75 to 100 mg/kg/day in divided doses, every six hours. Folinic acid, 6 to 10 mg/day orally or intramuscularly should be given to prevent megaloblastic anemia. Therapy usually is continued for one month.

As toxoplasmosis is most often a mild self-limited illness, therapy should not be routinely given. Treatment should be considered only for life-threatening or sight-threatening infection or infection in the newborn.

Prognosis The vast majority of toxoplasmosis is asymptomatic or a mild illness. The exceptions are congenital toxoplasmosis and disseminated infection in the immunocompromised patient. When pneumonia occurs, it is part of disseminated infection which itself has a poor prognosis. In the infant, even with survival, there is a high rate of residual chorioretinitis or mental deficiency.

Prevention The major emphasis is prevention of congenital toxoplasmosis in infants of pregnant women with negative antibody tests. These women should be cautioned not to eat rare meat, and not to handle cats and particularly cat litter during the pregnancy. Women who enter pregnancy with antibody and who have had toxoplasmosis, are immune, and cannot transmit the disease to their infants. The same precautions should be applied to immunosuppressed susceptible patients.

Kala-Azar

Kala-azar is a systemic disease caused by the protozoan *Leishmania donovani.* The pulmonary infection is a very minor part of the disease.

Microbial characteristics *L. donovani* appears in two forms, the flagellate (promastigote) form in the insect vector, *Phlebotomus* (the sandfly) and the nonflagellar (amastigote) form in man and other mammals. The amastigote form is found only in cells and is round and 2 to 5 μm in diameter. It has a large peripheral nucleus with an oval parabasal body that is very close to a dot-like blepharoplast. While the parasite can be seen on hematoxylin and eosin stain, the morphology is best delineated with Giemsa or Leishman's stains.

The promastigote form is found in the digestive tract of the insect or in culture media and is elongated and flagellated (8 to 25 μm $\times$ 4 to 5 μm). The insect ingests the amastigote form on feeding on an infected mammal. It transforms into the promastigote form which multiplies. On feeding, the insect then introduces the parasite which enters reticuloendothelial cells, transforms into the amastigote form and multiplies.

Epidemiology Kala-azar is found worldwide but not in the United States or Canada. Infection follows the bite of an infected *Phlebotomus.* The *Phlebotomus* becomes infected from biting infected man, dog, rodents, foxes and other mammals. Man-to-man transmission via feces, urine and saliva rarely may occur. Children or young adults are most often infected. Infection usually is asymptomatic and, following recovery, long-standing immunity develops.

Following inoculation of a flagellated form of *L. donovani* (promastigotes) into the skin, the protozoa enter reticuloendothelial cells where they lose their flagella and multiply by binary fission. Following dissemination in the blood, cells of the reticuloendothelial system become infected all over the body, including those of the lung.

Pathology The liver and spleen are enlarged, with marked proliferation of macrophages (Kupffer cells in the liver) which are filled with *L. donovani.* Many other organs also are involved and, in the lung, interstitial alveolar cells (which are part of the reticuloendothelial system) are similarly parasitized. The fine structure of the intracellular parasites is best seen with Giemsa or Leishman's stains.

Clinical course After a two-week to 18-month incubation period, there is onset of fever. Gradually, hepatosplenomegaly and pancytopenia develop. After many weeks of illness, death results from secondary bacterial infection or hemorrhage. The pulmonary manifestations usually are only those of x-ray findings of infiltrates without clinical symptoms or signs. Circulating immune complexes develop and can cause glomerulonephritis.

Laboratory findings Pancytopenia usually is present in long-standing disease. Marked hyperglobulinemia occurs early in the disease and persists throughout the course.

The diagnosis is made by demonstrating *L. donovani* in reticuloendothelial cells. The procedure of choice is marrow aspiration which is positive in 90% of cases. Liver biopsy is less likely to be positive. While splenic aspiration is positive in over 90% of cases, the procedure is dangerous. Usually, hematoxylin and eosin stain is used. Cultures in NNN medium may be positive in one to four weeks.

Complement fixation, latex agglutination, and indirect immunofluorescent tests have been used to demonstrate serum antibody and become positive after several weeks of illness. However, there are cross-reactions with other diseases. The Montenegro skin test is negative during the active disease but becomes positive after cure.

Differential diagnosis The combination of prolonged fever, hepatosplenomegaly and pancytopenia may suggest lymphoma or miliary tuberculosis as well as kala-azar.

Therapy Antimony sodium stibogluconate (available from the Centers for Disease Control), 6 mL/day in adults, is the drug of choice. It is given for six to 30 days depending on the locale (eg, six days in India, 30 days in Africa). Pentamidine, 4 mg/kg every other day, is used for cases that are not responsive to antimony.

Prognosis Without therapy, the mortality is over 90%; with therapy, the mortality is under 5%. However, relapses do occur.

Prevention Control of the insect vector is the only means of prevention.

NEMATODES, TREMATODES, AND CESTODES

Pulmonary disease from worms may be due to deposition of ova (eg, schistosomiasis), larvae (eg, ascariasis) or adult worms (eg, paragonamiasis) in the lungs. With deposition, there usually is degeneration with an inflammatory process. The eosinophil plays an important role when multicellular organisms (ie, worms and larvae) are the source of the inflammation, but no or little role with single cell organisms.

Leoffler's syndrome With larvae and worms, the eosinophilic reaction may be local and/or systemic. The eosinophilic pneumonia that results is identical to what has been called Leoffler's syndrome. This consists of fever, cough, hemoptysis, bronchospasm and peripheral eosinophilia associated with migratory pulmonary infiltrates which histologically contain many eosinophils. This syndrome can be caused by drugs, vasculitis, and fungi as well as by worms or their larvae.

NEMATODES

Ascariasis (Ascaris lumbricoides)

A. lumbricoides, an intestinal nematode of man, may produce pulmonary manifestations during the phase of larval migration through the pulmonary capillaries into the alveoli.

Characteristics The adult worm is white, 15 to 35 cm in length and has a life span of one to two years. The worms live in the small intestine. The female passes about 200,000 eggs per day. The eggs are about 60 μm

× 40 μm, with a thick shell, the outer portion of which is albuminous and mammillated.

The eggs mature outside the body and become infectious after about 10 days. They are very hardy and can remain viable for months. During this period, the eggs have gone through two larval stages.

Epidemiology *Ascaris lumbricoides*, the most common helminthic infection of man, is found all over the world wherever human feces contaminate food. Only humans are affected. In the United States most infections occur in the Southeast. Young children are affected most often. After ingesting the egg, larvae are released in the small intestine. They bore through the mucosa, entering lymphatics or venous channels. When they reach the pulmonary capillaries they pass through the vessel walls and enter the alveoli. After moulting in the alveoli, the larvae, now 1 to 2 mm in length, ascend through the tracheobronchial tree being swept up by the ciliated epithelium. They are either coughed out or swallowed. After reaching the small intestine, they grow to maturity. Female worms are then fertilized by male worms. The entire process from egg to egg-laying female is about two months.

Pathology Knowledge of the pulmonary pathology is based on very few cases. When the larvae break into the alveoli, they cause damage with hemorrhage and an inflammatory reaction consisting of polymorphonuclear leukocytes and eosinophils. Consolidation may occur with heavy infestation.

Clinical course A small proportion of those with ascariasis have pulmonary sysmptoms (fever, cough, hemoptysis, and bronchospasm), which occur during the migration of larvae through the lungs. The symptoms resolve after a few days to a week or more.

Although intestinal symptoms are also uncommon, intestinal obstruction may occur secondary to a mass of worms. The worms may also cause intestinal perforation or biliary tract obstruction or appendicitis secondary to migration of a worm into the biliary tree or appendix.

Laboratory findings During the pulmonary phase, there frequently is peripheral eosinophilia and eosinophils may be found in the sputum of symptomatic patients. The sputum is often bloody. The presence of larvae in the sputum or gastric aspirate is diagnostic. Ova in the stools of a patient with possible pulmonary ascariasis indicate old exposure and suggest that exposure has occurred again with active pulmonary infection. The x-ray demonstrates migratory pulmonary infiltrates which may be patchy or show an area of consolidation.

Differential diagnosis The pulmonary manifestations of *A. lumbricoides* must be differentiated from other eosinophilic pneumonias caused by drugs, fungi, vasculitis, or other worms.

Therapy The treatment of pulmonary ascariasis is supportive as antihelminthic drugs are not effective against the larvae. Antibiotic therapy is given if secondary bacterial pneumonia occurs. Corticosteroids are used for severe allergic manifestations (ie, serious asthmatic symptoms).

The intestinal phase with adult *Ascaris* can be treated with mebendazole, 100 mg twice a day for three days.

Prognosis The pulmonary manifestations of ascariasis usually are mild and self-limited. The intestinal manifestations such as perforation or obstruction are potentially serious.

Prevention Ascariasis is best prevented by sanitary disposal of human feces and avoidance of ingestion of food contaminated with feces.

Visceral Larva Migrans (Toxocara canis or cati)

Visceral larva migrans is the syndrome produced in man when larvae of *Toxocara canis* or occasionally *T. cati* (dog or cat ascarids) become trapped in various organs including the lungs. Other animal ascarids rarely cause the syndrome.

Characteristics *T. cati* has the same life cycle in the cat (the definitive host) as *A. lumbricoides* does in man. However, the life cycle of *T. canis* differs in the dog (the definitive host). Eggs are passed by adult *T. canis* in the intestine of puppies and pregnant or recently pregnant female dogs. The eggs take two to three weeks to become infective, but can remain viable for months. When dogs ingest eggs of *T. canis*, the eggs hatch in the intestine and larvae penetrate the intestinal mucosa to be carried to many organs; they do not break into the alveoli in the lungs. The larvae become encysted in various organs where they evoke a granulomatous reaction. The larvae remain infective for years, but will only develop further in a female. With pregnancy, the larvae are activated to cross the placenta; many enter the fetus and some may complete their cycle in the pregnant female. The larvae then follow their usual ascarid pathway in both fetus and mother. That is, they migrate through the pulmonary vessels into alveoli, move up the bronchi and trachea, are swallowed and then develop into egg-laying adults in the intestine. These animals can pass eggs in the stool for up to six months. If dogs ingest larvae by eating meat from noncanines infected with *T. canis*, the tracheal migration and final maturation of the worm can occur. However, the usual host for egg laying *T. canis* is a puppy.

The parasite has substances closely related to the antigens of blood groups A and B. Therefore, anti-A and anti-B antibody titers become markedly elevated in infected patients who do not have these antigens on their red cells. Antibodies to the larvae also form in infected animals and people.

Epidemiology Viceral larva migrans is found worldwide wherever there is the opportunity for humans to ingest feces from infected dogs (usually puppies) or occasionally cats. Young children are most often affected as they are most likely to put soil contaminated with feces in their mouths.

Following ingestion of ova of *T. canis* or *T. cati*, larvae are released in the intestine. As with *A. lumbricoides*, the larvae penetrate through the intestinal mucosa and reach the lungs through the blood. However, unlike *A. lumbricoides*, the larvae of *Toxocara* do not break out through capillaries in the lungs but rather are carried to many organs in which they migrate. The liver, brain, eye and heart are involved as well as the lung.

Pathology The pathology in the lungs is that of focal granulomas surrounding larvae. The granulomas are composed of giant cells, histiocytes, and many eosinophils. There may be widespread disease resulting in bronchopneumonia that may be hemorrhagic. Similar granulomas are found throughout the body wherever larvae lodge.

Clinical course The patients may be asymptomatic with only peripheral eosinophilia. Fever is common and there may be evidence of multiorgan involvement such as hepatitis, retinitis, cerebritis, etc. Enlargement of the liver is common. The pulmonary manifestations are those of cough, wheezing, rales, and chest x-ray findings of patchy or diffuse penumonitis. The illness, if untreated, can continue for months. Symptoms subside as the larvae become encapsulated. Eosinophilia can persist for years.

Laboratory findings There is striking peripheral eosinophilia ($> 3000/mm^3$). The chest x-ray findings are of migratory areas of infiltration. Liver chemistries often show evidence of hepatitis (eg, elevated SGOT). Liver or lung biopsy may show the granuloma or larva. Finding of larva on biopsy is diagnostic; however, liver biopsies are positive for larvae in only 20% of cases. Isoagglutinin titers (anti-A and anti-B) usually are elevated in visceral larva migrans as are other antibody titers (eg, indirect hemagglutination or precipitins against the worm), but these are nonspecific. A test using the enzyme-linked immunosorbent assay (ELISA) and *T. canis* larval antigen seems to be both specific and sensitive. Stool examinations for ova are valueless as no adult *Toxocara* are in the intestine.

Differential diagnosis A similar syndrome with fever, eosinophilia and multiorgan involvement can be seen with eosinophilic leukemia, vasculitis and infections with some other worms (eg, strongyloidiasis and trichinosis).

Therapy Thiabendazole, 50 mg/kg/day for one to two weeks is the treatment of choice. In life-threatening infections, corticosteroid therapy should be added.

Prognosis The illness is self-limited and death is rare. However, damage may be permanent in organs such as the eye.

Prevention The best way of preventing the disease is to deworm pet dogs and cats, especially puppies. Sanitary disposal of pet feces should be enforced (eg, pets kept out of sandboxes). Pica should be discouraged in children.

Hookworm Disease (Necator americanus and Ancylostoma duodenale)

Hookworms, intestinal nematodes of man, may produce pulmonary manifestations during the phase of larval migration through the pulmonary capillaries into the alveoli.

Characteristics The adult worm is thin and about 1 cm long. The adults live in the upper small intestine of humans attached to the mucosa. They suck blood (about 0.03 mL daily for each *N. americanus* and about 0.2 mL daily for each *A. duodenale*). The life span of the worm is two to five years. The female passes about 7000 eggs per day. The eggs are oval and about 60 × 40 μm with a thin, clear shell. At temperatures above 55°F the eggs hatch into infective larvae. The larvae can survive in warm soil for months.

Epidemiology Hookworms are found in tropical and subtropical areas where infestation is very common. Infection is found in the southeastern part of the United States. Only humans are affected. Infection is acquired when larvae, which have hatched from eggs deposited on the ground, come in contact with skin. They penetrate the skin, are carried in the blood to the lungs and penetrate through the capillaries into the alveoli. The larvae are carried up the tracheobronchial tree by the movement of ciliated epithelium and then are either expectorated or swallowed. The swallowed larvae develop into adults in the small intestine. The adult worms attach to the mucosa and suck blood which can result in iron deficiency anemia. The females mature and start laying eggs. The entire cycle from skin penetration to egg laying takes four to six weeks.

Pathology The pathology of hookworm disease in the lung is not known, but is probably very similar to what has been described in ascariasis.

Clinical course Pulmonary manifestations are uncommon in hookworm disease and are caused by migration of larvae through the capillaries into the alveoli. The pulmonary clinical syndrome is identical to that observed in ascariasis. The only other manifestations of hookworm disease are occasional pruritus and rash at the site of larval penetration, abdominal pain and diarrhea at time of worm attachment to the intestinal mucosa, and iron deficiency anemia if the worm burden is large and dietary intake of iron inadequate.

Laboratory findings These are identical to those of ascariasis. In hookworm disease, depending on the worm burden and dietary intake, iron deficiency anemia and hypoalbuminemia may result from fecal blood loss. The finding of larvae in the sputum or gastric aspirates is diagnostic. The stool is often positive for occult blood.

Differential diagnosis, therapy and prognosis The differential diagnosis of the pulmonary manifestations of hookworm disease is the same as for pulmonary manifestations of ascariasis. Hookworm disease is treated the same as ascariasis. However, ferrous sulfate should be administered if iron deficiency anemia is present. The prognosis of hookworm disease is good; anemia rarely is severe except in the malnourished.

Prevention Hookworm disease is best prevented by sanitary disposal of human feces and wearing of shoes.

Cutaneous Larva Migrans (Ancylostoma braziliense)

A. braziliense, the dog and cat hookworm, has an incomplete life cycle in man. The larvae penetrate the skin but become trapped in and migrate in the subcutaneous tissue.

Characteristics *A. braziliense*, the dog and cat hookworm has the same life cycle in dogs and cats as described for *A. duodenale* and *N. americanus* in humans.

Epidemiology *A. braziliense* is found worldwide, and in the United States is most common in the South. The definitive host is the dog or cat. Humans acquire the infection when the skin comes in contact with soil in which infected dog or cat feces have been deposited. The larvae which have developed from the eggs penetrate the skin and migrate in the subcutaneous tissue for months, producing very pruritic, raised erythematous serpiginous lesions. Some larvae may reach the lungs and cause symptoms.

Pathology The pulmonary pathology is unknown.

Clinical course The pulmonary manifestations are mild and of short duration and consist of bronchospasm, cough and peripheral eosinophilia. These symptoms are overshadowed by the severely pruritic lesions where the larvae are migrating.

Laboratory findings There may be peripheral eosinophilia, and eosinophils are present in the skin lesion. Tissue biopsy may reveal the larvae but is unreliable as the larvae move in unpredictable directions. On rare occasions, larvae may be recovered from sputum.

Differential diagnosis The skin lesion is so distinctive as to be essentially diagnostic. Patients will also often recall the exposure, as they will have been in contact with the ground at an unusual location, and they may have had tingling skin sensations at the time of larval penetration.

Therapy Thiabendazole, 25 mg/kg of body weight for two days, usually is curative.

Prognosis If untreated, spontaneous recovery will take place.

However, the skin lesions can persist for months without therapy.

Prevention Prevention depends on avoidance of skin contact with ground contaminated with animal feces (eg, wearing shoes, not lying unprotected on the ground).

Strongyloidiasis (Strongyloides stercoralis)

S. stercoralis are intestinal nematodes primarily of man and may produce pulmonary manifestations during the phase of larval migration through pulmonary capillaries into the alveoli.

Characteristics *S. stercoralis* females are about 2 mm in length with the male about one-third as long. The worm can live and reproduce in the small intestine of man or in the soil as a free-living form that can reproduce sexually. Thus, with proper soil conditions and no low temperatures, the ground can remain contaminated indefinitely.

Epidemiology *S. stercoralis* is found in the tropics and subtropical areas and to a minor degree may occur in temperate areas. In the United States infection is most common in the South. The infection rate is particularly high (up to 35%) among residents of institutions for the mentally defective in the southern United States. Humans are the principal host.

The life cycle in the human host is very similar to that of the hookworm. Infection is acquired when skin comes in contact with larvae (usually on the ground). The larvae penetrate through the skin and are carried through the blood to the lungs where they break out of the capillaries into the alveoli. The larvae are then carried up the tracheobronchial tree and swallowed. They grow to adulthood in the small intestine where they burrow into the mucosa and begin to lay eggs. Females start laying eggs four weeks after larval penetration of the skin. Unlike hookworm, however, the eggs tend to hatch rapidly, and larvae often emerge in the intestine. The larvae can develop into the infective forms either in the ground or in the intestine. When this occurs in the intestine, larvae can penetrate the intestinal mucosa or the skin of the perianal area and repeat the pulmonary cycle. Because of the reinfection cycle, patients can remain infected for many years. By means of autoinfection, the worm burden can become very large despite only minimal initial exposure. In addition, fecal contamination of bedsheets can spread strongyloidiasis among bedmates.

Pathogenicity The pathogenicity of *S. stercoralis* is very much related to the immune status of the host. Autoinfection is enhanced in patients with conditions that compromise the immune system and may lead to overwhelming lethal strongyloidiasis. Lymphoma, leukemia, lepromatous leprosy and administration of immunosuppressive agents or corticosteroids are some of the conditions that have been associated with severe strongyloidiasis.

Pathology The pulmonary pathology of strongyloidiasis in the normal host is the same as that of ascariasis. However, the possibility of massive pulmonary involvement is much greater with strongyloidiasis (because of autoinfection) than with ascariasis. With massive infection, larvae are found in many organs with a widespread inflammatory reaction. The intestinal mucosa can become denuded with a very large worm burden. In the immunocompromised host, who is most likely to develop overwhelming strongyloidiasis, eosinophilia and an eosinophilic response in tissues may be absent. In fact the pulmonary lesion may be hemorrhagic with little inflammation.

Clinical course About one third of patients with strongyloidiasis are asymptomatic. Intestinal symptoms (eg, diarrhea, cramps, malabsorption) and pruritic skin rash over the perianal and lower abdominal areas, thighs, and buttocks (areas of larval penetration) are the most common symptoms. Pulmonary manifestations (fever, cough, hemoptysis and bronchospasm) are uncommon and are related to the number of larvae reaching the pulmonary circulation. With massive infection, there is multiorgan involvement and symptoms from larvae becoming lodged at many sites. Bacteremia caused by gram-negative bacilli is a common cause of death and results from ulceration in the intestine.

Laboratory findings High peripheral eosinophilia is common in severe disease, but may not occur in the immunocompromised host. The diagnosis of strongyloidiasis is made by demonstration of larvae in *fresh* stool or aspirates of duodenal contents. Larvae also may be isolated from sputum or gastric aspirates and occasionally from pleural effusions.

Tests for occult blood in the stool may be positive. In overwhelming infection there may be multiorgan dysfunction related to larvae becoming trapped in the organs.

Differential diagnosis A similar syndrome with fever, eosinophilia and multiorgan involvement can be seen with eosinophilic leukemia, vasculitis and infection with some other worms (eg, visceral larva migrans and trichinosis).

Therapy All patients with strongyloidiasis should be treated even if asymptomatic, as it is potentially a very dangerous infection. Thiabendazole, 25 mg/kg twice a day for three days, is the therapy of choice.

Prognosis With massive infection, death is common, not infrequently caused by gram-negative rod bacteremia. Disseminated severe infection is most likely to occur in those with lymphomas or leukemias and in those receiving corticosteroids or immunosuppressive therapy.

Prevention Sanitary disposal of human feces and avoidance of skin contact with areas of human fecal contamination are the major approaches to prevention. It must be remembered that there is a free-living form of *S. stercoralis*. Therefore, contaminated soil may remain contaminated indefinitely. In regions where strongyloidiasis is endemic, examination of the stool for *S. stercoralis* should be considered before starting patients on steroids or immunosuppressants as untreated asymptomatic infection carries the danger of disseminated disease in this situation.

Tropical Pulmonary Eosinophilia (TPE)

Tropical pulmonary eosinophilia is a syndrome of pulmonary symptoms associated with peripheral eosinophilia. It is presumably caused by filarial worms (*Wuchereria* and *Brugia*) of animal origin and results from microfilariae becoming trapped in pulmonary capillaries.

Characteristics The exact filarial species producing TPE is not known. Larvae are introduced into the definitive host (not the human) via a mosquito bite. The larvae reach lymph nodes where they grow to worms 4 to 10 cm in length. After several months, fertilized females begin discharging microfilariae into the lymphatics. Microfilariae eventually reach the blood where they circulate until ingested by a mosquito to complete the cycle. Microfilariae of the human type are 250 × 7 μm in size, but those of TPE have not been characterized. In the definitive host, the worms live for many years.

TPE seems to occur when an animal filaria is unable to complete its life cycle in humans and microfilariae become trapped in pulmonary capillaries.

Epidemiology TPE occurs mainly in South Asia but also in Africa, South America and the Far East. This distribution is similar to that of *Wuchereria bancrofti* and *Brugia malayi* which cause human disease. It also has been reported in the United States where *Dirofilaria* infection of dogs occurs. TPE is probably transmitted from infected animals to humans by a mosquito bite.

Pathology There is little pathological data available on lung tissue in this syndrome. What has been described are pulmonary nodules scattered throughout the lungs. Microscopically there is interstitial fibrosis with alveoli containing hemosiderin-laden macrophages. Many eosinophils are seen in alveoli and interstitial areas. Granulomas are seen with foreign body giant cells surrounding the remains of microfilariae. Also, in the granulomas are many eosinophils, lymphocytes and plasma cells. On very rare occasions an adult filarial worm has been found in a pulmonary artery resulting in pulmonary infarction.

Clinical course The patient has fever, anorexia, a paroxysmal dry cough that is worse at night, and attacks of bronchospasm associated with peripheral eosinophilia and nodules in the lung fields on chest x-ray. Physical findings may be absent, except for wheezes, or there may be scattered rales. Hematomegaly and lymphadenopathy have been reported. Patients usually improve after several weeks to many months.

Laboratory findings There is high eosinophilia (up to 80% of the white blood cell count). The erythrocyte sedimentation rate is high. Chest x-ray shows generalized nodules up to 0.5 cm in diameter. A complement fixation test with *Dirofilaria immitis* as the antigen is positive in over 90% of cases but is not specific. There are no circulating microfilariae in blood smears.

Differential diagnosis The differential diagnosis is between TPE and pulmonary disease caused by vasculitis, drugs or other worms. The response to therapy is a useful diagnostic tool.

Therapy The therapy of choice is diethylcarbamazine, 2 mg/kg body weight three times a day for two weeks.

Prognosis Death is rare, with the vast majority of patients recovering spontaneously after weeks to months of illness.

Prevention The most effective preventive measure is avoiding mosquito bites with screen and insect repellants.

Dirofilariasis (Dirofilaria immitis)

Dirofilaria immitis is the dog heartworm. Man becomes infected as an accidental host. Manifestations occur when worms embolize to pulmonary arteries.

Characteristics The adult worm is 12 to 30 cm long and lives in the right side of the heart or in the pulmonary artery. The female releases microfilariae which are 315 μm in length. They circulate in the blood and are ingested by mosquitoes and perhaps fleas. Subsequent larval stages develop in the insects which can then infect dogs. Following the insect bite, the larvae develop in the animal's subcutaneous tissue. After 80 to 120 days, they migrate to the right heart where over a period of six months they mature.

Epidemiology *D. immitis* is found all over the world. *D. immitis* infection in the United States is found mainly on the east coast from New Jersey south and also in the Gulf states. As may as 40% of nonprotected dogs in this area are infected. The infection occurs in man when an infected mosquito injects the larval form. The dirofilarial larvae mature in the subcutaneous tissue and after several weeks to months, they enter the bloodstream. Unlike the situation in the definitive host where they migrate to and live in the heart or pulmonary arteries, they may grow for a while in the heart but eventually embolize to the lungs causing an infarct.

Pathology There is a 2- to 3-cm diameter pulmonary nodule, which microscopically is infarcted lung with a zone of lymphocytic infiltration on the periphery. The dead worm usually is seen in the artery. There is evidence of endarteritis in the artery and there may be a granulomatous response with eosinophils.

Clinical course Most patients are asymptomatic. The lesions, discovered on chest x-ray usually taken for other reasons, show one or more coin lesions. In a minority of patients, cough, hemoptysis, chest pain and fever may occur.

Laboratory findings Eosinophilia is uncommon. The chest x-ray shows one or more coin lesions.

Differential diagnosis The usual differential diagnosis is that of coin lesions in the lung. Resection is both diagnostic and curative.

Therapy The diagnosis and treatment usually is removal of the coin lesion.

Prognosis The prognosis is excellent.

Prevention Control of the disease in dogs and control of the mosquito vectors are the keys to prevention.

TREMATODES

Schistosomiasis (Schistosoma mansoni, haematobium, and japonicum)

Schistosomes are blood flukes that live in veins in close proximity to the intestines and/or urinary bladder. The pulmonary disease is produced mainly by embolization of eggs to the lungs.

Characteristics The adult schistosome is 1 to 2 cm long. The male is folded around the female to form a groove which holds her. *S. mansoni* and *S. japonicum* live in the mesenteric veins and *S. haematobium* live in the veins around the distal colon and in the vesical plexus. After mating, a female *S. mansoni* produces 300 eggs each day and *S. japonicum* 3000 eggs daily. The eggs are about 145 × 55 μm; eggs of *S. mansoni* have a lateral spine and eggs of *S. haematobium* have a terminal spine. The eggs penetrate through the walls of the vessels and into the lumen of the intestine or bladder. (Some eggs are swept by the venous flow to the liver or lung and these produce most of the clinical manifestations of schistosomiasis.) Eggs reaching fresh water hatch, and ciliated miracidia are released. These penetrate into the snail that is the appropriate intermediate host. There is a strict requirement for specific snail hosts for each of the schistosoma.

In the snail the larvae multiply and emerge as cercariae in four to six weeks. Cercariae have forked tails and are motile. Cercariae penetrate intact skin by means of lytic secretions and lose their tails.

Epidemiology *S. mansoni* is found in Africa, South America and the Caribbean Islands, including Puerto Rico. *S. haematobium* is found in Africa and *S. japonicum* is found in the Far East. The geographic distribution is related to the habitat of the specific intermediate host snails as well as the need for disposal of human feces or urine into fresh water. Although other species can be infected, man is the principal definitive host. The prevalence and intensity of infection is greatest in the young; this is probably related to immunological defense mechanisms limiting more infection as worms die after five to 10 years.

Man is infected when he comes in contact with fresh water containing cercariae which have been released from snails, the intermediary hosts. The cercariae penetrate the skin and migrate to liver and lungs where they mature to adult worms. The worms then move through the venous system to their final location. Egg laying starts about six to 10 weeks after the cecariae penetrate the skin. Worms can live up to 30 years, but most die within 10 years.

Pathology Most of the damage done in the lungs as well as in the liver is from the eggs. When eggs are deposited in these tissues, granulomas develop which consist of macrophages, lymphocytes and eosinophils. Healing is accompanied by fibrosis (called "pipe stem" fibrosis in the liver). The areas of fibrosis around where eggs had been deposited cause obstruction to blood flow in liver and lungs. This results in portal venous hypertension and pulmonary artery hypertension (with eventual cor pulmonale).

As the pathological process continues in the lungs, shunts open between the pulmonary artery and bronchial arteries. With *S. mansoni* and *S. japonicum*, the lungs are protected from egg deposition initially, as all eggs not shed into the intestine embolize to the liver. With development of portal hypertension, collateral venous circulation develops and eggs can then pass into the systemic veins and into the lungs. Cor pulmonale also can develop in patients with *S. haematobium* infection due to direct egg embolization from vesical veins. With obstruction of pulmonary arteries and pulmonary hypertension, plexiform lesions form. These are dilated endothelial channels at the sites of the obstruction which connect with the distal part of the artery.

The worms living in vessels cause little or no reaction. Occasionally, adult worms live in the pulmonary arteries and deposit their eggs into the pulmonary circulation. This results in an even heavier egg burden to the lungs and causes focal pneumonia. When a worm in the pulmonary artery dies and embolizes, there is endarteritis, infarction and an intense inflammatory reaction, containing many eosinophils and macrophages at the site of impaction. This can result in a coin lesion in the lung on chest x-ray.

The immunologic reactions of the host play an important role in the manifestations and progression of the disease. In early schistosomiasis granulomas are large; later the granulomatous response is much less intense. Circulating immune complexes may also cause some of the damage seen.

Pathogenicity Immunological mechanisms seem to be important in schistosomiasis. In endemic areas most infection occurs in the young, and degenerating eggs cause large granulomas. As exposure continues, defense mechanisms apparently mediated by eosinophils appear against cercarial survival after penetration of skin. Also the size of granulomas in response to egg degeneration tends to decrease. Therefore, as the child reaches adulthood and worms begin to die after five to 10 years, the rate of acquisition of new worms and the amount of damage resulting from egg deposition tends to decrease.

Clinical course Most patients with schistosomiasis are asymptomatic. A pruritic rash, "swimmer's itch," may occur following cercarial penetration of the skin; this is seen only in sensitized patients who have been infected before.

With massive infection, there may be a reaction, called "Katayama fever," at the time of initiation of egg laying in the venous circulation. There is fever, cough, wheezing, hepatosplenomegaly, lymphadenopathy and high eosinophilia lasting for several weeks; however, death may occur.

The likelihood of chronic disease developing depends on the magnitude of the worm burden and therefore the number of eggs deposited. *S. japonicum* lays many more eggs than *S. mansoni* or *S. haematobium* and thus also is more likely to produce chronic disease which develops over a period of years.

The major target organs are the intestine (diarrhea, ulceration), liver (hepatomegaly and presinusoidal obstruction, with portal hypertension resulting in massive splenomegaly and esophageal varices) and urinary tract (papillomatous reactions in the bladder and ureteral obstruction).

Ova are found in the lungs of up to one half of patients with schistosomiasis. One percent to 2% of these develop cor pulmonale. Cor pulmonale is seen mainly in patients with hepatosplenic schistosomiasis following development of portal-systemic venous anastomosis. For some reason, this complication is less common in *S. japonicum* infection.

Patients develop cough and progressive dyspnea. Hemoptysis, cyanosis and clubbing are rare. Presence of a dead worm in the pulmonary arterial system can result in a large granuloma giving the impression of a coin lesion on chest x-ray (as with *Dirofilaria immitis*).

Laboratory findings Finding of ova in the stool or urine (*S. haematobium*) is diagnostic of schistosomiasis. In more chronic disease, the intestinal mucosa may become thickened from the passage of many eggs, and ova may become trapped in the mucosa; rectal biopsy may be necessary to demonstrate eggs in these patients. Eggs may occasionally be found in the sputum. Eosinophilia usually is low grade except in those with acute massive infection (Katayama fever) where there is high eosinophilia. Circulating immune complexes have been observed in schistosomiasis and are responsible for the nephrotic syndrome that develops in some patients; they may also cause Katayama fever.

Liver function is preserved and liver chemistries tend to be normal in hepatosplenic schistosomiasis.

Immunological tests are available for schistosomiasis. However, many are not specific and even a true positive test may only indicate old infection.

With cor pulmonale, pulmonary artery pressures are high (eg, 70/20 mmHg). Hypoxemia is uncommon and, if present, can be eliminated by breathing 100% oxygen. Pulmonary function studies show evidence of restrictive disease (ie, decreased lung volumes).

Chest x-ray may show patchy areas of consolidation from egg deposition. When worms in the pulmonary artery lay large numbers of eggs in one area, a large area of consolidation may result. A dead worm may cause a coin lesion on x-ray. With development of cor pulmonale, there is right ventricular and pulmonary artery enlargement. Diffuse pulmonary fibrosis may be seen. Angiography may show obstruction of distal branches of the pulmonary artery or may show the lacework pattern of the plexiform lesions.

Differential diagnosis The major pulmonary differential diagnoses involve other causes of cor pulmonale such as chronic obstructive pulmonary disease and idiopathic pulmonary hypertension. Diffuse small patchy infiltrates on chest x-ray from egg granulomas may be confused with miliary tuberculosis, histoplasmosis or sarcoid. An infarct from a dead worm yielding a coin lesion on x-ray must be differentiated from carcinoma.

Therapy Therapy is aimed at decreasing the worm burden. Niridazole is effective against *S. mansoni* and *S. haematobium* at doses of 25 mg/kg body weight orally daily in two divided doses for seven days. However, this agent should not be used in the presence of hepatosplenic schistosomiasis and collateral circulation as central nervous system complications are common. *S. japonicum* is less responsive to niridazole and therapy with antimony potassium tartrate, which is much more toxic, may be necessary. Although treatment should be given, it does not seem to affect the course of cor pulmonale once it is established.

Praziquantel, an isoquinoline-pyrazine derivative, is a new oral antiparasitic agent that seems to show great promise in early trials in patients with schistosomiasis and will probably become the drug of choice. Praziquantel has apparently no major toxicity and is well-tolerated as well as being highly effective. The dose is either 40 mg/kg in a single dose or 60 mg/kg divided into three doses on the same day.

Prognosis Most patients with schistosomiasis are asymptomatic. Even after portal hypertension develops and bleeding from esophageal varices has occurred, patients may live for many years as liver function remains relatively normal. Eventually, liver failure may occur. Renal failure secondary to ureteral obstruction is a common cause of death in *S. haematobium* infection. Cor pulmonale has a bad prognosis.

Prevention Prevention is accomplished by avoiding contact with fresh lake or river water in endemic areas. Public health measures involve sanitary disposal of feces. The snails have been very resistant to attempts at eradication.

Paragonimiasis (Paragonimus westermani, uterobilateralis and africanus)

Paragonimus lives in the lungs of humans or other carnivorous mammals and produces local damage. The major cause of paragonimiasis is *P. westermani.*

Characteristics The hermaphroditic adult worms are reddish-brown, flattened and about 1 cm in length and 0.5 cm in width. The eggs are golden-brown and are 90 μm $\times$ 60 μm. They are operculated.

Epidemiology *Paragonimus* is found in the Far East, West Africa, and Central and South America. These are regions where water temperature supports miracidia (ie, above 10°C and optimally between 25° and 30°C, and where people eat uncooked fresh water crustaceans, and spit or defecate into fresh water). In the United States paragonimiasis has been reported recently among refuges from Indochina.

The adult fluke lives in cysts in the lung and lays many eggs which are coughed up in the sputum or swallowed and excreted in the feces. Egg laying starts five to six weeks after infection. The adult worms live for about five years and continue to pass eggs. When eggs reach fresh water, they hatch and miracidia are released which can penetrate into a variety of snails. After multiplying in the snail, cercariae emerge which can infect fresh water crabs or crayfish. When man ingests these crustaceans or water, which contains decomposing crustaceans, encysted larval forms (metacercariae) are released in the small intestine. They penetrate through the intestine into the peritoneal cavity. After further development, they penetrate through the diaphragm into the lungs where they mature into adults. Many larvae fail to reach the lungs and remain at ectopic sites.

Pathology After the initial invasion of the lung, there is tissue destruction accompanied by hemorrhage and inflammation. Cyst formation with fibrosis follows. The major lesions in the lung are destructive and result in nodules, cysts, and bronchiectatic cavities. The nodules actually are abscesses consisting of necrotic material containing the worm and degenerating ova in the center. At the edge of the necrotic material is granulation tissue with lymphocytes, plasma cells and relatively few eosinophils. There may be scattered free eggs in the parenchyma surrounded by macrophages and giant cells. Cysts may communicate with each other and may form bronchiectatic cavities. Calcification may occur.

Clinical course Paragonimiasis, although chronic, usually is a mild illness. There may be recurrent hemoptysis and slight dyspnea, but weight loss or severe manifestations are rare. Chronic bronchitis and bronchiectasis may result.

Paragonimiasis frequently is associated with pulmonary tuberculosis which can be severe. Also, flukes and eggs may reach the brain and cause encephalitis. Physical findings usually are minimal.

Laboratory findings The diagnosis is made by finding the eggs in sputum or feces. Charcot-Leyden crystals in the sputum are suggestive of the diagnosis. Eosinophilia is uncommon.

Chest x-ray may reveal a lung abscess or thin-walled cysts in areas of infiltration. It frequently looks like pulmonary tuberculosis. Pleural effusion also may be present. Complement-fixing antibodies are often present in serum.

Differential diagnosis The major differential diagnostic problem is with tuberculosis. However, the lack of systemic illness and progression in paragonimiasis is helpful in differentiating it from tuberculosis.

Therapy Bithionol, 30 mg/kg body weight every other day for 14 doses is effective. Praziquantel administered orally, 60 mg/kg divided into three doses on the same day, has been reported to be more effective. Antibiotics are required for secondary infection. Surgical excision may be required for localized cystic disease.

Prognosis The prognosis is excellent.

Prevention Prevention is based on cooking crabs or crayfish before eating and avoidance of ingestion of untreated water (potentially contaminated with degenerated crustaceans) in an endemic area. Pickling or soaking crustaceans in brine or wine does not kill the larvae.

CESTODES

Hydatid Disease (Echinococcus granulosus and Echinococcus multilocularis)

Hydatid disease develops when man ingests eggs from *Echinococcus* (a tapeworm) and becomes an accidental intermediate host with development of the larval cyst form.

Characteristics The adult tapeworm is about 0.5 cm long and has a head and three proglottides. The scolex (or head) has four suckers and hooklets by which it attaches to the small intestine. The last of the proglottides produces many ova which are passed in the feces.

Epidemiology Echinococcosis or hydatid disease caused by *E. granulosus* is found worldwide. *E. multilocularis* is found only in Canada, Alaska, and Russia. Dogs, wolves, foxes and jackals are hosts for the adult worm and often have many worms. The adult worm lives for about six months. The necessary intermediate hosts usually are herbivores (most often sheep) for *E. granulosus* and rodents (eg, mice and rats) for *E. multilocularis.* However, man can also become an accidental intermediate host and develop hydatid disease.

In order for the disease to occur, organs or meat of intermediate hosts must be eaten by definitive hosts and man must be in close contact with the definitive hosts. This is most likely to occur in sheep-raising areas where dogs (eg, sheep dogs) live with man and are fed parts of slaughtered animals. The disease has been particularly important in

Australia, New Zealand, South America, Africa and the Mediterranean areas (especially Lebanon and Greece).

Patients become infected when they ingest eggs from dog feces. With *E. granulosus*, this usually occurs from handling dogs. With *E. multilocularis*, infection mostly occurs from eating low-growing wild berries or vegetables that have been contaminated with feces.

Larvae hatch from the eggs and penetrate the mucosa of the small intestines and are carried in the blood to the liver (most often the right lobe). Most become trapped in the liver where they develop into cysts, but some pass through the liver and may reach the lungs, and less often other organs where they can develop into cysts. The *E. granulosus* cyst has an outer layer and an inner germinal layer, and is filled with fluid. The cyst enlarges as daughter cysts develop from invaginations of the germinal layer. Each daughter cyst develops more daughter cysts, and scolices develop from invaginations of the cysts. These eventually fall loose into the cysts where they remain as "hydatid sand." With *E. multilocularis*, cysts lack a continuous outer layer and tend to grow by evagination as well as by invagination. Adjacent structures may be invaded and, in fact, there may be metastases to distant sites.

If a carnivore such as a dog ingests scolices, the adult worm will develop in the intestine. These scolices will not develop further if ingested by man.

Pathology Most cysts are in the liver, with the lung as the next most common site. About 10% to 30% of *E. granulosus* cysts are in the lungs. However, cysts of *E. multilocularis* are rarely in the lungs. The cyst usually causes very little tissue reaction. However, the pressure of the expanding cyst can produce tissue atrophy. When a cyst ruptures, fluid in the cyst leaks and initially produces acute inflammatory changes followed by granulomatous changes. New cysts can develop from parts of the existing cyst including the scolices.

Clinical course The major manifestations of the cyst regardless of organ involved relate to pressure phenomena as the cyst enlarges over many years. It grows about 1 cm in diameter per year but can grow much faster.

In the lung, cysts usually are located in the lower lobes or occasionally on the pleural surfaces. There often are no symptoms at all, but there may be cough, dyspnea, dysphagia, superior vena caval syndrome or Horner's syndrome. Rupture of a cyst into a bronchus can result in the patient drowning in the fluid. The fluid release with rupture can cause anaphylaxis with a 25% mortality. Rupture of a cyst also can cause hemoptysis. Dissemination of the contents of a cyst throughout the lung or pleural space can result in development of new cysts.

E. multilocularis looks and acts like an infiltrating carcinoma. Microscopically, there is a granulomatous reaction around the areas of infiltration. Cysts can become secondarily infected forming pyogenic abscesses.

Laboratory findings With hydatid disease of the lungs, the chest x-ray shows one or more round lesions. Ultrasound, computed tomography or arteriography may be helpful in demonstrating the cystic nature of the lesions. Old cysts have a calcified border. Eosinophilia may occur, especially with leakage of cyst contents.

The diagnosis is proven by demonstrating scolices in the cyst or in sputum, or a pleural space if rupture has occurred. Needle aspiration of the cyst is a dangerous procedure and should not be attempted as rupture or spillage of the cyst contents may occur.

There are serological tests available to detect circulating antibody, but there are false positives and false negatives. Some of these are the indirect hemagglutination, latex agglutination, complement fixation and bentonite flocculation tests. The Casoni test, an intradermal test, gives an immediate reaction in over 75% of patients with hydatid cyst disease, but it may also be positive in patients with other parasitic diseases. A delayed reaction is positive in 25% to 30% of patients.

Differential diagnosis The cyst usually presents as a tumor mass. If the edge is calcified, it is very suggestive of a hydatid cyst. Presence of a cyst, together with a positive serological test, is highly suggestive of echinococcosis.

Therapy The treatment of choice is surgical removal of the intact cyst. If removal is impossible, marsupialization of the cyst with sterilization of the contents with formalin or 30% NaCl solution may be the best approach. Spillage of the cyst fluid is dangerous and great care must be taken to avoid this. Injection of formalin or hypertonic saline solution into the cyst before removal lessens the danger of spread from spillage but injection carries the danger of rupture of the cyst. Cysts that are not enlarging may best be left alone. Cysts that bud externally rather than internally (particularly *E. multilocularis*) may be very difficult to remove surgically.

Mebendazole in very large doses has been used experimentally to halt the growth of cysts and kill scolices. It may be useful when spill of cyst contents has occurred or when resection is impossible or inadvisable.

Prognosis The prognosis of the nonleaking cyst is good unless the cyst causes pressure in vital areas.

Prevention Avoiding feeding dogs uncooked meat from slaughtered animals, preventing carnivores from having access to livestock, and worming dogs may break the cycle.

SELECTED READINGS

Adickman M, Tuthill TM: Pulmonary infiltrates and eosinophilia. *Postgrad Med* 1976;60:143.

Barrett-Connor E: Parasitic pulmonary disease. *Am Rev Respir Dis* 1982;126: 558–563.

Gelpi AP, Mustafa A: Ascaris pneumonia. *Am J Med* 1968;44:377.

Mahmoud AAF: Current concepts. Schistosomiasis. *N Engl J Med* 1977;297:1329.

Mandell GL, Douglas RG, Bennett JE: *Principles and Practice of Infectious Diseases.* New York, John Wiley and Sons, 1979.

Markell EK, Voge M: *Medical Parasitology.* Philadelphia, WB Saunders Co, 1976.

Melvin DM, Brooke MM: *Laboratory Procedures for the Diagnosis of Intestinal Parasites.* Atlanta, U.S. Department of Health, Education and Welfare (CDC 75-8282), 1974.

Olsen WO: *Animal Parasites*, ed 3. Baltimore, University Park Press, 1974.

Praziquantel – A new antiparasitic drug. *Medical Letter* 1982;24:108–109.

Purtilo DT, Meyers WM, Connor DH: Fatal strongyloidiasis in immunosuppressed patients. *Am J Med* 1974;56:488.

Schantz PM, Glickman LT: Toxocaral visceral larva migrans. *N Engl J Med* 1978;298:436.

Shaba JK: Protozoan and metazoan infections, in Fishman AP (ed): *Pulmonary Diseases and Disorders*, New York, McGraw-Hill, 1980, pp 1182–1200.

Spencer H: Pulmonary parasitic diseases, in *Pathology of the Lung*, ed 3. Philadelphia, WB Saunders, 1977, pp 327–370.

Vik R, Tansusat P, Marquez-Monter H, et al, in Marcial-Rojas RA (ed): *Pathology of Protozoal and Helminthic Diseases with Clinical Correlation.* Baltimore, Williams and Wilkins, 1971.

Index